NEW, EXPANDED, UPDATED EDITION

A CONSUMER'S
DICTIONARY OF
MEDICINES

ALSO BY THE AUTHOR

Poisons in Your Food
Beware of the Food You Eat
How to Reduce Your Medical Bills
A Consumer's Dictionary of Cosmetic Ingredients
A Consumer's Dictionary of Food Additives
A Consumer's Dictionary of Household, Yard, and Office Chemicals
Ageless Aging
Cancer-Causing Agents
A Consumer's Guide to Medicines in Food

NEW, EXPANDED, UPDATED EDITION

A CONSUMER'S DICTIONARY OF MEDICINES

Prescription, Over-the-Counter, Homeopathic, and Herbal Plus MEDICAL DEFINITIONS

RUTH WINTER, M.S.

Crown Trade Paperbacks
New York

To my best friend, constant consultant,
and beloved husband,
Arthur Winter, M.D., F.I.C.S.

Copyright © 1993, 1996 by Ruth Winter, M.S.

Published by Crown Trade Paperbacks, 201 East 50th Street, New York, New York
10022. Member of the Crown Publishing Group

Random House, Inc. New York, Toronto, London, Sydney, Auckland

http://www.randomhouse.com/

CROWN TRADE PAPERBACKS and colophon are trademarks of Crown Publishers, Inc.

Originally published in different form by Crown Trade Paperbacks in 1993.

Printed in the United States of America

Library of Congress Cataloging-in-Publication Data
    A consumer's dictionary of medicines : prescription, over-the-counter, homeopathic,
and herbal, plus medical definitions / Ruth Winter.—New, expanded, updated ed.
    p. cm.
    1. Drugs—Dictionaries.   2. Drugs, Nonprescription—Dictionaries.
3. Herbs—Therapeutic use—Dictionaries.   I. Title.
RM300.W56   1996
615'.1'03—dc20   95-31382
                                                                  CIP

ISBN 0-517-88534-4
10 9 8 7 6 5 4 3 2 1
Revised Edition

INTRODUCTION

You must be more knowledgeable about the medicines you take. Your life may depend upon it!

Suppose you have a cold. Would you spray your nose with a decongestant and then down an over-the-counter cold pill? By doing that, you could skyrocket your blood pressure. Both spray and pill contain an ingredient that relieves nasal congestion but also raises blood pressure.

If your cold progresses to bronchitis and your doctor prescribes an antibiotic, would you swallow the medication with a glass of milk or juice? If so, you could make the antibiotic ineffective.

Your stomach is upset. Do you reach into your medicine chest for a prescription drug, an over-the-counter antacid, or an herbal remedy such as chamomile? Is your nose stuffy from a cold? An allergy? What pill do you down?

A Consumer's Dictionary of Medicines—Prescription, Over-the-Counter, Homeopathic, and Herbal is the first book that covers all four categories in an easy-reference format. The following symbols are used to designate the most common use of a medication or therapeutic ingredient:

Rx For prescription medication.
OTC For over-the-counter or nonprescription medication.
H For herbal or homeopathic medicines.

The text describes:

- Why a medication is used.
- The medicine's reported benefits and side effects.
- The medicine's known interactions with other drugs and foods.

Our need to know about medications is burgeoning because:

- We are becoming more and more responsible for our own health care due to the increasing cost of medical services and the decreasing amount of time that health professionals have to explain things to us.
- We may go to more than one physician and receive multiple prescriptions, which can lead to overdosing or underdosing should the drugs interact.
- We are increasingly buying medications at discount pharmacies and by mail so that a professional may not be available to advise us about when and how to use a drug.
- Many of us are purchasing herbal or homeopathic medications prescribed by proselytizers, media personalities, and health-food-store clerks.

The result of the above changes in consumer habits is that Rx, OTC, homeopathic, and herbal medications' overuse, misuse, and abuse have reached almost epidemic proportions. People experiencing acute drug reactions ranks seventh among the causes of hospitalization at a cost of more than $21 billion per year.[1] Rx and OTC nonsteroidal anti-inflammatory drugs (NSAIDs) alone are used by 13 million Americans and cause 7,600 deaths each year.[2] An estimated 40 percent of patients don't take their medications as directed.[3]

We, as consumers, have to recognize that if an Rx, OTC, or H remedy has a systemic effect, chances are that it will also have a side effect. A side effect is an unintended feeling or condition caused by a medication.

What Is a Prescription Drug?

The United States Food and Drug Administration (FDA) defines a prescription medication as a drug that is habit-forming or unsafe for use except under a doctor's supervision. The most commonly prescribed medicines are:

- Cardiovascular drugs (heart and circulation related).
- Anti-infectives (antibiotics such as penicillin).
- Mental-health medications (antidepressants, antipsychotics, and antianxiety drugs).
- Analgesics (painkillers).
- Diuretics (sometimes called water pills).[4]

RX DRUG APPROVAL

The drug approval process began in 1938 with the Food, Drug, and Cosmetic Act passed by Congress. For the first time, manufacturers were required to document the safety of their products, and the FDA had sixty days to object to a new drug before it was marketed. Following the thalidomide tragedy in Europe (thousands of severely deformed babies were born after their mothers used the sedative during pregnancy), Congress passed the Kefauver-Harris Amendment in 1962. That amendment requires drug companies to produce substantial evidence—in the form of patient testing—to prove that their products are both safe and effective. The U.S. system of new-drug approval is now perhaps the most rigorous in the entire world. It takes an average of 15 years and $359 million to get one prescription medicine from the laboratory to your medicine chest.[5]

Before a prescription drug can be marketed, it must pass through the following process:

1. "University of Rhode Island Study on Significant Misuse of Prescription Medications by the Elderly," survey published by University of Rhode Island, Kingston, R.I., March 5, 1990.

2. J. F. Fries, "Assessing and understanding patient risk," *Scandinavian Journal of Rheumatology Supplement* 92 (1992): 21–24.

3. "Prescription Drugs: A Guide to Safe Use of Medicines," *The University of Texas Lifetime Health Letter* 4, no. 6 (June 1992): 4–6.

4. Brochure published by National Council on Patient Information and Education, Washington, D.C., 1991.

5. John F. Beary, III, M.D., "The Drug Development and Approval Process," Office of Research and Development and Approval, Pharmaceutical Research and Manufacturers Association analysis, Washington, D.C., January 1996, 1.

Preclinical Testing. Laboratory and animal studies are done to show biological activity against a targeted disease, and the compounds are evaluated for safety. These tests take approximately three and a half years.

Investigational New Drug Application (IND). After completing preclinical testing, the company files an IND with the FDA to begin to test the drug's effects in people. The IND becomes effective if the FDA does not disapprove it within thirty days. The IND shows results of previous experiments; how, when, where, and by whom the future studies will be conducted; the chemical structure of the compound; how the compound is thought to work in the body; any toxic effects found in animal studies; and how the compound is manufactured. In addition, the IND must be reviewed and approved by the Institutional Review Board at the medical facility where the studies will be conducted, and progress reports on clinical trials must be submitted at least annually to the FDA.

Clinical Trials, Phase I. These tests take about a year and involve from about twenty to eighty normal, healthy volunteers. The tests study a drug's safety profile, including the safe dosage range. The studies also determine how a drug is absorbed, distributed, metabolized, and excreted, and the duration of its action.

Clinical Trials, Phase II. In this phase, controlled studies of approximately one hundred to three hundred volunteer patients (people with the disease the drug is being tested against) assess the drug's effectiveness, which takes about two years.

Clinical Trials Phase III. This phase lasts about three years and usually involves one thousand to three thousand patients in clinics and hospitals. Physicians monitor patients closely to determine efficacy and identify adverse reactions. A new development in drug testing has appeared. Private "study centers" are replacing university research facilities for testing new pharmaceuticals. The private centers, which advertise for patients over the radio, offer a more rapid, less expensive means of clinical trials. Questions about the selection of substances to be tested and the quality of research by nonuniversity investigators remain to be answered.

New Drug Application (NDA). Following the completion of all three phases of clinical trials, the company files an NDA with the FDA if the data demonstrate safety and effectiveness. The NDA must contain all the scientific information that has been gathered. NDAs typically run one hundred thousand pages or more. By law, the FDA is allowed six months to review an NDA. In almost all cases, the period between the first submission of an NDA and final FDA approval exceeds that limit; the average NDA review time for new molecular entities approved in 1994 was 19.5 months down from 26.5 months in 1993.[6] This reduction came at the end of the first year of the agency's new User Fee Program, under which its drug-approval system was redesigned and more reviewers were being trained, financed by fees paid by pharmaceutical companies.

Expedited Process. Under a plan implemented by the FDA early in 1989, Phases II and III may be combined to shave two to three years from the development time for those

6. FDA Report "New Drugs Approvals," Washington, D.C., January 20, 1996.

medicines that show sufficient promise in early testing and are targeted against serious and life-threatening diseases such as AIDS and cancer. Approval time for these drugs in 1994 averaged 5.9 months.[7]

Approval. Once the FDA approves an NDA, the new medicine may be prescribed by all physicians. The drug manufacturer is required to continue to submit periodic reports to the FDA, including any cases of adverse reactions and appropriate quality-control records. For some medicines, the FDA requires additional studies to evaluate long-term effects.

WHAT IS AN OVER-THE-COUNTER (NONPRESCRIPTION) DRUG?

Over-the-counter medicines are sold for the prevention, treatment, and symptomatic relief or cure of disease, injuries, or other conditions—acute or chronic—that you can identify and treat alone or with professional advice. An OTC product is not permitted to bear claims for serious disease conditions that require the continual attention and supervision of a licensed practitioner. Nonprescription medicines, therefore, are by legal definition safe for use without medical supervision and do not constitute a hazard to health. Label directions must be written in understandable language. The FDA has informed manufacturers that over-the-counter drugs must have simplified labels, similar to those required for foods since the early 1990s. The new labels were just beginning to come onto the market as of this writing, but eventually you should be able to tell at a glance how to properly use nonprescription drugs, the side effects, and when to see your physician.

An estimated three hundred thousand nonprescription products are marketed in the United States, containing one or more active ingredients from a selection of seven hundred to eight hundred. We treat, according to recent surveys, four times as many common health problems ourselves with OTC medications as those ailments we ask our doctors to treat.[8] Statistics show that six out of every ten of the medicines in our homes are OTC drugs, and about two cents of every health-care dollar goes to nonprescription remedies.[9] Self-medication is a growing part of our health care system because:

- Self-treatment with OTC medications costs less.
- The availability of more OTC medicines is broadening the range of self-treatable problems.
- We want to take part in our own health care when we can.[10]

The following table shows the most common ailments for which we treat ourselves with OTC products rather than seek professional service and how often we do so (percentage) for each product:

7. Ibid.

8. Frank E. Young, M.D., Ph.D., commissioner of Food and Drugs, *FDA Consumer* 22, no. 10 (December 1988-HB, 1989M): 6–7; William Soller, Ph.D., "Outlook for OTC Switches," *American Pharmacy* NS31, no. 2 (February 1991): 38–40.

9. "Facts about OTC Medicines," Nonprescription Drug Manufacturers Association Fact Sheet, Washington, D.C., July 1991; Marian Segal, "Rx to OTC: The Switch Is On," *FDA Cibsyner* (March 1991): 9–11.

10. "Self-Medication in the '90s: Practices and Perceptions, Highlights of a Survey on Consumer Uses of Nonprescription Medicines," prepared by the Nonprescription Drug Manufacturers Association, May 1992.

Top Ten Problems Most Likely
to Be Treated by OTC Medications[11]

Problem	Percentage
Headache	76
Athlete's foot	69
Lip problems	68
Common cold	63
Chronic dandruff	59
Premenstrual	57
Menstrual	57
Upset stomach	57
Painful dry skin	56
Sinus problems	54

The onslaught of new remedies on the market is expected to boost the outlay for OTC products to $19 billion by the year 2000, up 72.7 percent from 1990.[12] The market for OTC products is growing at a rate of 9 percent annually, compared to 7 percent for prescription drugs.[13]

FROM PRESCRIPTION TO OVER-THE-COUNTER

There had been no statutory requirement that a drug be sold by prescription until the Durham-Humphrey Amendment to the FDA Act passed in 1951. The amendment defined Rx medications as primarily those unsafe for use except under professional supervision, and OTC remedies as those safe for consumers to use by following directions and warnings on the label. Ten of the top 20 selling OTC medications in 1994 were products switched from Rx status.[14]

More than four hundred OTC products today employ ingredients or dosages available only through prescription fifteen years ago, and another fifty are candidates to be switched from Rx to OTC.[15] (At least thirty-four medicines that are sold without prescription in other countries are available only by prescription or not at all in the United States.[16])

A major impetus for switching drugs from Rx to OTC status has been the FDA's comprehensive review, begun in 1972, of the active ingredients in OTC drugs. The review grew out of those 1962 drug-law amendments that said drugs cannot be marketed unless they are proven effective. Before Congress passed this legislation, drugs had to be proven safe, but

11. Ibid.
12. Patricia Winters and Laurie Freeman, "New OTC Drugs to Flood Market," *Advertising Age* 72 (September 26, 1990): 107.
13. "100 Leading National Advertisers," *Advertising Age* 72 (September 26, 1990): 107.
14. "From Rx to OTC: The Switch Process," Nonprescription Drug Manufacturers Association, Washington, D.C., February 12, 1996.
15. *Facts & Figures,* Nonprescription Drug Manufacturers Association, Washington, D.C., 1991, 26.
16. Ibid.

proof of their effectiveness was not required by law. Thus, the FDA was obliged to reexamine all drugs—both prescription and OTC—that had previously been approved solely on the basis of safety.

The FDA reviews an application to switch a drug from Rx to OTC. The review includes data about studies of interactions that might occur if the drug is taken with prescription medication, and its potential for overuse.

When an Rx drug becomes available as an OTC, it is sometimes sold for different ailments and at different strengths than its Rx counterpart. For example, Rx ibuprofen was prescribed for chronic arthritis in 400-mg doses. When it became OTC in 1985, it was marketed as a general pain reliever in smaller doses, such as in Advil's 200-mg tablets for pain relief and fever reduction. Motrin and Advil were approved for OTC in even lower doses for sale for children.

Once a drug is available without a prescription, insurance plans do not pay for it. But an increased cost is offset by not having to pay a physician in order to obtain a prescription. One study found that consumers saved up to $750 million a year as a result of OTC cough-cold medications that were once available only by prescription; while another study found that doctor visits for the common cold fell by 110,000 a year between 1976 and 1989.[17] According to a survey of OTC uses by Scott-Levin associates in 1995, 45 percent of the obstetric/gynecological physicians who took part recommended OTC products for their patients. The reason for the increase was attributed to the Rx-to-OTC switches of antifungal medications, such as miconazole and clotrimazole (*see both*).

From a drug company's perspective, some of the most likely candidates for the switch from Rx to OTC are drugs whose patents are due to expire within the next few years. It is a way to extend the market. Some giant drug companies have recently organized divisions to handle the increasing Rx-to-OTC changes.

Pharmaceutical companies are also aware that prescription drug prices may be limited under new government health care plans.

From your point of view, proceed with care when opting for a switched drug. Some patients who were once given a prescription for Motrin® (*see* ibuprofen), found Advil® or Nuprin® on their supermarket shelves. They thought that if they took two or three of the Advil® or Nuprin®, they would obtain the same effect as the Rx drug. The result, instead, was a bleeding stomach ulcer. The same holds true for the newer Aleve® (*see* Naproxen) which is longer lasting in the system than the other OTC anti-inflammatory medications.

Don't be lured into buying a product that has a health-association name tacked on. Johnson and Johnson and the Arthritis Foundation started the ball rolling in the 1990s by launching a line of pain relievers aimed at the 40 million people who suffer from the crippling disease arthritis. Under a royalty agreement, the Foundation reportedly receives a million dollars a year for research in return for the use of the Foundation's imprint. Tylenol by any other name is still Tylenol!

---

17. "Transfer of Ingredients from Rx to OTC Status 1994–1996," Nonprescription Drug Manufacturers Association, Washington, D.C., February 14, 1996.

WHAT IS AN HERBAL MEDICATION?

A great deal of enthusiasm is occurring, at this writing, about a drug, Taxol (paclitaxel), that is proving successful in treating ovarian, breast, and lung cancers. Taxol is derived from the bark of the Pacific yew tree.

Plants have been a primary source of medicinal agents for centuries. Aspirin, digitalis, and quinine are a few of the many drugs with natural origins. And some of the most effective medications used in cancer chemotherapy are derived from the Madagascar periwinkle plant and the mayapple, a common woodland plant. In fact, approximately 25 percent of the pharmaceuticals on the market today are derived from plant sources.[18] But, some researchers say, the medicinal potential of plants remains virtually untapped: of the world's estimated 265,000 plants species, less than 5 percent have been studied for their therapeutic value. Estimates from the Institute of Economic Botany at New York Botanical Gardens are that as many as 40,000 plants may be useful in developing new medicines.[19]

One of the promising means of identifying medicinal plants lies in the field of ethnobotany, a science that combines the studies of anthropology and botany to learn the ways native healers use plants. The Plant Collection Program sponsored by the National Cancer Institute (NCI) sends scientists from the Institute of Economic Botany, the Missouri Botanical Gardens, and the University of Illinois, Chicago, searching the tropics in Asia and Africa to collect plant species for treating cancer and AIDS. They generally work by observing native healers— shamans or medicine men—to see which plants they use to treat a wide variety of ailments. Among plants showing promising screening results are Saint-John's-wort (*see*), which is a folk remedy for diarrhea, depression, bladder problems, and other ailments, and cranesbill root (*see*), also called wild or spotted geranium, which is used externally as a folk cancer remedy.[20]

In Samoa, native healers use the leaves of a small tree, *Homalanthus acuminatus,* to treat back pain and abdominal swelling. They use the roots to treat diarrhea and the wood to treat yellow fever. The bark of this Samoan tree has shown potent activity against the AIDS virus according to chemists and biologists with the NCI.[21]

In addition to the NCI-sponsored project, a number of pharmaceutical companies are conducting searches for natural products from around the world.[22] A plant extract may contain thousands of compounds that have to be separated out to determine which is responsible for the targeted chemical activity. New screening techniques are allowing drug researchers to screen thousands of substances a year, including everything from snake venom to leech saliva. One of the modern drugs, for example, ivermectin (*see*), prescribed to combat an ancient problem, river blindness, came from a microorganism found in the soil of a Japanese golf course.[23]

18. "Scientists Turn Plants into New Drugs," *Lahey Clinic Health Letter* (Burlington, Mass.) 3, no. 1 (January 1992): 5.
19. Ibid.
20. Lea McLees, "Folk Medicine Gets a Fresh Look," *Research Horizons,* (Georgia Institute of Technology) (Summer 1991): 3–5.
21. Dori Stehlin, "Harvesting Drugs From Plants," *FDA Consumer* 24, 8 (October 1990): 20–23.
22. "Scientists Turn Plants Into Drugs," *Lahey Clinic Health Letter* (Burlington, Mass.) 3, no. 1 (January 1992): 5–6.
23. Andrew Pollack, "Drug Industry Going Back to Nature," *New York Times,* March 5, 1992, LD 1.

What about the herbal products available to you right now on store shelves and by mail? Herbs are promoted in the modern marketplace as:

- Cleansers and purifiers of the body.
- Glandular tonics.
- Compounds rich in nutrients that build the body.
- Energizers of the body.
- Stimulators of the body's immune system.

Herbal products are regarded as food by the FDA and are not permitted to be sold with medical claims, although some may have medicinal benefits. If a health claim is made for an herbal product, it is then regarded as a drug and is supposed to be submitted for approval by the FDA.

Catalogs and, in many cases, pharmacies and health food stores, get around this prohibition of making medical claims by advertising the claims but not putting such claims on the label. The Federal Trade Commission regulates advertising, and the FDA is in charge of safety. Both agencies are understaffed and underfunded for their regulatory functions and are not inclined to go through the time-consuming, extremely expensive process of hauling offenders into court unless the product is a considerable danger to health.

As in the case of OTC products, some unscrupulous people produce questionable herbal products and/or make unsubstantiated claims. An FDA spokesperson admits the problem is overwhelming, but says the agency has to concentrate on situations where the greatest health risks are involved.[24]

While there may be doubts about some herbal products on the market, there is no doubt that plants have provided and are providing great benefits in therapeutics. One of the most fascinating aspects of researching this book was uncovering information about medications that are in all three categories, such as ephedra, which is in many herbal medicines under the name ephedra, ma huang, or Mormon tea. About forty species of this herb are mentioned in ancient scriptures of India, and the Chinese have used it for more than five thousand years. Ephedra is an H drug used to treat arthritis, asthma, emphysema, bronchitis, hay fever, and hives. The stems of ephedra contain ephedrine. Ephedrine is used as an OTC bronchodilator and to treat a stuffy nose, and as an Rx drug to raise blood pressure.

Ephedrine is also prescribed for bed-wetting in children, stress incontinence of the bladder in adults, and delayed ejaculation. Ephedra and ephedrine have actions similar to epinephrine, the "fight or flight hormone" in the human body that is used as an Rx drug to treat life-threatening allergic reactions. Its herbal versions are subject to abuse by people looking for a "high."

You will also discover in the book H, OTC, and Rx remedies to treat the same symptom. For instance, under the definition for sedative:

SEDATIVE • A compound that calms the nervous system and reduces stress and anxiety. Phenobarbital is an example of a prescription (Rx) drug for this purpose. Diphenhydramine is an example of a nonprescription (OTC) sedative, and the herbs valerian and skullcap are examples of herbs (H) used for this purpose.

What about efficacy? Herbalists maintain that plant materials should never be judged in

24. Mike Schaffer, United States Food and Drug Administration spokesperson, personal communication, September 16, 1992.

direct comparison to modern, concentrated drugs. The effects of using plants are often extremely slow, but frequently—but certainly not always—without the side effects experienced from modern preparations.

HOMEOPATHIC MEDICATIONS

Homeopathy abides by the ideas of Samuel Hahnemann, a German doctor of the late 1700s who believed that "like treats like." The name is derived from the Greek words *homos* meaning similar and *pathos* meaning disease or suffering. Dr. Hahnemann maintained you could treat an ailment by giving a patient an extremely diluted amount of a drug that caused the same symptoms in healthy persons. So, if you are nauseated, you might be given an extremely dilute solution of ipecac (*see*), a drug that in greater concentration causes nausea. A homeopath may prescribe a preparation made from an onion (*see Allium cepa*) if you have a burning, watery nasal discharge and frequent sneezing, because an onion may affect you the same way when you peel it. The remedy may or may not work, but it will not harm you.

Dr. Hahnemann believed that symptoms are actually efforts of the body to reestablish homeostasis or balance, and that therefore one should seek a medicinal substance that would support, rather than suppress, the body's inherent efforts to heal itself.

Homeopathy is undergoing a renewed interest among certain segments of the population. According to the FDA, sales of homeopathic medicines in the United States grew by 1,000 percent between the 1970s and the 1980s and 50 percent between 1988 and 1990.[25] The fact is that the "law of similars" purported by homeopaths is used in conventional medicine with immunizations and allergy treatments aimed at stimulating the body's immunity. Homeopathic medicines are exempted from premarketing scientific testing and reviews for safety and effectiveness. This loophole dates back to 1938 when Sen. Royal Copeland, the chief sponsor of the Food, Drug, and Cosmetic Act, saw to it that homeopathic medicines were not included. Dr. Copeland was a homeopathic physician.

Prescribed homeopathic products are prepared by repeatedly diluting active ingredients by a factor of ten—generally noted on labels by the Roman numeral X. A "6X" preparation means that a one-to-ten dilution was done six times—leaving the active ingredient as one part per million.

While the law gives the FDA no premarket review of true homeopathic dilutions, the FDA and traditional homeopaths have been concerned about instances of unlicensed, untrained practitioners treating people for cancer or other serious ailments—and about attempts by companies to produce nonprescription products under the homeopathic umbrella to avoid FDA regulations. Many of the traditional homeopathic medicines, as you will read in this book, are made from highly diluted, deadly poisons.

Some states regulate the practice of homeopathy, and the FDA has now ruled that homeopathic drugs cannot be offered without prescription for such serious conditions as cancer,

25. "Herbal and Homeopathic Remedies: Finally Starting to Reach Middle America?" *OTC Market Report,* July 1993, 223–38; "Herbal and Homeopathic Remedies: Enhanced Status for Alternative Medicines," *OTC Market Report,* July 1990, 245–64; "Riding the Coattails of Homeopathy," *FDA Consumer,* March 1985, 31.

AIDS, or any other condition requiring diagnosis and treatment by a licensed practitioner. Nonprescription homeopathic medicines may be sold, as other OTC drugs, only for self-limiting (definite and limited) conditions recognizable by the consumer.

MAKING A CHOICE

Before you make a decision about taking any drug—Rx, OTC, or H—you should be as knowledgeable as possible. This book is not a substitute for medical advice from a professional. Its aim is to help you gather information about medications so that you can ask the right questions of your physician and pharmacist about an Rx drug or consider the pros and cons of an OTC or H medication urged upon you by an advertisement, well-meaning friend, or clerk. As you refer to the information in this book, you should become more aware of the potential benefits and side effects of all chemicals you ingest, inhale, inject, or place on your body.

HOW A DRUG DOES ITS JOB

How you take a drug can affect how well it works and how safe it will be for you. Sometimes it can be almost as important as what you take. Timing, what you eat and when you eat, proper dosage, and many other factors can mean the difference between feeling better, staying the same, or even feeling worse.

Pharmacokinetics concerns the movement of a drug within your body (*see* Drug Delivery Systems). Under typical conditions, once you swallow a medication, it travels through your digestive tract to your small intestine, where it is absorbed into your bloodstream. It is then carried to your liver, where, in many cases, it is broken down into a form that can be better used by your body. The drug (or the product that has been broken down from the drug) circulates throughout your system to achieve its desired effects, and then, as with most drugs, it is rapidly eliminated by your kidneys. Your age, sex, size, diet, and existing health problems may all have an effect on this process.

Recommended doses of a particular drug are based on premarket clinical testing (*see* page 2), which evaluated the drug's effectiveness in a few thousand people. Until recently, most medications were tested in young or middle-aged males. The scientific community, recognizing the differences of drugs' effects between the sexes and between various age groups, has now added some older persons and some women in studies.

WHAT'S DIFFERENT ABOUT OLDER PEOPLE?

The 10 percent of the population over sixty-five now consumes about 25 percent of the medications taken in the United States.[26] Elderly patients are more sensitive than younger adult patients to the therapeutic actions of drugs and more likely to show altered, unexpected, and even bizarre responses.[27] In a study of 1,160 hospitalized patients, the incidence

26. "Using Your Medicines Wisely: A Guide for the Elderly," United States Department of Health, Education and Welfare Public Health Service, Washington, D.C., 1985 (PF 1436(1185), D317), 1.
27. "Physiologic and Pharmacokinetic Factors as Determinants of Drug Response in the Elderly," Sandoz Pharmaceuticals, East Hanover, N.J., 1980, 2.

of adverse effects rose from 3 percent in patients twenty to twenty-nine years old to 21 percent in patients seventy to seventy-nine years old—a sevenfold increase![28]

Why? Beginning in middle age, the liver becomes progressively and proportionally smaller, until by the tenth decade it may represent 1.6 percent of the total body weight, as compared to 2.5 percent during midlife.[29] Blood flow through the liver also decreases with advancing age. Thus, in persons sixty-five years old, liver blood flow may be about 40–45 percent less than in persons twenty-five years old. Changes in the enzyme system also affect the liver's capacity to metabolize drugs and break them down into a form that enables the kidneys to excrete them. The kidneys are the major route of elimination for many drugs. However, between the ages of twenty and ninety years, blood flow through the kidneys declines by about 53 percent. During these same years, the kidneys' filtration rate declines about 46 percent, and their ability to excrete chemicals decreases approximately 44 percent. Thus, in terms of actual kidney output, the older person's kidneys filter only about 120 liters/day producing 1.0 liters of urine, whereas the younger adult's kidney filters approximately 200 liters/day, forming about 1.5 liters of urine.[30] The decrease in liver enzyme activity and the changes in the kidneys lead to the prolongation of drug action and a reduction of drug elimination, leading to drug accumulation, and thus possibly contributing to the high incidence of adverse reactions among aged patients. Therefore, while a 10-mg dose of Valium (diazepam) may make a thirty-five-year-old man relax his muscles, the same dose might make a seventy-five-year-old woman so relaxed that her muscles lose coordination, causing her to fall and break a hip. A therapeutic dose of many medications for a younger person may be too strong for an older person.[31]

Adding to the problem, elderly patients, in contrast to younger patients, often have multiple ailments for which they may take from three to ten drugs or more each day. Obviously, the simultaneous use of multiple medications, even when monitored, carries a high risk of toxic reactions and drug interactions (*see* Drug Interaction, page 198). This risk may be further increased by patients' use of analgesics, laxatives, antacids, cold remedies, and other OTC preparations that are taken without a physician's knowledge or approval and can change the action of prescribed medications. In some cases, confusion and failing memory may lead to dosage errors, and thus to modified responses, because patients cannot comprehend even simple instructions. In others, diminished vision or hearing may result in improper dosage because patients are unable to hear instructions or read directions on the prescription label.

A study of more than six thousand people aged sixty-five and over by researchers at Harvard University and Australian health services, reported in the *Journal of the American Med-*

28. N. Hurwitz, "Predisposing Facts in Adverse Reactions to Drugs," *British Medical Journal* 1 (1969): 315–536.

29. Bender, A. D., "The Effect of Increasing Age on the Distribution of Peripheral Blood Flow in Man," *Journal of the American Geriatric Society* 13 (1968): 192–98.

30. S. Vernon, "Nocturia in the Elderly Male," *Journal of the American Geriatric Society* 6 (1958): 411–14.

31. Judy Fokenberg, "Testing Drugs in Older People," *FDA Consumer* (DHHS Publication (FDA) 91-3185), November 1990.

ical Association in 1994,[32] concluded that physicians prescribe potentially inappropriate medication for nearly a quarter of all older people, placing them at risk for adverse drug effects such as cognitive impairment and sedation. Among the inappropriate medications were long-acting tranquilizers and sleeping pills and certain pain remedies that are more likely to cause internal bleeding than others.

One out of ten hospital admissions for older people is drug related. Two-thirds of those admissions are caused by patients' misuse of drugs, and one-third are caused by drug interactions or overdosing. Each year, an estimated 32,000 older Americans sustain hip fractures caused by drug-induced falls; 163,000 have mental impairment caused or worsened by medication.[33]

WHAT'S DIFFERENT ABOUT WOMEN?

It is understandable that drug researchers were and still are reluctant to include females in clinical trials. Women have more adverse reactions to drugs than men and die from these adverse reactions more often. Furthermore, women of childbearing age may become pregnant, and the drug being tested may harm the fetus.[34]

To assess how well the research-based pharmaceutical industry was meeting the medical needs of women, the Pharmaceutical Manufacturers Association (PMA) took a survey in 1991 of companies to identify the medicines that were either in human clinical trials or at the FDA for review.[35] They found that virtually every major pharmaceutical company is now taking into account the special medical needs of women, especially in the areas of heart and blood-vessel disease, cancer, and gynecological diseases.

The companies were asked how often they detected differences between men and women in clinical-trial data. In the key areas of cardiovascular, central nervous system, and non-steroidal anti-inflammatory medicines, among others, such differences were detected.

These differences may be caused by two main factors, according to the PMA:

• There are essential differences between the speeds at which men and women metabolize certain prescription drugs.

• Hormone levels and other biological systems within a woman vary because of the effects of menstrual cycles, pregnancy, and menopause. These variations may influence how well a drug works for a woman and the adverse reactions it causes.

WHAT ABOUT PREGNANCY?

In 1979, the FDA instituted labeling categories for prescription drugs that may be given to pregnant women.

32. Sharon Wilcox et al., "Inappropriate Drug Prescribing for the Community-Dwelling Elderly," *Journal of the Amerian Medical Association* 272, no. 4 (July 27, 1994): 292–96.

33. "The Elderly and Drug Use," Inspector General's 1989 Report, United States Department of Health and Human Services, Washington, D.C., 1989.

34. Diane Rehm, "Is There Gender Bias in Drug Testing?" *FDA Consumer* no. 3 (April 1991): 10–13.

35. "Survey New Medicines for Women in Development," Pharmaceutical Manufacturers Association, Washington, D.C., 1991.

In *Category A* are drugs for which both human and animal studies have failed to demonstrate a risk to the fetus.

In *Category B* are drugs for which no controlled studies in women are available, and animal studies have not demonstrated a risk. The same classification applies to drugs for which clinical experience shows no risk, but animal studies have demonstrated teratogenic effects.

In *Category C* are drugs for which controlled studies in women are not available and animal studies have shown adverse effects, as well as drugs for which controlled studies in women and in animals are not available. B and C drugs, the FDA says, should be used during pregnancy only when clearly needed.

Category D is for drugs for which there are no animal data, but clinical experience shows they cause birth defects. These drugs generally will be used in life-threatening situations where the benefits may be acceptable despite known risks.

Category X is reserved for those drugs for which both animal and clinical studies show teratogenic effects. In these cases, pregnancy information is included under the "contraindications" section of the labeling with the advisory that if the drug is used during the patient's pregnancy, or if she becomes pregnant, she should be told of the potential harm to the fetus.

The author has deliberately left out the A, B, C, D, and X listings for drugs because she strongly feels that no woman should take any medication—Rx, OTC, or H—while pregnant unless absolutely necessary, and then only under the supervision of a physician who is knowledgeable about the remedy. You can now, however, with your knowledge about the existence of the A, B, C, D, and X categories, ask your doctor about the pregnancy category of a prescription drug and then discuss the risks to your unborn child.

Scientific information about the effects of chemicals on unborn children is, for the most part, inadequate. As sparse as the data is about prescription drugs, the information about the effects in pregnancy of over-the-counter and herbal medications is even more uncertain. The labels of some over-the-counter products are required to advise women who are pregnant or nursing to seek the advice of a health professional before using them. The information about the risk of herbal remedies is folklore, supplied mostly by laypersons.

You may decide it is wiser to suffer an ache, an anxiety attack, or insomnia than to use a medication that may harm the baby, as women who took the tranquilizer thalidomide discovered so tragically.

CHILDREN ARE NOT JUST LITTLE ADULTS

Is a lower dose of an adult medication appropriate for a child?

The FDA says that the vast majority of prescription drugs lack adequate information on their pediatric use. One of the major roadblocks to the right medicine in the proper amount for children is the reluctance by pharmaceutical researchers for legal and ethical reasons to use youngsters to test experimental medications.

Currently 80 percent of prescription drugs lack full pediatric approval and are labeled with such disclaimers. Nevertheless, physicians routinely prescribe these drugs for youngsters. They base use and dose decisions on studies, personal experience, and prevailing medical practice. That's not always good enough.

A new rule published in the Federal Register on December 13, 1994, requires manufacturers to reexamine existing information to determine whether the pediatric labeling of products currently on the market can be modified based on adult studies and other data. If so, the manufacturers must submit an application for supplemental labeling.[36]

The FDA says it will ensure that necessary pediatric data are included for new products that will be widely used by children.

Parents, as well as pharmaceutical manufacturers and the FDA, have to take responsibility for the medications given to boys and girls, especially when it comes to the common cold.

A report from the National Center for Health Statistics published in the October 5, 1994, issue of the *Journal of the American Medical Association* found that nearly 54 percent of a representative group of 8,145 three-year-old children had been given some sort of nonprescription medicine during the previous thirty days.[37]

"Evidence that these [cold] medications are inefficacious and may, in some circumstances, have adverse effects has apparently done little to dampen enthusiasm for their use," the report stated. "Although the vast majority of over-the-counter medications are used in accordance with the manufacturers' directions, the use . . . may be harmful in some cases and adverse reactions and overdoses can occur. Parents need to be more realistic about what to expect from the management of the common cold."

During the five-year period from 1985 through 1989, the authors note that about 670,000 reports were received by poison control centers for children under six years of age involving either analgesic agents, cough/cold preparations, or gastrointestinal preparations.

"Everyone has a log of problems that occurred because we didn't have adequate labeling or information," said Cheston Berlin, Jr., M.D., chair of the American Academy of Pediatrics' committee on drugs, quoted in the *American Medical News.*[38]

Dr. Berlin expressed uneasiness about the new rule that states pediatric-use information can be based on adult studies, pharmacokinetics, and safety data only if the course of the disease and the drug's effects are sufficiently similar for children and adults.

"But who is going to determine that?" Dr. Berlin asks. "Is childhood depression, for example, the same as adult depression? And will treatment be the same with kids as with adults?"

PRESCRIPTION DRUG SAFETY

Of the more than two thousand prescription drugs deemed safe and effective by the FDA, virtually all carry some risks. This means that they may fail to work or have harmful side effects under certain circumstances. Makers of prescription drugs are required to list all potential adverse reactions. Manufacturers have options. Adverse reactions can be categorized by organ system (heart, lungs, liver, etc.), by severity or frequency, by toxicological mechanisms, or by a combination of these. However, listing adverse reactions does not nec-

36. Greg Borzo, "Physicians to get more data on pediatric drug dosages," *American Medical News,* January 29/30, 1994, 4.
37. "When Kids Have Colds, Parents Reach for OTC Meds," *American Medical News,* October 10, 1994, 23.
38. Borzo, "Physicians to get more data."

essarily mean that they occur frequently. Pharmaceutical manufacturers sometimes list a reaction if it happened in one or two persons out of tens of thousands taking the drug worldwide. On the other hand, you may have a reaction that is not listed.

When safety concerns force a drug off the market, many people recognize that the FDA has done exactly what it's supposed to do. For example, when reports of liver failure associated with the blood-pressure drug ticrynafen (Selacryn), and allergic shock caused by the pain reliever zomepirac sodium (Zomax), led to their removal from the market in the early 1980s, the general reaction was that the FDA had taken the only appropriate action to protect the public.[39]

But market withdrawal is certainly not the only way the FDA addresses such problems. More often, the agency resolves the situation through changes in the warnings and other information in a product's labeling.

Before the FDA approves a new drug for marketing, agency scientists and health professionals work with the product's manufacturer to develop its official labeling. The labeling summarizes the results of scientific research on the product, including studies in humans to assess safety and effectiveness. But these studies, which seldom involve more than a few thousand people, can't generate a perfect picture of how a drug will behave when it's used by hundreds of thousands or millions of people. As a result, it's often hard to anticipate all adverse effects—those that may occur only once in ten thousand or more uses.

The FDA has in place systems to continue to monitor the safety of approved drugs after they come into general use. As those systems disclose safety problems, the agency takes corrective action.

Since 1962, sponsors of drugs newly approved for marketing have been required to notify the FDA of all reports of adverse reactions to their products. Since 1985, serious adverse reactions that are not mentioned in the approved labeling must be reported. In 1995, the agency proposed a new regulation requiring manufacturers to submit safety reports every six months for the life of all their drugs and biologics.

In 1993, the FDA established a new program that encourages health professionals to report serious side effects or defects in a broad range of medications. The MEDWatch program is aimed at increasing the amount of available information. In the past, physicians have not consistently reported adverse effects, if they recognize them at all. Reporting is still voluntary, but the process has been greatly simplified for busy practitioners. MEDWatch is particularly important for postmarketing information.

In one year, the FDA receives some 52,000 reports of adverse reactions to drugs, about 10 percent of which come directly from health professionals. Each of these reports is checked against the agency's computerized Adverse Reaction Reports Data Base.

The FDA determines if the problem is occurring frequently, and whether the adverse reaction is described in the product labeling but is being seen more often than expected, or is one that the labeling doesn't even mention.

39. Frank E. Young, M.D., Ph.D., "Product Labels: First Line of Protection from Harm," *FDA Consumer* 23, no. 5 (June 1989): 5–6.

If adverse-reaction reports tied to a specific product accumulate, the FDA is faced with an important question: Is the problem so serious that the product has to come off the market, or can it be dealt with responsibly by adding a warning to the labeling or taking other steps to inform doctors and patients of the need to guard against the hazard?

When isotretinoin (Accutane) was approved in 1982 for treating severe cystic acne unresponsive to other therapy, the labeling warned against its use by pregnant women. Animal studies had shown that the drug could cause birth defects. Soon after it came into general use, the FDA began to receive reports of human birth defects associated with the drug. One of every four fetuses exposed to the drug was injured by it. Clearly, the warning against use by pregnant women was not being well heeded.

The labeling for Accutane was changed several times to strengthen the warning against use in pregnancy. Manufacturers sent letters to physicians emphasizing the risk of fetal damage.

Adverse-reaction monitoring and evaluation has identified problems with drugs, required relabeling and that safety problems be publicized, and enabled valuable drugs to stay on the market.

In addition to labeling, how else do physicians find out about a drug? Much of it comes from pharmaceutical-company sales personnel, medical journals, and direct-mail advertisements.

In a federally funded study, prescription drug advertisements targeted for physicians were found to be misleading in 66 of the 109 drug advertisements reviewed. It was determined that drug advertising for doctors sometimes has misleading headlines and insufficient information on side effects.[40]

Of the 19,000 prescription drug advertisements publicized in 1991, the FDA took action against drug companies 217 times. Of that total, only 39 advertisements were canceled, and legal action was taken in only two instances.[41]

How can you, as a layperson, obtain more information about a prescription drug? In addition to reading books such as this and talking to professionals, you can request a "package insert." The FDA tried to get a mandatory patient-package insert program in the early 1980s for ten classes of drugs. But companies and pharmacists complained that the inserts would require considerable storage space and constant reprinting due to changes in medical knowledge. These complaints are no longer valid, according to the FDA, because of the rapid expansion of computer technology. Easily updated software could allow pharmacists to print needed patient information while filling a prescription.[41]

OTC Safety

In 1972, the FDA began reviewing ingredients contained in an estimated three hundred thousand nonprescription drug products sold in this country. Under this ongoing review, the

---

40. Lawrence Altman, "Study Says Drug Ads in Medical Journals Frequently Mislead," *New York Times,* June 1, 1992, 1.
41. "Patients Want to Know More About Prescriptions," *FDA Consumer* 26, no. 2 (March 1992): 7.

FDA evaluates reports prepared by advisory panels of outside experts together with comments from industry and the public. Ultimately, the agency issues a final regulation that is, in effect, a standard or recipe of acceptable ingredients, doses, formulations, and instructions as well as permitted claims.

Most of the ingredients have been in use since before 1962, when a change in the law required that manufacturers submit proof of effectiveness for new drug products as well as for drug products already on the market.

The FDA in August 1992 proposed banning 415 ingredients from seven categories of prescription drugs because they had not been shown safe and effective as claimed. In similar actions, the FDA banned 223 ineffective ingredients from nineteen categories of products in November 1990, and 111 ineffective weight-control ingredients in August 1991. Most of the ingredients named had already been discontinued, but several products containing one or more of the ingredients remain on the market, and manufacturers are being required to reformulate or remove them from the market.

The ban on some ingredients is not total, however; an ingredient banned for one use may be allowed for another. For example, salicylic acid (*see*) is banned as an external pain reliever in insect-bite and sting treatment drugs, but has been found effective for removal of warts, corns, and calluses. In some cases ingredients known to be safe, but that would not be allowed for certain claims, may be used as inactive ingredients. For example, peppermint, while not effective as a digestive aid, may be used as a flavoring agent.

There are OTC monographs—standards or recipes—that list the ingredients allowed, the claims permitted, and requirements for labeling. Most OTC products are produced in accordance with monographs, and the manufacturers do not have to apply for premarket testing. If, on the other hand, a firm applies for approval of an "innovator" OTC product—one for which there is no monograph—a New Drug Application must be filed, just as with a prescription drug, and it may take just as long to obtain marketing approval.

The FDA does sometimes require supplemental information for OTC products on the market. OTC labeling for aspirin was updated when an association was discovered between the use of aspirin in children with viruses and Reye's syndrome, a potentially fatal brain disease. New combinations are allowed. Adjustments are made. Monographs are revised. The FDA will usually not take enforcement action against marketed OTC drugs provided the producer follows the guidelines and does not exaggerate the benefits of the remedy to the public.

This does not mean OTC drugs have no potentially dangerous side effects!

The labels on certain OTC products must carry warnings. For example, phenyl-propanolamine (PPA) (*see*) is a common ingredient in diet aids. It can induce rapid heartbeat and high blood pressure, a major concern for people already prone to high blood pressure. In extreme cases, the drug's stimulants can induce dangerously rapid and erratic heartbeats.

Digestive aids such as antacids can interfere with the way the body absorbs other substances. Overuse of antacids can cause digestive problems, primarily diarrhea or constipation.

Sodium bicarbonate contains a lot of salt and shouldn't be used by people with high blood pressure or a history of heart failure.

Those who use certain OTC antihistamines need to be warned of possible drowsiness or insomnia. Dr. Fran Gengo, associate professor of neurology and pharmacy at the State University of New York at Buffalo, tested the ability of healthy, young males to drive two to four hours after a common antihistamine had been administered.

"The change in reaction on the average went from 0.8 seconds to 2 seconds," Dr. Gengo noted, "which can mean the difference between life and death if a young child or dog runs out in front of your car."[42]

Recent studies have shown that regular use of ibuprofen and the painkiller acetaminophen can cause further damage in people who already have mild kidney disease.[43]

Even vitamins, if used improperly, can be harmful. At this writing, most researchers seem to agree that acetaminophen is safe for most people if they stick with the recommended dosage—4 grams or eight extra strength tablets a day. There were 102,619 cases of acetaminophen overdose in long-acting products in one year with 100 deaths, according to a notice in the March 6, 1996, issue of *The Journal of the American Medical Association.*[44]

The FDA is aiming to have manufacturers put the sodium content of drugs on labels, and to make certain the print used on all labels is optimum size and style so that it can easily be read by purchasers. A large portion of the public cannot accurately read the labels on OTC products because the print is too small.

In the meantime, how far we can go with the diagnosis and treatment of our own illnesses is still a matter of debate among professionals and consumer advocates. For example, when vaginal yeast-infection remedies changed from Rx to OTC, there was a question about the self-diagnosis. But the FDA advisory board ruled vaginal yeast symptoms are so specific that once a woman is diagnosed and treated by a physician, there is no need to return should those symptoms recur. As of this writing, the self-diagnosis and treatment of vaginal yeast infections seems to be working well.

HERBAL AND HOMEOPATHIC SAFETY

Herbal and homeopathic medications, for the most part, do not list potential adverse reactions. Herbs are considered to be food, and homeopathic medications are exempted from the Food, Drug, and Cosmetic Act. This does not mean they are absolutely harmless. Just as with Rx and OTC remedies, if they have an effect, chances are they also have a side effect.

Herbalists claim their compounds are safer than most Rx and OTC drugs because they are natural and have a long history—sometimes thousands of years of use. But herbal remedies, just as Rx and OTC drugs, can produce serious adverse reactions.

Pennyroyal oil, which contains a potent ingredient that causes abortion, has been found to induce serious bleeding, liver and kidney damage, and death. A tea brewed from tonka

---

42. Fran Gengo, personal communication with author, March 14, 1990.

43. "Over-the-Counter Drugs: Non-Prescription Doesn't Mean Harmless," *Lifetime Health Letter* (University of Texas Health Science Center at Houston) 2, no. 12 (December 1990): 1–3.

44. Cetaruk, Edward et al., "Extended-Release Acetaminophen Overdose." *Journal of the American Medical Association,* March 6, 1996, 686.

beans, sweet clover, and woodruff, all of which are natural sources of the anticoagulant coumarin (*see*), resulted in an almost fatal hemorrhage. An herbal laxative containing podophyllin (*see*), which is toxic to cells, caused severe neurological problems and coma. For those who are sensitive to it, even the popular aloe vera (*see*) products can cause hives and rashes.

Ma huang, promoted as a stimulant and "energizer," when taken with other stimulants or combined with them in a compound, can cause severe adverse reactions including death. The FDA issued a warning in 1995 that the agency had received more than one hundred reports of adverse reactions ranging from heart attacks to hepatitis and several deaths. Among the stimulants that can add to the adverse reactions is caffeine, contained in colas and coffee.[45]

Herbal teas, which became a modern commercial bonanza as part of the back-to-earth movement, are sold in supermarkets as well as in health food stores. The FDA takes a cautious view of herbal teas, maintaining that there is not enough information to conclude they are safe or to predict their effects, in varying concentrations, on the human body.[46] Most of the problems, however, according to the FDA's Center for Food Safety and Applied Nutrition, are reported from people making their own herbal teas, not from the commercial variety.[47] The FDA officially regards herbal teas as being consumed for their taste and aroma only—and not for medicinal purposes. Although no regulations govern herbal teas per se, any herb that is considered safe by the FDA for use in food is presumed to be safe in tea as well.[48]

Mail order catalogs may make all sorts of claims for herbal medications. If the United States Postal Service or the Federal Trade Commission should catch up with them and charge them with fraudulent advertising—and those chances are slim—the promoters can pay the fines and open up under another name.

Since most herbal remedies are considered harmless and ineffective by federal regulators, they are not high on the priority list unless an obvious health hazard is brought to the regulators' attention.

Canada, on the other hand, established an advisory committee on herbs in 1984. As a result, Canada banned the sale of some fifty-seven herbs and required warning labels on five others that, though generally not considered harmful, could pose a health risk if used during pregnancy.

As to the safe use of herbal remedies, you would do well to pay heed to the saying, "There are old mushroom hunters. And there are bold mushroom hunters. But there are no old, bold mushroom hunters."

For example, nux vomica, a homeopathic medicine, is derived from *Strychnos nux-vomica*, a small evergreen tree native to India, Sri Lanka, and Malaysia. The seeds contain strychnine, the poison. Nux vomica (*see*) is used—greatly diluted, of course—to treat indigestion.

---

45. Jane Brody, "A Note of Caution in Exploring the World of Medicinal Herbs: It's a Jungle Out There," *New York Times*, February 15, 1990, B19.
46. Sharon Snider, "Herbal Teas and Toxicity," *FDA Consumer* 25, no. 4 (May 19, 1991): 31–33.
47. Ibid.
48. Ibid.

Whether you choose to use an Rx, OTC, or H remedy, or any combination of these, you should be aware of potentially hidden pitfalls. Just because an herbal or homeopathic remedy is "all natural" does not mean it is "all harmless." It may certainly be so, but proceed with caution, especially if you are thinking of giving it to a child or a pregnant woman.

INACTIVE INGREDIENTS

Inactive or inert ingredients such as binders, fillers, and preservatives may cause allergic reactions in those who are sensitive to them. An adverse reaction to a remedy may actually be a response to an artificial or "inert" ingredient. You may have developed a rash when taking penicillin as a child and avoided this potentially lifesaving medication ever since. The cause of the rash, according to experts in the field, may have been the flavoring agent, not the antibiotic.[49]

Colorings in medications also are a not uncommon source of adverse reactions for those who are allergic or hypersensitive. In this book you will find listed under FD&C and D&C colorings the colorings permitted in drugs. FD&C Yellow No. 5 and FD&C Yellow No. 6 must be listed on labels because many people who are allergic to aspirin and other salicylates are often allergic to these two colorings as well. If a coloring you suspect may be a problem is not listed on a label, look under FD&C colorings in this book. If you are still not sure of the compound used, you may check with the manufacturer or ask your physician to call to obtain the name of the exact coloring chemical used.

SEXUAL DYSFUNCTION

While inert ingredients may cause hidden problems, another common occult side effect of drugs may be sexual dysfunction. As you will see in the listings, a number of medications affect sexual interest and performance. Among the drugs you may not suspect as causing sexual dysfunction, for example, are blood pressure medications, antidepressants, and antiulcer drugs.

And perhaps the biggest problem of all, one that affects all of us at one time or another, concerns drug interactions.

DRUG INTERACTIONS

Many of us do not consider telling a physician we are taking a vitamin, an herbal remedy, an antacid, or a drink of wine. Yet these chemical compounds may interfere with prescribed medications or with each other.

When two or more drugs are taken, the combined effects can increase the chances for adverse reactions by 30 percent, yet patients over sixty-five years of age receive an average of thirteen prescription drugs per year, according to the National Council on Patient Information and Education.[50]

49. Julius Goepp, M.D., Johns Hopkins University news release, August 1992.
50. "Seniors Warned About Mixing Drugs," *Health State* (University of Medicine and Dentistry of New Jersey), summer 1991.

Drug interactions may cause:

Altered absorption. Use of multiple drugs can interfere with their being absorbed into the bloodstream. If, for example, antacids are taken in conjunction with antibiotics from the tetracycline family, the antacids interfere with the absorption of the antibiotics into the blood, thereby diminishing their effect.

Rapid breakdown. When one drug stimulates the body to break down another drug faster than normal, the result is reduced effectiveness of the drug whose breakdown has been hastened. For example, a number of blood-thinning (anticoagulant) medications will be broken down rapidly in people who are also using certain types of sleeping pills.

Rapid elimination. Since many drugs are eliminated by the blood through the kidneys, any drug that interferes with the kidneys' filtration will also affect the elimination of the drug. Aspirin and other drugs from the salicylate family, for example, will interact with some antigout medications by speeding their elimination times—and therefore reducing their effectiveness.

Opposing results. Two drugs can counteract one another, thereby destroying the positive effects of both medications. A number of common antidepressant drugs can counteract and be counteracted by high blood pressure medications, as can certain over-the-counter diet pills and decongestants.

Potentiation. Drugs can interact in a number of ways to increase the levels of medication in a person's blood. But in this situation more is not better.

In fact, this is the case with the interactions between Seldane and ketoconazole, and Seldane and erythromycin. In both instances, according to the FDA, increased levels of Seldane can build up in the blood and, through a little-understood process, disrupt the heart's electrical system, resulting in irregular heart rhythm. Patients with liver disease who use either Seldane or Hismanal can experience the same type of reaction—because their damaged livers are unable to properly metabolize the antihistamines, the drugs build up in their blood.

Among other common drug interactions are the following:

• Alcohol interacts with many Rx, OTC, and H remedies, and the adverse effects may worsen with age because tolerance for alcohol decreases as years increase.

• Antihistamines taken with sleeping pills or narcotics can cause oversedation.

• Aspirin used while taking oral anticoagulants can lead to a hemorrhage.

• Aspirin taken while using diuretics may cause fluid retention and blood pressure hikes.

• Pain relievers used with diabetes medications may lower blood sugar levels too much.

• Laxatives interfere with the action of many medications.

DRUG-FOOD INTERACTIONS

Medicines also interact with food. The use of MAO inhibitor drugs (*see*) for depression, and any foods containing tyramine, such as herring and red wine, can cause a dangerous rise in blood pressure and sometimes lead to a stroke. Eating a dairy product while taking the antibiotic erythromycin (*see*), makes the drug ineffective. The use of potassium-sparing diuretics such as spironolactone (*see*) can cause a heart-affecting overdose of potassium if oranges, bananas, or salt substitutes are ingested. Certain vegetables may make thyroid medication ineffective. When such information is available, it is given in the listings in addition to whether or not a medication should be taken with food.

Now that you know more about how a medication gets to market, its safety aspects, benefits, and risks, you can consider costs. No matter how miraculous an Rx, OTC, or H remedy may be, if you can't afford it, it does you no good.

The following provides some insights into how you may be able to reduce the costs of your medications.

WHAT IS A GENERIC DRUG?

A generic drug is a copy of a brand-name, "innovator" drug that is no longer protected by a patent. Generic drugs generally cost 30 to 50 percent less, and because generic-drug manufacturers compete against each other, the prices of their drugs usually remain low.[51] The number of applications submitted by generic-drug manufacturers to the FDA averages about twenty to twenty-five a month, and the median review time is now about four months. This review time compares to a peak of fifteen months in the late 1980s.

A generic drug must contain the same amount of the active ingredient present in a brand-name product. The inactive ingredients—fillers and coatings that bind the active chemicals—can differ. The generic drug must deliver the active ingredients to the proper site in sufficient quantity to produce the same effect as the original or innovator drug.

About 37 percent of the applications by generic-drug companies to manufacture a copycat product are turned down. Stability concerns are by far the most common reason for field inspectors to withhold approval from generic manufacturers. Other reasons include poor test methods, the plant is not capable of producing the product, and other product-equivalency problems.[52]

Ninety-two percent of new drugs are developed by researched-based pharmaceutical companies, which spend more than $11 billion a year on research and development.[53] Because of their great developmental expense, innovator drugs are protected by patent for seventeen years. That period begins, however, when the company applies for the patent rather than when it receives market approval, which may be years later. Patent protection is designed to allow companies to recoup the cost of developing a new drug before competitors can copy and sell it at a lower price.

The Drug Price Competition and Patent Term Restoration Act of 1984 ensured that new drugs have at least five years of exclusive market protection following approval. It also

---

51. "Seven Quick Facts to Remember About Generic Drugs," brochure from the Generic Pharmaceutical Association, New York, N.Y., 1992.

52. Food and Drug Administration Generics Office report, February 16, 1995.

53. Paul E. Freiman, chairman of the Pharmaceutical Manufacturers Association, 1992 Pharmaceutical Manufacturers Association annual meeting, White Sulphur Springs, W.V., May 12, 1992.

streamlined the approval process for generic drugs. A new 1995 federal law to match practices of other nations, the Uruguay Round Table Agreement Act, opened the door for many drugs to get months and even years of added patent protection, delaying the introduction of generic versions. A generic drug firm is no longer required to repeat all the safety and efficacy studies that were done for the "innovator" drug. Instead, it must prove that its version is equivalent to the original drug and works just as well.

A scandal rocked the generic industry in 1989 when thirteen generic-drug firms were accused of irregularities. Some of the generic drugs were recalled and a few companies were suspended for either submitting false data in their applications or for violations in their manufacturing processes. Three FDA employees pleaded guilty to accepting illegal gifts given by drug-company executives in hopes of speeding marketing approval of their products.[54]

In 1990, the FDA instituted product-specific preapproval inspections of manufacturing sites listed in a generic sponsor's application. Agency inspectors also review on-site product records, examine exhibit batches, and determine whether the plant is capable of properly producing the drug.

Some drug companies will market an identical product both as a brand-name and a generic drug. In 1992, one of the largest and most prestigious brand-name pharmaceutical companies announced that it would market lower-priced versions of its own products and was creating a generic drug division to do so.

It is also common for one manufacturer to produce a drug that is distributed by other firms under many different product names.

Generic drugs account for one-third of all prescriptions filled in the United States. In many states, pharmacists are required to fill a prescription with a generic version of a brand-name drug unless the physician has specified "no substitution." The reason is that generic drugs cost less, on average, about half the price of the brand-name product.

There is no doubt that most generic pharmaceuticals are the same quality as the brand-name. With certain drugs, however, the therapeutic range is narrow because relatively minor changes in circulating levels can affect how well they work. For people with epilepsy or congestive heart failure, the result of any deviation is potentially devastating. Patients with these conditions should consult their physicians before substituting a generic drug for the brand-name version.

Not all drugs are available in generic form. About fifteen innovator drugs lose patent protection annually. These drugs, however, are often protected in their labeling by several patented indications for use. Labeling for generic products reflects only approved indications that are not patent protected.

Companies are also seeking to protect their patents by producing a variety of forms of an innovator drug. For example, Ciba-Geigy's Voltaren was one of the world's best-selling non-steroidal anti-inflammatory drugs for the treatment of arthritis, earning $1.2 billion a year. As its patent protection was running out, Ciba-Geigy produced Voltaren as eyedrops, intra-

---

54. Jeffrey Yorke, "FDA Ensures Equivalence of Generic Drugs," *FDA Consumer,* September 1992, 11–15.

venous solutions, time-released pills, and emulgel, a cross between a cream and an ointment so novel that it earned Ciba-Geigy a new cycle of patent coverage.

MANAGED CARE

The practice of medicine is changing rapidly and thus the prescribing of medications. In the recent past, your physician learned about a drug from a pharmaceutical representative who came to the office, doled out samples, and explained the benefits of the product. Physicians also learned about the pros and cons of medications from medical journals and by attending conferences often infused with pharmaceutical companies' promotion money.

Committees belonging to "managed care" organizations now select a list of medications physicians on staff may prescribe. The committees, concerned with price, are increasingly opting for generic drugs (*see* page 22), which are less expensive than brand-name, and for those medications in a category that are the least costly. This is cost-effective and not necessarily bad. If your doctor, however, wants to try a new medication or one that he or she thinks may be more effective, permission may not be granted. Your busy physician, on the other hand, may not even be aware that a new medication for a particular problem is on the market because pharmaceutical advertising and promotion to the individual doctor and to many medical journals and conferences are disappearing along with the formerly large profit margins of pharmaceutical companies.

From 1984 through 1989—when the inflation rate for all goods and services was no more than 3 or 4 percent annually—prescription drug prices rose at an average annual rate of 9 percent, according to the Bureau of Labor Statistics. In 1993, drug price inflation slowed to the rate of inflation in general. For much of 1994, the producer price index for drugs lagged slightly behind the general rate of inflation. Meanwhile, research and development costs continued to soar.

The U.S. pharmaceutical industry has led the world in the support of the development of new medications. Its future is cloudy, however. Between 1994 and 1998, the federal government will drain $14.5 billion from the brand-name drug industry's profits through rebates, taxes, and user fees. According to the accounting firm Price Waterhouse, the average annual cost of those charges will represent more than 30 percent of the industry's after-tax profits of $9.5 billion.

OTC DRUGS

It is, of course, less costly to treat yourself for a minor ailment with an over-the-counter drug than it is to have a professional prescribe a drug for you. The Nonprescription Drug Manufacturers Association maintains we saved $770 million in one year (1989) through the recent switch of thirteen cough/cold medicines from Rx to OTC status—in the cost of doctors' fees, prescription drugs, and time lost from work.[55]

And just as buying generics over brand names may save money, choosing house brands or

---

55. "Nonprescription Drug Manufacturers Association Fact Sheet," Washington, D.C., August 7, 1991; Peter Temin, Ph.D., "Costs and Benefits in Switching Drugs from Rx to OTC," *Journal of Health Economics* 2 (1983): 187–205.

nonadvertised OTC products may save money as well. Since the FDA requires OTC producers of a drug for a certain category to follow a recipe, many cough-control products, for example, with a variety of names, may contain exactly the same ingredients. You can check the back of labels for product comparison, and if the percentages of the ingredients are the same or close, you may opt for the less expensive product. Of course, one compound may taste or look better than the other, and you have to keep in mind that enforcement of standards is spotty, so you may still wish to choose a brand name over a less well-known manufacturer's product.

HERBAL AND HOMEOPATHIC REMEDIES

There is little regulation of herbal or homeopathic products, so you are probably safest opting for those produced by well-respected companies. Buying mixtures produced by a local shaman or concocting your own herbal remedies may be costly if they make you sick.

Check with your supermarket and discount drugstore. They often sell herbal products at prices less (although sometimes more) than your local health food store or mail order catalog.

If you look up certain homeopathic medicines in this book, you may be surprised. Natrum muriatricum, also called nat. mur. and nat-m. in homeopathy, is, as you will find in the listing in this book, sodium chloride. So is the salt on your table.

YOUR RESPONSIBILITY

We are a medicated society. Each year Americans take 1.6 billion prescriptions, and often, improper use of those drugs leads to severe health problems. According to the National Council on Patient Information and Education, an estimated 125,000 Americans die each year because they do not take their prescription drugs properly.[56]

Among the reasons for medication problems found by a University of Rhode Island survey are:

- Duplication of drug products.
- Drug interaction or contraindicated use.
- Patient confusion over drugs whose names sound alike.
- Problems from changes in dosage directions not recorded on label.
- Improper drug administration.
- Outdated or expired medicine.
- Lack of sufficient patient understanding of drug therapy.[57]

When your doctor writes a prescription, ask questions. Ninety-six percent of patients don't ask and, according to a survey by the FDA, seven out of ten doctors never tell their patients about the risks of drugs prescribed.[58] Ask!

56. "Seniors Warned About Mixing Drugs," *Health State* (University of Medicine and Dentistry of New Jersey), summer 1991, 34.

57. University of Rhode Island College of Pharmacy Study on Significant Misuse of Prescription Medications Among the Elderly," Kingston, R.I., March 5, 1990, 1–5.

58. "Prescription Drugs: A Guide to Safe Use of Medicines," *University of Texas Newsletter* (Houston, Tex.) 4, no. 6 (June 1992): 4–6.

Ask your pharmacist about a prescription or OTC drug. Pharmacists have to offer counseling to anyone having a Medicaid prescription filled. At least twenty-one states have adopted a requirement that pharmacists offer to counsel all patients. When prescribed a drug, gather the following information:

- What is the name of the medicine, and what is it supposed to do?
- How and when do I take the medicine, and for how long?
- What foods, drinks, other medicines, or activities should I avoid while taking this medication?
- Tell your physician all the medications you are taking, including over-the-counter drugs and vitamin and mineral supplements, and ask if there will be any adverse interactions.
- Relate any problems you or your family members have had with specific medications, such as an allergic reaction, and ask if the prescription may cause such side effects.
- Discuss health problems that might put you at special risk, such as kidney or liver dysfunction.
- Be sure to inform your doctor if you are pregnant or plan to become pregnant soon, and ask to which pregnancy category the particular drug belongs.
- Ask about the side effects and what you should do if they occur.
- Request available written information about the medication.

IN YOUR HOME

When you are in your home, you also have responsibilities concerning your medications. First of all, you have to remember to take them on time. This is often a problem when you have to take a number of remedies, or when the drugs have to be taken at different times. If you are an older person or have a busy schedule, you may forget to take a dose or even forget whether or not you took it. A number of "reminder" devices are available, the least expensive of which is a calendar to record your medications on a day-by-day basis or a checkoff list. Once you have a routine down pat, there are other considerations:

- If you experience what you think might be a serious side effect, notify your physician immediately.
- Don't skip taking a drug just because you feel better: most drugs, especially antibiotics, need the fully prescribed time to work.
- Don't raise or lower the dose on your own. If one pill is good, two are not better and, in fact, might be dangerous. Taking too little may render a medication ineffective.
- Don't stop taking a medicine abruptly without the doctor's advice. Some drugs, such as corticosteroids, must be tapered.
- Don't mix alcohol and medication unless your doctor tells you that it is okay to do so.

PROPER STORAGE AND DISPOSAL OF MEDICATIONS

Store your medicines properly. Since heat and humidity harm pharmaceuticals, store them in a cool, dry place. If you're traveling, keep in mind that the glove compartment or trunk of your car gets hot and is not a good place to store medicines. An insulated thermos is better.

• Don't transfer a medication from its original bottle to another container.

• Discard any Rx, OTC, or H medicines that are no longer being taken, and any medicine that has a noticeable change in color or odor. Chemical changes occur with age, light, heat, air, or water and may cause a drug to break down into useless or harmful substances. Evaporation of water or alcohol may cause a drug to become much stronger per dose. Microbes may breed in a drug, causing contamination. Water may make it cake or destroy its protective coating. Consumers expect expiration dates and, when they don't find them, assume incorrectly that the medicine may be good indefinitely. Ask your pharmacist to place an expiration date on your medication label if it is not on the container.

• Get rid of medicines for which the label or package instructions are missing or cannot be read clearly.

• Remember, in addition to the potential harm to you of old medications, keeping them around creates an unnecessary safety hazard for curious children.

• Dispose of medicines properly. Flush the contents down the sink or toilet and place only the empty container in the trash.

How to Use This Book

While unique in content, this dictionary follows the format of most dictionaries. The following are examples of entries with any explanatory notes that may be necessary:

TERFENADINE (Rx) • Seldane. Seldane-D (with pseudoephedrine). Introduced in 1977, it is used to relieve symptoms associated with seasonal allergic rhinitis such as sneezing, runny nose, itching, and tearing. Promoted as a nonsedating antihistamine. Relief begins in one hour. Contraindicated in patients with known hypersensitivity to terfenadine or any of its ingredients. Should be used cautiously in patients with liver dysfunction, low potassium, or irregular heartbeat. In July 1992, the FDA instructed the makers of terfenadine to strengthen the warning about the risk of patients developing life-threatening, abnormal heart rhythms if they have liver dysfunction or if they take one of three antibiotics—erythromycin, ketoconazole, or troleandomycin—concurrently with terfenadine. Reports received by the company of severe adverse cardiovascular effects include, in addition to irregular heartbeat, low blood pressure, heart palpitations, and fainting. Nine cases of serious side effects including one death have been reported in Japan in association with terfenadine. The adverse drug reactions were related to heart problems in patients receiving certain antibiotics, or in those with liver problems. Other potential adverse terfenadine effects include drowsiness, headache, fatigue, dizziness, nervousness, weakness, appetite increase, abdominal distress, nausea, vomiting, a change in bowel habits, dry mouth, nose, and throat, cough, sore throat, nosebleed, hair loss, menstrual irregularity, female breast enlargement with milk production, sweating, muscle ache, tingling of hands and feet, visual disturbances, liver dysfunction, itching, and rash. Unlike other antihistamines, terfenadine reportedly does not interact with alcohol and other central nervous system depressants. Medication should be discontinued four days before taking a skin allergy test because it can lead to inaccurate results. Terfenadine may be taken on an empty stomach. A candidate for OTC status, as of this writing. Also a candidate for production as a less costly generic drug.

From this listing you learn that terfenadine is the generic name of a prescription drug, the brand name of which is Seldane. It was introduced in 1977, so you know it has been on the market for a number of years. Its purpose—as a nonsedating antihistamine—is given as well as its potential adverse side effects, including a recent warning that it can cause severe heart and blood-vessel side effects when taken at the same time as certain other medications. Terfenadine's interaction with other drugs, including alcohol, is given, and it is noted that it can make skin allergy tests inaccurate and may be taken on an empty stomach. You also learn that it is a candidate for a switch to OTC status, and for production as a less expensive generic drug.

If you are not certain of a term in the listing, such as *contraindicated,* just look it up in the dictionary:

CONTRAINDICATED • Means that a medication may hold a risk for an individual because of heredity, other medications being taken, kidney or liver problems, or other reasons that may lead to an adverse reaction.

The following is a listing for an herbal remedy:

UVA-URSI (H) • *Arctostaphylos uva-ursi.* **Bearberry.** An astringent used to treat bladder problems, its action is believed due to the high concentration of the antiseptic arbutin. Arbutin, in passing through the system, yields hydroquinone (*see*), a urinary disinfectant. Uva-ursi leaves contain anesthetic principles that numb pain in the urinary system, and the herb has been shown to have antibiotic activity. Crude extracts of uva-ursi reportedly possess some anticancer property. In 1992, the FDA proposed a ban on uva-ursi extract in oral menstrual drug products because it had not been shown to be safe and effective as claimed. Regular use of this plant may lead to constipation.

From this entry you learn that the herb has several names, contains certain ingredients that are in other medications, and that its main use is as a urinary disinfectant. Information is given that the herb has been shown to have some antibiotic and anticancer activity. It is also noted that the FDA proposed a ban on using uva-ursi in oral menstrual drugs because it had not been shown to be safe and effective as claimed. It remains in herbal formulations for other purposes.

The following is an OTC listing:

CHLORPHENIRAMINE (OTC) • **Alka-Seltzer Plus Cold Medicine. Aller-Calor. Allerest. A.R.M. Allergy Relief. BC Cold Powder. Cerose-DM. Cheracol. Chloramine. Chlorate. Chlor-100. Chlor-Pro. Chlorspan. Chlortab. Chlor-Trimeton. Comtrex. Contac. Coricidin. Dorcol. Dristan. 4-Way Cold Tablets. Genallerate. Isoclor. Medi-Flu Caplets. Novahistine. Orthoxicol. PediaCare. Pfeiffer's Allergy. Phenetron. Pyranistan.**

Pyrroxate. Rhyna. Sinarest Extra Strength. Sine-Off. Singlet. Sinulin. Sinutab Sinus. Sudafed Plus. Telachlor. Teldrin. TheraFlu Flu and Cold Medicine. Triaminic. Trymegen. Tussi-Organidin. Tylenol Allergy Sinus. Tylenol Cold & Flu. Vicks Children's NyQuil. Vicks Formula 44. An antihistamine recategorized from Rx to OTC, first in low dosage in 1976, and in stronger strengths in 1981. It is used to treat stuffy nose and other allergy symptoms. Potential adverse effects include stimulation, sedation, drowsiness (in the elderly), excitability (in children), low blood pressure, palpitations, stomach distress, dry mouth, urine retention, rash, hives, and thick bronchial secretions. Central nervous system depressants, including alcohol, increase sedation, and MAO inhibitors may increase blood pressure. Contraindicated in acute asthmatic attacks. Use cautiously in elderly patients, those with glaucoma, overactive thyroid, heart or kidney disease, high blood pressure, bronchial asthma, enlarged prostate, bladder-neck obstruction, and peptic ulcer. Coffee or tea may reduce drowsiness. Medication should be discontinued four days before taking a skin allergy test because it can lead to inaccurate results. In 1992, the FDA issued a notice that chlorpheniramine maleate had not been shown to be safe and effective as claimed in OTC products for poison ivy, poison oak, and poison sumac drug products.

We can determine that this OTC antihistamine that was once sold only as an Rx drug has many names. The adverse reactions are given and it is noted that in 1992 the FDA determined it was not shown to be safe and effective for treatment of poison ivy, poison oak, and poison sumac. Chlorpheniramine remains one of the most widely used OTC ingredients on the market for other uses.

There is a listing elsewhere that will add more information when you read "(*see*)." As much as possible, explanations of medical terms are listed in the dictionary. Since many medical terms are literally Greek, there are listings to help you understand many formerly mysterious words. For example, the *dys-, dis-* prefix you will read means "bad" or "difficult," and thus you can better understand why dysmenorrhea means painful menstruation, dyscrasia means bad blood, dyspepsia signifies disturbed digestion, and dyslexia means difficulty in reading and/or understanding written material.

There are also definitions of medical conditions. For example:

EMBOLUS • A blood clot or other material such as a fragment of fat carried along in the bloodstream.

FIBROCYSTIC BREAST DISEASE • A benign condition that is the most common disorder of the female breast. The fact that new cysts usually do not appear after menopause suggests that ovarian hormones are involved in this disease.

GOUT • **Arthritis Nodosa.** An inherited disorder of purine metabolism, occurring mostly in men. Involves a high level of uric acid and sudden, severe onset of arthritis resulting from deposits of crystals of sodium urate in connective tissue and cartilage. The feet, ankles, and knees are commonly affected.

There are even definitions of common herbal and homeopathic terms such as:

EMMENAGOGUE • An agent that induces or increases menstrual flow. Among the herbs used for this purpose are motherwort, cramp bark, and fenugreek (*see all*).

SUCCUSSION • Vigorous shaking while a homeopathic remedy is being diluted.

Terminology has generally been kept to a middle road between what is understandable to a professional and to the average interested consumer, while at the same time avoiding oversimplification of data. If in doubt, look up alphabetically any term listed that seems unfamiliar or whose meaning has been blunted by overuse.

With *A Consumer's Dictionary of Medicines—Prescription, Over-the-Counter, Homeopathic, and Herbal,* you will be able to work with your physician and pharmacist and with OTC and herbal labels to determine the benefits and risks of a particular remedy. The knowledge you gain may not only save you money, it may save your health and your life.

A

AZLINA-, AN- • Prefixes meaning absent or lacking, deficient or without, such as anorexia: without appetite; or anemia: deficient in blood.

A AND D OINTMENT (OTC) • *See* Vitamin A and Vitamin D.

ABBOCILLIN-VK (Rx) • *See* Penicillin V.

ABBOKINASE (Rx) • *See* Urokinase.

ABCIXIMAB (Rx) • **Reopro.** A biotech product, a monoclonal antibody (*see*) for the reduction of acute heart complications in patients undergoing angioplasty and who are at high risk for abrupt artery closure by blood clots. It is the first of a new class of agents that targets the platelet IIb/IIIa receptors. It has been dubbed a "superaspirin" because it blocks the final common pathway of platelet activation and so is more effective than current agents. Bleeding, as in the case of aspirin and other similar drugs, is of concern. It was approved after a twelve-month review by the FDA and its first market is the United States.

ABDRONATE (Rx) • *See* Testosterone.

ABELCET (Rx) • A suspension of Amphotericin B (*see*) encapsulated in a fatty carrier for IV administration.

ABORTIFACIENT • Medicine that causes abortion.

ABRADE • Scrape or erode a covering such as skin or the lining of the intestines.

ABSCESS • A circumscribed collection of pus.

ABSENCE SEIZURE • **Petit Mal Epilepsy.** Attacks of impaired consciousness, occasionally accompanied by spasm or twitching of the muscles of the head.

ACACIA GUM (OTC) (H) • *Acacia vera.* **Black Catechu. Gum Arabic. Egyptian Thorn.**
Acacia is the odorless, colorless, tasteless dried exudate from the stem of the acacia tree, grown in Africa, the Near East, India, and the southern United States. Its most distinguishing quality among the natural gums is its ability to dissolve rapidly in water. The use of acacia dates back four thousand years. Used today in denture adhesive powder and to give shape to tablets, as a demulcent to soothe irritations, particularly of the mucous membranes, and by herbalists to treat burns. Can cause allergic reactions such as skin rash and asthmatic attacks. Oral toxicity is low. In 1992, the FDA issued a notice that catechu tincture had not been shown to be safe and effective as claimed in OTC digestive aid products.

ACARBOSE (Rx) • **Precose.** Isolated from the strains of *Actinoplanes,* it belongs to a new class of drugs that reduce sugar absorption in the gastrointestinal tract. An oral medication, it is prescribed for patients with Type II (non-insulin dependent) diabetes, whose high blood sugar cannot be managed on diet alone. It significantly reduces after-meal blood sugar levels. In addition, unlike sulfonylurea (*see*) drugs and insulin, acarbose reportedly does not cause low blood sugar, high blood sugar, or weight gain. Potential side effects include flatulence, abdominal distention, and diarrhea due to fermentation of undigested carbohydrates.

ACCUPRIL (Rx) • *See* Quinapril.

ACCURBRON (Rx) • *See* Theophylline.

ACCUTANE (Rx) • *See* Isotretinoin.

ACE • Abbreviation for angiotensin-converting enzyme (*see*), an effective treatment for high blood pressure and heart failure.

ACEBUTOLOL (Rx) • **Sectral.** Introduced in 1985, acebutolol is a beta-blocker (*see*) that is most commonly used to treat high blood pressure, angina, and abnormal heart rhythms. It is also used to relieve anxiety, and palpitations and tremor caused by overactivity of the thyroid gland. Unlike some similar drugs that act on both the heart and the lungs, acebutolol acts mainly on the heart. This allows it to be used for asthmatics and those who suffer from bronchitis or other lung problems. It also, reportedly, does not raise blood fats. Potential adverse reactions include lethargy, cold hands and feet due to reduced circulation, nausea, nightmares, rash, breathlessness, and fainting. May adversely affect asthma and heart problems. As with other beta-blockers, acebutolol affects the body's response to low blood sugar, which can trigger problems in diabetics. When Nifedipine is used with acebutolol, blood pressure may fall too low. Antiarrhythmic drugs may cause a further reduction in heart rate. Indomethacin (see) reduces the blood pressure-lowering effect of acebutolol. Cimetidine can increase the levels of acebutolol in the blood. Acebutolol should not be discontinued abruptly since this could worsen symptoms and may even result in a heart attack. May be taken with or without food.

ACE INHIBITORS (Rx) • Angiotensin-Converting Enzyme Inhibitors.

A class of drugs that acts by blocking an enzyme in the blood responsible for converting angiotensin 1 to angiotensin 2. Angiotensin 2 induces sodium retention and constriction of peripheral blood vessels, raising blood pressure. Birth defects and fetal deaths have been associated, however, with the use of ACE inhibitors during pregnancy, and in 1992, the FDA issued an advisory to physicians against prescribing it for women in the second and last trimester of pregnancy. Among the ACE inhibitors available: benazepril, captopril, enalapril, fosinopril, lisinopril, quinapril, and ramipril.

ACEMANNAN • Carrisyn. See Aloe Vera.

ACEPHEN (OTC) • See Acetaminophen.

ACETAMINOPHEN (OTC) • Paracetamol Sedapap-10.

An ingredient introduced in the early 1900s, now in more than one hundred over-the-counter medications. The following are among the products that have acetaminophen as the main ingredient: **Acephen, Aceta, Actamin, Actifed Plus Caplets, Allerest, Allergy-Sinus Comtrex, Amphenol, Anacin-3, Anuphen, APAP, APF Arthritis Pain Formula, Aspirin-Free Anacin Acetaminophen, Banesin, Benadryl Cold Tablets and Nighttime Formula, Bromo-Seltzer, Bufferin A/F Nite Time, Capital and Codeine, Cold Control + Intense Cold Medicine, Conacetol, Congespirin for Children, Contac Cough and Chest Cold, Coricidin, Dapa, Datril, Dolanex, Drixoral, Excedrin PM Analgesic/Sleeping Aid, Feverall, Genagesic, Genapap, Genebs, Halenol, Histosal, Hydrocet, Hydrogesic, Hy-Phen, Liquiprin, Lorcet Plus, Lortab, Meda Tab, Medi-Flu, Medigesic, Midol, Midrin, Myapap, Neopap Suppretes, Oraphen-PD, Ornex, Pamprin, Panadol, Panex, Pedric Wafers, Peedee, Percocet, Percogesic, Premsyn PMS, Phenaphen, Phenaphen with Codeine, Pyrroxate Capsules, Rid-A-Pain, Robitussin Night Relief, St. Joseph Aspirin-Free Fever Reducer for Children, Sinarest, Sine-Aid, Sine-Off, Singlet Tablets, Sinubid, Sinulin, Sinus Excedrin Analgesic, Sinutab Sinus Allergy Medication, Sominex Pain Relief Formula, Sudafed Severe Cold Formula, Sudafed Sinus Tablets, Suntab Sinus Medication, Suppap, Tapanol, Tapar, Tempra, Tenol, TheraFlu Flu and Cold Medicine, Triaminicin, Tylenol, Tylenol Acetaminophen Children's Chewable Tablets, Tylenol Allergy Sinus Medication, Tylenol with Codeine, Tylox, Ty-Pap, Ty-Tabs, Unisom with Pain Relief, Valadol, Valorin, Vanquish Analgesic Caplets, Vicks DayCare, Vicks Formula 44M Multi-Symptom Cough & Cold Medicine, and Vicks NyQuil Nighttime Cold/Flu Medicine.** A coal tar (see) derivative, this pain reliever and fever reducer is believed to work by blocking pain impulses, due to inhibition of the manufacture of prostaglandin or other substances that sensitize pain receptors to mechanical or chemical stimulation. Unlike aspirin, it does not affect prostaglandins elsewhere in the body or relieve the redness or swelling caused by rheumatoid arthritis. It can be used by persons allergic to aspirin. Considered one of the safest painkillers, it usually does not irritate the stomach or cause allergic reactions. However, it may affect the kidney or liver if taken in large amounts over a prolonged period, especially if alcohol is ingested. Acetaminophen is derived from phenacetin (*see*), but is associated with less toxicity. Phenacetin, which was removed from the market in the 1980s because of its serious and sometimes fatal side effects, turned into acetaminophen in the body. Side effects of acetaminophen may include diarrhea, skin rash, loss of appetite, increased sweating, swelling, pain or tenderness in the upper abdomen or stomach area, painful urination, nausea, vomiting, stomach cramps, and sodium depletion. Persons with kidney or liver damage should not use this drug nor should people who are anemic. Also not prescribed for persons who drink large quantities of alcohol, because alcohol may increase acetaminophen's toxic potential, and vice versa. Should not be taken for more than ten consecutive days unless directed by a physician. Should not be used with AZT (*see*) because it causes higher blood levels of AZT and increases the chance of serious side effects. Acetaminophen should not be taken with aspirin or other salicylates or NSAIDs (*see*) because it will increase the side effects of such drugs, including gastrointestinal upsets and bleeding. Acetaminophen may cause false results in blood-sugar tests. A study by researchers at the University of Pittsburgh Medical Center found that as little as five grams or ten tablets a day could injure the liver if patients were not eating or if they were drinking heavily. An Alexandria, Virginia, federal court awarded $8.8 million to a Virginia man who said the recommended dose of Tylenol —combined with three or four glasses of wine a night—destroyed his liver. There were 102,619 cases of acetaminophen-containing products in one year with 100 deaths, according to a notice in the March 6, 1996, issue of *The Journal of the American Medical Association*. At this writing, most researchers seem to agree that acetaminophen is safe for most people if they stick with the recommended dosage—4 grams or eight extra-strength tablets a day.

ACETAZOLAMIDE (Rx) • Ak-Zol. Dazamide. Diamox.
Introduced in 1953, it inhibits an enzyme in the body, carbonic anhydrase, which allows the drug to be used as a weak diuretic and as part of the treatment of glaucoma by helping to reduce pressure inside the eye. Potential adverse reactions include nausea, vomiting, drowsiness, anemia, numbness, confusion, tingling in the limbs, transient nearsightedness, loss of appetite, kidney stones, low blood potassium, acidosis caused by high blood chloride, and rash. May activate gout or cause syndromes similar to lupus or hepatitis. Contraindicated as long-term therapy for certain types of glaucoma and in persons with low blood sodium, low blood potassium, kidney, liver, or adrenal dysfunction, or high blood chloride. Should be used cautiously in patients with lung disease, and in patients receiving other diuretics. It may cause allergic reactions in people allergic to sulfa drugs, interact with over-the-counter products containing stimulants, and cause problems for those with heart disease or glaucoma. Aspirin may increase its effects. To prevent an upset stomach when ingested, acetazolamide may be taken with food. Foods rich in potassium such as apricots and bananas should be in the diet since acetazolamide may deplete the body of potassium. However, if a physician prescribes a potassium supplement, such a high-potassium diet may cause a dangerous potassium overload. Check with your doctor.

ACETIC ACID (OTC) • Domeboro Otic. Star-Otic Ear Solution. Tridesilon. VoSol Otic.
The acid found in vinegar. Used in douches and ear drops. It inhibits or destroys bacteria present in the ear canal and the vagina. Potential adverse reactions include irritation or itching, hives, and overgrowth of nonsusceptible organisms.

ACETIC ESTER • *See* Ethyl Acetate.

ACETOHEXAMIDE (Rx) • Dymelor.
Antidiabetic. A member of the sulfonylurea (*see*) family, introduced in 1963, it is prescribed to reduce blood glucose levels by stimulating the pancreas to produce insulin. Adjunct to diet to lower the blood sugar in patients with noninsulin-dependent diabetes. Potential adverse reactions include nausea, vomiting, heartburn, sodium loss, low blood sugar, rash, itching, facial flushing, and hypersensitivity reactions. Anabolic steroids (*see*), chloramphenicol, clofibrate, guanethidine, MAO

inhibitors, oral blood thinners, salicylates, and sul-fonamides increase blood-sugar-lowering activity. Beta-blockers (*see*) and clonidine prolong the low blood sugar effect and may mask symptoms of low blood sugar such as fast heartbeat or high blood pressure. Because of this, a diabetic may not take steps to immediately correct blood sugar levels. Corticosteroids, glucagon, rifampin, and thiazide diuretics decrease blood-sugar-lowering effect. Contraindicated in treating insulin-dependent diabetes, in diabetes adequately controlled by diet, and in Type II diabetes complicated by ketosis, acidosis, diabetic coma, Raynaud's disease, gangrene, liver or kidney dysfunction, or thyroid or other endocrine dysfunction. The possibility of increased heart disease deaths is associated with the use of sulfonylureas.

ACETOHYDROXAMIC ACID (Rx) •
Lithostat. A drug that prevents formation of kidney stones and is also used to treat infections related to kidney stones. Potential adverse reactions include nausea, vomiting, diarrhea, anemia, mild headache, depression, anxiety, phlebitis, palpitations, loss of appetite, constipation, rash, hair loss, and malaise. Oral iron supplements reduce absorption. Acetohydroxamic acid is contraindicated in patients who are candidates for urinary tract surgery or are responsive to antibiotics, and those with poor kidney function. Alcohol may cause a rash if consumed while taking acetohydroxamic acid. Acetohydroxamic acid works best on an empty stomach.

ACETONE (OTC) •
A colorless, ethereal liquid derived by oxidation or fermentation. Used as a solvent. Inhalation may irritate the lungs. It is narcotic in large amounts, causing symptoms of drunkenness similar to those of alcohol. In 1992, the FDA proposed a ban on acetone in astringent (*see*) drug products because it had not been shown to be safe and effective as claimed.

ACETOPHENAZINE MALEATE (Rx) •
Tindal. A piperazine (*see*) phenothiazine that increases dopamine (*see*) in the brain. Used to treat psychotic disorders. Potential adverse reactions include low white blood cell count, uncontrolled movements, dizziness, drop in blood pressure when rising from seated or prone position, vision changes, dry mouth, constipation, urine retention, menstrual irregularities, breast enlargement in men, inhibited ejaculation, liver dysfunction, mild photosensitivity, skin rashes, weight gain, increased appetite, fever, irregular heartbeat, and profuse sweating. Abrupt stoppage of the drug may cause gastritis, nausea, vomiting, dizziness, tremors, feeling of warmth or cold, sweating, irregular heartbeat, headache, and insomnia. Alcohol and other central nervous system depressants should not be used with it. Antacids inhibit absorption, thus acetophenazine should not be taken within three hours of taking them. Barbiturates may decrease phenothiazine's effects. Contraindicated in central nervous system depression, bone-marrow suppression, and brain damage. Also contraindicated with use of spinal or epidural anesthetic, or adrenergic-blocking agents (*see*). Should be used cautiously in the elderly or in debilitated patients, and in persons with liver disease, cardiovascular disease, exposure to extreme heat or cold, respiratory disorders, high blood calcium, seizures, glaucoma, or enlarged prostate. Tardive dyskinesia (*see*) may occur after prolonged use. The drug should not be withdrawn suddenly. Should be taken at bedtime to facilitate sleep. Decrease sedation during daytime.

ACETOXYMETHYLPROGESTERONE • *See*
Medroxyprogesterone.

ACETYLCHOLINE (Rx) • Miochol.
A chemical neurotransmitter that is released by nerve cells and stimulates other nerve cells and muscles and organs throughout the body. This neurotransmitter is believed to be involved in memory function. Acetylcholine also dilates the blood vessels and helps to move food through the intestines. In a chloride solution for the eye it causes contraction of the iris, resulting in contraction of the pupil. Used after eye surgery. No adverse reactions reported for a 1 percent solution.

ACETYLCHOLINESTERASE •
An enzyme that breaks down the neurotransmitter, a chemical messenger between nerve cells in the brain. In-

hibitors of this enzyme may be useful in treating Alzheimer's disease.

ACETYLCYSTEINE (Rx) • Mucomyst. Mucosil. A mucolytic (*see*) used to relieve mucous congestion of the nose, sinuses, and airways in pneumonia, bronchitis, tuberculosis, cystic fibrosis, emphysema, atelectasis, and complications of chest and heart surgery. The drug is administered in a spray. Because it alters the action of mucus in the stomach, acetylcysteine may cause digestive problems, especially in people with peptic ulcers. May also cause nausea and vomiting, rash, breathing difficulties, and excessive and bloody mucus. Has a foul taste. Should be used cautiously in asthma or severe respiratory insufficiency, and in elderly or debilitated patients.

ACETYLSALICYLIC ACID • *See* Aspirin.

ACHEMILLA VULGARIS (H) • *See* Lady's Mantle Extract.

ACHES-N-PAINS (OTC) • *See* Ibuprofen.

ACHROMYCIN • *See* Tetracyclines.

ACID • An acid can be liquid, solid, or gas. Although there are a great variety of acids, properties are common to most of them. When dissolved, acids taste sour, and they neutralize bases, react with metals to form salts and water, turn blue litmus paper red, and can conduct electric current. An acid solution has a pH (*see*) of less than 7.

ACIDOSIS • A buildup of too much acid in the blood or body tissues. *See* Acidulants.

ACID, GASTRIC • A corrosive and bitter substance—hydrochloric acid—that enables the enzyme pepsin to digest food and is secreted by cells in the lining of the stomach.

ACID MANTLE CREME (OTC) • *See* Aluminum Acetate.

ACIDOPHILUS (OTC) (H) • *Lactobacillus acidophilus.* A type of bacterium that ferments milk and is used to treat intestinal disorders. It changes the intestinal flora. Yogurt that has live cultures of this bacteria reportedly decreases by a third the number of vaginal yeast infections in women. Acidophilus is also widely used to prevent and to relieve diarrhea, especially when taking antibiotics. *See* Yogurt.

ACID STOMACH • A burning or gnawing pain in the upper abdomen. The stomach is naturally acidic, but may become overacidic due to slow emptying, oversecretion, or other causes.

ACIDULANTS • Acidulants are acids that make a substance more acidic and function as a flavoring agent to acidify taste, to blend unrelated flavoring characteristics, and to mask any undesirable aftertaste. Acidulants are also used as preservatives to prevent germ and spore growths that spoil foods and pharmaceutical compounds. Acidulants control the acid-alkali (pH) balance. *See* pH. *See* Acid.

ACIDULATED PHOSPHATE (OTC) • An .02 percent fluoride solution used as a dental rinse. In 1980, it was recategorized Rx to OTC.

ACIDULIN • *See* Glutamic Acid.

A-CILLIN • *See* Amoxicillin.

ACINETOBACTER • A gram-negative (*see*) bacterium that occurs frequently in tissue, especially in the genitourinary tract.

ACLOVATE • *See* Alclometasone.

ACNE • Skin pores become plugged with an oily substance, sebum, and other materials such as pigment, dead cells, and bacteria. If the plug (comedo) remains just beneath the surface, it appears as a small, round, whitish bump, a "whitehead." If it reaches the skin surface, it looks like a black dot, a "blackhead." In some cases, the plugged pore may burst, thereby releasing its oily contents into the surrounding tissue and causing inflammation. This results in the formation of pimples, pus-filled lesions, or even cysts, cavities containing a sticky fluid.

ACO • Homeopathic medicine's abbreviation for aconite (*see*).

ACON • *See* Vitamin A.

ACONITE (OTC) (H) • *Aconitum napellus.* **Aco. Friar's-Cowl. Monkshood. Mousebane. Wolfsbane. Hyland's Cough Syrup with Honey.** Dried tuberous root of *Aconitum napellus,* found in the mountain regions of Europe, Asia, and North America. Among its constituents are aconitine, a toxic alkaloid that can be absorbed through the skin, aconitic acid, itaconic acid, succinic acid, fat, and levulose (fruit sugar). It is used to reduce fever, as a sedative, and externally to relieve sciatica and neuralgia. Can be toxic in large amounts and was used by the ancient Greeks as a poison. Homeopaths used it to treat coughs, abdominal complaints, fevers, and sore ears and eyes. It is used only in great dilution in homeopathic medicines because of it potential toxicity. In large doses, it can be fatal. Symptoms of poisoning include numbness of the mouth and throat, speech difficulty, nausea, vomiting, blurred vision, muscular paralysis, convulsions, and respiratory paralysis. Even topical application may cause poisoning if put on abraded skin. *See* Monkshood.

ACONITUM NAPELLUS • *See* Aconite and Monkshood.

ACORNS (H) • **Akarn.** The nut of the oak. The name means "fruit of the forest trees." Acorn is used in teas and food as a nutrient, and to soothe skin. It contains tannins, flavonoids, sugar, starch, albumin, and fats. Was used by American Indians to treat diarrhea, and as a food staple.

ACORUS CALAMUS • *See* Calamus.

ACRIVASTINE (Rx) • Nonsedating antihistamine. Used to treat hives and allergic rhinitis. *See* Semprex D.

ACROCYANOSIS • **Crocq's Disease.** A circulatory disorder in which the hands and, less commonly, the feet are persistently cold and blue; some forms are related to Raynaud's disease (*see*).

ACT (OTC) • *See* Sodium Fluoride.

ACT (Rx) • *See* Dactinomycin.

ACTAGEN • *See* Pseudoephedrine and Triprolidine.

ACTAMIN • *See* Acetaminophen.

ACTH (Rx) • Abbreviation for adrenocorticotropic hormone. This hormone emanates from the pituitary gland, which stimulates the adrenal gland to produce cortisonelike hormones. *See* Corticotropin.

ACTHAR • *See* Corticotropin.

ACTIBINE • *See* Yohimbine.

ACTICORT • *See* Hydrocortisone.

ACTIDIL • *See* Triprolidine.

ACTIDOSE (OTC) • *See* Activated Charcoal.

ACTIDOSE-AQUA (OTC) • *See* Activated Charcoal.

ACTIFED (OTC) • *See* Pseudoephedrine and Triprolidine.

ACTIGALL • *See* Ursodiol.

ACTIMMUNE (Rx) • Interferon gamma-1b. Produced by Genentech, Inc., it is used in the management of chronic granulomatous disease (*see*).

ACTINEX • *See* Masoprocol Cream.

ACTINIC KERATOSES • **AK.** Roughness and thickening of the skin caused by overexposure to the sun's ultraviolet rays. AK can degenerate into a squamous cell cancer of the skin.

ACTION POTENTIAL • An electric burst that travels the length of the nerve cell and causes the release of a neurotransmitter.

ACTIVASE • *See* Alteplase.

ACTIVATED CHARCOAL (OTC) • **Acti-dose-Aqua. Charcoaid. Charcocaps. Flatulex. Liqui-Char. SuperChar.** An adsorbent, detoxicant, and soothing agent. The charcoal is obtained by distillation of organic material such as vegetables or animal bones and activated by heating with steam or carbon dioxide, resulting in a porous material. It is used to relieve intestinal gas discomfort and diarrhea and is recognized by the FDA for the treatment of swallowed poisons. It adheres to many drugs and chemicals, inhibiting their absorption from the GI tract. Potential adverse reactions include black stools and nausea.

ACTIVE IMMUNITY, IMMUNITY • Produced by the body in response to stimulation by a disease-causing organism or a vaccine.

ACTIVE INGREDIENTS • Ingredients in medicine that provide therapeutic benefit. *See* Inert.

ACTRON • *See* Ketoprofen.

ACUTE • Describing a disease of rapid onset, with severe symptoms of brief duration.

ACUTRIM (OTC) • *See* Phenylpropanolamine.

ACV • Abbreviation for acyclovir (*see*).

ACYCLOVIR (Rx) • **ACV. Zovirax.** An antiviral drug introduced in 1979, it reduces the rate of growth of the herpes simplex virus, Epstein-Barr virus, cytomegalovirus, and herpes varicella-zoster (*see all* under "Herpes" and individually). It reduces the severity of cold sores and shingles. It does not, however, prevent herpes from recurring or decrease contagion from an infected person to another individual. May be taken by mouth, given by injection, or applied topically. Potential adverse reactions include headache, menstrual irregularities, lethargy, tremors, confusion, hallucinations, agitation, seizures, coma, low blood pressure, nausea, vomiting, diarrhea, and when applied to the skin, rash, itching, pain, burn-ing, and inflammation at injection site. Any drugs that affect the kidney may increase the adverse kidney effects of acyclovir. Probenecid may increase acyclovir blood levels to the point of toxicity, and acyclovir may increase the adverse side effects from interferon and methotrexate. Acyclovir should not be used for herpes of the eye, nor should it be used if an allergy exists to any component of the ointment, such as polyethylene glycol (*see*). Acyclovir should be taken with food. A great effort has been made to make a version of acyclovir over-the-counter for the treatment of cold sores (herpes virus 1). The FDA's advisory committee recommended against its being OTC in 1994 lest people misdiagnose their skin lesions and get into serious problems. Acyclovir is over-the-counter in Australia and New Zealand. The committee had another concern: prescription acyclovir is paid by third-party payers but an OTC version would not be. The members felt that many AIDS patients would not be able to afford OTC acyclovir for treatment of herpes infections. The American Society of Hospital Pharmacists testified before the FDA. Its members opposed OTC acyclovir because they felt it has limited effectiveness for the proposed OTC medication, potential for drug resistance, and potential for misuse.

ADALAT • *See* Nifedipine.

ADAMANTANAMINE HYDROCHLO-RIDE • *See* Amantadine.

ADAPETTES (OTC) • An artificial-tear (*see*) preparation.

ADAPIN • *See* Doxepin.

ADDERALL • *See* Amphetamines.

ADDER'S-TONGUE (H) • *Ophioglossum vulgatum.* **Dogtooth Violet. Rattlesnake Violet. Serpent's-Tongue. Yellow Snakeleaf. Yellow Snowdrop.** A plant that derives its name from the shape of its leaf and grows in woods and other shady places throughout the northern and middle United States. Used by herbalists to produce vomiting and for gout. Related to the compound colchicine (*see*), used in traditional medicine to treat gout. Has also been reported to be a remedy for scurvy. Can be toxic.

ADDISON'S DISEASE • A chronic disease characterized by weakness, easy fatigability, skin pigmentation, low blood pressure, and other symptoms. The underlying cause is atrophy or disease of the outer layer of the adrenal gland, creating an insufficient supply of adrenocorticosteroids. Pres. John F. Kennedy reportedly suffered from this condition.

ADEFLOR (OTC) • A multivitamin with fluoride.

ADEN- • Prefix denoting a gland. An adenoma (*see*) is a glandular tumor.

ADENINE ARABINOSIDE • *See* Vidarabine Monohydrate.

ADENOCARCINOMA • Cancer of glandular tissue.

ADENOCARD • *See* Adenosine.

ADENOMA • A benign growth formed of glandular tissue.

ADENOSINE (Rx) • **Adenocard. 9-Beta-D-Ribofuranosyladenine.** A white, crystalline powder derived from yeast. Introduced in 1989, it is used to treat irregular heartbeat. Also an orphan drug (*see*) for treatment of brain tumors.

ADENOVIRUSES • A group of viruses responsible for respiratory infections such as the common cold, intestinal infections, and various other ailments, especially in the young.

ADHESIONS • Abnormal cohesion of tissues that should slip or slide freely over each other.

ADIPEX-P • *See* Phentermine.

ADIPOST • *See* Phendimetrazine.

ADIXPIX-P • *See* Phentermine.

ADJUNCT • A substance, treatment, or a drug that aids another substance in its action.

ADJUVANT • A substance or drug that aids another substance in its action. Adjuvant usually means "in addition to" initial treatment.

ADJUVANT CHEMOTHERAPY • One or more anticancer drugs used in combination with surgery or radiation therapy as a part of the treatment of cancer.

ADPHEN • *See* Phendimetrazine.

ADR • *See* Doxorubicin.

ADREN-COMP NO. 827 P.S.E. (H) • Herbal formula with extracts of licorice, curcuma, and ginseng (*see all*).

ADRENAL CORTEX • The outer layer of tissue of the adrenal gland (*see*), which produces hormones.

ADRENAL GLAND • About the size of a grape, an adrenal gland lies on top of each of the kidneys. Each adrenal gland has two parts. The first part is the medulla, which produces epinephrine and norepinephrine, two hormones that play a part in controlling heart rate and blood pressure. Signals from the brain stimulate production of these hormones. The second part is the adrenal cortex, which produces three groups of steroid hormones. The hormones in one group control the levels of various chemicals in the body. For example, they prevent the loss of too much sodium and water into the urine. Aldosterone is the most important hormone in this group. The hormones in the second group have a number of functions. One is to help convert carbohydrates, or starches, into energy-providing glycogen in the liver. Hydrocortisone is the main hormone in this group. The third group consists of the male hormone androgen and the female hormones estrogen and progesterone.

ADRENALIN • *See* Epinephrine.

ADRENERGIC • Secreting epinephrine (*see*) or substances with similar activity.

ADRENERGIC-BLOCKING AGENTS (Rx) • Drugs blocking receptors that receive the neurotransmitters norepinephrine and epinephrine, which activate the contraction of artery walls, relax muscles in the lungs, increase heart rate, and stimulate other involuntary actions.

ADRENOCORTICOIDS (Rx) (OTC) • Hormones necessary to good health, produced by the adrenal glands (*see*). Certain adrenocorticoids are used to provide relief of inflammation, and as part of the treatment for a number of diseases including asthma and arthritis. *See also* Cortisone and Corticosteroids.

ADRENOCORTICOTROPIC HORMONE • *See* Corticotropin.

ADRIAMYCIN • *See* Doxorubicin.

ADRUCIL • *See* Fluorouracil.

ADSORBOCARPINE • *See* Pilocarpine.

ADSORBONAC OPHTHALMIC • *See* Sodium Chloride.

ADSORBOTEAR (OTC) • *See* Artificial Tears.

ADVANCE (OTC) • A diagnostic test for pregnancy.

ADVERSE REACTION • Side effect. Any unintended, abnormal reaction to a medicine taken at normal doses.

ADVIL (OTC) • *See* Ibuprofen.

AEROBIC • Requiring oxygen for survival.

AEROBID • *See* Flunisolide.

AEROLATE • *See* Theophylline.

AEROLONE • *See* Isoproterenol.

AEROSEB-DEX • *See* Dexamethasone.

AEROSPORIN • *See* Polymyxin B.

AEROZOIN (OTC) • *See* Benzoin.

AFRICAN RUE • *See* Rue.

AFRIN (OTC) • *See* Oxymetazoline.

AFRINOL (OTC) • *See* Pseudoephedrine.

AFTATE • *See* Tolnaftate.

AGAR • Homeopathic abbreviation for agaricus.

AGAR (H) • *Gelidium polyporus.* **Purging Agaric.** Obtained from various seaweeds, it is used by herbalists to treat night sweats and diarrhea and to dry the breast milk of nonnursing mothers. In large doses, it is a purgative. In May 1992, it was banned by the FDA as an ingredient in laxatives.

AGARICUS (H) • **Fly Agaric. Fly Mushroom.** A homeopathic medicine (*see*) derived from a mushroom with a characteristic bright scarlet cap covered with thick, white, wartlike spots. It is native to Europe, Siberia, and North America and contains muscimol, ibotenic acid, and muscazone. It is used to lower blood pressure and stimulate the heart. It has hallucinogenic and narcotic properties. Recent research has shown that the muscimol found in the mushroom has distinct blood-pressure-lowering and heartbeat-slowing effects. It is also used as a pesticide to kill flies. It is toxic, and in severe cases of poisoning, delirium is followed by convulsions, coma, and death.

AGAVE (H) • *Agave americana.* **Century Plant.** A succulent perennial native to tropical America. The leaves and juice contain saponins, volatile oil, gums, and proteins. It is used by herbalists as a diuretic, laxative, antiseptic, and emmenagogue (*see*). It is used internally for digestive disorders, liver ailments, pulmonary tuberculosis, and veneral disease. It is also used for skin diseases and to treat burns and cuts. Agave may be toxic in large doses. It can cause irritation of the mucous membranes of the stomach, nausea, vomiting, and hemorrhage. Large and frequent doses can lead to liver damage.

AGEUSIA • Lack of taste.

AGONIST • A drug, hormone, or neurotransmitter that binds to a receptor site and triggers a response.

AGORAL (OTC) • A laxative preparation containing mineral oil and phenolphthalein (*see* both). *See also* Laxative.

AGORAL PLAIN (OTC) • *See* Mineral Oil.

AGRANULOCYTOSIS • An acute, frequently fatal illness associated with extreme reduction or complete absence of granular white blood cells from the bone marrow. Absence of cells that protect against infection results in weakness, rapid onset of high fever, sore throat, prostration, and ulcerations of the mouth and mucous membranes.

AGRIMONY (H) • *Agrimonia eupatorin.* **Cocklebur. Sticklewort.** A common weed, it contains tannins, glycosides, coumarins, flavonoids, nicotinic acid amide, silicic acid, polysaccharides, vitamins B and K, iron, and essential oil. Mentioned in medical literature as early as 63 B.C., it has been used in American folk medicine as an astringent, an analgesic, to stop bleeding, and to treat inflammations. It is also used in ointments and boluses to shrink hemorrhoids, as a tonic, and to treat abscesses and gout.

AHF • *See* Antihemophilic Factor.

AIDS • Abbreviation for Acquired Immune Deficiency Syndrome (*see* HIV). Breakthrough drugs called protease inhibitors (*see*) were announced in 1996. They increased defensive cells in the immune system while lowering the number of HIV viruses. In combination with other drugs, they seem highly effective and many researchers were saying that AIDS could become a chronic disease controlled by medication much as diabetes is controlled by insulin. (*See* Crixivan, Ritonavir, Iamivudine, and invirase.)

AK • Abbreviation for actinic keratoses (*see*).

AKARPINE • *See* Pilocarpine.

AK-CHLOR • *See* Chloramphenicol.

AK-CIDE • *See* Prednisolone and Sulfacetamide.

AK-CON • *See* Naphazoline.

AK-DEX • *See* Dexamethasone.

AK-DILATE • *See* Phenylephrine.

AK-FLUOR • *See* Fluorescein.

AK-HOMATROPINE • *See* Homatropine.

AKINETON • *See* Biperiden.

AK-METHOLONE • *See* Fluorometholone.

AK-NEFRIN • *See* Phenylephrine.

AKNE-MYCIN • A topical antibiotic. *See* Erythromycin.

AK-PENTOLATE • *See* Cyclopentolate.

AK-POLY-BAC • *See* Bacitracin and Polymyxin B.

AK-PRED • *See* Prednisolone.

AK-SPORE • *See* Bacitracin, Neomycin, and Polymyxin B.

AK-SPORE H.C. • *See* Neomycin, Polymyxin B, and Hydrocortisone.

AK-SULF • *See* Sulfacetamide.

AK-TAINE • *See* Proparacaine.

AK-TATE • *See* Prednisolone.

AK-TRACIN • *See* Bacitracin.

AK-TROL • *See* Dexamethasone, Neomycin, and Polymyxin B.

AK-ZOL • *See* Acetazolamide.

ALBA-DEX • *See* Dexamethasone.

ALBALON (OTC) • *See* Naphazoline and Antazoline.

ALBALON LIQUIFILM • *See* Naphazoline.

ALBUTEROL (Rx) • **Proventil. Salbutamol. Ventolin.** Introduced in 1968, it is a bronchodilator prescribed for asthma, bronchial spasms, and premature labor. It does not stimulate the heart as much as some other drugs used to treat these conditions and is longer-acting than isoproterenol (*see*). The most common potential adverse reaction is fine tremor of the hands. Other potential reactions include anxiety, tension, restlessness, nausea, increase in cholesterol and sugar levels in the blood, headache, and heart palpitations. The side effects from inhalation of albuterol sprays may be more pronounced than from ingestion of the tablets, so follow directions carefully. Albuterol interacts with other stimulants and may increase the risk of adverse effects. Beta-blockers (*see*) may inhibit the effects of albuterol and vice versa. Monoamine oxidase inhibitors (MAOIs) (*see*) can interact with albuterol and quickly raise blood pressure to dangerous levels, even within two weeks after discontinuing use of MAOIs. In some cases, albuterol can worsen asthma instead of relieving it. Should be used cautiously in persons with heart problems, high blood pressure, an overactive thyroid, or diabetes. Sometimes prescribed fifteen minutes before exercise to prevent exercise-induced bronchospasm. Most effective

when taken on an empty stomach one to two hours before or after meals.

ALCAINE • *See* Proparacaine.

ALCLOMETASONE (Rx) • **Alclovate. Logoderm.** An ointment or cream used to treat skin inflammation. Potential adverse reactions include burning, itching, irritation, dryness, inflammation of the hair follicles, acne, rash around the mouth, spots of pigment loss, hairiness, allergic contact dermatitis, and if covered with a dressing, secondary infection, atrophy, streaks, and blisters. Should be used cautiously in skin problems caused by viruses such as herpes, and in fungal or bacterial skin infections. Should not be used for more than two weeks due to potential absorption into the system, consequently causing an effect on the hypothalamus, and pituitary and adrenal glands. Should not be applied near the eyes or mucous membranes, under the arms, on the face, groin, or under the breast unless medically specified.

ALCLOVATE • *See* Alclometasone.

ALCOHOL (Rx) (OTC) (H) • **Ethanol. Ethyl Alcohol.** Alcohol is a solvent and is manufactured by the fermentation of starch, sugar, and other carbohydrates. It is found in plants, sterols and volatile oils, and waxes. Medicinally, used externally as an antiseptic and internally as a stimulant and hypnotic. An added ingredient in many drugs for sedative or solvent purposes. Alcohol interacts with a wide variety of drugs. It increases the sedative and respiratory effects and may be fatal if taken with sleeping medications, tranquilizers, antidepressants, pain relievers, some muscle relaxants, antihistamines, motion-sickness pills, allergy medications, some cough and cold products, and some high blood pressure medications. May cause dizziness, fainting, light-headedness, and loss of consciousness if used while taking antianginal medication (for chest pain), and some high blood pressure medications. If used while taking aspirin, antiarthritic medications, potassium tablets, or blood thinners, it may increase stomach irritation and bleeding. If taken while using

Flagyl (*see*), oral antidiabetic medications, and some antifungal and antibiotic agents, it can cause Antabuse-like (*see*) reactions including weakness, headache, vomiting, flushing, rapid heartbeat, and difficulty breathing. The FDA issued a notice that alcohol is ineffective in treating digestive problems, insect bites, poison ivy, poison oak, and poison sumac, and such claims should not be made for it in OTC products. The FDA banned the use of alcohol in oral menstrual products. Alcohol may also interfere with the effectiveness of many drugs including blood thinners, antidiabetes medications, epilepsy medications, and gout medications. Taken, particularly in the form of red wine, with MAO inhibitors (*see*), alcohol may cause a dangerous rise in blood pressure. Since serious side effects can occur with drug and alcohol interactions, do some research before drinking alcohol while taking a medication. Read the label and package insert. Check the medication's listing in this book. If you have any doubt at all, check with your physician and/or pharmacist.

ALCOHOL, RUBBING (OTC) • Ethyl Alcohol. Contains not less than 68.5 percent and not more than 71.5 percent by volume of absolute alcohol, and the remainder denaturants that are added to make it poisonous to drink. Used as a rubefacient (*see*) and an antiseptic.

ALCONEFRIN (OTC) • *See* Phenylephrine.

ALDACTAZIDE (Rx) • A combination of hydrochlorothiazide and spironolactone (*see both*), used as a diuretic (*see*).

ALDACTONE • *See* Spironolactone.

ALDECIN • *See* Beclomethasone.

ALDER BUCKTHORN (OTC) (H) • *Rhamnus frangula*. **Black Dogwood. Frangula.** A shrub that produces globular fruit and is native to Europe, Central Asia, and North America. It is cultivated in Europe. It is used by herbalists and sold in stores as a laxative. The bark may cause severe vomiting. Chronic use of alder buckthorn can cause abdominal cramps and discoloration of urine and the mucous membranes of the colon. It is contraindicated in pregnancy and in persons suffering from intestinal inflammation or hemorrhoids.

ALDESLEUKIN • Interleukin-2. Proleukin. Used to treat malignancies of the kidney and immunodeficiency diseases.

ALDOCLOR (Rx) • A combination of chlorothiazide and methyldopa (*see both*), used as a treatment for high blood pressure.

ALDOMET • *See* Methyldopa.

ALDORIL (Rx) • A combination of hydrochlorothiazide and methyldopa (*see both*), used to lower blood pressure.

ALDOSE REDUCTASE • An enzyme that converts glucose to sorbitol and has been cited as contributing to nerve damage and cataracts in diabetics.

ALDOSTERONE • A hormone produced by the cortex of the adrenal gland. The hormone is a powerful regulator of salt and water balances.

ALENDRONATE (Rx) • Fosamax. The first non-hormonal medication introduced in 1995 for the treatment of osteoporosis (*see*) in postmenopausal women and for Paget's disease, a chronic skeletal disorder. The drug builds healthy bone, restoring some of the bone loss as a result of osteoporosis. It reportedly cut new spinal fractures by up to 63 percent. Should be taken first thing in the morning with a full glass of water, at least 30 minutes before the first food, beverage, or other medication. You should not lie down for at least 30 minutes after taking the drug. Potential side effects have been reportedly mild, and include abdominal pain, nausea, constipation, and musculoskeletal pain.

ALEVE (OTC) • Naproxen sodium was introduced in 1994; this is a weaker version of Naprosyn (*see*) for use as a pain reliever. It is indicated for the same conditions as aspirin, ibuprofen, and acetaminophen but is longer acting.

Should not be taken more than ten days for pain, or more than three days for fever, unless directed by your physician. Not more than three tablets should be taken in twenty-four hours. Should not be taken in the last three months of pregnancy unless directed to do so by a physician because it may cause problems in the unborn child or complications during pregnancy. *See* NSAIDs and Naproxen.

ALFACALCIDOL • *See* Vitamin D.

ALFALFA (H) • **Herb and Seed. Lucerne. Muxu.** Extract of *Medicago sativa*. The name comes from the Arab *al-fasfasah*, meaning father. A natural cola, liquor, and maple flavoring agent for beverages and cordials. The leaves contain beta-carotene, vitamins C, D, E, and the coagulating vitamin, K. It also contains various mineral salts including calcium, potassium, iron, and phosphorous. Used as a tonic, to fight fever, to build red blood cells, to stop hemorrhaging, and as a diuretic. Also used to improve digestion, for weight gain, and to treat cystitis and prostate inflammation. A folk medicine for lower-back pain, arthritis, increasing mother's milk, insomnia, and to regulate the bowels. Alfalfa is widely cultivated for forage and is a commercial source of chlorophyll. Excessive doses can cause intestinal gas and diarrhea. May also cause an estrogenlike response because it contains a phytoestrogen (*see*). In 1992, the FDA proposed a ban on alfalfa maleate in oral menstrual drug products because it had not been shown to be safe and effective as claimed.

ALFENTA • *See* Alfentanil Hydrochloride.

ALFENTANIL HYDROCHLORIDE (Rx) • **Alfenta.** An injectable narcotic altering both perception of and emotional response to pain through an unknown mechanism. Given as an adjunct to general anesthesia. Potential adverse reactions include low or high blood pressure, irregular heartbeat, nausea, vomiting, itching, muscle spasms, and respiratory depression. Alcohol and central nervous system depressants may add to the effects. Must be used cautiously in patients with head injury or lung problems.

ALFERON N INJECTION • *See* interferon.

ALG-, -ALGIA • Prefix and suffix signifying pain, as in *neuralgia*, nerve pain.

ALGICON (OTC) • An antacid combination of aluminum hydroxide and magnesium carbonate (*see both*).

ALGINIC ACID (OTC) (H) • Obtained from brown seaweed gel. It is used as a stabilizer in drugs and cosmetics. It has a laxative effect.

ALGLUCERASE (Rx) • **Ceredase. Glucocerebrosidase.** An orphan drug (*see*) introduced in 1991 to treat Gaucher's disease, a rare, hereditary metabolic disorder characterized by anemia, enlargement of the liver and spleen, bone erosion, and pain. This, the only treatment for the disease, is reputed to be the world's most expensive drug, costing $380,000 for the first year of treatment for an adult. In 1992, researchers at Scripps Institute in La Jolla, California, reported that if the drug was given in smaller doses more frequently, the cost could be greatly reduced. The drug is so expensive because it is derived in tiny quantities from human placentas.

ALKABAN-AQ • *See* Vinblastine Sulfate.

ALKALI • The term originally covered the caustic and mild forms of potash and soda. Now a substance is regarded as an alkali if it gives hydroxyl ions in solution. An alkaline aqueous solution is one with a pH (*see*) greater than 7. Sodium bicarbonate is an example of an alkali.

ALKALINE • Having a pH (*see*) of more than 7. The opposite of acidic.

ALKALOIDS • Compounds of vegetable origin, some of which have great dietary importance. Usually derived from a nitrogen compound such as pyridine, quinoline, isoquinoline, or pyrrole, designated by the ending *-ine*. Examples are atropine, morphine, nicotine, quinine, codeine, caffeine, cocaine, and strychnine. The alkaloids are potent and include the hallucinogen mescaline and the deadly poison brucine. There are alkaloids that act on the liver, nerves, lungs, and digestive systems.

ALKALOSIS • Increased alkalinity of the blood.

ALKA-MINTS • *See* Calcium Carbonate.

ALKA-SELTZER (OTC) • A combination of aspirin, sodium bicarbonate, and citric acid (*see all*) used to relieve an upset stomach.

ALKA-SELTZER EFFERVESCENT ANTACID • *See* Citric Acid.

ALKERAN • *See* Melphalan.

ALKYLATING AGENTS • Drugs to treat cancer that act within the cell nucleus to damage the cell's genetic material, DNA. This prevents the cell from growing and dividing.

ALLANTOIN (OTC) • **Herpecin-L Cold Sore Lip Balm.** A uric-acid derivative. Applied topically, it is used in skin preparations because of its ability to help heal wounds and skin ulcers, and to stimulate the growth of healthy tissue.

ALLBEE C-800 (OTC) • A multivitamin preparation.

ALLBEE WITH C (OTC) • A multivitamin preparation.

ALL-C • Homeopathic abbreviation for *Allium cepa* (*see*).

ALLER-CHLOR • *See* Chlorpheniramine.

ALLEREST (OTC) • A combination of chlorpheniramine and naphazoline (*see both*) used to relieve cold or allergy symptoms.

ALLEREST 12-HOUR NASAL (OTC) • *See* Oxymetazoline.

ALLERFRIN • *See* Triprolidine.

ALLERGEN • A substance that provokes an allergic reaction in the susceptible, but does not normally affect other people. Plant pollens, fungi spores, and animal danders are some of the common allergens.

ALLERGEN EAR DROPS (OTC) • *See* Benzocaine and Antipyrine.

ALLERGIC REACTION • Abnormal bodily response to an ingredient in a medication or a natural substance such as pollen, molds, foods, cosmetics, and drugs. Symptoms vary widely, but may include rash, hives, sneezing, wheezing, runny nose, or a life-threatening reaction leading to collapse. *See* Anaphylaxis.

ALLERGY • An altered immune response on re-exposure to a specific substance such as ragweed or pollen.

ALLERGY DROPS (OTC) • *See* Polyethylene Glycol.

ALLERHIST (OTC) • *See* Brompheniramine and Phenylpropanolamine.

ALLERMAX (OTC) • *See* Diphenhydramine.

ALLERPHED (OTC) • *See* Triprolidine and Pseudoephedrine.

ALLERSONE (OTC) • A combination of hydrocortisone, diperodon, and zinc oxide (*see all*) used for the relief of skin inflammation and itching.

ALLIUM CEPA (H) • A homeopathic medicine (*see*) for allergies, especially allergy to cats and dogs. Derived from onions, it causes a runny, irritated nose similar to what happens when you peel an onion. It is also used to treat colds. A study by the National Cancer Institute showed diets high in allium vegetables, such as onion (*Allium cepa*) and garlic (*Allium sativum*), suffer from less stomach cancer. Both contain sulfides, which probably explains their actions as strong disinfectants. The team of Michael Wargovich, Ph.D., at the University of Texas MD Anderson Cancer Center in Houston, has shown that sulfides, the substances that give garlic and onions their strong odor, inhibit cancers of the colon and esophagus in animals. Other researchers have found that the substances also inhibit stomach cancer. Sulfides work in two ways: they block the action of cancer-causing substances, and they slow tumor development.

ALLIUM SATIVUM • *See Allium cepa* and Garlic.

ALLOGENIC MARROW • Bone marrow used for transplantation, from a tissue-type-matched donor.

ALLOPATHY • From the Greek words *allo,* meaning "other," and *pathos,* meaning "suffering." It was coined by Dr. Hahnemann (*see* page 9) to describe orthodox medicine as distinguished from homeopathy.

ALLOPURINOL (Rx) • **Lopurin. Zurinol. Zyloprim.** A drug used since 1963 in the prevention of recurrent attacks of gout. It acts by halting the formation in the joints of uric acid crystals, which cause the inflammation associated with gout. At first, it may increase the gout attacks. Also used to lower uric acid levels caused by other drugs, especially anticancer drugs. Other antigout drugs reduce uric acid levels by increasing its excretion in urine, but allopurinol does not, thus reducing the risk of kidney stones. Potential adverse reactions include allergic rash, nausea, drowsiness, headache, tingling in hands and feet, metallic taste, liver dysfunction, cataracts, diarrhea, fever, and chills. Iron supplements, including vitamin compounds with iron, are contraindicated with allopurinol because iron salts may be deposited in the liver. Allopurinol may increase the adverse effects of mercaptopurine, azathioprine (*see both*), and anticoagulants. Thiazide diuretics reduce the benefits of allopurinol. Alcohol, bumetanide, diazoxide, ethacrynic acid, furosemide, triamterene, mecamylamine, pyrazinamide, ampicillin, and amoxicillin increase the risk of adverse effects with allopurinol. Contraindicated in hypersensitivity to allopurinol and in hemochromatosis (*see*). Should be used cautiously in those with cataracts or liver or kidney disease. Vitamin C may increase the possibility of kidney stone formation. Each dose should be taken with a full glass of water, and at least ten to twelve full glasses of fluid should be drunk each day while on this medication.

ALLYLIC SULFIDES • Found in garlic and onions, these compounds may protect against cancer-causing agents by stimulating production of a detoxification enzyme, glutathione-S-transferase.

ALLYL ISOTHIOCYANATE (OTC) • The salt of a strong acid used to treat fever blisters and cold sores. The FDA proposed banning it because allyl isothiocyanate had not been shown to be safe and effective as claimed on OTC products.

ALMOND (H) • *Prunus amygdalus.* The oil is obtained from a small tree grown in France, Spain, and Italy. Almond oil has been reported by researchers to lower cholesterol. It is used as a flavoring agent in the United States. It is distilled to remove hydrocyanic acid (prussic acid), which is toxic. Almond meal is used to create soothing skin preparations. Almond paste was a favorite early European cleanser. Almonds also contain amygdalin, which served as the basis of laetrile, a controversial anticancer drug that has not been permitted on the market by the FDA.

ALOE VERA (Rx) (OTC) (H) • *Aloe peryi. Aloe barbadensis.* **Cortaid Cream and Ointment. First-Aid Plant. Lu Hui. Nature's Remedy Natural Vegetable Laxative Tablets.** A compound expressed from the aloe plant leaf. There are more than two hundred species of this lilylike plant. Aloe contains aloins, anthraquinones, glycoproteins, sterols, saponins, albumin, essential oil, silica, phosphate of lime, a trace of iron, organic acids, and polysaccharides including glucomannans. Used medicinally for more than three thousand years, it is referred to in the Bible.

Ancient Egyptian women, just as women today, used it for softening benefits in skin creams. In the West, aloe gel is considered an effective healing agent for the treatment of burns and injuries. A diluted liquid is taken daily for its enzyme-promoting activity. It is used to regulate menstruation and female hormones, ease liver problems, and counteract wrinkles. Aloe was used as a cathartic, but was found to cause severe intestinal cramps and sometimes kidney damage. An injectable derivative of aloe, acemannan, is being tested against HIV. It reportedly prevents HIV from entering uninfected cells in the laboratory, and early clinical studies are about to get under way at this writing. Cross-reacts with benzoin and balsam of Peru in those who are allergic to these compounds. In 1992, the FDA proposed a ban on aloes in oral menstrual drug products because it had not been shown to be safe and effective as claimed. Aloe is contraindicated in pregnancy, hemorrhoids, kidney disease, and appendicitis. Aloe should also not be used while breastfeeding because it may cause diarrhea in the infant. Some species of the aloes, particularly those in Kenya, the Middle East, and Madagascar, may contain toxic alkaloids.

ALOIN (OTC) • Banned by the FDA, May 1992, as an ingredient in laxatives.

ALOPHEN • *See* Phenolphthalein.

ALPHA ADRENERGIC RECEPTORS • Receptors in the autonomic nervous system that react to norepinephrine and epinephrine (*see both*) and that cause effects such as contraction of blood vessels, the pupil of the eye, and the skin muscles that move hair. A-adrenergic blockers are drugs that mimic norepinephrine and epinephrine and block the receptors. Phenoxybenzamine and methoxamine (*see both*) are examples of A-adrenergic blockers.

ALPHA BLOCKERS • Drugs, such as labetalol, that block the alpha andrenergic receptors (*see*) in the body and thus reduce blood pressure.

ALPHADERM • *See* Hydrocortisone.

ALPHA KERI (OTC) • A mineral oil and lanolin bath additive for dry, itchy skin. *See* Mineral Oil and Lanolin.

ALPHAMOX • *See* Amoxicillin.

ALPHAMUL (OTC) • *See* Castor Oil.

ALPHA-1 PROTEINASE INHIBITOR (Rx) • **Prolastin.** A human-derived enzyme inhibitor that replaces alpha-1 proteinase in emphysema patients with alpha-1 antitrypsin deficiency. Potential adverse reactions include possible viral transmission from the human blood from which it is derived. However, at this writing there have not been reports of hepatitis developed by patients receiving this medication.

ALPHAREDISOL • *See* Hydroxocobalamin.

ALPHA-RUVITE • *See* Vitamin B_{12}.

ALPHA TOCOPHEROL ACETATE • *See* Vitamin E.

ALPHATREX • *See* Betamethasone.

ALPHOSYL • *See* Coal Tar.

ALPIDINE • *See* Apraclonidine.

ALPRAZOLAM (Rx) • **Xanax.** Introduced in 1982, alprazolam belongs to the family of benzodiazepines, used to treat anxiety and insomnia, and as muscle relaxants. Alprazolam is specifically used to treat panic disorders and anxiety accompanied by agitated depression. It is also prescribed for phobias, including agoraphobia, fear of crossing or being in open spaces. The first of a new type of benzodiazepine, alprazolam is more rapidly metabolized and excreted than other drugs in the family and causes less of a hangover. Potential adverse effects include addiction, daytime sleepiness, dizziness, loss of balance, blurred vision, memory problems, confusion, headache, and rash. The drug is not prescribed for everyday stress. Contraindicated in glaucoma, and in psychoses, as it may cause depression. Should not be combined with caffeine, alcohol, or other antidepressants. Alprazolam should not be discontinued suddenly. Most effective when taken on an empty stomach, but can be taken with food if stomach upset is a problem. May interact with fluvoxamine (*see*).

ALPROSTADIL (Rx) • **PGE_1. Prostin VR.** Introduced in 1981, alprostadil is used to treat newborns with congenital heart defects that impair the flow of blood between the heart and lungs. Alprostadil is a synthetic prostaglandin (*see*) that keeps open the ductus arteriosus, a blood vessel that links a newborn's heart and lungs. The drug is given by injection and closely monitored until the condition is corrected. Contraindicated in newborns with respiratory distress syndrome. The drug, under the name Caverject, was approved in 1995 to treat impotence by injection into the penis shortly before sexual intercourse. It is not recommended for use more than three times a week or more than once in 24 hours. It is contraindicated in persons with sickle-cell anemia, multiple myeloma, leukemia (*see all*), or penile implants. Potential adverse effects include fever, flushing, seizures, diarrhea, and difficulty breathing.

AL-R • *See* Chlorpheniramine.

ALREDASE • *See* Tolrestat.

ALS • Abbreviation for Amyotrophic Lateral Sclerosis (*see*).

ALSEROXYLON (Rx) (H) • A fat-soluble alkali extracted from the root of *Rauwolfia serpentina,* containing reserpine. Used as a sedative in psychoses, in mild high blood pressure, and as an adjunct to more potent blood pressure drugs.

ALT • **Autolymphocyte Therapy.** An orphan drug (*see*) for kidney-cancer therapy approved in 1994. A patient's own white blood cells are extracted, treated to make them attack tumor cells, then reintroduced into the patient.

ALTACE • *See* Ramipril.

ALTEPLASE (Rx) • *See* T-PA.

ALTERATIVE • A term used in herbal medicine to signify herbs that are tonics or blood cleansers. Such herbs include yellow dock, goldenseal, and buckbean (*see all*).

ALTERNAGEL (OTC) • *See* Aluminum Hydroxide.

ALTHAEA ROOT (H) • *Hibiscus moscheutos.* **Hollyhock. Marshmallow Root. Rose of Sharon.** A natural substance from a plant grown in Europe, Asia, and the United States. The dried root is used in flavorings. The boiled root is used in ointment to soothe skin and mucous membranes. The roots, flowers, and leaves are used externally as a poultice. Nontoxic.

ALTRETAMINE (Rx) • **Hexamethylmelamine. HMM. Hexalen.** An anticancer agent used in the palliative treatment of patients with persistent or recurrent ovarian cancer. Potential adverse reactions include nausea, vomiting, nerve damage, loss of appetite, fatigue, seizures, anemia, and kidney dysfunction. Cimetidine (*see*) may increase the toxicity of altretamine. MAO inhibitors (*see*) may cause a severe drop in blood pressure.

ALU-CAP (OTC) • *See* Aluminum Hydroxide.

ALUDROX (OTC) • *See* Aluminum Hydroxide and Magnesium Hydroxide.

ALUDROX ORAL SUSPENSION (OTC) • *See* Aluminum Hydroxide.

ALUM (OTC) • **Aluminum Ammonium. Potash Alum. Potassium Sulfate.** A crystalline, water-soluble solid used in astringent lotions and as a styptic to stop skin bleeding. In concentrated solutions alum has produced gum damage, kidney damage, and fatal intestinal hemorrhages. The FDA issued a notice in 1992 that potassium alum and ammonium alum had not been shown to be safe and effective as claimed in OTC products, including astringent drug products.

ALUMINUM ACETATE (OTC) • Acid Mantle. Bluboro. Burow's Solution. Domeboro Astringent Solution Effervescent Tablets and Astringent Solution Powder Packets. Pedi-Boro.
A mixture including acetic acid and boric acid (*see both*), with astringent and antiseptic properties. It is applied to soothe the skin or outer ear. Used prophylactically against swimmer's ear. Prolonged and continuous exposure can produce severe sloughing of the skin. Also causes skin rashes in some persons. Ingestion of large doses can cause nausea and vomiting, diarrhea, and bleeding.

ALUMINUM CARBONATE (OTC) • Basaljel Capsules and Suspension.
A carbonate of varying formula, formerly used as a mild astringent and styptic. Currently used as an antacid and to lower phosphate in the blood. Aluminum carbonate is not found as an individual compound.

ALUMINUM CHLORHYDROXY COMPLEX (OTC) •
An antiperspirant. May be irritating to abraded skin and may also cause allergic reactions. In 1992, the FDA proposed a ban on aluminum chlorhydroxy complex in astringent (*see*) drug products because it had not been shown to be safe and effective as claimed.

ALUMINUM CHLORIDE (OTC) • Drysol.
The first antiperspirant salt to be used for commercial antiperspirant products. Still the most effective available. It is also an antiseptic, but can be irritating to sensitive skin and causes allergic reactions in susceptible people.

ALUMINUM CHLOROHYDRATE (OTC) • Desenex Foot & Sneaker Deodorant Spray Powder.
The most frequently used antiperspirant in the United States. Causes occasional infections of the hair follicles. May be irritating to abraded skin and may also cause allergic reactions, but is considered one of the least irritating of the aluminum salts. In spray form, inhaling the contents can be fatal. Spraying in the eyes or near a source of fire should be avoided.

ALUMINUM HYDROXIDE (OTC) • ALTernaGEL. Alu-Cap. Alu-Tab. Amphojel. Cama Arthritis Pain Reliever. Dialume. DiGel. Fermalox. Gaviscon Extra Strength Relief Formula Liquid Antacid. Gelusil. Gelusil Liquid and Tablets. Nephrox Suspension. Silain Gel. WinGel Liquid. In combination: Ascriptin. Gaviscon. Kolantyl. Kudrox. Maalox. Mylanta.
In use for more than half a century, it is a mild astringent and alkali, with water-absorbing properties, and prolonged action. Used for the treatment of acid stomach, diarrhea, peptic ulcers, and reflux esophagitis. Also used to lower high blood phosphate in people suffering from kidney dysfunction. Aluminum compounds can interfere with the absorption of phosphate from the diet, causing weakness and bone damage if taken in high doses over a long period. Potential adverse reactions may also include nausea, vomiting, bone pain, and muscle weakness. Aluminum hydroxide interferes with the absorption or excretion of antibiotics, digitalis, anticoagulants, antipsychotic drugs, phenytoin, and corticosteroids. May cause constipation unless combined with a laxative. In 1992, the FDA proposed a ban and issued a notice on aluminum hydroxide in diaper-rash drug products and OTC digestive-aid products, respectively, because it had not been shown to be safe and effective as claimed. *See* Antacid.

ALUMINUM NICOTINATE (OTC) •
Used as a source of niacin in special diet foods; also as a medication to dilate blood vessels and combat fat. Tablets of 625 mg are a complex of aluminum nicotinate, nicotinic acid, and aluminum hydroxide. Potential adverse reactions include flushing, rash, and gastrointestinal distress.

ALUMINUM OXIDE •
The mineral corundum is natural aluminum oxide, and emery, ruby, and sapphire are impure crystalline varieties. It is mixed with water to produce an antacid.

ALUMINUM PHOSPHATE • Phosphaljel.
White crystals, insoluble in water, used in ceramics, dental cements, and cosmetics as a gelling agent. Also used to reduce fecal excretion of phosphates. Corrosive to tissue.

ALUMINUM SILICATE • Obtained naturally from clay or synthesized, it is used as an anticaking and coloring agent in powders. Essentially harmless when given orally and when applied to the skin.

ALUMINUM SUCROSE SULFATE • *See* Sucralfate.

ALUMINUM SULFATE (OTC) • **Cake Alum.** Colorless crystals used as antiseptics, astringents, and detergents in antiperspirants, deodorants, and skin fresheners. In 1992, the FDA issued a notice that aluminum sulfate had not been shown to be safe and effective as claimed in OTC products.

ALUPENT • *See* Metaproterenol.

ALURATE • *See* Aprobarbital.

ALU-TAB (OTC) • *See* Aluminum Hydroxide.

ALZAPAM • *See* Lorazepam.

ALZHEIMER'S DISEASE • A deterioration of the brain with severe memory impairment.

AMALAKI (H) • *Phyllanthus emblica.* An herb used for thousands of years in India to treat coughs, eating disorders, and to normalize bowel function. Also used currently to treat skin diseases and tumors.

AMANTADINE (Rx) • **Symadine. Symmetrel.** An antiviral used to prevent or treat certain influenza infections, and to treat Parkinson's disease (*see*). In use since the 1960s, it is sometimes combined with levodopa, another anti-Parkinson's drug. This drug has a narrow margin of safety, so directions must be followed exactly. Potential side effects include depression, fatigue, confusion, dizziness, psychosis, anxiety, irritability, insomnia, loss of balance, weakness, heart failure, low white blood count, headache, water retention, low blood pressure, loss of appetite, nausea, nightmares, constipation, vomiting, dry mouth, urinary retention, and skin changes. Alcoholic beverages, stimulants including caffeine, appetite suppressants, and medications for asthma may increase side effects. Should be used with caution in patients with heart disease or other circulation problems, kidney disease, epilepsy, eczema, or mental or emotional illnesses. This medicine has to be taken at evenly spaced doses to maintain protective blood levels.

AMARANTH (H) • *Amaranthus hybridus.* **Love-Lies-Bleeding. Red Cockscomb.** Used for digestion, bleeding, diarrhea, menstrual pain, as a douche for vaginal discharge, dysentery, and as a food. It has astringent, nutrient, styptic (*see*), and diuretic properties and is high in vitamins A and C.

AMARYL • *See* Glimepiride.

AMBENONIUM (Rx) • **Mytelase.** Introduced in 1956 to treat myasthenia gravis (*see*), it increases the stimulant neurotransmitter acetylcholine in the brain. Potential adverse reactions include headache, dizziness, muscle weakness, discoordination, seizures, mental confusion, jitters, sweating, slow heartbeat, blurred vision, low blood pressure, nausea, vomiting, diarrhea, abdominal cramps, increased salivation, urinary frequency, incontinence, bronchospasm, muscle cramps, and breathing paralysis. Atropine, corticosteroids, magnesium, procainamide, and quinidine may make ambenomium less effective. Contraindicated in intestinal obstruction, urinary tract problems, and slow heartbeat or low blood pressure. Must be used with extreme caution in patients with bronchial asthma. Weakness occurring thirty to sixty minutes after taking the medication is a warning sign of drug toxicity. Should be taken with food or milk.

AMBENYL (Rx) • A codeine phosphate and bromodiphenhydramine combination (*see both*) used to treat coughs.

AMBI- • Prefix meaning both, such as in *ambidextrous,* using both hands equally well.

AMBIEN • *See* Zolpidem Tartrate.

AMCILL • *See* Ampicillin.

AMCINONIDE (Rx) • **Cyclocort.** A corticosteroid ointment or cream used to treat skin inflammations. Potential adverse reactions include burning, itching, irritation, dryness, inflammation of the hair follicles, acne, rash around the mouth, spots of pigment loss, hairiness, allergic contact dermatitis, and if covered with a dressing, secondary infection, atrophy, streaks, and blisters. Should be used cautiously in skin problems caused by viruses such as herpes, and in fungal or bacterial skin infections. Should not be used for more than two weeks because of the potential for absorption into the system, causing an effect on the hypothalamus, and pituitary and adrenal glands. Should not be applied near eyes or mucous membranes, under the arms, or on the face, groin, or under the breast unless medically specified.

AMCORT • *See* Triamcinolone.

AMDINOCILLIN • *See* Penicillins.

AMEBIASIS • *See* Amebic Dysentery.

AMEBIC DYSENTERY • **Amebiasis.** Caused by *Entamoeba histolytica,* it is a protozoan infection that primarily affects the colon, but may affect other organs, especially the liver. Severe amebiasis is characterized by diarrhea with blood and/or pus and mucus in the water discharges. Infection is generally caused by the drinking of water contaminated with sewage containing amoebas.

AMEBICIDES • Any agent that causes destruction of amoebas, single-celled organisms abundant in soil and organic debris. Among the common amebicides are chloroquine hydrochloride, chloroquine phosphate, emetine hydrochloride, iodoquinol, metronidazole, and pentamidine isethionate (*see all*).

AMEN • *See* Medroxyprogesterone.

AMENORRHEA • Absence of cyclic menstrual periods, often due to failure to ovulate.

AMERICAINE • *See* Benzocaine.

AMERICAN MISTLETOE • *See* Mistletoe.

AMERICAN WORMSEED • *See* Epazote.

AMESEC • *See* Aminophylline, Amobarbital, and Ephedrine.

A-METHA-PRED • *See* Methylprednisolone.

AMETHOCAINE • *See* Tetracaine.

AMGEN • *See* G-CSF.

AMICAR • *See* Aminocaproic Acid.

AMIDATE • *See* Etomidate.

AMIFOSTINE (Rx) • **Ethyol.** A chemotherapy protectant used during treatment of breast, cervical, lung, and ovarian cancer. Introduced in 1995, it is an agent that selectively protects healthy cells from the damaging effects of the chemotherapy. It is indicated for the reduction of cumulative kidney toxicity associated with repeated administration of cisplatin (*see*) in patients with advanced ovarian cancer.

AMIKACIN (Rx) • **Amikin.** An injectable aminoglycoside (*see*) used against serious infections caused by *Pseudomonas aeruginosa, Escherichia coli, Proteus, Klebsiella, Serratia, Enterobacter, Acinetobacter, Providencia, Citrobacter,* and *Staphylococcus* (*see all*). Among potential adverse side effects: headache, lethargy, neuromuscular problems; ear problems including dizziness, ringing, and hearing loss; kidney dysfunction, liver damage, and hypersensitivity reactions. Use with cephalothin may increase liver damage, with dimenhydrinate may affect the ear, and with general and local anesthetics may increase nerve problems.

AMIKIN • *See* Amikacin.

AMILORIDE (Rx) • **Midamor. Moduretic.** A potassium-sparing diuretic introduced in 1967, used to treat high blood pressure and fluid retention. It inhibits sodium reabsorption. Potential adverse reactions include digestive disturbance, lethargy, muscle weakness, decreased libido, impotence, and rash. Because it spares potassium, it may be contraindicated in patients with kidney dysfunction. As with other potassium-conserving agents, amiloride may cause dangerously high potassium levels that may be fatal. Amiloride may increase the blood levels of lithium, leading to an increased risk of lithium poisoning. ACE inhibitors and NSAIDs (*see both*) may decrease amiloride's effects. Contraindicated in patients with elevated blood potassium levels, or who are taking other potassium-sparing diuretics. If you take this drug, you should be careful about ingesting too many potassium-rich foods or potassium-containing salt substitutes. Most effective when taken on an empty stomach, but amiloride may be taken with food to prevent nausea.

AMINO ACIDS • Marlyn Formula 50. Building blocks of proteins and neurotransmitters. There are about twenty amino acids, nine of which are called essential because the body cannot synthesize them and they must be obtained from food. Combinations with B_6 are used to treat splitting, peeling nails. Arginine, lysine, and phenylalanine were banned by the FDA from over-the-counter diet pills, February 10, 1992, as being ineffective.

AMINOBENZOIC ACID (OTC) • Part of the vitamin B complex and found in brewer's yeast, it is sold under a wide variety of names as a sunscreen lotion to prevent sun damage. Also used as a local anesthetic in sunburn products, and medicinally, to treat arthritis. In susceptible people it can cause a sensitivity to light. In 1992, the FDA proposed a ban on aminobenzoic acid in internal analgesic products because it had not been shown to be safe and effective as claimed.

AMINOBENZYLPENICILLIN • *See* Ampicillin.

AMINOCAPROIC ACID (Rx) • Amicar. Introduced in 1964, it is used to control bleeding by limiting the action of plasmin (*see*), a natural blood thinner. Prescribed after surgery, for bleeding disorders, aplastic anemia, and for certain cancers. Particularly effective in urinary tract bleeding. Sometimes used to halt brain hemorrhages. Potential adverse effects include nausea, vomiting, diarrhea, headache, dizziness, stuffy nose, irritated eyes, fatigue, itching, and rash. Aminocaproic acid interacts with oral contraceptives, increasing the risk of blood clots. Should be used cautiously in patients with blood-clotting problems, and heart, kidney, or liver dysfunctions.

AMINO-CERV VAGINAL CREAM • *See* Urea.

AMINOGLUTETHIMIDE (Rx) • Cytadren. In use since 1960 to treat Cushing's syndrome, a condition caused by the overproduction of corticosteroids in the adrenal glands, resulting in the swelling of the torso and face. It inhibits the function of adrenal glands. Also used to treat adrenal cancer, and metastatic breast cancer. Potential adverse effects include deepening of the voice and increased body hair in women, drowsiness, loss of balance, rash, headache, numbness of the hands and feet, fever, muscle pain, and low blood pressure. Alcohol may potentiate the effects of aminoglutethimide. Dexamethasone, medroxyprogesterone, digitoxin, and theophylline may make it less effective. Allopurinol may increase the blood levels of aminoglutethimide, leading to toxicity. Oral blood thinners may be less effective if taken with aminoglutethimide.

AMINOGLYCOSIDES • Antibiotics derived from a species of streptomyces, or from micromonospora, bacteria that kill other, harmful bacteria. They are effective against gram-negative (*see*) bacilli and mycobacterium tuberculosis. Some common aminoglycosides are streptomycin, kanamycin, neomycin, tobramycin, amikacin, and gentamycin. Aminoglycosides are given by injection to treat serous bacterial infections in many parts of the body. Some aminoglycosides are applied in solution to the skin or mucous membranes, and others are given by inhalation. Potential adverse reactions include nausea, vomiting, increased thirst, dizziness, loss of appetite, numbness, tingling, or burning of face or mouth, convulsions, ringing in the ears, rash, loss of hearing, and clumsiness. If vancomycin hydrochloride, captopril, or NSAIDs (*see all*) are given at the same time, the risk of hearing, balance, or kidney side effects is increased.

AMINOPHYLLIN • *See* Aminophylline.

AMINOPHYLLINE (Rx) (OTC) • **Amesec. Aminophyllin. Amoline. Phyllocontin. Somophyllin. Truphylline Suppositories.** In combination: **Asmacol. Dainite KL.** An antiasthmatic drug belonging to the xanthine family of bronchodilating drugs that widen the airways and stimulate the respiratory center in the brain. Has been allowed in some OTC products in combination since 1976. Prescribed to ease breathing in asthmatics and those suffering from other bronchial diseases. Also used to dilate blood vessels and increase the output of the heart in congestive heart failure, and to treat apnea, temporary interrupted breathing, in the newborn. Potential adverse effects include nausea, vomiting, headache, irritability, insomnia, seizures, dizziness, and palpitations. A number of drugs increase the effect of aminophylline, such as beta-blockers and erythromycin, and others reduce its effects, such as anticonvulsants, barbiturates, phenytoin, tobacco (smoking), rifampin, and sulfinpyrazone. Aminophylline may increase the effects of anticoagulants. Should be taken with a full glass of water at meals, even though this may delay absorption.

AMINOSALICYLATE • *See* Aminosalicylic Acid.

AMINOSALICYLIC ACID (Rx) • **Pamisyl. Para-Aminosalicylic Acid (PAS).** Tebacin. Derived from phenol (*see*), it was introduced in 1948 to treat tuberculosis, but is usually not the drug of first choice due to its side effects. Potential adverse effects include nausea, vomiting, diarrhea, rash, itching, fever, sore throat, weakness, fatigue, and jaundice. Aminosalicylic acid may impair absorption of rifampin taken by mouth and may increase the effects of oral anticoagulants. Probenecid and sulfinpyrazone may increase the blood levels of aminosalicylic acid. Ethionamide may increase the risk of adverse effects with aminosalicylic acid. May be taken with food to reduce stomach upset.

AMIODARONE (Rx) • **Cordarone.** An antiarrhythmic for abnormal heart rhythms. In use since 1986, it is similar in structure to natural thyroid hormone. It slows down the transmission of nerve impulses through the heart muscle. Side effects are common, and potential adverse reactions include headache, malaise, nerve damage, low blood pressure, irregular heartbeat and congestive heart failure, eye problems, nausea, vomiting, increased breast size in men, thyroid problems, lung problems, liver dysfunction, and muscle weakness. Sunblock should be worn outdoors because amiodarone increases skin sensitivity to sunlight. Amiodarone increases the effects of procainamide, quinidine, phenytoin, and warfarin. It can interact with beta-blockers and calcium channel blockers (*see both*) to cause the heart to beat slowly. Most effective when taken on an empty stomach, but may be taken with a small amount of food if stomach upset is a problem. An IV form of this medication, which has been available in ninety-nine countries to treat life-threatening abnormal rhythms, was approved for the United States market by the FDA in 1994.

AMIPAQUE • *See* Metrizamide.

AMIPRILOSE • **Therafectin.** Medication for rheumatoid arthritis expected to be approved soon.

AMITONE (OTC) • *See* Calcium Carbonate.

AMITRIL • *See* Amitriptyline.

AMITRIPTYLINE (Rx) • **Amitril. Elavil. Emitrip. Endep.** In combination: **Etrafon. Limbitrol. Triavil.** An antidepressant introduced in 1961, belonging to the family of tricyclics (*see*). Elevates mood, increases physical activity, improves appetite, and restores interest in everyday activities. Because it has some sedating properties, it is often used when anxiety accompanies depression. Taken at night, it helps induce sleep.

Potential adverse effects include drowsiness, sweating, flushing, blurred vision, dizziness, fainting, rash, difficulty urinating, impotence, changes in libido, sensitivity to sunlight, and palpitations. An overdose may cause coma and death from abnormal heart rhythms. Sedatives may increase the sedative effects of amitriptyline. Barbiturates may reduce its antidepressant benefits, but may increase its toxic effects. Heavy smoking may reduce the antidepressant effect of amitriptyline. Serious side effects may occur, including seizures and delirium, if monoamine oxidase inhibitors (MAOIs) (*see*) are given with it. Contraindicated in persons recovering from heart attacks and used with caution in those with epilepsy, difficulty in urinating, glaucoma, heart disease, or thyroid disease. Amitriptyline may be taken on an empty stomach, but may be taken with food if stomach upset is a problem.

AMLODIPINE BESYLATE (Rx) • **Norvasc.** A once-a-day calcium channel blocker (*see*) used to treat high blood pressure and angina. Introduced in 1992. In rare cases it has been found to worsen blocked-coronary-artery disease. The most common adverse reaction is fluid retention and headache. A greater incidence of adverse reactions was reported in women than in men. They include flushing, palpitations, and sleepiness. Other potential adverse reactions include constipation, heartburn, irregular heartbeat, diarrhea, gas, vomiting, muscle cramps, sexual dysfunction, insomnia, nervousness, depression, rash, abnormal vision, red eyes, thirst, and rarely, amnesia. Drug interactions have not been reported to be a problem. Must be used with caution in patients with liver dysfunction or heart failure.

AMMONIA SPIRIT, AROMATIC (Rx) • **Smelling Salts. Aromatic Ammonia Aspirols.** Used as a respiratory and circulatory stimulant, and treatment for fainting.

AMMONIATED MERCURY (OTC) (Rx) • An ointment used to treat psoriasis and minor skin infections. Ointment strength depends on whether it is sold OTC or Rx. Should not be used on deep burns or open wounds, or mercury poisoning may result. Potential adverse reactions include nausea, cloudy urine, dizziness, headache, irritation, soreness, or swelling of gums and rash. The use of iodine- or sulfur-containing preparations at the same time may increase the possibility of adverse reactions.

AMMONIUM CHLORIDE (Rx) • A drug used to increase the acidity of urine and to speed the excretion of certain poisons in the urine. Potential adverse reactions include nausea, vomiting, drowsiness, headache, confusion, excitement alternating with coma, hyperventilation, calcium deficiency, twitching, slow heartbeat, gastric irritation, rash, pallor, and irregular breathing. Contraindicated in severe liver or kidney dysfunction. Should be used cautiously. The oral form should be taken after meals to decrease GI effects, but it should not be taken with milk or other alkaline solutions due to incompatibility. Spironolactone may cause systemic acidosis if used with ammonium chloride.

AMMONIUM HYDROXIDE (OTC) • **Ammonia Water.** A weak alkali formed when ammonia dissolves in water; exists only in solution. Irritating to the skin and mucous membranes. In 1992, the FDA proposed a ban on ammonium hydroxide in insect-bite and -sting drug products because it had not been shown to be safe and effective as claimed.

AMMONIUM LACTATE • *See* Lactic Acid.

AMMONIUM PHOSPHATE (OTC) • **Monobasic and Dibasic. Ammonium Salt.** An odorless, white or colorless, crystalline powder with a cooling taste, used in mouthwashes. Used also as an acidic constituent of baking powder and medically for its saline action. Has a diuretic effect (reducing body water) and makes urine more acidic.

AMOBARBITAL (Rx) • **Amytal.** A barbiturate sleeping drug that probably interferes with transmission of impulses from the thalamus to the cortex of the brain. Used for preoperative anesthesia. Potential adverse reactions include drowsiness, lethargy, hangover, paradoxical excitement in elderly patients, nausea, vomiting, rash, hives, and swelling. Contraindicated in uncontrolled severe pain, respiratory disease, allergy to barbiturates, history of drug abuse, or porphyria. It must also be used with caution in patients with liver or kidney disease. Elderly patients are more sensitive to the drug's side effects. Long-term use may lead to dependence.

AMONIDRIN (OTC) • *See* Guaifenesin.

AMOXAPINE (Rx) • **Asendin.** An antidepressant, introduced in 1970, belonging to the family of tricyclics. Prescribed for depression combined with anxiety, it elevates mood, increases physical activity, improves appetite, and restores interest in daily life. A weaker sedative than some other tricyclic antidepressants (*see*), it interferes less with tasks that require alertness. Potential adverse reactions include drowsiness, dry mouth, constipation, nipple discharge, rash, swelling of the testicles, menstrual irregularities, decreased libido, painful or inhibited ejaculation, palpitations, and seizures. It also may cause irregular heartbeat. Serious side effects such as seizures and delirium may occur if it is used with monoamine oxidase inhibitors (MAOIs) (*see*). Prolonged use may cause tremors and abnormal movements. Heavy smoking may reduce amoxapine's benefits, and use with sedatives may increase depression of the central nervous system. Most effective when taken on an empty stomach, but may be taken with a small amount of food if stomach upset is a problem.

AMOXICILLIN (Rx) • **Alphamox. Amoxidil. Amoxil. Apo-Amoxi. Augmentin. Axicillin. Cilamox. Clavulin. Ibiamox. Larotid. Moxacin. Novamoxin. Polymox. Sumox. Trimox. Utimox. Wymox.** Introduced in 1969, it is a penicillin-type antibiotic. When combined with clavulanate, it is used to treat lower-respiratory infections, ear infections, sinusitis, and skin and urinary-tract infections caused by susceptible strains of gram-positive and gram-negative (*see both*) organisms. Amoxicillin trihydrate is used to treat systemic infections, and acute and chronic urinary-tract infections caused by susceptible strains of gram-positive and gram-negative organisms. Potential adverse reactions include anemia, a decrease in blood platelets and white blood cells, nausea, vomiting, diarrhea, hypersensitivity including potentially fatal allergic reactions, and overgrowth of nonsusceptible organisms. Amoxicillin may reduce the effectiveness of the contraceptive pill and also increase the risk of breakthrough bleeding. May be taken with food.

AMOXIDIL • *See* Amoxicillin.

AMOXIL • *See* Amoxicillin.

AMOXYCILLIN • *See* Amoxicillin.

AMPHETAMINE (Rx) • **Adderall.** A brain stimulant used to treat attention deficit disorder with hyperactivity. Potential adverse reactions include restlessness, tremor, hyperactivity, talkativeness, insomnia, irritability, dizziness, headache, chills, overstimulation, palpitations, irregular heartbeat, low blood pressure, high blood pressure, nausea, vomiting, cramps, dry mouth, diarrhea, constipation, metallic taste, loss of appetite, weight loss, hives, impotence, and altered libido. Ammonium chloride, phenothiazines, haloperidol, and vitamin C make it less effective. Antacids, caffeine, sodium bicarbonate, and acetazolamide may increase its effectiveness. MAO inhibitors (*see*) may cause a severe rise in blood pressure. Must be taken at least six hours before bedtime to avoid insomnia. May alter insulin needs.

AMPHOCIL • *See* Amphotericin B.

AMPHOJEL • *See* Aluminum Hydroxide.

AMPHOTERICIN B (Rx) • **Amphocil. Fungilin Oral. Fungizone. Mysteclin-F.** Used to combat systemic fungal infections such as histoplasmosis, coccidioidomycosis, blastomycosis, cryptococcosis, disseminated moniliasis, aspergillosis, phycomycosis, and meningitis. It is used topically for eye and ear infections and is applied to the skin to combat candida (thrush) infections of the skin or nails. Amphocil is an injectable agent used to treat life-threatening systemic fungal infections. Potential side effects of intravenous methods for treating systemic infections include anemia, headache, nerve damage, low blood pressure, irregular heartbeat, loss of appetite, weight loss, nausea, vomiting, diarrhea, and stomach cramps. May cause kidney dysfunction, joint pain, muscle pain and weakness, fever, chills, malaise, and generalized pain. May interact with other kidney-affecting antibiotics increasing the potential for kidney damage. Topical application may cause skin reactions at the site of application. Amphotericin increases the toxicity of digitalis, and with diuretics, it increases the risk of low potassium levels. If used with aminoglycoside antibiotics, the risk of kidney damage is increased. When applied topically, the skin should not be tightly covered. Potential adverse reactions to skin application may be dryness, rash, burning, or itching.

AMPICILLIN (Rx) • Amcill. Ampicillin Trihydrate. D-Amp. Novo Ampicillin. Omnipen. Omnipen-N. Penamp. Penbritin. Polycillin. Principen. Supen. Totacillin. A penicillin antibiotic introduced in 1961 to treat systemic infections, and acute and chronic urinary tract infections caused by susceptible strains of gram-positive and gram-negative (*see both*) organisms. Also used to treat meningitis and gonorrhea (*see both*). Potential adverse reactions include anemia and other blood problems, nausea, vomiting, diarrhea, sore throat, pain at injection site, and hypersensitivity including rash, hives, and potentially fatal allergic reactions. Also may cause an overgrowth of nonsusceptible organisms. Should not be used with antibiotics such as erythromycins or tetracyclines. Ampicillin is most effective when taken on an empty stomach one to two hours before or after meals. If stomach upset is a problem, it can be taken with a small amount of food.

AMPLICOR CHLAMYDIA TRACHOMATIS TEST • A fast test for chlamydia, a sexually transmitted disease, approved in 1993 by the FDA. In men, the test is done on a sample of urine or with a swab sample of the urethra. In women, it is carried out with a swab sample of the cervix. According to the FDA, detecting and treating chlamydia, which affects 4 million people a year in the United States, can significantly prevent future reproductive problems in young women.

AMRINONE LACTATE (Rx) • Inocor. Used in the treatment of a heart that is not putting out sufficient blood such as in heart failure or certain infections. Potential adverse reactions include irregular heartbeat, vomiting, cramps, nausea, low blood pressure, upset stomach, diarrhea, liver dysfunction, and allergic reactions. It is given by infusion.

AMSTAT • *See* Tranexamic Acid.

AMVISC • *See* Sodium Hyaluronate.

AMYGDALIN (H) • A glycoside (organic compound) found in bitter almonds, peaches, and apricots. It has been a controversial substance due to claims that it can fight cancer in the compound laetrile. Such claims have not been accepted by mainstream scientists in the United States and the FDA, but the compound is widely available in Mexico.

AMYLASE (Rx) • An enzyme prepared from the hog pancreas or vegetable extracts, used to treat nutritional deficiencies and to combat inflammation. The FDA issued a notice in 1992 that amylase had not been shown to be safe and effective as claimed in OTC digestive-aid products. Nontoxic, but may cause an allergic reaction in persons sensitive to pork.

AMYL NITRITE (Rx) • The crushable ampules reduce cardiac oxygen demand by decreasing pressure in the heart and systemic blood-vessel resistance. They also increase blood flow through the collateral coronary vessels and are used to treat angina pectoris (*see*), and for relief of kidney or gallbladder colic. Amyl nitrite is effective within thirty seconds, but acts only for three to five minutes. Also used to treat cyanide poisoning. Potential adverse reactions include lack of oxygen in the blood, headache, dizziness, weakness, a drop in blood pressure upon rising from a seated or prone position, irregular heartbeat, flushing, fainting, nausea, vomiting, and hypersensitivity reactions. Contraindicated in those with sensitivity to nitrites, and during an acute heart attack. Also must be used with caution in patients with stroke, head injury, glaucoma, and low blood pressure. Cigarettes must be extinguished before use because ampules may ignite.

AMYOTROPHIC LATERAL SCLEROSIS
• **ALS.** A degenerative disease that is of unknown cause and leads to muscular weakness and atrophy.

AMYTAL • *See* Amobarbital.

ANABOLIC STEROIDS (Rx) • **Sex Hormones.** Drugs related to male hormones, sometimes given to "build up," to stimulate growth, weight gain, strength, and appetite. They are given to patients to help them gain weight after a severe illness, injury, or continuing infection, or when, for unknown reasons, patients fail to gain or maintain normal weight. Anabolics are also used to treat certain types of anemia, breast cancer, and hereditary angioedema, which causes swelling of the face, arms, legs, and throat. Abuse of these drugs has caused problems, especially among young athletes who wish to build muscle and strength. Uncontrolled use can cause liver damage and cancer. On February 27, 1991, anabolic steroids became controlled drugs requiring prescriptions and record keeping. The list of anabolic steroids includes boldenone, clostebol, dehydrochlormethyltestosterone, dihydrotestosterone, dromostanolone, ethylestrenol, fluoxymesterone, formebolone, mesterolone, methandienone, methandranone, methandriol, methandrostenolone, methenolone, methyltestosterone, mibolerone, nandrolone, Neo-Durabolic, norethandrolone, oxandrolone, oxymesterone, oxymetholone, stanolone, stanoxol, testolactone, testosterone, trenbolone, and any salt, ester, or isomer of these drugs. Anabolic steroids may alter many laboratory studies during therapy, and for two to three weeks after therapy has ceased.

ANABOLIN • *See* Nandrolone.

ANACIN (OTC) • Aspirin and caffeine (*see both*). Anacin contains 32 mg of caffeine per tablet.

ANACIN 3 (OTC) • *See* Acetaminophen.

ANACOBIN • *See* Vitamin B_{12}.

ANADROL • *See* Oxymetholone.

ANAEROBIC • Able to grow in the absence of oxygen.

ANAFRANIL • *See* Clomipramine Hydrochloride.

ANAGALLIS ARVENSIS (H) • *See* Pimpernel, Scarlet Kea.

ANALGESIA • Loss of sensibility to pain; loss of response to a painful stimulus.

ANALGESIC • Medication that relieves painful symptoms, especially headache, and muscle soreness and stiffness. Some analgesics may be applied topically to relieve itching or muscle pain.

ANALGESIC LINIMENT • Liquid rubbed on the skin that mildly stimulates nerve endings for warmth, coolness, or relief of pain.

ANALGESICS • Agents that relieve pain.

ANAMINE (OTC) • A combination of chlorpheniramine and pseudoephedrine (*see both*) used to alleviate cold and allergy symptoms.

ANANDRON • *See* Nilutamide.

ANAPHYLACTIC SHOCK • A severe and sometimes fatal allergic reaction to a sensitizing substance such as a drug, food, or chemical.

ANAPHYLAXIS • Severe hypersensitivity reaction to an allergen. Symptoms may include rash, swelling, breathing difficulty, and collapse. A severe form is anaphylactic shock.

ANAPROX • *See* Naproxen.

ANASPAZ (Rx) • A combination of phenobarbital and hyoscyamine (*see both*).

ANASTROZOLE (Rx) • **Arimidex.** The first in a new class of selective oral drugs for the treatment of advanced breast cancer in postmenopausal women, whose disease has progressed following treatment with tamoxifen (*see*). It lowers estrogen. Among side effects are nausea, headache, numbness, swelling, and bone pain.

ANATUSS (OTC) • A cough medication that is a combination of acetaminophen, chlorpheniramine, dextromethorphan, phenylephrine, phenylpropanolamine, and guaifenesin (*see all*).

ANAVAR • *See* Oxandrolone.

ANBESOL (OTC) • A combination of benzocaine and ethyl alcohol (*see both*) used to treat sore gums in babies and adults.

ANCEF • *See* Cefazolin Sodium.

ANCOBON • *See* Flucytosine.

ANDRO- • Prefix meaning male, as in the male hormone androgen.

ANDRO • *See* Testosterone.

ANDRO-CYP • *See* Testosterone.

ANDRODERM • Testosterone patch that supplies the hormone for 24 hours after application. *See* Testosterone.

ANDRO/FEM • *See* Estradiol and Testosterone.

ANDROGENS (Rx) • **Andro. Android-F. Cypionate. Delatest. Everone. Fluoxymesterone. Halotestin. Histerone. Metandren. Methyltestosterone. Ora-Testryl. Oreton. Testex. Testosterone. Testred. Testrin. Virilon.** Male hormones produced naturally in the body for normal sexual development. Natural and synthetic androgens are used to replace natural hormones when the body is unable to produce enough on its own, to stimulate the beginning of puberty in boys who are late starting puberty naturally, and to treat certain types of breast cancer in women. Androgens are banned and tested for in athletes by the U.S. Olympic Committee and National Collegiate Athletic Association, because they have been used to build muscle strength. When used for this purpose, they are dangerous to health and may lead to liver cancer. Contraindicated in breast cancer (in males), diabetes, fluid retention, kidney disease, liver disease, enlarged prostate, prostate cancer, and heart or blood-vessel disease. Androgens can increase the effects of blood thinners. May also interact with many other medications, including oral contraceptives, making these medications less effective or increasing their side effects. Should be taken with food to lessen stomach upset.

ANDROID • *See* Methyltestosterone.

ANDROID-F • *See* Fluoxymesterone.

ANDRO-L.A. • *See* Testosterone.

ANDROLAN • *See* Testosterone.

ANDROLONE-D • *See* Nandrolone.

ANDRONAQ • *See* Testosterone.

ANDROPOSITORY • *See* Testosterone.

ANDRYL • *See* Testosterone.

ANECTINE • *See* Succinylcholine.

ANEMIA • A below-normal level of red blood cells and/or hemoglobin resulting in fatigue, breathlessness, and low resistance to infection.

ANEMONE (H) • *Anemone ranunculaceae.* **Lily of the Field. Pulsatilla. Windflower.** Common throughout Europe, these small herbs of the buttercup family are referred to in ancient Greek and Chinese medicinal literature. Anemone is still used today as a homeopathic remedy for various emotional ills and the common cold. *See* Hepatica.

ANEMONE HEPATICAS • *See* Hepatica.

ANERGAN • *See* Promethazine.

ANESTACON • *See* Lidocaine.

ANESTHETIC • Medication that deadens sensations or feeling.

ANEURINE HYDROCHLORIDE • *See* Thiamin.

ANEURYSM • Sac formed by the dilation of an artery. If the sac ruptures, a hemorrhage can result.

ANEXSIA • *See* Hydrocodone and Acetaminophen.

ANGELICA (H) • *Angelica archangelica. Angelica officinalis.* **Archangel. Masterwort.** The benefits of this northern-European wild herb were said to have been revealed by an angel to a monk during a time of plague. Medicinally, herbalists use it as an astringent, a tonic to improve the circulation and warm the body, and for arthritis pain. The stems, if chewed, reduce flatulence. A beverage of dried leaves with lemon and honey is used as a cure for coughs and colds. Angelica is contraindicated in pregnancy and during menstruation, in cases of acute gastritis, peptic ulcers, and kidney inflammations. It may also cause photosensitivity. *See* Dong Quai.

ANGELICA TREE • *See* Zanthoxylum.

ANGI-, ANGIO- • Prefixes meaning blood or lymph vessel, as in *angiogram,* X-ray visualization of blood vessels.

ANGINA PECTORIS • Severe pain, usually in the chest and/or arm, often brought on by exertion or stress, and caused by inadequate blood flow to the heart muscle due to obstructions in the heart arteries.

ANGIOEDEMA • **Angioneurotic Edema.** Acute local swelling, like giant hives, under the skin. The swelling can be very serious if it occurs around the tongue and larynx, causing potential suffocation.

ANGIOGRAPHY • Radiography of vessels after the injection into a feeding artery of material opaque to X rays.

ANGIOPLASTY • A technique to open up blocked coronary arteries with a catheter.

ANGIOTENSIN • A powerful elevator of blood pressure produced by the action of renin, an enzyme made in the kidneys. All of the components of the renin-angiotensin system have been found in the brain. There are indications that they are part of the brain's mechanism for regulating blood pressure, as well as signaling thirst to the body and the need to take in fluids.

ANGIOTENSIN-CONVERTING ENZYME INHIBITORS (Rx) • **ACE Inhibitors. Capozide. Captopril. Enalapril. Lisinopril. Prinzide. Vaseretic. Zestoretic.** The exact way ACE inhibitors work is unknown, but it is known that they block an enzyme in the body necessary to produce a substance that causes blood vessels to tighten. As a result, they relax blood vessels. This lowers blood pressure and increases the supply of blood and oxygen to the heart. ACE inhibitors, while effective and popular blood-pressure-lowering drugs, have serious side effects: birth defects and fetal deaths. The FDA has issued a warning that they not be used in the second or third trimester of pregnancy.

ANHYDRON • *See* Cyclothiazide.

ANILINE • A colorless to brown liquid derived from coal tar that darkens with age. Used in the manufacture of dyes and medicines.

ANISEED (H) • *Pimpinella anisum.* **Anise. Umbelliferae.** A native of Asia and India, it is a medicinal plant used in Egypt as early as 1500 B.C. Greek physicians recommended it to warm the abdomen, prevent and expel gas, aid digestion, and relieve belching, nausea, and abdominal pains. Herbalists use it in a tea for intestinal gas, indigestion, bloating, and nausea. In 1992, the FDA issued a notice that aniseed had not been shown to be safe and effective as claimed in OTC digestive-aid products.

ANISOTROPINE (Rx) • **Valpin 50.** An anticholinergic, antispasmodic drug used to relieve irritable bowel syndrome and peptic ulcer. Potential adverse reactions include headache, insomnia, drowsiness, dizziness, confusion or excitement in elderly patients, nervousness, weakness, palpitations, rapid heartbeat, blurred vision, increased pressure in the eye, sensitivity to light, dry mouth, trouble swallowing, heartburn, loss of taste, nausea, vomiting, paralytic intestine, constipation, urinary retention, impotence, hives, decreased sweating, fever, and allergic reactions. Contraindicated in glaucoma, urinary obstruction, severe ulcerative colitis, myasthenia gravis (*see*), hypersensitivity to anticholinergics (*see*), heart problems, hemorrhage, and toxic megacolon. Must be used with caution in hot or humid environments because heatstroke can develop. Should be given thirty minutes to one hour before meals.

ANISOYLATED PLASMINOGEN-STREP-TOKINASE ACTIVATOR COMPLEX • *See* Anistreplase.

ANISTREPLASE (Rx) • **Anisoylated Plasminogen-Streptokinase Activator Complex. APSAC. Eminase** (*see*). An enzyme derived from human blood plasma that dissolves blood clots in acute heart attack. Anistreplase is given only under the direct supervision of a doctor. Potential adverse reactions include severe spontaneous bleeding, stroke, low blood pressure, irregular heartbeat, hypersensitivity, and hives. Aspirin, dipyridamole, heparin, and coumarin (*see all*) increase the risk of bleeding.

ANNUAL MERCURY • See Mercury Herb.

ANODYNE • Any medicine that allays pain.

ANOGENITAL • Relating to the body's anal and genital regions.

ANOREX • *See* Phendimetrazine.

ANOREXIA • Prolonged loss of appetite that leads to significant weight loss.

ANOSMIA • Lack of sense of smell.

ANOXINE-AM • *See* Phentermine.

ANSAID • *See* Flurbiprofen.

ANSPOR • *See* Cephradine.

ANSWER (OTC) • A diagnostic test for pregnancy.

ANTABUSE • *See* Disulfiram.

ANTACID • A compound that neutralizes hydrochloric acid found in the stomach. Over-the-counter antacids are one of the most widely used medications in this country. It has been estimated that over 25 percent of adult Americans take antacids more than twice a month, usually for heartburn or indigestion. Heartburn is the symptom usually associated with acid regurgitation, where acid from the stomach passes upward into the esophagus. The most common antacids contain magnesium, which may cause loose bowel movements, or aluminum, which may cause constipation. Antacids can interfere with the absorption of other medications such as digoxin, tetracycline, and ketoconazole (*see all*).

ANTAGONIST • A drug, hormone, or neurotransmitter that blocks a response from a receptor site on a cell. It is similar to blocking a keyhole so a key cannot enter.

ANTAZOLINE (Rx) • **Albalon.** An antihistamine used in decongestants for the eyes.

ANT-C • Homeopathic abbrevation for antimonium crudum (*see*).

ANTHELMINTIC • A medication that will destroy or expel worms from the digestive system. Among those in use: mebendazole, niclosamide, oxamniquine, piperazine, praziquantel, pyrantel, quinacrine, and thiabendazole. Herbs used for this purpose include aloe vera and wormwood (*see both*).

ANTHEMIS NOBILIS • See Chamomile.

ANTHRACYCLINE ANTIBIOTICS • An important class of antitumor agents exhibiting activity against a variety of neoplasms.

ANTHRA-DERM • See Anthralin.

ANTHRALIN (Rx) • **Anthra-Derm. Drithocreme. Drithocreme-HP. Lasan Cream. Lasan HP.** Derived from coal tar (*see*). On the market since 1936, it is used topically to treat severe psoriasis. To boost its beneficial effects, anthralin is sometimes used with ultraviolet light. Potential adverse effects include irritation, redness, and rash. Any drug that increases sensitivity to light may increase the irritative effects of anthralin.

ANTHRAQUINONES • Plants containing anthraquinones, such as yellow dock and buckthorn, are often used as gentle laxatives. Applied topically, anthraquinones may cause skin irritation and allergic reactions. Anthraquinone coal-tar colors are produced industrially from phthalic anhydride and benzene. Anthraquinones also are used as organic inhibitors to prevent growth of cells and as repellents to protect seeds from being eaten by birds. Caused tumors when given orally to rats in doses of 72 mg per kg of body weight.

ANTHRISCUS CEREFOLIUM • See Chervil.

ANTI- • Prefix meaning against, such as *antibiotics,* against live germs.

ANTIANGINALS (Rx) • Drugs to treat angina pectoris (*see*). These include bepridil, diltiazem, erythrityl tetranitrate, isosorbide, nadolol, nicardipine, nifedipine, nitroglycerin, pentaerythritol tetranitrate, propranolol, and verapamil.

ANTIARRHYTHMICS (Rx) • Drugs that restore the rhythm of the heartbeat when it becomes irregular (*see* Arrhythmia). Antiarrhythmic drugs either impede the flow of electrical impulses to the heart muscle or inhibit the ability of the muscle to contract. Beta-blockers (*see*) reduce the ability of the natural pacemaker in the heart to pass electrical signals to the atria, the upper right side of the heart. Digitalis (*see*) drugs reduce the passage of signals from the atrioventricular node in the upper center of the heart. Calcium channel blockers (*see*) interfere with the flow of calcium into muscle cells. Drugs such as quinidine and disopyramide (*see*) reduce the sensitivity of muscle cells to electrical impulses. In addition to the drugs mentioned above, other antiarrhymics in current use include mexiletin, procainamide, pirmenol, propafenone, and imipramine. Sotalol, a drug widely used in Europe for arrhythmia, was expected soon on the American market at this writing.

ANTIARTHRITIC • Medication that helps relieve arthritis symptoms, such as swelling, redness, and pain.

ANTIBILIOUS • A medication that helps the body remove excess bile in cases of gallbladder disease or jaundice.

ANTIBIOTIC • A chemical compound that kills or inhibits the growth of bacteria; usually produced from living organisms such as other bacteria or fungi.

ANTIBODY • A protein in the blood formed to neutralize or destroy foreign substances or organisms (antigens). Each antibody is tailor-made for an antigen (*see*).

ANTICATARRHAL • A medication to soothe mucous membranes. Herbs used for this purpose include boneset, bearberry, and goldenseal.

ANTICHOLINERGIC DRUGS (Rx) • Drugs that block the action of acetylcholine, a neurotransmitter that signals the relaxation or constriction of some involuntary muscles. These medicines include the natural belladonna alkaloids—atropine, belladonna, hyoscyamine, and scopolamine (*see all*). Such drugs are used to treat urinary incontinence, because they relax the bladder muscles while tightening those of the sphincter that shuts off the bladder. Anticholinergics are also used to relax the muscles of the intestines, helping to relieve stomach cramps and to prevent seasickness.

ANTICHOLINESTERASE • A drug, such as physostigmine (*see*), that inhibits or inactivates acetylcholinesterase, the enzyme that breaks down the neurotransmitter acetylcholine (*see*), involved in sending messages between cells that involve memory. Acetylcholinesterase is believed to play a part in the development of Alzheimer's disease (*see*).

ANTICOAGULANTS • Drugs, such as warfarin and dicumarol (*see both*), that slow the blood-clotting process of the body. Vitamin E supplements may increase tendency to bleed and should not be taken with anticoagulants without medical advice.

ANTICONVULSANTS • Drugs that are primarily used to reduce the number and severity of epileptic seizures. The choice of drug depends upon the type of seizure.

ANTIDEPRESSANTS • A wide range of medications used principally to prevent or relieve the symptoms of depression. These medications include the benzodiazepines, beta-blockers, monoamine oxidase inhibitors (MAOIs), and tricyclics (*see all*).

ANTIDIARRHEAL • Medication that lessens or controls an increase in the fluidity and frequency of bowel movements. Among the drugs used for this purpose are belladonna, kaolin, and loperamide (*see all*).

ANTIDIURETIC HORMONE (ADH) • A hormone produced in brain areas that are linked with the pituitary gland. Antidiuretic hormone is stored in the posterior pituitary gland. Its secretion reduces urine output. *See* Vasopressin.

ANTIEMETIC • A drug or treatment that stops or prevents nausea or vomiting.

ANTIFIBRINOLYTICS • Medications used to treat serious bleeding. They are sometimes given before operations to prevent hemorrhaging. Aminocaproic acid (*see*) is an example.

ANTIFLATULENT • A compound that reduces intestinal gas. Antiflatulents are sometimes combined with antacids in a single product to relieve gas and other symptoms of indigestion.

ANTIFUNGAL • A compound that destroys or prevents the growth of fungi. Usually applied topically. Fungal infections include jock itch, athlete's foot, and ringworm. Among antifungal drugs in common use are amphotericin B, fluconazole, griseofulvin, ketoconazole, miconazole, and nystatin (*see all*).

ANTIGEN • A foreign protein that can cause an immune response by stimulating the production of antibodies in the body.

ANTIESTROGEN • Any substance that prevents the full biological effects of estrogen (*see*) on responsive tissues, either by producing antagonistic effects on the target tissue or by blocking the effects of estrogen.

ANTI-FATIGUE (H) • A homeopathic formula. *See* Acidum Phosphoricum.

ANTIHEMOPHILIC FACTOR • **AHF. Hemofil M. Koate-HS. Monoclate.** Directly replaces deficient blood-clotting factor. Used to prevent hemorrhage in patients with hemophilia. Potential adverse reactions include headache; pins and needles in limbs, loss of consciousness, rapid heartbeat, low blood pressure, visual disturbances, nausea, vomiting, rash, hives, chills, fever, back-ache, flushing, and hypersensitivity reactions.

ANTIHISTAMINE • A drug minimizing allergy symptoms by blocking the action of histamine, a substance in the body that affects nasal and other tissues and may cause runny nose, congestion, sneezing, and itching. Some antihistamines are also used as sleep aids because they induce drowsiness. Antihistamines may diminish mental alertness in both children and adults. MAO inhibitors (*see*) prolong and intensify the drying effects of antihistamines; alcohol increases their drowsiness-producing effect. In young children particularly, antihistamines produce excitation. In infants and children, high doses of antihistamines may cause hallucinations, convulsions, or death. Antihistamines are more likely to cause dizziness, sedation, and high blood pressure in the elderly.

ANTIHYPERTENSIVES • These are prescribed when blood pressure cannot be lowered by losing weight, reduction in salt intake, and increased exercise. There are several classes:

• Centrally acting antihypertensives target the brain's mechanism for controlling blood-vessel size.

• Beta-blockers block the force of the heartbeat.

• Diuretics act on the kidneys to reduce blood volume.

• ACE inhibitors act on enzymes in the blood to dilate blood vessels.

• Calcium channel blockers act on the muscles to prevent constriction of the blood vessels.

• Sympatholytics block the nerve signals that trigger constriction of blood vessels.

Some people with high blood pressure suffer from headache or palpitations, but most have no symptoms, hence high blood pressure is called "the silent killer." The use of medications to lower blood pressure is believed to be one of the major reasons for the decline of strokes in the United States in recent years. Combinations of drugs may be used in severe hypertension. However, antihypertensive drugs may cause adverse reactions, especially at the beginning, causing a problem with compliance.

ANTILEPROTIC • A drug to treat leprosy, or Hansen's disease, an infection caused by *Mycobacterium leprae* and affecting the cooler parts of the body such as the skin.

ANTILIRIUM • *See* Physostigmine.

ANTILITHIC • A medication to prevent formation or aid in removal of stones or gravel in the urinary system. Rx drugs to treat the condition include chenodiol and pancrelipase (*see both*). Among the herbs used for this purpose are gravel-root and stoneroot (*see both*).

ANTIMALARIALS • Drugs to treat a disease characterized by chills and intermittent or remitting fever, caused by parasites transmitted to humans by the bites of mosquitoes. Among the drugs used: chloroquine, hydroxychloroquine sulfate, mefloquine hydrochloride, primaquine phosphate, pyrimethamine, and quinine.

ANTIMETABOLITES • A diverse group of compounds that interfere with normal cellular functions. Their primary benefit is their ability to disrupt the control center in the cell. They are most effective on rapidly multiplying tumors.

ANTIMICROBIAL • Medications that can help the body destroy or resist germs. Soaps containing an ingredient that kills or inhibits the growth and reproduction of bacteria are considered antimicrobial. Herbs that are reputed to be antimicrobial include balsam of Peru, echinacea (*see both*), and myrrh (*see* Myrrh Gum).

ANTIMINTH • *See* Pyrantel.

ANTIMONIUM CRUDUM (H). • **Ant-c. Black Antimony. Sulfuret of Antimony.** Occurs as a chemical compound and in crystalline form as the mineral stibnite, which is found in Europe and the United States. Legend has it that a German monk threw some antimony to his pigs and found, after purging them violently, it fattened them. He decided to give his fellow monks a dose so that they would put on some weight. The experiment failed and the monks died—hence the name *antimonk,* or antimony. Homeopaths use it for people who overeat or are sluggish. It is also used for nausea.

ANTIMONIUM TARTARICUM (H). • A homeopathic medicine used for chest complaints and gastric or bowel disorders. Made from the metal antimony, which can be irritating to the skin and mucous membranes. Antimonium tartrate was used in conventional medicine to get rid of intestinal parasites and to cause vomiting. Tartrate is made from grapes.

ANTIPRURITIC • A product to curb itching. Corticosteroids (*see*) are used for this purpose.

ANTIPYRETIC • A drug used to treat fever.

ANTIPYRINE (Rx) • Auralganotic Solution. Tympagesic Ear Drops. An analgesic drug used in ear drops for outer-ear inflammation. In 1992, the FDA proposed a ban on antipyrine in internal analgesic products because it had not been shown to be safe and effective as claimed.

ANTIRABIES SERUM, EQUINE (Rx) • An injection that provides passive immunity to rabies after rabies exposure. Potential adverse reactions include serum sickness within six to twelve days. Symptoms are skin eruptions, joint pain, itching, swollen glands, fever, headache, malaise, abdominal pain, or severe allergic reactions. Corticosteroids and immunosuppressants (*see both*) interfere with the serum's effectiveness.

ANTISCORBUTIC • A substance that prevents or treats scurvy, a disease caused by lack of vitamin C.

ANTISENSE DRUGS • One of the hottest areas of research in the 1990s, these substances are aimed at preventing the release of specific proteins by cells critical to the replication of viral or cancer cells. In simple terms, tumors and viruses make their own chemicals to keep themselves growing. Antisense technology identifies the individual tumor's or virus's growth compound and blocks it so that the tumor or the virus cannot continue to grow and eventually dies. The results will be more effective cures of malignancies and viruses without the terrible side effects of many of the poisonous drugs now in use.

ANTISEPTIC • An agent that slows or stops the growth of bacteria, but may not actually kill them. Often used to reduce bacteria in a wound and lessen the chance of infection.

ANTISEROTONIN EFFECT • A result of a drug that suppresses serotonin, a chemical present in relatively high concentrations in some areas of the brain and nervous tissue. Serotonin is also present in some tumors. *See* Serotonin.

ANTISPAS • *See* Dicyclomine Hydrochloride.

ANTISPASMODIC • A drug that reduces muscle spasms of the gastrointestinal tract, airways, and genitourinary tract such as the Rx drug dicyclomine (*see*) or the herbs cramp bark and eucalyptus (*see both*).

ANTITHROMBOTIC • A drug that breaks up or prevents the formation of blood clots. *See* Anticoagulants.

ANTITOXIN • A substance that neutralizes a specific bacterial, animal, or plant toxin.

ANTI-TUSS • *See* Guaifenesin.

ANTITUSSIVE • A medication that suppresses or inhibits coughing. Most suppressants act directly to inhibit the brain's cough-control center.

ANTIVERT • *See* Meclizine.

ANTIVIRALS • Common viral illnesses include colds, influenza, mumps, chicken pox, hepatitis, herpes, and AIDS. Viruses live by penetrating body cells. The invaded cell eventually dies and new viruses are released, spreading to and infecting other cells. An antiviral drug acts to prevent a virus from using the cell's genetic material, DNA, to multiply. Unable to divide, the virus dies and the spread of infection is stopped. There are topical and systemic antiviral drugs. Most antivirals act against only one type of virus. Some antiviral drugs can harm normal cells, particularly those in bone marrow. Topical antivirals can cause irritation of the skin. Systemic antivirals may cause dizziness and nausea. Among the antiviral medications available are acyclovir, amantadine, ganciclovir, idoxuridine, ribavirin, trifluridine, vidarabine monohydrate, and zidovudine (*see all*).

ANTRENYL • *See* Oxyphenonium.

ANTRIZINE • *See* Meclizine.

ANTUITRIN • *See* Gonadotropin, Human Chorionic.

ANTURANE • *See* Sulfinpyrazone.

ANUJECT (Rx) • *See* Procaine and Isobutyl-benzoate.

ANUPHEN • *See* Acetaminophen.

ANURIA • Absence of urine formation.

ANUSOL (OTC) • Cream and suppositories containing pramoxine HCL, phenylephrine HCL, benzyl benzoate, zinc oxide, and other ingredients for the relief of anal irritation. Potential adverse reactions include burning and allergic reactions to ingredients in the product. Contraindicated, unless directed by a physician, in persons with thyroid disease, diabetes, or difficulty in urination due to enlarged prostate. People taking drugs for high blood pressure or depression should consult a physician before using Anusol. Children may absorb proportionally large amounts and be more susceptible to systemic toxicity.

ANXANIL • *See* Hydroxyzine.

ANXIETY • Anxiety and fear are often used to describe the same emotion. Anxiety refers to an unpleasant and overriding inner emotional tension that has no apparent identifiable cause. Fear, on the other hand, causes emotional tension due to a specific, external reason. Anxiety disorders include phobias, panic disorder, obsessive-compulsive disorder, and post–traumatic stress disorder. These disorders are severe enough to interfere with social or occupational functioning.

ANXIOGENIC • Causing anxiety; a drug that produces such an effect.

ANXIOLYTIC • An antianxiety drug.

AORTA • The main trunk artery from which the systemic arterial system proceeds.

AP • Homeopathic abbreviation for apis mellifica (*see*).

APACET (OTC) • *See* Acetaminophen.

APAP • *See* Acetaminophen.

APERIENT • A term used in herbal medicine referring to herbs that are mild laxatives.

APF ARTHRITIS PAIN FORMULA • *See* Acetaminophen.

APHRODYNE • *See* Yohimbine.

APIS MELLIFICA (H) • A homeopathic (*see*) mixture of bee honey for bee and insect stings and for rashes. It is also prescribed after a fright, rage, vexation, jealousy, or hearing bad news. It is also used to treat cystitis, diarrhea, earache, eye inflammation, fever, and headache. Folk-medicine practitioners claim bee stings help ease rheumatism. Apis is prepared from the sting of the live common hive bee.

A.P.L. • *See* Gonadotropin, Human Chorionic.

APLASTIC ANEMIA • Bone-marrow disorders that cause insufficient production of red blood cells. About 50 percent of cases of aplastic anemia are due to drug or chemical side effects. Among the drugs known to induce aplastic anemia: acetazolamide, anticancer drugs, aspirin, carbamazepine, chlordiazepoxide, chloromycetin, chlorothiazide, chlorpheniramine, chlorpromazine, chlorpropamide, colchicine, indomethacin, lithium, mephenytoin, meprobamate, methimazole, oxyphenbutazone, penicillin, phenacetin, phenytoin, primidone, promazine, quinacrine, sulfonamides, tetracyclines, thiouracil, tolbutamide, triflupromazine, trimethadione, and tripelennamine.

APNEA • Cessation of respiration; inability to catch one's breath.

APO-AMOXI • *See* Amoxicillin.

APO-CLOXI • *See* Cloxacillin Sodium.

APO-METRONIDAZOLE • *See* Metronidazole.

APOMORPHINE (Rx) • A drug to induce vomiting in poisoning. Potential adverse reactions include depression, euphoria, restlessness, acute circulatory failure, rapid heartbeat, and depressed breathing. Contraindicated in patients with hypersensitivity to narcotics, impending shock, corrosive poisoning, or those who have overdosed on alcohol or narcotics.

APPETITE SUPPRESSANTS • Medications for short-term use to treat obesity. Among the drugs available: benzphetamine, diethylpropion, mazindol, phendimetrazine, and phentermine (*see all*).

APPG • *See* Penicillin.

APPLICATION SUBMITTED • An application for marketing that has been submitted by a company to the U.S. Food and Drug Administration (FDA).

APRACLONIDINE (Rx) • **Lopidine.** An eye solution to prevent or control pressure within the eye after laser surgery. Potential adverse reactions include nausea, vomiting, diarrhea, insomnia, irritability, nightmares, headache, slow heartbeat, low blood pressure, a drop in blood pressure when rising from a seated or prone position, raised eyelid, constriction of the pupil, burning, discomfort, foreign-body sensation, eye dryness and itching, blurred vision, allergic response, nasal burning or dryness, itching, sweaty palms, body-heat sensation, decreased interest in sex, and pain or numbness in the extremities. Contraindicated in patients with hypersensitivity to apraclonidine or clonidine.

APRESAZIDE (Rx) • **Apresodex. Hydral. Hydralazine. Hydra-zide.** A combination of hydralazine and hydrochlorothiazide (*see both*), used to treat high blood pressure. It is not for initial therapy and must be reevaluated periodically. May cause systemic lupus erythematosus–like symptoms. Signs and symptoms usually regress when the drug is stopped. Thiazides (*see*) have to be used with caution in patients with impaired liver function. Potential adverse reactions include headache, loss of appetite, nausea, vomiting, difficulty in urinating, irregular heartbeat, and angina.

APRESODEX • *See* Apresazide.

APRESOLINE • *See* Hydralazine.

APROBARBITAL (Rx) • **Allurate.** A barbiturate sleeping drug that probably interferes with transmission of impulses from the thalamus to the cortex of the brain. Potential adverse reactions include drowsiness, lethargy, hangover, paradoxical excitement in elderly patients, nausea, vomiting, rash, hives, and swelling. Alcohol or other central nervous system depressants including narcotic analgesics may cause central nervous system and respiratory depression. Aprobarbital may cause a decreased absorption of griseofulvin. MAO inhibitors (*see*) inhibit metabolism of barbiturates and may cause prolonged central nervous system depression. Aprobarbital may make oral blood thinners, estrogens, oral contraceptives, doxycycline, and corticosteroids less effective. Rifampin may decrease blood levels of aprobarbital. Contraindicated in uncontrolled severe pain, respiratory disease, allergy to barbiturates, history of drug abuse, or porphyria. Also must be used with caution in patients with liver or kidney disease. Elderly patients are sensitive to the drug's side effects. Long-term use may lead to dependence.

APRODINE (OTC) • *See* Triprolidine and Pseudoephedrine.

APSAC • *See* Anistreplase.

AQUACHLORAL SUPPRETTES • *See* Chloral Hydrate.

AQUAMEPHYTON • *See* Phytonadione.

AQUASOL A (OTC) • *See* Vitamin A.

AQUASOL E (OTC) • *See* Vitamin E.

AQUATAG • *See* Benzthiazide.

AQUATAR (OTC) • *See* Coal Tar.

AQUATENSEN • *See* Methyclothiazide.

AQUAZIDE-H • *See* Hydrochlorothiazide.

AQUEOUS PROCAINE PENICILLIN G • *See* Penicillin.

ARA-A • *See* Vidarabine Monohydrate.

ARABINOSYLCYTOSINE • *See* Cytarabine.

ARA-C • *See* Cytarabine.

ARACHIS OIL • Refined peanut oil applied topically to treat scaly skin conditions.

ARALEN • *See* Chloroquine.

ARALEN HCL • *See* Chloroquine.

ARALEN PHOSPHATE • *See* Chloroquine.

ARAMINE • *See* Metaraminol Bitartrate.

ARBUTIN (H) • A diuretic and anti-infective derived from the dried leaves of the heath family, genus *Vaccinium,* including blueberries, cranberries, and bearberries (*see* Uva-Ursi), and most pear plants. This may explain why cranberry juice is reputed to ward off and treat urinary tract infections.

ARBUTUS (H) • *Arbutus unedo.* **Strawberry Tree.** An erect evergreen shrub or small tree with creamy white flowers and scarlet fruit. Native to southern Europe and cultivated elsewhere for its fruit, arbutus contains arbutin, bitter principle, hydroquinones, and tannins (*see all*). Has astringent, diuretic, antiseptic, and anti-inflammatory actions. It is used to treat diarrhea and cystitis. Externally, it has been used as a gargle for sore throats. It is nontoxic but can cause constipation.

ARC • Abbreviation for AIDS-related complex.

ARCTIUM LAPPA • *See* Burdock.

ARECA NUT • *Areca cathecu.* **Betel Nut. Pinang.** An erect, slender palm native to Malaysia, Laos, and Vietnam. Among its ingredients are volatile oils, mucilage, resin, and tannins. The main alkaloid in this plant, arecoline, causes cancer in experimental animals. Folk-medicine practitioners have long used areca nut to get rid of worms, to stimulate the brain, and to stop spasms. Areca is toxic. Danish scientists have developed a medication from betel nuts to treat epilepsy.

AREDIA • *See* Pamidronate.

AREOLA • The circular pigmented area surrounding the nipple.

ARFONAD • *See* Trimethaphan Camsylate.

ARGENTUM NITRICUM (H) • A homeopathic remedy used as a fungicide. It is also used to treat diarrhea, eye inflammation, gas, headache, hoarseness, indigestion, and sore throat. *See* Silver Nitrate.

ARGESIC-SA • *See* Salsalate.

ARGININE (Rx) (OTC) • L-Arginine. **R-Gene 10 Injection.** An essential amino acid (*see*), strongly alkaline, that plays an important part in urea excretion. It has been used for the treatment of liver disease. Banned as unsafe by the FDA, February 10, 1992, for use in over-the-counter diet pills.

ARG-N • Homeopathic abbreviation for argentum nitricum (*see*).

ARGYROL (OTC) • *See* Silver Protein.

ARIMIDEX Rx • *See* Anastrozole.

ARISTOCORT • *See* Triamcinolone.

ARISTOSPAN • *See* Triamcinolone.

ARM-A-MED ISOETHARINE • *See* Isoetharine.

ARM-A-MED METAPROTERENOL • *See* Metaproterenol.

ARN • Abbreviation used for arnica (*see*) in homeopathic medicine.

ARNICA (H) • *Arnica montana.* **Leopard's Bane. Mountain Tobacco.** An herbal and popular homeopathic medicine (*see*), arnica contains sesquiterpene lactone helenalin, which is an anti-inflammatory. It contains volatile oil, helenalin esters, flavonoids, and triterpenoids. Arnica flowers have been used in herbal medicines as emollients and vulneraries (*see*), and to reduce inflammation in the nasal passages. Internally, herbal arnica preparations have been used for high blood pressure, various heart disorders, and stomach ailments, but it is now used mostly topically. Homeopaths use it to treat bruises and swollen joints. It should not be applied to broken skin. Arnica may be toxic. Should not be taken internally.

AROMATIC • The term is used in herbal medicine to signify essential oils that have a strong and often pleasant odor. They are reputed to stimulate the digestive system and are used in medicines to add aroma and taste. In 1992, the FDA issued a notice that aromatic powder had not been shown to be safe and effective as claimed in OTC digestive-aid products.

AROMATIC AMMONIA ASPIROLS • *See* Ammonia Spirit, Aromatic.

ARRHYTHMIA • Abnormal rhythm of the heart. *See* Atrial Fibrillation, Tachycardia, Ventricular Arrhythmia, Supraventricular Tachycardia, and Heart Block.

ARROWROOT (H) • *Maranta arundinacea.* The mashed rhizomes were once used by Central and South American Indians as an antidote for poisons used on arrowheads. When mixed with hot water, the root starch becomes gelatinous and serves as an effective demulcent for irritated mucous membranes.

ARS • *See* Arsenicum Album.

ARSEN. ALB • *See* Arsenicum Album.

ARSENICUM ALBUM (H) • A homeopathic medicine used for anxiety, restlessness, and weakness. It is given to children who are anxious and unable to breathe properly. It is used to treat colds, boils, burns, cystitis, diarrhea, and exhaustion. Arsenic compounds, which occur in the earth's crust, were described and used in antiquity. Most forms of arsenic are toxic.

ARTANE • *See* Trihexyphenidyl.

ARTEMISIA ABROTANUM • *See* Southernwood.

ARTERIOSCLEROSIS • A thickening and hardening of the walls of arteries and capillaries, leading to a loss of their elasticity.

ARTERY • A blood vessel that carries blood from the heart to body tissues.

ARTHR- • Prefix meaning joint, as in *arthritis,* inflammation of the joint.

ARTHRA-G • *See* Salsalate.

ARTHRALGEN (OTC) • A combination of acetaminophen and salicylamide (*see both*), used as a pain killer and fever reducer.

ARTHROPAN (OTC) • *See* Choline Salicylate.

ARTICULOSE • *See* Primaquine.

ARTIFICIAL TEARS (OTC) • **Adsorbotear. HypoTears. Isopto Alkaline. Isopto Plain. Isopto Tears. Lacril. Lacri-Lub. Lacrisert. Liquifilm Forte. Liquifilm Tears. Lyteers. Moisture Drops. Neo-Tears. Nethulose. Refresh. Tearisol. Tears Naturale. Tears Plus. Ultra Tears. Visculose.** Products used to relieve dryness of the eyes. They contain salt, mimic natural tears, and coat and lubricate dry mucous membranes. They help the eye hold moisture and/or thicken the tear fluid. Potential adverse reactions include eye discomfort, burning, pain on instillation, blurred vision—particularly with Lacrisert—and crust formation on eyelids and eyelashes—particularly with oily products such as Adsorbotear, Isopto Tears, and Tearisol. Contraindicated in patients with hypersensitivity to active product or preservatives. Should not be used with contact lenses in place unless product is specifically for that use.

ARUM (H) • **Cuckoopint. Lords-and-Ladies.** A hairless perennial native to Europe and cultivated in India. Its rhizome contains alkaloids and salt of oxalic acid. It is used as an expectorant, to induce sweating, and to get rid of worms. It is also used by herbalists to treat flatulence, indigestion, and rheumatism. Externally, arum ointment is used to treat sores, swellings, and ringworms. It is poisonous and should not be taken internally.

ASA (OTC) • *See* Aspirin.

ASAFETIDA (H) • *Ferula assafoetida.* **Devil's Dung. Gum Asafetida.** Routinely used as a carminative and as a substitute for garlic in many Asian countries, it is recommended by herbalists as a digestant, carminative, aromatic, antispasmodic, and expectorant. In 1992, the FDA issued a notice that asafetida had not been shown to be safe and effective as claimed in OTC digestive-aid products. May be toxic, especially to infants.

ASARABACCA (H) • **Hazelwort. Wild Nard.** A creeping perennial native to Europe and parts of Asia, it contains volatile oil, tannins, resin, and mucilage. It was formerly used as a substitute for ipecac (*see*) but is rarely used now. It has been used in homeopathic medicine to treat gastroenteritis and rheumatism. Can be toxic.

ASBRON • *See* Guaifenesin and Theophylline.

ASCARIASIS • Infestation with a species of roundworms that inhabit the small bowel.

ASCITES • Accumulation of fluid in the abdominal cavity, indicative of impaired circulation often related to heart failure, cirrhosis of the liver, malignancy, or kidney disease. Diuretic drugs or sodium and fluid restriction may control this condition, depending upon the underlying disease.

ASCLEPIAS TUBEROSA (OTC) • In 1992, the FDA proposed a ban on the herb *Asclepias tuberosa* in oral menstrual drug products because it had not been shown to be safe and effective as claimed.

ASCORBIC ACID • *See* Vitamin C.

ASCORBICAP • *See* Vitamin C.

ASCRIPTION A/D • Buffered aspirin with Maalox (*see*).

ASENDIN • *See* Amoxapine.

ASH BARK • *See* Zanthoxylum.

ASHWAGANDHA (H) • *Withania somniforal.* An herb used in India as a sedative and to heal broken bones.

ASMACOL • *See* Aminophylline.

ASPARAGINASE (Rx) • **L-Asparaginase. Elspar.** An anticancer drug that destroys the amino acid asparagine, which is needed to manufacture protein in acute lymphocytic leukemia. This leads to death of the leukemic cell. Potential adverse reactions include nausea, vomiting that may last up to twenty-four hours, bleeding, a drop in white blood cells, lethargy, loss of appetite, cramps, weight loss, kidney dysfunction, liver dysfunction, rash, hives, pancreatitis, chills, fever, and severe allergic reaction. Asparaginase decreases methotrexate's (*see*) effectiveness. Vincristine and prednisone (*see both*) increase the toxicity of asparaginase.

ASPARAGUS (H) (OTC) • *Asparagus officinalis.* **Sparrowgrass.** The root is used in Chinese medicine as a tonic. In India, it is used as a hormonal tonic for women, prescribed to promote fertility, relieve menstrual pains, increase breast milk, and generally nourish and strengthen the female reproductive system. It is also used as a tonic for the lungs in consumptive diseases and for AIDS wasting. Asparagus contains glycosides, asparagine, sucrose, starch, and mucilage. In 1992, the FDA proposed a ban on asparagus in oral menstrual drug products because it had not been shown to be safe and effective as claimed.

ASPARTIC ACID • A nonessential amino acid.

ASPERCREME (OTC) • A lotion or cream containing trolamine salicylate as well as glycerin, mineral oil, and a number of other alcohols. Used as a rub for temporary relief of minor aches and pains of muscles associated with simple strains and sprains. Advertised as containing no aspirin, but its major ingredient is a salicylate, related to aspirin.

ASPERGILLOSIS • Infection caused by aspergillus, a fungus found in old buildings or decaying plant matter.

ASPERGILLUS ORYZA ENZYMES (OTC) • In 1992, the FDA issued a notice that aspergillus oryza enzymes had not been shown to be safe and effective as claimed in OTC digestive-aid products.

ASPERGUM • *See* Aspirin.

ASPIRIN (OTC) (Rx) • **ASA. Acetylsalicylic Acid.** OTC products include: **Alka-Seltzer, Anacin, Arthritis Strength Bufferin, Arthritis Strength PC, Ascriptin A/D Caplets, Bayer Aspirin, Cama Arthritis Pain Reliever, Dasin, Ecotrin, Empirin, Excedrin Extra Strength, Fiogesic, 4-Way Cold Tablets, Halfprin Low Strength Aspirin, Maximum Strength Arthritis Pain Formula, Mobigesic, Arthropan Liquid, BC Tablets and Powder, Buffinol, Doan's Pills, Duoprin, Duradyne, Momentum Muscular Backache Formula, Norwich Maximum Strength Aspirin, Norwich Regular Strength Aspirin, P-A-C Analgesic, Pepto-Bismol Tablets and Suspension, Persistin Tablets, Sine-Off Sinus Medicine, St. Joseph Adult Chewable Aspirin, Ursinus Inlay-Tabs,** and **Vanquish Analgesic Caplets.** Rx medications include: **Argesic, Ascription with Codeine, Axotal Tablets, Buff-A-Comp No. 3, Darvon with A.S.A., Disalcid, Easprin, Empirin with Codeine, Equagesic Tablets, Fiorinal with Codeine, Gemnisyn, Lanorinal, Magan, Magsal, Marnal, Measurin, Micrainin, Mobidin, Noregisc Forte, Pabalate-SF, Percodan, Robaxisal, SK-65, Synalgos-DC, Talwin, Trilisate,** and **ZORprin.** Aspirinlike medicines have been used for more than two thousand years. The aspirin used today was introduced in 1899. Americans reportedly take 80 million aspirins a day and 29 billion yearly. One of the most versatile drugs, aspirin is used as an anti-inflammatory, fever reducer, and blood-thinner medication. It inhibits the body's production of hormonelike substances called prostaglandins, which trigger fever, pain, and inflammation. Aspirin, used in many compounds, is the most inexpensive of the common pain relievers. Aspirin is now recommended to prevent blood clots, heart attacks, and strokes, as well as "multi-infarct dementia," loss of mental ability due to multiple ministrokes in the small blood vessels of the brain. Aspirin can irritate the lining of the stomach. Thus, abdominal pain is a common side effect. As a result, aspirin is taken with food or milk, or purchased with an enteric coating that does not dissolve until it reaches the intestines. Prolonged use and high doses of aspirin can cause stomach bleeding or interfere with the blood's ability to clot. High doses of aspirin may cause ringing in the ears, dizziness, deafness, and rapid breathing. Other side effects include hypersensitivity reactions such as rash and bronchospasm in susceptible individuals. In elderly people, such effects may occur without warning. Aspirin should not be given to a child under sixteen years of age with a viral infection, especially the flu or chicken pox. A link has been reported between aspirin use in such circumstances and an inflammatory disease of the brain and liver, Reye's syndrome. Pregnant or nursing women should not take aspirin. Anyone with gout or ulcers should avoid it, and those on blood thinners should take it only with a doctor's supervision. Discontinue using aspirin at least five hours before visiting a physician, as it can mask symptoms and lead to an inaccurate diagnosis. Because of aspirin's effect on blood clotting, do not take it for at least a week or two before surgery. Aspirin should not be mixed with acidifying agents, alcohol, coumarin anticoagulants, fenoprofen, ibuprofen, methotrexate, naproxen, probenecid, sulfinpyrazone, tolmetin, urinary alkalinizers, or warfarin. In combination with vitamin C or foods high in vitamin C, aspirin may cause dizziness, ringing in the ears, impaired hearing, nausea, vomiting, diarrhea, fatigue, and mental confusion. In the *New England Journal of Medicine,* July 16, 1992, researchers from the University of Texas, surveying the latest literature on aspirin, reported that people with chest pain caused by blockage of one or more coronary arteries may prevent heart attacks by taking low-dose aspirin (one regular-strength tablet every other day). For people with no outward symptoms of heart disease, however, the researchers reported, the risks of bleeding and other side effects of aspirin may outweigh its prophylactic benefits. In 1992, the FDA proposed a ban for the use of aspirin to treat fever blisters, cold sores, poison ivy, poison oak, and poison sumac, because it had not been shown to be safe and effective as claimed in OTC products. Aspirin aluminate was also on the banned list for internal analgesic products. The FDA, at this writing, is proposing new labeling on over-the-counter products containing aspirin, buffered aspirin, or aspirin in combination with an antacid. The agency is concerned that people reading about new uses of aspirin such as reducing the risk of heart attack will begin long-term use without being aware of potential side effects. The label would point out that you should see your physician before taking aspirin products for your heart or for other unlabeled uses because serious side effects may occur.

ASPROJECT • *See* Sodium Thiosalicylate.

ASTEMIZOLE (Rx) • **Hismanal.** A once-a-day antihistamine introduced in 1989, used to relieve symptoms associated with hives and hay fever. Contraindicated in persons allergic to astemizole. Potential adverse reactions include headache, nervousness, dizziness, drowsiness, dry mouth, sore throat, irritated eyes, nausea, diarrhea, abdominal pain, increased appetite, joint pain, and weight gain. Should be used cautiously in persons with asthma because its drying effects can increase mucous plug formation. Should also be used with caution in those with liver or kidney dysfunction. In 1992, the FDA issued a warning that astemizole taken in quantities greater than the manufacturer's recommended dosage can cause dangerous heart rhythm disturbances and, in severe cases, lead to cardiac arrest. Astemizole should be discontinued four days before taking a skin allergy test because it can lead to inaccurate results. It should be taken on an empty stomach at least one hour before or two hours after a meal. A candidate for OTC status.

ASTHMA • A condition of difficult, labored, wheezy breathing.

ASTHMA & ALLERGY FORMULA (H) • A homeopathic formula to relieve shortness of breath, tight chest, and wheezing. It contains adrenalinum 6x, ipecacuanha 4x, and yerba santa 3x. *See* Adrenalin, Ipecac, and Yerba Santa.

ASTHMA PLANT (H) • **Asthma Weed.** *Euphorbia hirta* or *pilulifera.* An annual native to India and Australia widely grown in tropical regions. It has long been used to treat asthma, hence its name. It is also used to treat hay fever, emphysema, bronchitis, and cough. No toxicity has been reported, but related plants have been shown to be tumor promoting.

ASTRAGALUS (H) • *Astragalus membranaceus.* **Bok Kay. Gum Tragacanth. Huang Chi.** A plant found in Iran, Asia Minor, and Syria and used in Chinese medicine for centuries as an aphrodisiac and stimulant. It also is used by herbalists as a tonic for the spleen, kidneys, lungs, and blood. The dried gummy exudate, gum tragacanth, is widely used as a food additive, in the compounding of drugs, and in makeup and hand lotions. One of the oldest-known natural emulsifiers, its history predates the Christian era by hundreds of years; it has been recognized in the *USP* (*see*) since 1829. In recent scientific experiments, astragalus has been found to increase immunity and aid cancer patients in fighting their disease. Can cause allergic reaction, diarrhea, gas, or constipation.

ASTRAMORPH/PF • *See* Morphine Sulfate or Hydrochloride.

ASTRINGENT • A substance that causes skin or mucous membranes to pucker and shrink by reducing their ability to absorb water. Often used in skin cleansers, and to help stop bleeding. Tannins and witch hazel are astringents used in herbal and conventional medicine.

ASTROCYTES • Cells that support the neurons (*see*), nerve cells of the brain and spinal cord.

ATABRINE • *See* Quinacrine.

ATARACTICS • Tranquilizers (*see*).

ATARAX • *See* Hydroxyzine.

ATAXIA • Loss of muscle coordination.

ATENOLOL (Rx) • **Tenoretic. Tenormin.** Introduced in 1981, belonging to the family of beta-blockers (*see*), it decreases the heart's requirement of oxygen, allowing it to beat more slowly. Thus, it is used for treating high blood pressure, heart attack, and angina pectoris (*see*). Atenolol is prescribed for diabetics, and those with lung problems and poor circulation, because, unlike other beta-blockers, it acts mainly on the heart rather than other parts of the body. It may be given right after a heart attack to protect the heart from further damage. Atenolol is reportedly the least likely of the beta-blockers to cause confusion, hallucinations, nervousness, and nightmares, but has been associated with emotional depression. Potential adverse effects include muscle ache, dizziness, cold hands and feet, nightmares, sleeplessness, rash, digestive disturbances, male impotence, breathing difficulties, and confusion. Atenolol has the potential hazard of further depressing heart contractions and precipitating more severe failure in patients with congestive heart failure controlled by digitalis and/or diuretics. Should be used with caution in patients with asthma, impaired kidney function, and diabetes. Antacids reduce its effect. Catecholamine-depleting drugs such as reserpine may have an additive effect and may cause a drop in blood pressure and a slowing of the heartbeat, dizziness, and fainting. Allergic patients may react more to their allergies while taking atenolol. The drug should not be discontinued abruptly. Can be taken with food. *See* Catecholamines. A generic version was approved in 1995.

ATGAM • *See* Lymphocyte Immune Globulin.

ATHEROMA • Fatty deposits that develop in arterial walls and narrow arteries.

ATHEROSCLEROSIS • A condition in which arteries are clogged by fatty deposits on their inner walls.

ATHLETE'S FOOT • **Tinea Pedis.** A fungus infection in which the skin between and under the toes, especially the fourth and fifth toes, becomes irritated, red, flaky, and itchy. Sweat or water makes the top layer of the skin white and soggy. Other parts of the foot may also be affected.

ATIVAN • *See* Lorazepam.

ATOPIC DERMATITIS • A chronic form of eczema characterized by an intensely itchy skin rash, occurring in people who have an inherited tendency toward allergies. It is common in babies, often appearing between two and eighteen months.

ATOVAQUONE (Rx) • An AIDS drug rushed to market in 1992. It is used for the treatment of mild to moderate *Pneumocystis carinii* pneumonia (*see*) in patients who cannot tolerate trimethoprim or sulfamethoxazole.

ATOZINE • *See* Hydroxyzine.

ATRIAL FIBRILLATION • A common form of arrhythmia (*see*) involving rapid irregular contraction of the atria, the upper chambers of the heart, so that the ventricles, the lower chambers of the heart, cannot keep pace. It is often treated with digoxin, sometimes in combination with quinidine (*see both*). *See also* Antiarrhythmics.

ATROMID-S • *See* Clofibrate.

ATROPAIR • *See* Atropine.

ATROPHY • Wasting away or shrinking in size of an organ or tissue.

ATROPINE SULFATE (Rx) • **Atropisol. Atropoine. Barbidonna. Bellergal. BufOpto. Dey-Dose Atropine. Donnagel. Donnatal. Haponal. Hexalol. Hyonatal. Hyosophen. Isopto Atropine. I-Tropine. Kinesed. Lofene. Logen. Lonox. Lo-Trol. Ocu-Tropine. Spasmolin. Spasquid. Wigraine.** An anticholinergic (*see*) drug introduced in 1831 that inhibits transmission between certain nerves and is used to treat irregular heart rhythms. It also is used in eye ointments and solutions to dilate the pupil for the treatment of eye irritations. Potential adverse reactions, systemically, include increase in white blood cell count, headache, restlessness, disorientation, hallucinations, coma, insomnia, dizziness, irregular heartbeat, visual changes, dry mouth, thirst, constipation, nausea, vomiting, urine retention, and hot flushed skin. In eye preparations, potential adverse reactions include eye redness and congestion, contact dermatitis, swelling, blurred vision, eye dryness, and sensitivity to light. *See also* Belladonna, Hyoscyamine, and Scopolamine.

ATROPISOL • *See* Atropine.

ATROPOINE • *See* Atropine.

ATROVENT • *See* Ipratropium Bromide.

A/T/S • *See* Erythromycin.

ATTAPULGITE (OTC) (H) • **Fuller's Earth. Diar-Aid. Diasorb. Donnagel Liquid. Kaopectate Concentrated. Reaban Maximum Strength.** A white or brown, naturally occurring, earthy substance that is a variety of kaolin (*see*). Contains aluminum magnesium silicate. Used as an absorbent in medications to treat diarrhea.

ATTENUATION • A reduction in the severity or virulence of a disease or organism.

ATTENUVAX • Measles vaccine.

A-200 PEDICULICIDE (OTC) • *See* Pyrethrins.

A-200 PYRINATE (OTC) • *See* Pyrethrins.

AUGMENTIN (Rx) • A combination of amoxicillin and clavulanic acid, this antibiotic is used to treat sinus, urinary, ear, lung, and skin infections. Clavulanic acid augments the effects of ampicillin. It cannot be taken by penicillin-sensitive persons. Potential adverse reactions include upset stomach, diarrhea, skin rash, and allergic responses. Use with other antibiotics will make it less effective. Probenecid increases its side effects. Can cause false readings in tests for sugar in urine. May be taken with food.

AURALGAN (OTC) • **Allergen Ear Drops. Auromid. Auroto. Earocol. Oto.** An analgesic for earaches, a combination of antipyrine, benzocaine, glycerin, and oxyquinoline sulfate. Potential adverse reactions may cause irritation of the ear canal.

AURANOFIN (Rx) • Ridaura. An antiarthritic medication introduced in 1985, it is a gold compound that can be taken by mouth instead of by injection. Gold is believed to arrest or slow the progression of rheumatoid arthritis. Since gold drugs are toxic, they are used only after other drugs have failed to prevent disease progression and deformity. The main side effect is diarrhea. Other potential adverse reactions include rashes, nausea, conjunctivitis, mouth ulcers, and kidney dysfunction. Use of nonsteroidal anti-inflammatory drugs (NSAIDs) and penicillamine (*see both*) with auranofin may increase the risk of kidney dysfunction. Penicillamine may also increase the risk of blood disorders. Phenytoin may be increased to toxic levels if used with auranofin. Contraindicated in patients with a history of severe enterocolitis, lung problems, bone-marrow disorders, and skin diseases that cause flaking. Should also be used cautiously in patients who have kidney or liver dysfunction, inflammatory bowel disease, or skin rash. Most effective when taken on an empty stomach, but may be taken with food if stomach upset is a problem.

AUREOMYCIN • *See* Chlortetracycline.

AUROCANINE-2 • *See* Boric Acid.

AURO-DRI (OTC) • *See* Boric Acid.

AURO EAR DROPS (OTC) • *See* Carbamide Peroxide.

AUROMID • *See* Antipyrine and Benzocaine.

AUROTHIOGLUCOSE (Rx) • Gold-50. Gold Sodium Thiomalate. Myochrysine. Solganal. A gold-based drug to treat rheumatoid arthritis that has not responded to salicylates, rest, and physical therapy. Potential adverse reactions include nausea, vomiting, blood disorders, dizziness, fainting, sweating, slow heartbeat, low blood pressure, deposits of gold in the cornea, metallic taste, sore mouth, difficulty swallowing, kidney

dysfunction, liver dysfunction, rash (that can lead to fatal sloughing of the skin), angioneurotic edema, and severe allergic reactions. Contraindicated in severe uncontrollable diabetes, kidney and liver dysfunction, high blood pressure, heart failure, systemic lupus erythematosus, Sjogren's syndrome (*see*), skin rash, drug allergies, and other hypersensitivities. Should be used cautiously with other drugs that affect the blood.

AUROTO • *See* Antipyrine and Benzocaine.

AURUM ANALGESIC LOTION • *See* Camphor.

AUSTRASTAPH • *See* Cloxacillin Sodium.

AUTOIMMUNE • A condition in which the body manufactures antibodies against its own tissues and damages itself. Arthritis and lupus are examples of autoimmune diseases.

AUTOLOGOUS MARROW • Bone marrow taken from a patient's body and later reimplanted in that patient.

AUTOLOGOUS TRANSFUSION • A blood transfusion with one's own blood.

AUTOLOGOUS TRANSPLANTATION • A graft from one part of one's body to another.

AUTOLYMPHOCYTE THERAPY • *See* ALT.

AUTONOMIC NERVOUS SYSTEM • The division of the nervous system that regulates involuntary vital functions, such as the activity of the heart and breathing. Governs the excitation and relaxation of muscles. One part of the system, the sympathetic, widens airways to the lung, increases the flow of blood to the arms and legs, and prepares the body for fight or flight. The other part, the parasympathetic, slows the heart rate and stimulates the flow of digestive juices. Although the sympathetic and parasympathetic cooperate in the functional rhythm of most organs, the muscles surrounding the blood vessels are affected only by the signals from the sympathetic system. The trigger for constriction or relaxation of the blood vessels involves two sets of receptors, the alpha and beta. Among the compounds that act on the sympathetic nervous system are the alpha blockers, beta-blockers, epinephrine, and norepinephrine (*see all*). Among the compounds that act on the parasympathetic system are acetylcholine, cholinergic drugs, and anticholinergic drugs (*see all*).

AVC • *See* Sulfanilamide.

AVEENO ANTI-ITCH CONCENTRATED LOTION • *See* Camphor.

AVENA SATIVA • *See* Oat Fiber.

AVENS (H) • *Geum urbanum.* **Clove Root. Colewort. Herb Bennet. Wild Rye.** A perennial herb deriving its name from the Spanish word for antidote. It contains essential oils, tannins, bitter principle, flavone, resin (*see all*), and organic acids. Used as an astringent tonic for stomach problems, diarrhea, and leukorrhea, and as a gargle for sore throats.

AVENTYL • *See* Nortriptyline.

AVLOSULFON • *See* Dapsone.

AVOBENZONE (OTC) • **Filteray Broad Spectrum Sunscreen Lotion.** Derived from alcohol; used in sunscreens and as an anti-inflammatory.

AVONEX (Rx) • A new drug for the treatment of multiple sclerosis. It has been recommended for approval by the FDA's Expert Committee and, at this writing, approval was pending. The medication reportedly reduced MS progression by 37 percent.

AXICILLIN • *See* Amoxicillin.

AXID • *See* Nizatidine.

AXOTAL (Rx) • A combination of aspirin (*see*) and butalbital (*see* Butalbital Compounds) used to treat mild to moderate pain.

AXSAIN (OTC) • *See* Capsaicin.

AYGESTIN • *See* Norethindrone.

AYURVEDIC MEDICINE • A system of medicine in India based upon Hindu scriptures.

AZACTAM • *See* Aztreonam.

AZALIDES • A newer class of antibiotics, azalides are chemically related to erythromycin but possess unique pharmacologic properties. Zithromax (*see*) is the first on the market.

AZATADINE MALEATE (Rx) • **Optimine.** An antihistamine introduced in 1977, it is used to treat allergic reactions to insect bites and chemicals, relieving the symptoms of allergies such as itching, swelling, and redness of the skin and runny eyes and nose. With a strong sedative effect, it is useful to induce sleep at night. Potential adverse reactions include drowsiness, dry mouth, blurred vision, nausea, loss of appetite, dizziness, loss of balance, difficulty passing urine, and rash. Sedatives may increase the central nervous system depressive effects of azatadine. If taken within two weeks of taking a monoamine oxidase inhibitor (MAOI) (*see*), blood pressure may shoot up. Anticholinergic drugs (*see*) may increase the smooth-muscle-relaxing effects of azatadine, including some anti-Parkinson's drugs, antipsychotics, and tricyclic antidepressants.

AZATHIOPRINE (Rx) • **Imuran.** An immunosuppressant introduced in 1968, it is used to prevent rejection of transplanted organs, and to treat rheumatoid arthritis and other autoimmune diseases including systemic lupus erythematosus, polymyositis, dermatomyositis, myasthenia gravis (*see*), and chronic inflammatory bowel disease. It acts on dividing stem cells, from which all white blood cells develop. Potential adverse reactions include digestive disturbances, jaundice, unusual bleeding and bruising, fever and chills, sore throat, nausea, vomiting, weakness, fatigue, thinning hair, and rash. Drugs that affect the breakdown of other drugs in the liver or kidneys may alter the blood levels of azathioprine. These include phenytoin, phenobarbital, rifampin, allopurinol, and a number of antibiotics. If taking this drug, be sure to report even a cold or mild infection to your physician.

AZEDERACH (H) • *Melia azederach.* **China Tree.** A tree with purple flowers native to southwestern Asia and widely cultivated as an ornamental tree. The root bark contains cardiac glycosides, alkaloids, tannins, and volatile oils. In folk medicine it is used as a bitter tonic to increase the appetite and improve digestion. Also used as a laxative and to treat delayed menstruation. It is highly toxic and should not be used.

AZELAIC ACID CREAM (Rx) • A cream introduced in 1995 for the treatment of mild-to-moderate inflammatory acne vulgaris. It is a naturally occurring substance found in whole grain cereals and animal products.

AZELEX CREAM • *See* Azelaic Acid.

AZIDE • *See* Chlorothiazide.

AZIDOTHYMIDINE • *See* Zidovudine.

AZITHROMYCIN (Rx) • **Zithromax.** The first of the azalides, substances related to erythromycin (*see*). Introduced in 1991, it is an oral antibiotic used to treat mild to moderate infections in patients at least sixteen years of age, or adults with mild to moderate acute bacterial exacerbations of infections. It also is used to treat chronic bronchitis, pharyngitis, tonsillitis in patients who cannot use penicillin, skin infections, urethritis, and cervicitis due to trachomatis. One publicized benefit is that it need be taken only once a day for just five days. Potential adverse reactions include gastrointestinal upsets, such as vomiting, heartburn, and gas, palpitations and chest pain, monilia vaginitis, kidney inflammation, headache, sleepiness, fatigue, rash, photosensitivity, hives, dizziness, and pain. Aluminum- and magnesium-containing antacids decrease its effectiveness. Azithromycin may increase cyclosporine, hexobarbital, carbamazepine, and triazolam levels in the blood. If taken while on azithromycin, ergotamine may cause acute ergot toxicity. Because azithromycin is principally eliminated by the liver, it must be used with caution in patients with impaired liver function. Should be taken at least one hour before or two hours after meals.

AZLIN • *See* Azlocillin.

AZLOCILLIN (Rx) • **Azlin. Azlocillin Sodium. Securopen.** A penicillin antibiotic, used to treat serious infections caused by susceptible strains of gram-negative (*see*) organisms, including *Pseudomonas aeruginosa* (*see*). Potential adverse reactions include bleeding (with high doses), neuromuscular irritability, headache, dizziness, nausea, diarrhea, low potassium, local pain at injection site, hypersensitivity including potentially fatal allergic reactions, and overgrowth of nonsusceptible organisms.

AZMACORT • *See* Triamcinolone.

AZO DYES • A large class of dyes made from diazonium compounds and phenol, with an extensive category of colorings, used in the food, drug, and cosmetics industries. The dyes are characterized by the way they combine with nitrogen. They usually contain a mild acid, such as citric or tartaric acid. Azo dyes can cause allergic reactions, particularly hives. People who become sensitized to permanent hair dyes containing paraphenylene diamine (*see*) also develop a cross-sensitivity to azo dyes. If you are allergic to "penny" candy colored with azo dyes, you may also be allergic to a drug colored with an azo dye.

AZO-GANTANOL (Rx) • A combination of phenazopyridine hydrochloride and sulfisoxazole (*see both*).

AZO GANTRISIN (Rx) • **Azo-Sulfisoxazole.** A combination of phenazopyridine and sulfisoxazole, used to treat urinary-tract infections. Contraindicated in persons allergic to sulfa. Potential adverse reactions include nausea, vomiting, stomach pains, fatigue, hallucinations, dizziness, ringing in the ears, chills, and malaise. It increases the side effects of blood thinners, including aspirin and probenecid. Should be taken with a full glass of water.

AZO-STANDARD • *See* Phenazopyridine Hydrochloride.

AZO-SULFISOXAZOLE • *See* Azo Gantrisin.

AZT • *See* Zidovudine.

AZTREONAM (Rx) • **Azactam.** The first member of a new class of antibiotics classified as monobactams, aztreonam is a totally synthetic bactericidal antibiotic with activity against a wide spectrum of gram-negative (*see*) aerobic bacteria. It is used to treat infections caused by a variety of gram-negative organisms, including urinary tract, lower respiratory tract, skin, intra-abdominal, and gynecologic infections, and septicemia. May be used in penicillin-allergic patients. Potential adverse effects include anemia, seizures, headache, insomnia, low blood pressure, diarrhea, cramps, muscle aches, rash, nausea, vomiting, halitosis, altered taste, severe allergic reactions, and blood clots at the IV site. Should be used with caution in patients with impaired liver or kidney function. Furosemide and probenecid (*see both*) increase levels of aztreonam in the blood.

AZULFIDINE • *See* Sulfasalazine.

B

BABEC TEETHING LOTION • *See* Benzocaine.

BAC • *See* Benzalkonium Chloride.

BACAMPICILLIN (Rx) • **Spectrobid.** A penicillin antibiotic introduced in 1979, used to treat upper- and lower-respiratory-tract infections due to streptococci, pneumococci, staphylococci, gonorrhea, *Hemophilus influenzae;* urinary-tract infections due to *Escherichia coli, Proteus mirabilis,* and *Streptococcus faecalis;* and skin infections due to streptococci and susceptible staphylococci. Bacampicillin turns into ampicillin in the stomach. Its advantage is that it can be taken every twelve hours instead of every six as required with ampicillin. Potential adverse reactions include anemia, low white blood cell count and platelet count, nausea, vomiting, diarrhea, sore throat, and hypersensitivity, including potentially fatal allergic reactions and overgrowth of nonsusceptible organisms. When given with allopurinol (*see*) incidence of skin rash increases. Bacampicillin is most effective when taken with a full glass of water on an empty stomach.

BACARATE • *See* Phendimetrazine.

BACID (OTC) • *See* Acidophilus.

BACIGUENT (OTC) • *See* Bacitracin.

BACILLI • Cylindrical, rod-shaped bacterial cells. Bacilli may exist as single cells, in pairs, or in chains.

BACILLUS ACIDOPHILUS (OTC) • In 1992, the FDA issued a notice that bacillus acidophilus had not been shown to be safe and effective as claimed in OTC digestive-aid products. *See* Acidophilus.

BACILLUS CALMETTE-GUERIN (Rx) • **BCG. TheraCys. TICE BCG.** Instillation of live bacteria causes a local inflammatory response. Used in the treatment of cancers of the urinary bladder, and to promote active immunity to tuberculosis. Potential adverse reactions include nausea, vomiting, diarrhea, anemia, loss of appetite, painful and frequent urination, urinary incontinence, bladder spasms and pain, urinary-tract infection, kidney toxicity, malaise, fever, chills, mild abdominal pain, genital pain, and muscle and joint pain. Antibiotics taken concurrently for other infections may make BCG less effective. Immunosuppressants, bone-marrow depressants, and radiation therapy may impair the response to BCG, because these treatments can decrease the patient's immune response and may also increase the risk of infection. Contraindicated in patients with compromised immune systems.

BACITRACIN (Rx) (OTC) • **AK-Tracub. Aquaphor Antibiotic Ointment. Baciguent. Bactine First Aid Antibiotic. Campho-Phenique Triple Antibiotic. Foille. Mycitracin. Neosporin. Neotal. Neotricin. Polysporin.** Introduced in 1948, it is used systemically to treat pneumonia or abscesses caused by staphylococci, and topically to treat staphylococcic and streptococcic infections of the skin, outer ear, and eyelids. It is combined with other drugs into ointments that have a wide spectrum of bacteria-killing action. Some bacitracin preparations contain a corticosteroid (*see*) to reduce inflammation. In an ointment, it is used to treat eye infections. Topical bacitracin rarely causes adverse effects. Potential side effects of systemic bacitracin include blood problems, ear problems, nausea, vomiting, loss of appetite, diarrhea, rectal itching or burning, kidney dysfunction, hives, rash, pain at injection side, overgrowth of other infectious agents, fever, and severe allergic reactions. In eye ointments it may slow wound healing and cause temporary visual haze and an overgrowth of resistant organisms.

BACLOFEN (Rx) • **Lioresal.** A muscle-relaxant drug introduced in 1978 that acts on the brain and spinal cord. It relieves spasms, cramping, and rigidity of muscles characteristic of such conditions as cerebral palsy, multiple sclerosis, and stroke or brain injury. Also used for the severe facial pain known as tic douloureux or trigeminal neuralgia. Baclofen increases mobility and makes physical therapy easier to perform. It is less likely to cause muscle weakness than similar drugs. Elderly people, however, are more likely than younger people to suffer excitement, confusion, or hallucinations. Other potential adverse reactions include dizziness, drowsiness, nausea, constipation, and headache. Baclofen may increase blood sugar levels, so the dosage for antidiabetic drugs may have to be adjusted. It may also increase blood pressure, lowering the effects of antihypertensive medications. Sedatives may increase central nervous system depression in baclofen users. Take the drug with meals or milk to prevent GI distress. The drug should not be abruptly discontinued.

BACTEREMIA • Presence of bacteria in the bloodstream.

BACTERIA • Microscopic single-cell organisms. Bacteria are among the most common microorganisms responsible for diseases in humans.

BACTERICIDAL • A compound that kills bacteria. *See* Antibiotic.

BACTERIOSTATIC • An agent that stops the growth or multiplication of bacteria. *See* Antibiotic.

BACTERIUM • A microscopic organism composed of a single cell. Many but not all bacteria cause disease.

BACTINE • *See* Hydrocortisone.

BACTOCILL • *See* Oxacillin Sodium.

BACTOPEN • *See* Cloxacillin Sodium.

BACTRIM (Rx) • **Septra.** A combination of sulfamethoxazole and trimethoprim (*see both*), it is an inexpensive antibiotic useful in treating *Pneumocystis carinii* pneumonia (PCP), the most common, life-threatening, opportunistic infection affecting persons with AIDS. Also used for urinary-tract infections, ear infections, acute exacerbations of chronic bronchitis in adults, and traveler's diarrhea. Contraindicated in persons hypersensitive to trimethoprim or sulfonamides—fatalities have occurred with sulfonamides, due to severe reactions. Also should not be used in patients with megaloblastic anemia due to folate deficiency, or in pregnancy at term and during the nursing period because sulfonamides pass the placenta and are excreted in the milk. Bactrim should be given with caution to patients with kidney or liver dysfunction, to those with possible folate (vitamin B) deficiency, and to those with severe allergies, or bronchial asthma. The most common adverse effects are gastrointestinal disturbances and allergic skin rashes. Bactrim should be discontinued at the first appearance of skin rash or any sign of adverse reaction. Symptoms such as rash, sore throat, fever, joint pain, cough, shortness of breath, pallor, itching, or jaundice may be early indications of serious reactions.

BACTROBAN • *See* Mupirocin.

BA DAN XING REN • *See* Almond.

BAKER'S P & S (OTC) • *See* Phenol.

BAKER'S YEAST (OTC) • The yeast you buy at the supermarket to make cakes and breads may contain an element that can prevent the common cold. When a molecule isolated from the yeast by a University of California professor is placed in a dish with the cold virus, it stops it dead. It can no longer spread to other cells. Dr. Asim Dasgupta, professor of microbiology and immunology at UCLA, says that it is possible that at the first sign of a cold, you could spray the yeast molecule into your nose and throat and prevent the virus from doing its dirty work. To be effective, according to Dasgupta, the yeast molecule must be highly purified, concentrated, and reduced in size.

BAKING SODA • *See* Sodium Bicarbonate.

BALDEX • *See* Dexamethasone.

BAL IN OIL • *See* Dimercaprol.

BALLOTA NIGRA • *See* Horehound.

BALM • A soothing or healing preparation applied to the skin.

BALM (H) • *Melissa officinalis.* **Lemon Balm. Sweet Balm.** A sweet-tasting herb introduced into Britain by the Romans, it has been used from early times in England for nervousness, menstrual irregularity, and for surgical dressings. The Greeks used it for fevers, scorpion stings, and the bites of rabid dogs. A hot balm tea causes perspiration and is said to stop the early symptoms of a cold.

BALMEX EMOLLIENT LOTION (OTC) • *See* Lanolin and Peruvian Balsam.

BALMEX OINTMENT (OTC) • *See* Bismuth and Zinc Oxide.

BALM MINT (H) • *Balsamodendron opobalsam.* **Balm of Gilead.** The secretion of any of several small evergreen African or Asian trees with leaves that yield a strong aromatic odor when bruised. Known in ancient Palestine as a soothing medication for the skin. Used in cosmetics as an unguent that is said to soothe and heal the skin.

BALM OF GILEAD (H) • *See* Balm Mint and Poplar Extract.

BALMONY (H) • *Chelone glabra.* **Scrophulariaceae. Turtlehead.** The dried herb is used to prevent vomiting and as a stimulant and laxative. It is particularly useful, according to herbalists, for liver problems.

BALNETAR • *See* Coal Tar.

BALSAM OF PERU • *See* Peruvian Balsam.

BANCAP HC • *See* Acetaminophen and Hydrocodone.

B AND 0 SUPPRETTES (Rx) • A combination of belladonna and opium (*see both*), rectal suppositories used for the relief of moderate to severe pain. Should not be used in patients with glaucoma, severe liver or kidney disease, bronchial asthma, respiratory depression, epilepsy, acute alcoholism, delirium tremens, or premature labor. May cause addiction. Potential adverse reactions include nausea, vomiting, drowsiness, dizziness, dry mouth, urinary retention, sensitivity to light, blurred vision, hives, and itching.

BANESIN (OTC) • *See* Acetaminophen.

BANFLEX • *See* Orphenadrine.

BANOFED • *See* Diphenhydramine.

BANTHINE • *See* Methantheline.

BAPT • Homeopathic abbrevation for baptisia (*see*).

BAPTISIA (H) • *Baptisia tinctoria.* **Indigoweed. Wild Indigo.** In ointment or tea, the roots and leaves are used by herbalists and homeopaths as an anti-inflammatory with antibiotic properties. It has been used to treat all sorts of infections, from tuberculosis to sore nipples and swollen glands.

BARBASED • *See* Butabarbital Sodium.

BARBERRY (H) • *Berberis vulgaris.* **Holy Thorn. Oregon Grape Root. Pipperidge Bush.** A thorny bush. Herbalists used a tincture made from barberry to treat kidney stones. In ancient Egypt, a syrup of barberry combined with fennel seed was reputedly of value in warding off the plague. Barberry roots have high berberine (*see*) content and, thus, may act as a purgative. Barberry root preparations are also used to halt diarrhea. It is contraindicated in pregnancy.

BARBIDONNA (Rx) • A combination of phenobarbital, atropine, hyoscyamine, and scopolamine (*see all*) used to treat gastrointestinal disorders.

BARBITA • *See* Phenobarbital.

BARBITURATES (Rx) • Central nervous system depressants acting on the brain to produce results that may be helpful or harmful. Some barbiturates may be used before surgery to relieve anxiety or tension, as anticonvulsants to help control seizures, or as sleeping medication. Barbiturates can be habit-forming. As sleeping medications, they are ineffective after two weeks. Potential adverse reactions include bleeding sores on lips, chest pain, muscle or joint pains, red, thickened, or scaly skin, rash, sores, sore throat, fever, swelling of eyelids, face, or lips, wheezing, confusion, mental depression, unusual excitement, hallucinations, loss of appetite, and weakness. Barbiturates should not be mixed with alcohol, coumarin anticoagulants, digitoxin, griseofulvin, or monoamine oxidase inhibitors (MAOIs) (*see all*).

BARC • *See* Pyrethrins.

BAR-C • Homeopathic abbreviation for baryta carbonica (*see*).

BARIDIUM • *See* Phenazopyridine Hydrochloride.

BARIUM • A silver-white earth metal widely used commercially in paints, textiles, and other products. Can be toxic.

BARIUM ENEMA • An enema containing the metallic chemical barium, which may be seen on X rays. A series of pictures, taken while the enema flows through the bowel, reveals the lining of the colon and rectum.

BARIUM SWALLOW • A procedure used to detect diseases of the digestive tract. A liquid containing the metallic chemical barium is ingested and then visible on X rays as it is digested.

BARLEY (H) • *Hordeum vulgares.* **Pearl Barley. Prelate.** The seed is used by herbalists to treat diarrhea and bowel inflammation. Chinese herbalists use it as an anti-inflammatory diuretic for relieving gallbladder ailments, reducing swelling and tumors, and treating jaundice. Barley contains proteins, prolamines, albumin, sugars, starch, fats, B vitamins, and alkaloids (*see*).

BAROPHEN (Rx) • A combination of hyoscyamine, atropine, scopolamine, and phenobarbital (*see all*) used to treat gastrointestinal disorders.

BAROSMA • *See* Buchu.

BARYTA CARBONICA (H) • **Bar-C. Barium Carbonate.** A homeopathic medicine for the common cold and sore throat. *See* Barium.

BASALJEL (OTC) • *See* Aluminum Carbonate.

BASAL METABOLISM • A baseline of the minimal rate of energy expenditure for maintaining basal activities such as heart action, breathing, and heat production when the body is at rest. Used in diagnosing certain diseases, especially those involving the thyroid gland.

BASAL NUCLEUS • A specific area deep in the brain that plays a critical role in memory and is one of the first areas to undergo degeneration in Alzheimer's disease.

BASIL (H) • *Ocimum basilicum.* **Luole. Sweet Basil.** Grown in Britain since the sixteenth century, its name comes from the Greek *basilikon,* meaning royal. It is used as an infusion (*see*) for all stomach problems including vomiting, constipation, and gastritis. The infusion, sweetened with honey, is used for coughs and as a tonic. It promotes perspiration, treats early symptoms of the common cold, and is also said to relieve pains caused by delayed menstruation.

BASOPHIL • A white blood cell that contributes to inflammatory reactions. Along with mast cells, basophils are responsible for the symptoms of allergy.

BATCH CODE OR LOT • The series of numbers and/or letters on over-the-counter medication labels indicating manufacturer and where and when a particular bottle of medicine was produced.

BAY (H) • *Laurus nobilis.* A tree of the laurel family, bay is native to southern Europe, where it can grow to a height of fifty feet. In Roman times, the aromatic quality of the leaves led the Romans to scatter it in buildings to ward off the plague. Bay was one of four hundred remedies used by Hippocrates, and through the centuries, herbalists have used it to treat hysteria, ague, sprains, earache, and many other illnesses. Every part of the tree has healing properties, according to herbalists. Not recommended for internal use.

BAYBERRY (H) • *Myrica cerifera.* **Myricaceae. Candleberry. Waxberry. Wax Myrtle.** The bark contains volatile oil, starch, lignin, albumin, gum, astringent resins, tannic and gallic acids, and an acid resembling saponin. Used by herbalists as a stimulant, astringent, expectorant, and to induce sweating. Has been used to treat uterine prolapse and excessive menstrual bleeding, in a douche for vaginal infections, and to stop bleeding from the bowel and gums. A famous patent medicine, Dr. Thompson's Composition Powder, was used by many physicians to treat colds, coughs, and flu. Several modern versions are used by herbalists. Bayberry may cause adverse effects because of its gallic acid and high tannin content. Tannic acid and gallic acid can lead to irritation and even damage of the kidneys when used internally over a long time.

BAYLOCAINE • *See* Lidocaine.

BAYTUSSIN • *See* Guaifenesin.

B CELL • **B Lymphocytes.** A type of white blood cell emanating from bone marrow that helps the body fight infections.

BCG • *See* Bacillus Calmette-Guerin.

BCNU • *See* Carmustine.

BEAN (OTC) • In 1992, the FDA issued a notice that bean had not been shown to be safe and effective as claimed in OTC digestive-aid products.

BEAN CURD (H) • **Dou Fu-Tofu.** A soft vegetable cheese cooked by the Chinese into a soup to treat colds. It is prepared by treating soybean milk with magnesium chloride, dilute acids, or other coagulants, then draining and pressing.

BEARBERRY • *See* Uva-Ursi.

BECAUSE • *See* Nonoxynol-9.

BECLOMETHASONE (Rx) • **Aldecin Aqueous Nasal Spray. Beclovent. Beconase. Beconase Nasal Inhaler. Ceconase AQ Nasal Spray. Vancenase. Vancenase AQ Nasal Spray. Vancenase Nasal Inhaler. Vanceril.** A synthetic corticosteroid (*see*) prescribed to relieve the symptoms of allergic stuffy nose, and to control asthma. Introduced in 1976, it controls nasal symptoms by reducing nasal inflammation and mucus production in the nose. Used to prevent recurrence of nasal polyps after surgical removal. Also helps to reduce wheezing and coughing by reducing inflammation in the lungs. Taken by oral inhaler or in a nasal spray, beclomethasone is prescribed to patients whose asthma does not respond to bronchodilators (*see*). Potential adverse effects include nasal irritation, cough, sore throat, watery eyes, nausea and vomiting, development of fungal infections, and nosebleed. During withdrawal, some patients may experience joint and muscle pain. This drug is used to prevent asthma attacks and is not intended to treat an attack as it occurs.

BECLOVENT • *See* Beclomethasone.

BECONASE • *See* Beclomethasone.

BEDOCE • *See* Vitamin B_{12}.

BEDSORES • **Decubitus Ulcer.** Sores or ulcers resulting from pressures on parts of the body in persons confined to bed for long periods.

BEEPEN-VK • *See* Penicillin V.

BEE POLLEN (H) • A popular compound among naturalists, it contains nineteen amino acids, up to 35 percent protein, twelve vitamins, calcium, phosphorus, magnesium, iron, copper, manganese, sodium, potassium, chlorine, and sulfur. It is said to increase stamina. Those who are allergic to bee stings may also be allergic to bee pollen. In 1994, the FDA ordered a company producing Bee-Sweet to cease and desist representing its bee pollen and bee propolis products as being "effective as a cure or in mitigating" certain physical ailments. Bee-Sweet, on the other hand, claimed that "for centuries people have been using nature's perfect food [bee pollen] as nutritional enhancement or as an aid in the treatment of anemia, sexual stamina, back pain, allergies, weight control, digestive problems, arthritic symptoms, and pulse-rate control."

BEESIX (OTC) • *See* Pyridoxine Hydrochloride.

BEGGAR'S BUTTONS (H) • *See* Burdock.

BELAP (Rx) • *See* Belladonna and Phenobarbital.

BELDIN (OTC) • *See* Diphenhydramine.

BELIX (OTC) • *See* Diphenhydramine.

BELL • Homeopathic abbreviation for belladonna (*see*).

BELLADENAL (Rx) • *See* Belladonna and Phenobarbital.

BELLADONNA (Rx) (OTC) (H) • *Atropa belladonna.* **Belladenal. Deadly Nightshade. Hyland's Bed Wetting Tablets. Hyland's Teething Tablets. Levorotatory Alkaloids of Belladonna. Supprettes.** A member of the potato family, the name, meaning beautiful lady, is attributed to its use as eyedrops by Spanish women to dilate or enlarge the pupils. In use as a drug since 1831, atropine is derived from belladonna to dilate the pupil during eye examinations and surgery. Belladonna also contains hyoscyamine and scopolamine (*see both*). Taken internally, belladonna can accelerate the heartbeat, but its main use is in preventing spasms of the stomach and inhibiting the production of mucus in the lungs and saliva. The generic name, *atropa,* is derived from Atropos, the daughter of Erebus and Night. Potential adverse reactions include blurred vision, dry mouth, constipation, difficulty passing urine, headache, eye pain, and palpitations. It has long been used in homeopathic medicines for sudden complaints including fever and congestion. Contraindicated in glaucoma, obstruction of the urinary or gastrointestinal tracts, slow-moving intestines, heartbeat irregularities, hiatal hernia, kidney or liver dysfunctions, and ulcerative colitis. Antacids may reduce absorption of belladonna; sedatives may increase its sedative properties. Should be given thirty minutes to an hour before meals and at bedtime. In 1992, the FDA issued a notice that belladonna alkaloids and the powdered extract of belladonna leaves had not been shown to be safe and effective as claimed in OTC digestive-aid products. It is used in homeopathic medicine to treat dry skin and mucous membranes, fever, and congestion. *See also* Bellafoline, Bellergal-S, and Atropine.

BELLAFOLINE • Alkaloids of belladonna used as an adjunctive therapy for peptic ulcer, irritable bowel syndrome, and functional gastrointestinal disorders. Blocks acetylcholine, which decreases GI movement and inhibits gastric acid secretion. Potential adverse reactions include headache, insomnia, drowsiness, dizziness, confusion or excitement in elderly patients, palpitations, irregular heartbeat, blurred vision, difficulty in urinating, impotence, hives, and allergic reactions. It also inhibits sweating, so it should be used cautiously in hot or humid weather. Should be taken one hour before meals. *See* Belladonna.

BELLERGAL-S (Rx) • *See* Belladonna, Ergotamine Tartrate, and Phenobarbital.

BELLIS PERENNIS • **White Daisy.** A homeopathic medicine (*see*) that is used for first aid, insomnia, bruises, joint pain, and pregnancy problems.

BELL-P. • Homeopathic abbrevation for *Bellis perennis* (*see*).

BELL'S PALSY • Paralysis of the facial muscles due to facial nerve dysfunction of unknown cause.

BEMINAL 500 (OTC) • A multivitamin preparation.

BEMOTE • *See* Dicyclomine.

BENACEN • *See* Probenecid.

BENACTYZINE (Rx) • **Deprol.** A mild antidepressant and anticholinergic (*see*) that reduces the response to emotion-provoking stress. Potential adverse reactions include dizziness, difficulty in thinking, disturbed sleep, blurred vision, dry mouth, upset stomach, euphoria, and loss of balance. Contraindicated in people with glaucoma.

BENADRYL (OTC) • *See* Diphenhydramine.

BEN-AQUA (OTC) • *See* Benzoyl Peroxide.

BENAZEPRIL (Rx) • **Lotensin.** A newer orally active, non-sulfhydryl-containing ACE inhibitor (*see*) used to treat high blood pressure. Potential adverse reactions include nausea, vomiting, drowsiness, cough, fatigue, dizziness, headache, liver dysfunction, constipation, rash, flushing, anxiety, decreased libido, insomnia, nervousness, numbness, angioedema (*see*), low blood pressure, high blood potassium, and a drop in white blood cells. Agranulocytosis (*see*) has occurred with other ACE inhibitors and may be a potential side effect of this drug. Contraindicated in patients with impaired kidney function, those hypersensitive to ACE inhibitors, and pregnant women. Potassium supplements may increase the risk of high levels of potassium in the blood with potentially serious consequences. Benazepril increases the toxicity of lithium. May be taken after breakfast.

BENDROFLUAZIDE • *See* Bendroflumethiazide.

BENDROFLUMETHIAZIDE (Rx) • **Bendrofluazide. Naturetin.** A thiazide diuretic that increases urine excretion of sodium and water and is used to treat edema and high blood pressure.

Potential adverse reactions include nausea, vomiting, anemia, a drop in blood platelets, dehydration, a drop in blood pressure when rising from a seated or prone position, loss of appetite, pancreatitis, liver dysfunction, low blood potassium, high blood sugar, fluid and electrolyte imbalances, gout, skin rash, sensitivity to light, and other hypersensitivity reactions such as lung and blood-vessel inflammations. Cholestyramine, colestipol hydrochloride, and NSAIDs (*see all*) decrease its effectiveness. Diazoxide (*see*) increases the blood-pressure-lowering effect and increases the levels of sugar and uric acid in the blood. Contraindicated in urinary retention or hypersensitivity to other thiazides or other sulfonamide-derived drugs. Use cautiously in severe kidney diseases and impaired liver function. If you are taking this drug, ask your physician whether you should avoid foods rich in potassium, including citrus fruits, bananas, tomatoes, dates, and apricots. Use a sunscreen to protect your skin against sun sensitivity.

BENDYLATE • *See* Diphenhydramine.

BENEMID • *See* Probenecid.

BEN-GAY (OTC) • A topical preparation containing methyl salicylate (oil of wintergreen), camphor, and menthol (*see all*). Both methyl salicylate and menthol are external analgesics that stimulate the skin receptors for warmth and cold. This produces a counterirritant (*see*) effect that, reportedly, alleviates minor aches and pains of muscles and joints associated with simple backache, arthritis, strains, and bruises. A heating pad should never be used with Ben-Gay. Toxic if swallowed. Since both methyl salicylate and menthol can be irritating (in solutions of more than 3 percent), keep the compound away from eyes, mucous membranes, and broken or irritated skin. If skin irritation develops, pain lasts ten days or more, redness is present, or with arthritislike conditions in children under twelve years of age, consult a physician.

BEN-GAY ULTRA STRENGTH PAIN RELIEVING RUB (OTC) • *See* Camphor and Ben-Gay.

BENIGN • Describes an abnormal growth that will neither spread to surrounding tissues nor recur after removal.

BENISONE • *See* Betamethasone.

BENN • *See* Probenecid.

BENOQUIN • *See* Monobenzone.

BENOXINATE (Rx) • Derived from benzoic acid (*see*), it is used in the eyes as a local anesthetic.

BENOXYL • *See* Benzoyl Peroxide.

BENTYL • *See* Dicyclomine.

BENTYL WITH PHENOBARBITAL (Rx) • *See* Dicyclomine and Phenobarbital.

BENYLIN (OTC) • *See* Diphenhydramine.

BENYLIN DM (OTC) • *See* Diphenhydramine and Dextromethorphan.

BENYLIN DME (OTC) • *See* Diphenhydramine, Dextromethorphan, and Guaifenesin.

BENZAC W (OTC) • *See* Benzoyl Peroxide.

BENZAGEL (OTC) • *See* Benzoyl Peroxide.

BENZALKONIUM CHLORIDE (OTC) • **Bactine Antiseptic/Anesthetic First Aid Liquid. BAK. Ionax. Orajel Mouth-Aid. Zephiran Chloride.** A skin antiseptic, it is a widely used ammonium detergent. Also used in eye lotions and preparations to soothe sore mouth. Allergic conjunctivitis may occur as a reaction to eye lotions. In 1992, the FDA proposed a ban for the use of benzalkonium chloride to treat insect bites and stings, and in astringent (*see*) drugs, because it had not been shown to be safe and effective as claimed in OTC products.

BENZAMYCIN (Rx) • Benzoyl peroxide and erythromycin (*see both*). Used to treat skin and infections.

BENZATHINE PENICILLIN G • *See* Penicillin G.

BENZEDREX (OTC) • *See* Propylhexedrine.

BENZENE HEXACHLORIDE • *See* Lindane.

BENZETHONIUM CHLORIDE (OTC) • **Clinical Care Dermal Wound Cleanser. Formula Magic Antibacterial Powder. Orchid Fresh II Perineal/Ostomy Cleanser.** A synthetic detergent, it is used as an antiseptic. An oral poison. In 1992, the FDA issued a notice that benzethonium chloride had not been shown to be safe and effective as claimed in OTC products, including those to treat poison ivy, poison sumac, and poison oak, and in astringent (*see*) drugs.

BENZOCAINE (OTC) • **Americaine. Anbesol. BiCozene Creme. Cepacol Anesthetic Lozenges. Chloraseptic. Dentapaine Gel. Dermoplast. Foille. Foille Plus. Ger-O-Foam. Hurricane. Legatrin Rub. Orajel. Oxipor. Rhulicaine. Rhulispray. Vicks Formula 44 Cough Control Discs. Ziladent Oral Analgesic.** In combination: **Allergen Ear Drops. Auralgan. Cetacaine. Kanalka. Semets. Tympagesic.** One of the earliest local anesthetics, it was introduced in 1905 and is widely used in topical preparations to relieve sunburn, itching, and pain of minor burns. A gel is used for relief of toothache and teething pain, and ointment formulations for treating hemorrhoids and other painful anal disorders. It also is used in ear drops, throat lozenges, and as a diet aid. Not absorbed readily through the skin or mucous membranes. Potential adverse effects include burning, stinging, itching, redness, swelling, and rash. In 1992, the FDA issued a notice that benzocaine (0.5 to 1.25 percent) had not been shown to be safe and effective as claimed in OTC products, including those to treat poison ivy, poison sumac, and poison oak, as well as in products to kill lice and in astringent (*see*) drugs.

BENZODIAZEPINES (Rx) • One of the most frequently prescribed classes of drugs, which includes minor tranquilizers, antianxiety drugs, muscle relaxants, and sleep-inducing medications.

There are more than twelve benzodiazepines on the market. Among these are chlordiazepoxide, clorazepate, flurazepam, oxazepam, and perhaps the best known, diazepam (Valium). They are relatively safe in overdose. Among the potential adverse reactions to these medications are impaired memory, hallucination, muscle weakness, unusual bleeding or bruising, and behavioral problems.

BENZOIC ACID (H) (OTC) • A preservative that occurs in nature in raspberries, tea, anise, cherry bark, and cassia bark. It was first described in 1608, when found in gum benzoin. Used as a topical antifungal drug. A mild skin irritant. In 1992, the FDA proposed a ban on benzoic acid in astringent (*see*) drug products because it had not been shown to be safe and effective as claimed.

BENZOIN (H) (OTC) • **AeroZoin. Gum Benjamin. Gum Benzoin.** An aromatic resin from spicebush, a plant grown in Thailand, Cambodia, Sumatra, and China. It is added to steam inhalations for the treatment of sinusitis and nasal congestion and is also used to protect irritated skin. May cause allergic reactions.

BENZONATATE (Rx) • **Tessalon Perles.** A cough suppressant used to treat nonproductive cough by acting directly on the lungs, breathing passages, and the cough center in the brain. In patients with unusually large amounts of mucus, medications such as benzonatate are not recommended because they suppress the cough. Potential adverse reactions include nausea, constipation, drowsiness, headache, dizziness, burning sensation in the eyes, nasal congestion, rash, and chills. A candidate for OTC status.

BENZOPHENONES • **Neutrogena Moisture SPF.** At least a dozen different benzophenones exist. Solubilized coal tar (*see*) for soothing the skin is used in the manufacture of antihistamines, hypnotics, and insecticides. Some benzophenones may cause allergic reactions.

BENZOYL PEROXIDE (OTC) • **Benzac W. Cepacol Dry Throat Lozenges. Itch-X Gel. PanOxyl. Rhuligel.** In combination: **Acne Aid.**

Acne Soap. Acne-10. Ben-Aqua 5. Benoxyl 10. Benzac W 5. BPO. Buf-Oxal 10. Clear by Design. Clearasil Maximum Strength. Cuticura Acne. Del Aqua 10. Desquam-E. Dry and Clear Double Strength. 5 Benzagel. Fostex 10%. Loroxide-HC. Oxyl-5. Oxy-10 Cover. Oxy-10 Wash. Panoxyl. PanOxyl 5. Persa-Gel. PhisoAc-BP. Propa P.H. Liquid. Sulfoxyl and Vanoxide-HC. Topex. Vanoxide. Xerac BP5. Zeroxin. A bleaching agent introduced for medical use in 1931, it is used for the topical treatment of acne. Available in varying strengths, it removes the top layer of skin and unblocks the oil glands. It also reduces inflammation of blocked hair follicles by killing bacteria that infect them. Side effects are less likely if treatment is started with a low-concentration preparation. Potential adverse reactions include stinging on application, warmth, painful irritation, dryness and peeling, redness, crusting, swelling, rash, itching, blisters, and allergic contact dermatitis. Toxic by inhalation. In 1992, the FDA began a three-year study of this medication because studies showed that it caused skin tumors in rats. Abrasives, medicated soaps and cleansers, acne preparations and preparations containing peeling agents, topical alcohol preparations including cosmetics, and aftershave lotions may increase skin irritation.

BENZPHETAMINE (Rx) • **Didrex.** An amphetamine used as a short-term adjunct to treat obesity. Potential adverse reactions include restlessness, tremor, hyperactivity, talkativeness, insomnia, irritability, dizziness, headache, chills, overstimulation, palpitations, irregular heartbeat, low blood pressure, high blood pressure, nausea, vomiting, cramps, dry mouth, diarrhea, constipation, metallic taste, loss of appetite, weight loss, hives, impotence, and altered libido. Ammonium chloride, phenothiazines, haloperidol, and vitamin C make it less effective. Antacids, sodium bicarbonate, caffeine, and acetazolamide may increase its effectiveness. MAO inhibitors (*see*) may cause a severe rise in blood pressure. Must be taken at least six hours before bedtime to avoid insomnia. May alter insulin needs. Dependence may occur, especially in patients with a history of drug addiction.

BENZQUINAMIDE (Rx) • Emete-Con. An antinausea, antivomiting drug used to treat those conditions, associated with anesthesia and surgery. Potential adverse reactions include drowsiness, insomnia, headache, excitation, tremors, twitching, dizziness, transient irregular heartbeats, hives, loss of appetite, dry mouth, salivation, blurred vision, nausea, muscle weakness, flushing, hiccups, sweating, chills, fever, and sudden jump in blood pressure.

BENZTHIAZIDE (Rx) • Aquatag. Exna. Hydrex. Marazide. Proaqua. A thiazide diuretic that increases urine excretion of sodium and water and is used to treat edema and high blood pressure. Potential adverse reactions include nausea, vomiting, anemia, dehydration, a drop in blood pressure when rising from a seated or prone position, loss of appetite, pancreatitis, liver dysfunction, low blood potassium, high blood sugar, electrolyte imbalances, gout, skin rash, photosensitivity, and hypersensitivity reactions such as lung and blood-vessel irritation. Contraindicated in absence of urine or hypersensitivity to other thiazides or sulfonamide-derived drugs. Should be used cautiously in severe kidney disease and impaired liver function. If taking this drug, eat foods rich in potassium such as citrus fruits, bananas, tomatoes, dates, and apricots. Use a sunscreen to avoid problems caused by skin sensitivity to the sun.

BENZTROPINE (Rx) • Cogentin. Introduced in 1954, it is used to relieve symptoms of Parkinson's disease (*see*), including rigidity, tremor, and excess salivation. Because it does not much improve the slow physical movements that also characterize the disease, it is often used in conjunction with other levodopa-based drugs. Potential adverse effects include dry mouth and eyes, difficulty in passing urine, constipation, nervousness, blurred vision, sensitivity to light, confusion, nausea, vomiting, rash, and palpitations. If taking the drug, limit activities in hot weather as it reduces sweating and may result in heatstroke. Take the drug after meals to reduce gastrointestinal problems. The drug may require two or three days to manifest beneficial effects. Antihistamines and anticholinergic drugs (*see both*) may increase the toxicity of this drug. Benztropine should not be discontinued abruptly.

BENZYL ALCOHOL (OTC) • A local anesthetic for topical application, with a faint, sweet odor, it is derived as a pure alcohol and is a constituent of jasmine, hyacinth, and other plants. Ingestion of large doses causes intestinal upsets. It may cross-react with Peruvian balsam (*see*). In 1992, the FDA proposed a ban on benzyl alcohol in lice-killing products and in poison ivy, poison oak, and poison sumac drug products because it had not been shown to be safe and effective as claimed.

BENZYL BENZOATE (OTC) • Scabanaca. Occurs naturally in balsams of Tolu and Peru, and various flower oils. In 1992, the FDA proposed a ban on benzyl benzoate in lice-killing products because it had not been shown to be safe and effective as claimed.

BENZYLPENICILLIN • *See* Penicillin G.

BENZYLPENICILLOYL-POLYLYSINE • Pre-Pen. A scratch test to determine sensitivity to penicillin in adults who have a history of penicillin allergy.

BEPRIDIL HYDROCHLORIDE (Rx) • Vascor. A calcium channel blocker (*see*), it is used to treat angina pectoris (*see*) in patients who fail to respond to or are intolerant to other agents. Potential side effects include a drop in white blood cells, dizziness, water retention, flushing, palpitations, heartbeat irregularities, nausea, diarrhea, rash, and shortness of breath. When fentanyl anesthesia is given to those taking bepridil, a severe drop in blood pressure may occur. Grapefruit juice may cause potentially dangerous, increased levels of this medication in the blood.

BERACTANT (Rx) • Survanta. A naturally derived surfactant for the prevention and treatment of respiratory distress syndrome (RDS) in premature infants. Introduced in 1991, it is an orphan drug (*see*).

BERBERINE (H) (OTC) • A mild antiseptic and decongestant used in eye lotions, and as a dressing for skin ulcers. Derived as yellow crystals, from various plants. *See* Berberis.

BERBERIS (H) (OTC) • *Berberis vulgaris.* **Holly-Leaved Barberry.** The dried roots of shrubs grown in the United States and British Columbia. Used medicinally to soothe skin ulcers and break up intestinal gas and lower fever. Used in creams as a mild antiseptic. *See* Oregon Grape Root and Berberine.

BERGAMOT (H) • *Citrus bergamia.* **Bergamot Orange or Red. Oswego Tea.** An orange flavoring extracted from a pear-shaped fruit whose rind yields a greenish brown oil. Used in a tea for digestive problems and as a tonic. Can stain skin and may cause sensitivity to sunlight.

BEROCCA C (OTC) • A multivitamin preparation.

BEROTEC • *See* Fenoterol.

BERUBIGEN • *See* Vitamin B$_{12}$.

BETA-BLOCKERS (Rx) • Drugs that slow heart activity and thus lower blood pressure: acebutolol, labetalol, nadolol, oxprenolol, propranolol, timolol, esmolol, atenolol, metoprolol, and others. They are used to treat angina (chest pain), high blood pressure, and irregular heart rhythms. Given after a heart attack, they reduce the likelihood of fatal irregular heartbeat or further damage to the heart muscle. These drugs are also prescribed to improve heart function in damaged hearts. Beta-blockers may also be used to prevent migraine headaches, to reduce anxiety, to control fluid pressure in the eye, and for an overactive thyroid. There are two types of beta-receptors. Beta-1 receptors are located mainly in the heart muscle, and beta-2 receptors are in the airways and blood vessels. Specific receptors on cells are tailor-made to receive specific chemicals in a lock-and-key fashion. Beta-blockers occupy the beta-receptors in these areas. By blocking these receptors, they block the stimulating action of the nerve-stimulating chemical norepinephrine. Thus, they reduce the force and speed of the heartbeat and prevent the dilation of the airways to the lungs and the blood vessels surrounding the brain and leading to the extremities. Drugs for the heart act mainly on beta 1 receptors. Beta-blockers are usually not prescribed for people who have poor circulation, particularly in the legs and arms. Beta-blockers should not be discontinued suddenly after prolonged use because this may worsen the symptoms of the disorders for which they were prescribed. They should not be taken with foods, beverages, or over-the-counter medications that contain caffeine or alcohol or are high in sodium content, because the combination may increase heart rate or elevate blood pressure.

BETA-CAROTENE (Rx) (OTC) (H) • **Provitamin A. Bugs Bunny Children's Vitamins. Flintstones Children's Chewable. One-A-Day Women's Formula. Solatene. Theragran-M Tablets.** Found in all plants and in many animal tissues, it is the chief yellow coloring matter of carrots. Oral doses of beta-carotene (180 mg/day) given for two weeks to normal volunteers significantly increased the T cells in their blood, which are involved in immunity. Low levels of beta-carotene in serum or plasma have been associated with subsequent development of lung cancer. There is no official recommended daily allowance (RDA) for adults, but 6 mg daily has been recommended. There are controversies over whether doses of beta-carotene may lower the risk of cardiovascular disease, and cancers of lung, stomach, and mouth. Some studies have shown it to be useless against lung cancer. Too much carotene in the blood can lead to carotenemia, a pale yellow-red pigmentation of the skin that may be mistaken for jaundice. It is a benign condition, and withdrawal of carotene cures it. Beta-carotene has less serious side effects than vitamin A. Animal studies have shown that regular drinking of alcoholic beverages while taking beta-carotene may cause liver damage.

BETADINE (OTC) • An antiseptic. *See* Povidoine-Iodine.

BETAGAN • *See* Levobunolol.

BETAINE (H) • Used as a coloring and as a dietary supplement, it occurs in common beets and in many other vegetables, as well as animal substances. Used in resins. Has been employed medically to treat muscle weakness. In 1992, the FDA issued a notice that betaine hydroxide had not been shown to be safe and effective as claimed in OTC digestive-aid products.

BETA INTERFERON (Rx) • **Betaseron. Avonex.** An interferon (*see*) that is being tested against Kaposi's sarcoma, AIDS, and ARC. It was approved in 1993 for the treatment of multiple sclerosis. In 1996, the FDA approved beta interferon 1a, which requires only once-a-week intramuscular injection. Although the cause of multiple sclerosis is unknown, it involves attacks on the body from its own immune system. The progressive nerve damage is caused by white blood cells destroying the myelin sheath that insulates nerves. Beta interferon seems to suppress the attacks of the white blood cells. The potential adverse reactions include flu-like symptoms and redness at the site of injection.

BETA-LACTAMS (Rx) • A large group of antibiotics, including the penicillins and cephalosporins, that contain a common structural component, the beta-lactam ring. This group of drugs acts by inhibiting the manufacture of bacterial cell walls. Beta-lactamase is an enzyme in bacteria that attacks the beta-lactam ring found in many antibiotics, reducing their effectiveness. A new class of antibiotics, the azalides, do not have the beta-lactam structure and are active against beta-lactamase-producing bacteria.

BETALIN S • *See* Thiamin.

BETALIN 12 • *See* Vitamin B_{12}.

BETAMETHASONE (Rx) • **Alphatrex. Benisone. Betatrex. Beta-Val. B-S-P. Celestone. Diprolene. Diprosone. Flubenisone. Maxivate. Uticort. Valisone. Valnac.** Combined: **Lotrisone.** Available since 1961, betamethasone is a corticosteroid for the treatment of steroid-responsive skin disorders caused by allergy or inflammation. It is related to prednisolone (*see*) and differs only in having a fluorine and methyl group in place of hydrogens. It can be applied topically or injected into the joints to relieve the pain and stiffness of arthritis and other joint inflammation. In an inhaler, the drug is used for asthma and sinus attacks. It may also be given by mouth to treat corticosteroid deficiency as a result of pituitary or adrenal gland disorders. Betamethasone by mouth or injection reduces the action of insulin, anticoagulants, and drugs for treating high blood pressure. Potential adverse effects include indigestion, peptic ulcer, weak bones, weight gain, acne, muscle weakness, mood changes, and bloody stools. It also may retard growth in children. Betamethasone should not be discontinued suddenly. The drug interacts with digoxin, increasing digoxin's adverse effects. Serious reactions such as infections may occur when vaccinations are given during betamethasone treatment. Contraindicated in persons who have a systemic fungal infection, and must be used cautiously in patients with GI ulceration, kidney disease, high blood pressure, osteoporosis, chicken pox, diabetes, Cushing's syndrome, blood-clotting disorders, seizures, myasthenia gravis, congestive heart failure, tuberculosis, herpes infections, or emotional problems. Older adults are more likely to develop high blood pressure while taking this medicine orally. The potential adverse reactions of betamethasone in an ointment or cream used to treat skin inflammations include burning, itching, irritation, dryness, inflammation of the hair follicles, acne, rash around the mouth, spots of pigment loss, hairiness, allergic contact dermatitis, and if covered with a dressing, secondary infection, atrophy, streaks, and blisters. Should be used cautiously in skin problems caused by viruses such as herpes, and in fungal or bacterial skin infections. Should not be used for more than two weeks due to potential absorption into the system, consequently causing an effect on the hypothalamus, and pituitary and adrenal glands. Should not be applied near the eyes or mucous membranes, under the arms, on the face, groin, or under the breast unless medically specified.

BETAPACE • *See* Sotalol.

BETAPEN-VK • *See* Penicillin V.

BETASERON • *See* Beta Interferon.

BETATREX • *See* Betamethasone.

BETA-2 BISORINE • *See* Isoetharine.

BETA-VAL • *See* Betamethasone.

BETAXOLOL HYDROCHLORIDE (Rx) • **Betoptic. Kerlone.** Introduced in 1983, a beta-blocker (*see*) that lowers blood pressure and is also used in the treatment of glaucoma. Potential adverse reactions include irregular heartbeat, chest pain, a severe drop in blood pressure, worsening of angina, congestive heart failure, water retention, fainting, fatigue, headache, anxiety, gas, decreased libido, impotence, menstrual irregularities, constipation, nausea, diarrhea, dry mouth, vomiting, and loss of appetite. Other potential adverse reactions include shortness of breath, wheezing, bronchospasm, insomnia, and skin rash. Must be used cautiously in patients with heart disease or lung dysfunction. When used with calcium channel blocking agents, the risk of low blood pressure and heart failure may increase. In eyedrops, it may cause sensitivity to light. When used with lidocaine, reserpine, and catecholamine-depleting drugs, the effects of these drugs may be additive. Cocaine may inhibit betaxolol's effects. Betaxolol should not be discontinued abruptly. May be taken with or without meals.

BETAZOLE (Rx) • **Histalog.** Compound related to histamine that stimulates stomach secretions and is used to test their flow.

BETHANECHOL (Rx) • **Duvoid. Myotonachol. Urabeth. Urecholine.** A drug that mimics the action of the neurotransmitter acetylcholine (*see*), it is used to treat urine retention, abdominal distension, megacolon, and backup of acid into the throat caused by low esophageal sphincter pressure. It produces a contraction of the muscles to empty the bladder and stimulates gastric motility. Its effects may appear within thirty minutes and last for as long as six hours. Contraindicated in persons hypersensitive to bethanechol, those with overactive thyroids, peptic ulcers, bronchial asthma, slow heartbeat, low blood pressure, coronary artery disease, epilepsy, or parkinsonism. Potential adverse reactions are rare after oral ingestion, but not after injection. These include malaise, abdominal cramps, colicky pain, nausea, belching, diarrhea, salivation, urinary urgency, headache, a drop in blood pressure, flushing, sweating, bronchial constriction, asthmatic attacks, and tearing of the eyes. Should be taken on an empty stomach. If not, nausea and vomiting may occur.

BETHROOT (H) • **Birthroot. Cough Root. Trillium.** From the root and rhizome of *Trillium pendulum,* native to eastern North America, it contains glycosides, alkaloids, resin, and tannins (*see all*). Used in folk medicine and by homeopathic physicians for the treatment of excessive menstruation and menopausal symptoms. It is also used as an ointment to treat skin diseases. The plant can affect the uterus and thus should not be taken in large doses and should be avoided during pregnancy. It is also contraindicated in heart disease because of its glycoside content.

BETONY • *See* Wood Betony.

BETOPTIC • *See* Betaxolol Hydrochloride.

BIAXIN • *See* Clarithromycin.

BICALUTAMIDE (Rx) • **Casodex.** A once-a-day tablet, introduced in 1995, for the treatment of advanced prostate cancer. It is used in combination with a luteinizing hormone-releasing hormone analogue.

BICARBONATE OF SODA • *See* Sodium Bicarbonate.

BICILLIN • **Bicillin L-A.** *See* Penicillin G.

BICILLIN C-R • *See* Penicillin G and Procaine.

BICITRA (OTC) • An antacid containing sodium citrate and citric acid (*see both*).

BICALUTAMIDE (Rx) • **Casodex.** A nonsteroidal antiandrogen with no other known endocrine activity. It is used in combination therapy with a lutenizing hormone-releasing hormone (LHRH) for the treatment of advanced prostate cancer. Among the potential adverse reactions include enlargement and pain in the breast, general body pain, flu-like symptoms, headache, anemia, urinary problems, impotence, dizziness, insomnia, and shortness of breath. It has to be used with caution in patients with liver problems. Should not be stopped suddenly and should be taken at the same time as LHRH. Can be taken with or without food.

BICNU • *See* Carmustine.

BICOZENE (OTC) • *See* Benzocaine.

BI-K • *See* Potassium.

BILBERRY (H) • *Vaccinium myrtillus.* **Blueberry.** Grown in the Alps and Scandinavia. Folk-medicine practitioners use this fruit to improve night vision. A number of modern studies have shown that bilberry anthocyanins (the blue-coloring chemicals) given orally improve vision in healthy people and also help treat those with eye diseases. The anthocyanins contained in bilberry act to prevent blood-vessel fragility and inhibit blood-clot formation. It has been reported that bilberry increases prostaglandin (*see*) release from arterial tissue, which dilates blood vessels. Bilberry also contains arbutin (*see*), a diuretic and anti-infective derived from the dried leaves.

BILE • A yellowish fluid continuously produced by the liver. An enzyme, it is stored and concentrated in the gallbladder and released as needed to process fats and to alkalinize the intestine. The bile duct connects the gallbladder and the duodenum, the first part of the small intestine. Bile acids and salts were banned as an ingredient in laxatives by the FDA, May 1992.

BILE SALTS • The salts of bile acids. They are powerful cleansing agents and aid in the absorption of fats from the intestines. *See* Bile.

BILIARY • Relating to bile (*see*).

BILIRUBIN • The principal pigment of bile (*see*).

BILTRICIDE • *See* Praziquantel.

BIOAVAILABILITY • The measurable properties of a drug that determine how rapidly, how much, and how long the drug's active ingredient is absorbed into the bloodstream and affecting the body.

BIOCA (OTC) • *See* Calcium Carbonate.

BIOCHEMICAL • A substance that is produced by a chemical reaction in a living organism. Some can also be made in the laboratory.

BIOCHEMIC CELL SALTS • *See* Tissue Salts.

BIOEQUIVALENCE • The ability of a drug product to produce its intended therapeutic effect; related to its bioavailability (*see*).

BIOFLAVONOIDS (OTC) (H) • **Vitamin P.** A group of water-soluble, brightly colored substances that are often found with vitamin C in fruits and vegetables. They contain citrin, hesperidin, rutin, flavones, and flavonols. Bioflavonoids are essential for the utilization of vitamin C. The bioflavonoids reportedly have an antihistamine action and reduce the fragility of blood vessels. There is no recommended daily allowance (RDA) (*see*) for bioflavonoids.

BIOFORCE BLADDER IRRITATION FORMULA (H) • A homeopathic medicine (*see*) for the relief of "simple" bladder irritation with mildly painful, insufficient urination. It contains solidago (*see* Goldenrod), pareira brava 2x, hellebore niger 3x, chimaphila umbellata 2x (*see* Pipsissewa Leaves Extract), lespedeza 3x (*see*), viola tricolor 3x (*see* Pansy, Wild), lamium album 1x (*see* Lamium), and berberis vulgaris 3x (*see* Berberis). Also contains about 66 percent alcohol. Bioforce has mild diuretic (*see*) action. Adults are supposed to take twenty drops on the tongue, three to five times daily, fifteen to thirty minutes before eating. In acute cases, hourly, gradually reducing frequency as improvement occurs. Or as directed by a physician. Children are supposed to be given half the dose. Carries a warning that if symptoms persist more than three to five days, or new ones occur, consult a physician. Also says to consult a physician before using the product if you are pregnant or nursing a child.

BIO-GAN • *See* Trimethobenzamide.

BIOGLAN • *See* Vitamin B$_{12}$.

BIOMAG + GINKGO (H) • A homeopathic formula for the relief of mental fatigue "and minor stress associated with activities that challenge mental acuity and memory." Contains magnesii chloridum 1x, magnesii phosphas 1x, and ginkgo biloba 1x. *See* Magnesium Chloride, Magnesium Phosphate, and Ginkgo.

BIOPLASMA (H) • A homeopathic remedy. *See* Tissue Salts.

BIOPSY • A procedure in which a piece of tissue or amount of fluid is taken from a person's body and examined with a microscope to determine whether or not the cells are normal.

BIOTECHNOLOGY • The collection of industrial processes that involve the use of biological systems. Some of these processes use genetically engineered organisms.

BIOTEL/UTI • A urinary-tract-infection test kit for home use.

BIOTIN (OTC) (H) • **Bio-Tn. Coenzyme R. Vitamin Bw. Vitamin H.** One of the vitamin B complex, it helps to metabolize protein, fat, and carbohydrate. The recommended daily allowance (RDA) (*see*) is 0.3 mg. The lack of biotin is rare.

However, if it occurs, it may lead to skin rash, loss of hair, high blood levels of cholesterol, and heart problems.

BIOTIS-D • *See* Neomycin, Polymyxin B, and Hydrocortisone.

BIO-TRIPLEX • *See* Neomycin, Polymyxin B, and Hydrocortisone.

BIOZYME C • *See* Collagenase.

BIPERIDEN (Rx) • **Akineton.** An anticholinergic drug (*see*) used in treatment of Parkinson's disease. Potential adverse reactions include disorientation, euphoria, restlessness, irritability, incoherence, dizziness, increased tremor, low blood pressure, blurred vision, constipation, dry mouth, nausea, vomiting, and difficulty in urinating. Phenothiazines and tricyclic antidepressants may increase its central nervous system effects. Should be used with caution in those with prostate problems, irregular heartbeat, glaucoma, or epilepsy. Tolerance may develop.

BIPOLAR DISORDER • **Manic Depression.** A major affective or mood disorder in which there are episodes of both mania and severe, disabling depression. Psychiatric researchers believe it is caused by a chemical imbalance in the brain.

BIRCH (H) • **Betulaceae. Sweet Oil. Tar Oil.** Derived from the bark and wood of trees common in the Northern Hemisphere, birch products have a long history of use in folk medicine. The medicinal properties of the plant tend to vary, depending upon which part of the tree is used. Birch extract has been used as a laxative, as an aid for gout, to treat rheumatism and fluid retention, and to dissolve kidney stones. It is supposedly good for bathing skin eruptions. Researchers at the University of Illinois reported in 1995 that a substance derived from birch bark shrank some human melanoma (*see*) tumors, but National Cancer Institute researchers said that while the Illinois data looked good, betulinic acid from the birch had not worked so far with strains of melanoma used at the Cancer Institute. Melanomas, the NCI researchers said, appear in many varieties and may vary in their response to treatment. *See* Birch, Silver.

BIRCH, SILVER (H) • *Betula pendula.* The young leaves and bark contain tannins, saponins, bitter principles, glycosides, essential oils, and flavonoids (*see all*). It is used by herbalists as a diuretic, antiseptic, and tonic and has also been used to treat gout and arthritic pain. *See* Birch.

BISACODYL (OTC) • **Bisac-Evac. Bisco-Lax. Carter's Little Pills. Dacodyl. Deficol. Dulcolax. Fleet Bisacodyl. Theralax.** Used in combination: **Clysodrast.** A strong laxative widely used to treat constipation, it stimulates muscle contractions and softens stools. Taken at nighttime with food, the effects will not be felt until morning. Tablets are enteric (*see*) coated to avoid stomach irritation. Rectal suppositories are faster acting. Regular long-term use of this laxative can lead to severe, prolonged diarrhea and disrupt the balance of potassium in the body. Potential adverse reactions include stomach and bowel irritation, nausea, vomiting, abdominal cramps, protein loss, and fluid imbalance. Other side effects include belching, and diarrhea. Contraindicated in persons with abdominal pain, nausea, vomiting, or other symptoms of appendicitis, or with rectal fissures or ulcerated hemorrhoids. Taken with dairy products, vegetables (except corn and lentils), almonds, chestnuts, coconuts, citrus fruits (except cranberries), plums, or prunes, it may cause abdominal cramping, nausea, and vomiting.

BISCO-LAX • *See* Bisacodyl.

BISHOP'S-WEED (H) • The fruit of *Ammi majus,* native to the Mediterranean regions, contains, among other ingredients, psoralen, flavonoids, and tannins (*see all*). It is used by herbalists to treat psoriasis and vitiligo. Potential adverse effects include general weakness, headache, nausea, and vomiting. Excessive doses can cause liver irritation and damage, inflammation of the pancreas, and mucosal irritation of the stomach. It can also cause photosensitivity.

BISHYDROXYCOUMARIN • *See* Dicumarol.

BISMUTH (OTC) • **Balmex Ointment. Devrom. Pepto-Bismol.** A metal whose salts are used to treat inflammatory diseases of the stomach and bowel. Has a mild water-binding capacity and may also absorb toxins and provide protective coating for mucosa. Potential adverse reactions include temporary darkening of the tongue and stools, dizziness, headache, anxiety, confusion, loss of hearing, constipation, stomach pain, trembling, and nausea. May cause salicylism (*see*) in high doses. There is an increased risk of adverse effects of oral blood thinners and drugs for diabetes following high doses of bismuth. Bismuth subsalicylate (Maximum Strength Pepto-Bismol) contains a large amount of salicylate and should be used cautiously in patients taking aspirin. Both the liquid and tablet forms of Pepto-Bismol are effective against traveler's diarrhea. In an ointment, it is used to soothe the skin. Those allergic to drugs such as fenoprofen, ibuprofen, indomethacin, tolmetin, or zomepirac, as well as many salicylates such as oil of wintergreen, may also be allergic to bismuth subsalicylate. In 1992, the FDA issued a notice that bismuth subcarbonate and bismuth subgallate had not been shown to be safe and effective as claimed in OTC digestive-aid products. Also in 1992, the FDA proposed a ban on bismuth subnitrate in fever-blister and cold-sore treatment products, and poison ivy, poison oak, and poison sumac OTC products because it had not been shown to be safe and effective as claimed.

BISOPROLOL FUMARATE-HYDROCHLOROTHIAZIDE (Rx) • **Ziac.** Indicated for the treatment of high blood pressure, it combines two antihypertensive agents in a once-daily dosage—a beta-blocker and an ace inhibitor, plus a diuretic. The low-dose composition reportedly lowers side effects. The drug is contraindicated in heart failure, heart block, urinary problems, and hypersensitivity to any of the components. The most common side effects are dizziness and fatigue. It has a low incidence of cough, fluid retention, and headache.

BISPECIFIC ANTIBODY • Two pieces of an antibody (*see*) linked together. One piece binds to a cancer cell and the other binds to a white blood cell that will attack the cancer cell. As of this writing, Medarex, Inc., of Princeton, New Jersey, has several bispecific antibody drugs being tested in patients, one for ovarian cancer, two for leukemia, and one for life-threatening autoimmune conditions.

BISSY NUT • *See* Kola Nut.

BISTORT (H) • *Polygonum bistorta. Polygonum bistortoides.* **Adderswort. Dragon Wort. Passion's Dock. Snakeweed. Twice-Twisted.** A common perennial weed native to Europe and the United States. The name means twice-twisted, referring to its underground stem. Containing up to 20 percent tannins, bistort has been used in the treatment of cholera, dysentery, measles, diarrhea, jaundice, and gonorrhea. It is also used for gargles, as a mouthwash for sore gums, and for clearing pimples and soothing stings. The powdered root is said to stop the bleeding of small wounds, and a bistort poultice is used for sores and hemorrhages. It was said to heal internal ulcers and was used as a cure for toothaches and to stop mucous discharges. Can be irritating and toxic.

BISTROPAMIDE • *See* Tropicamide.

BITOLTEROL (Rx) • **Tornalate.** An aerosol bronchodilator introduced in 1985 to prevent and treat bronchial asthma and bronchospasm. Potential adverse reactions include tremors, nervousness, headache, dizziness, light-headedness, palpitations, chest discomfort, rapid heartbeat, throat irritation, cough, nausea, shortness of breath, and allergic reaction. Should be used cautiously in those with insufficient blood supply to the heart, high blood pressure, overactive thyroid, diabetes, irregular heartbeat, and seizures. Beneficial effects last up to eight hours. The medication should not be overused. Side effects may be increased if bitolterol is taken with MAO inhibitors (*see*), antidepressants, thyroid drugs, antihistamines, and other bronchodilators. Bitolterol may make blood-pressure-lowering drugs less effective.

BITTER BARK • *See* Quinine.

BITTER MELON (H) • *Momordica charantia.* A species of Old World tropical herbal vine with a warty fruit. The seeds contain momordica anti-HIV protein. In 1991 researchers at New York University reported this protein effective against the AIDS virus. It is reportedly nontoxic to normal cells and may eventually be used in condoms, vaginal jellies, and toothpastes to minimize the risk of HIV transmission.

BITTER PRINCIPLES (H) • A group of bitter-tasting chemicals in plants. They differ chemically, but most belong to the iris or pine families. Bitter principles reputedly stimulate the liver and the secretion of digestive juices. They are being scientifically investigated today as antifungals, antibiotics, and anticancer agents. The bitter principle in mallow plants is being investigated as a male contraceptive. Other bitter principles in herbs are used as sedatives and to combat coughs.

BITTERSWEET • *See* Dulcamara.

BLACKBERRY (H) • *Rubus fruiticosus.* The berries, leaves, and root bark are used to treat fevers, colds, sore throats, vaginal discharge, diarrhea, and dysentery. The berries contain isocitric and malic acids, sugars, pectin, monoglycoside of cyanidin, and vitamins C and A. The leaves and bark are said to lower fever, act as astringents, and stop bleeding.

BLACK BRYONY (H) • **Blackeye Root.** A perennial herb, *Tamus communis,* native to Europe and North America, it contains steroidal saponins, histaminelike substances, alkaloids, mucilage, and calcium oxalate. It is used by herbalists as a diuretic and rubefacient. It was once popular as an asthma remedy. It is now used externally in plaster to relieve arthritis. The plant is toxic when ingested in large doses.

BLACK CATECHU • *See* Acacia.

BLACK COHOSH (H) • *Cimicifuga racemosa.* **Black Snakeroot. Bugbane. Cimicifuga.**

Rattleroot. The root contains various glycosides (*see*) including estrogenic substances and tannins. Herbalists have used it to relieve nerve pains, menstrual pains, and the pain of childbirth. Also used to speed delivery, and to reduce blood pressure. Black cohosh is also believed to have sedative properties. In 1992, the FDA proposed a ban on black cohosh in oral menstrual drug products because it had not been shown to be safe and effective as claimed.

BLACK DRAUGHT (OTC) • *See* Senna.

BLACK EXTRACT (H) • *See* Viburnum Extract.

BLACK HAW (H) • *Viburnum prunifolium.* **American Sloe. Stag Bush.** The stem and root bark contain coumarins (*see*), arbutin, salicin, and tannin (*see*). It was used by herbalists to treat spasms of the uterus and all forms of menstrual disorders.

BLACK HELLEBORE • *See* Lungwort.

BLACK MUSTARD • *See* Mustard, Black.

BLACK NIGHTSHADE • *See* Nightshade, Black.

BLACK RADISH POWDER (OTC) • In 1992, the FDA issued a notice that black radish powder had not been shown to be safe and effective as claimed in OTC digestive-aid products.

BLACK ROOT • *See* Culver's Root.

BLACK SNAKEROOT • *See* Black Cohosh.

BLACK TEA • *See* Tea.

BLACK WIDOW SPIDER ANTIVENIN (EQUINE) (Rx) • **Antivenin.** An injection that neutralizes and binds venom. Potential adverse side effects include severe allergic reactions and nerve damage.

BLADDER WRACK (H) • *Fucus vesiculosus.* **Bladder Fucus. Black-Tang. Cut-Weed. Kelpware. Sea-Oak. Sea Wrack.** An abundant seaweed, found in the Atlantic and Pacific Oceans, with little bladders on its fronds that contain a gel. Herbalists claim the gel strengthens weak limbs and relieves arthritis, sprains, and strains. They use it as a diuretic and as an aid in losing weight.

BLASTOMYCOSIS • A rare, noncontagious condition caused by a fungus found in wood and soil. The infection originates in the respiratory tract and usually disseminates to the lungs, skin, and bone.

BLENOXANE • *See* Bleomycin.

BLEOMYCIN (Rx) • **Blenoxane.** An antibiotic, anticancer drug used to treat cervical, throat, head, neck, and testicular cancers, and Hodgkin's disease. Potential adverse reactions include nausea, vomiting, prolonged loss of appetite, sensitivity of the scalp and fingers, headache, sore mouth, diarrhea, redness of the skin, blisters, discoloration and hardness of the skin on the palms and the soles of the feet, dark spots on the skin, acne, reversible hair loss, joint swelling, lung disorders, severe allergic reactions, fever up to 106° F, and shortness of breath.

BLEPH • *See* Sulfacetamide.

BLEPHAMIDE, BLEPHAMIDE S.O.P. (Rx) • *See* Prednisolone, Sulfacetamide, and Benzalkonium Chloride.

BLEPHAR-, BLEPHARO- • Prefixes meaning eyelid, as in *blepharospasm,* twitching of the eyelid.

BLEPHAROSPASM • Involuntary, prolonged contraction of an eyelid muscle that causes almost complete eye closure.

BLESSED THISTLE (H) • *Cnicus benedictus.* **Holy Thistle.** The thistle contains tannin (*see*), lactone, mucilage (*see*), and essential oil. Used by herbalists to treat stomach and liver complaints. It increases appetite, lowers fevers, and reputedly breaks up blood clots, relieves jaundice and hepatitis, and stops bleeding. In 1992, the FDA issued a notice that blessed thistle had not been shown to be safe and effective as claimed in OTC digestive-aid products or oral menstrual drugs.

BLINX • *See* Boric Acid.

BLOCADREN • *See* Timolol Maleate.

BLOOD-BRAIN BARRIER • The protective barrier that prevents the passage of various substances from the bloodstream to the brain.

BLOOD CELLS • Cells are produced in bone marrow and consist of:
   • Red blood cells, which bring oxygen to tissues and take carbon dioxide from them.
   • White blood cells, which fight invading germs, infections, and allergy-causing agents.
   • Platelets, which are responsible for clotting.

BLOOD COUNTS • The number values assigned to the major types of blood cells. Blood counts indicate the amount of blood cells circulating in the bloodstream.

BLOODROOT (H) • *Sanguinaria canadensis.* **Red Indian Paint. Redroot. Tetterwort.** The root contains isoquinoline alkaloids including sanguinarine and berberine (*see*). Herbalists use it to treat coughs, sore throats, skin eruptions, skin cancer, athlete's foot, and gum disease. The root is emetic and purgative in large doses. In smaller doses it is a stimulant, diaphoretic, and expectorant. Sanguinaria can cause glaucoma if taken over a long time.

BLOOD THINNERS • Any medicines, including aspirin and coumarin (*see both*), that make the blood more fluid and prevent clotting.

BLUBORO (OTC) • An astringent solution containing aluminum sulfate and calcium acetate (*see both*).

BLUEBERRY • *See* Bilberry.

BLUE COHOSH (H) • *Caulophyllum thalictroides.* **Papooseroot. Squawroot.** The rhizome contains fungicidal saponin, glycosides (*see*), gum, starch, salts, phosphoric acid, and a soluble resin. Herbalists use it for menstrual irregularities and pain, and to ease the pain of childbirth. It is also used to treat worms. It is toxic when ingested in large amounts and should be avoided during pregnancy and by individuals with high blood pressure.

BLUE FLAG (H) • *Iris versicolor.* **Flag Lily. Fleur-de-lis. Liver Lily. Poison Flag. Wild Iris.** The rhizome contains salicylic (*see*) and isophthalic acids, volatile oil, iridin, a glycoside (*see*), gum, resin, and sterols. Herbalists use it as a cathartic and emetic, and to treat liver complaints, swollen glands, hepatitis, jaundice, skin diseases, and loss of appetite. Promoted in herbal medicines as both relaxing and stimulating.

BNP • Abbreviation for brain natriuretic peptide (*see*).

BOGBEAN • *See* Buckbean.

BOLDO (H) • An evergreen shrub native to Chile and cultivated in North Africa and Italy, it contains alkaloids, flavonoids, and volatile oil. It has mainly been used in the treatment of liver and gallbladder diseases. It stimulates both the secretion of bile and contractions of the gallbladder. It has also been used for abdominal pain and gas. It is generally considered harmless in small doses, but it is contraindicated in acute inflammation of the gastrointestinal tract, internal hemorrhages, pregnancy, and heart disease.

BOLUS • A ball of chewed food as it passes from the mouth through the gastrointestinal tract.

BONE MARROW • The soft, spongy center of the bone that acts like a factory to produce white blood cells, the primary agents of the body's immune system.

BONE MARROW DEPRESSION • A serious reduction in the ability of the bone marrow to carry on its normal production of white blood cells. This can occur as a result of certain drugs and chemicals, as well as disease. Impairment of blood cell production can lead to a drop in immunity, lack of energy, intolerance to cold, and a host of other physical symptoms. *See* Bone Marrow.

BONE MASS • Total amount of bone tissue contained in bones.

BONESET (H) • *Eupatorium perfoliatum.* **Feverwort. Thoroughwort. Hyland's C-Plus Cold Tablets.** Native Americans introduced the settlers to this herb. Its name reflects its use for a severe strain of flu called breakbone fever (dengue fever). The herb contains flavonoids, quercetin, vitamin C, volatile oil, and sterol. Herbalists use it today to treat fevers, colds, flu, and liver complaints. It reportedly loosens phlegm, clears nasal passages, relieves constipation, and reduces fever.

BONINE • *See* Meclizine.

BONTRIL • *See* Phendimetrazine.

BOR • Homeopathic abbreviation for borax veneta (*see*).

BORAGE (H) • *Borago officinalis.* **Herb of Gladness.** A beautiful European plant with blue flowers, it was often cultivated in fifteenth-century gardens. The folk saying "borage for courage" has a basis in fact. The chemicals in the herb act upon the adrenal gland, which releases hormones needed to fight or flee during threat. Borage also contains potassium and calcium. The oil is one of three major sources of gamma-linolenic acid—a prostaglandin/eicosanoid precursor. The prostaglandins made from GLA contribute to widening blood vessels and keeping blood platelets from sticking together. They also inhibit cholesterol production and improve circulation. Borage is also used medicinally for its emollient properties, and for bronchial, lung, and chest disorders. Borage tea is used in a lotion for sore eyes, and by herbalists to reduce fevers. Borage is also used in a gargle for sore throats and ul-

cerated mouths, and as a nerve tonic. May cause liver damage.

BORAX VENETA (H) • **Bor. Natrum Biboracicum. Sodium Biborate. Sodium Borate. Sodium Tetraborate.** Hard, odorless crystals that absorb water from the air. Homeopathic preparations are made by fusing boracic acid and sodium carbonate and dissolving out the borax with warm water. The borax is then diluted. It is used for breast-feeding problems, diarrhea, thrush, and travel sickness. Sodium borate is toxic and as little as five to ten grams have caused severe vomiting, diarrhea, shock, and death in young children.

BORIC ACID (OTC) • **Aurocaine 2. Auro-Dri. Blinx. Borofax Ointment. Collyrium. Collyrium for Fresh Eyes. Dri-Ear. Ear-Dry. Neo-Flo. Star Optic Ear Solution. Swim Ear.** An antiseptic with bactericidal and fungicidal properties, now rarely used in skin and eye antiseptics because of risk of excessive absorption through the skin. It is used to irrigate the eye after removal of a foreign body or examinations with instruments, and to inhibit bacteria present in the ear canal in treating external ear-canal infection. It also is used for temporary relief of chapped, chafed, or dry skin, diaper rash, abrasions, minor burns, sunburn, insect bites, and other skin irritations. Severe poisonings have followed both ingestion and topical application to abraded skin. Contraindicated in perforated eardrum or broken skin. In 1992, the FDA issued a notice that boric acid had not been shown to be safe and effective as claimed in OTC products, including astringent (*see*) drug products, fever-blister and cold-sore treatments, and poison ivy, poison oak, and poison sumac drug products.

BOROFAX OINTMENT (OTC) • *See* Boric Acid.

BORON (OTC) • An element occurring in the earth's crust in compounds, never in its pure form. It is used in dietary supplements of up to 1 mg per day. Salts of boron are widely used as antiseptics even though toxicologists warn about possible adverse reactions. Borates are absorbed by the mucous membranes and can cause symptoms such as gastrointestinal bleeding, skin rash, and central nervous system stimulation. The adult lethal dose is one ounce. There is a preparation, promoted by one organization as "anti-aging," containing 2 mg of boron in a vitamin and mineral supplement that is claimed to increase the production of testosterone.

BOTULINUM TOXIN TYPE A (Rx) • Oculinum. A substance released by the organism that causes botulism, or severe food poisoning. Used to treat spasms of the eye and face, it has a paralytic effect. The peak of paralysis occurs five to seven days after injection. The patient recovers from the effects of the toxin in six to nine months. After recovery, the injected muscle may or may not resume the preinjection level of function. Ophthalmologists began experimenting with the toxin in the early 1970s when they realized botulism or systemic food poisoning paralyzes eye muscles. The clinical use of botulinum A toxin began in 1977 as an alternative to surgery for strabismus, or crossed eyes. The FDA approved the toxin for strabismus and blepharospasm (eyelid twitching) in 1989. It is now being used by doctors at Cornell Medical Center to treat writer's cramp (spasms of the hands and fingers) and spasmodic torticollis (neck and shoulder muscle spasms). It is also being tested at Stanford University to remove wrinkles.

BOTULISM ANTITOXIN, BIVALENT EQUINE (Rx) • A serum that neutralizes and binds toxin. Potential adverse reactions include severe allergic reactions and serum sickness, which may occur five to fourteen days afterward.

BOXWOOD (H) • Dogwood. Green Ozier. A small tree, *Buxus semperiverens,* found in all parts of the United States. The bark possesses astringent, stimulant, and tonic properties. The bark was used in the treatment of malaria. It is also used as a laxative, to induce sweating, to counteract fever, and to lower blood pressure. In excessive doses it may cause nausea, diarrhea, dizziness, convulsions, collapse, respiratory failure, and death.

BRACKEN (H) • Bracken Fern. An erect, treelike fern, *Pteridium aquilinum,* it contains glycosides and tannins (*see both*). It is used by herbalists to treat diarrhea and intestinal ailments. It is also used topically for wounds and ulcers. Bracken was formerly considered safe, but recent investigations have shown that bracken induces tumors of the stomach and intestinal tract when fed to experimental animals.

BRADY- • Prefix meaning slow, such as in *bradycardia,* slow heartbeat.

BRADYCARDIA • Slowing of the heartbeat to less than fifty beats per minute.

BRADYKINESIA • Slowness in movement.

BRADYPHRENIA • Sluggish mentality.

BRAHMI (H) • *Hydrocotyle asiatica.* An herb used in India to relieve anxiety, and to treat epilepsy and leprosy. Named for the ancient Indian Brahmi script.

BRAIN NATRIURETIC PEPTIDE • BNP. Natrecor. A naturally occurring hormone, it is predominantly produced in the ventricles of the heart. Studies show that BNP production in the heart increases dramatically in patients with congestive heart failure, indicating that it may be a natural corrective response to a failing heart. Research to date suggests that BNP has many biological effects including dilating blood vessels to improve cardiac function, getting rid of salt and water from the body, and decreasing the output of certain hormones that lead to blood-vessel constriction and elevated blood pressure. A genetically engineered product is being tested in patients at ten centers in the United States.

BRASIVOL • *See* Aluminum Oxide.

BRASSICA NIGRA • *See* Mustard, Black.

BREATHEASY • *See* Epinephrine.

BREOKINASE • *See* Urokinase.

BREONESIN • *See* Guaifenesin.

BRETHAIRE • *See* Terbutaline Sulfate.

BRETHINE • *See* Terbutaline Sulfate.

BRETYLIUM (Rx) • **Bretylol.** An antiarrhythmic drug used in immediately life-threatening, irregular-heartbeat problems. Potential adverse reactions include dizziness, fainting, nausea, vomiting, severe low blood pressure, irregular heart rhythm, and chest pain. Interacts with all high blood pressure drugs and may lower blood pressure too much.

BRETYLOL • *See* Bretylium.

BREVIBLOC • *See* Esmolol Hydrochloride.

BREVICON (Rx) • An oral contraceptive. *See* Ethinyl Estradiol, Norethindrone, and Oral Contraceptives.

BREVITAL SODIUM • *See* Methohexital Sodium.

BREXIN (OTC) • *See* Carbinoxamine and Pseudoephedrine, Guaifenesin, and Pseudoephedrine.

BRICANYL • *See* Terbutaline Sulfate.

BRIETAL SODIUM • *See* Methohexital Sodium.

BROMALINE (OTC) • *See* Brompheniramine and Phenylpropanolamine.

BROMAREST (OTC) • *See* Brompheniramine.

BROMASE (Rx) (OTC) • **Bromelain. Proteolytic Enzyme.** A prostaglandin (*see*) modulator, it is a supplement for inflammatory conditions resulting from prostaglandin metabolism, surgical procedures, sports activities, and other trauma. In 1992, the FDA issued a notice that stem bromelain had not been shown to be safe and effective as claimed in OTC digestive-aid products. It can react with papain, wheat, grass rye, and flour. It should not be used by persons with bleeding tendencies.

BROMATAPP • *See* Brompheniramine.

BROMBAY (OTC) • *See* Brompheniramine.

BROMELAIN • *See* Bromase.

BROMELIN (H) • A protein-digesting, milk-clotting enzyme found in pineapple. Orally administered in the treatment of inflammation and swelling of soft tissues associated with traumatic injury.

BROMFED • A combination of brompheniramine and pseudoephedrine (*see both*).

BROMFED-PD • *See* Brompheniramine and Pseudoephedrine.

BROMHIDROSIS • Foul-smelling perspiration.

BROMIDES, POTASSIUM and SODIUM (Rx) (OTC) • A group of sedative drugs now used only rarely. Potassium bromide has been used medically as a sedative and anticonvulsant. Sodium bromide has been used as a sedative and a sleep inducer. The bromides can cause skin rashes. Large doses can cause central nervous system depression, and prolonged intake may cause mental deterioration. The use of sodium or potassium bromide in OTC sleep aids was determined to be ineffective in 1991 by the FDA, and manufacturers had to reformulate their products or they were banned.

BROMINE • A dark, reddish brown liquid derived from seawater and natural brines by oxidation of bromine salts. Toxic by ingestion and inhalation. Bromine reacts with many metals to form bromides (*see*).

BROMOCRIPTINE (Rx) • **Parlodel.** Introduced in the 1970s, Parlodel inhibits the secretion of the hormone prolactin from the pituitary gland. Oversecretion of prolactin is involved in some types of infertility, impotence, premenstrual breast discomfort, and benign pituitary tumors that cause abnormal bone growth. Bromocriptine was sometimes used to suppress breast milk in women who did not wish to breast-feed their babies. The FDA withdrew approval of bromocriptine to prevent lactation, based on a reevaluation finding that the drug has not been shown to be safe for this use. The company had already withdrawn this indication. The drug is still approved to treat Parkinson's disease, acromegaly, and various hyperprolactinemia-associated dysfunctions. Potential adverse reactions include nausea, vomiting, confusion, dizziness, headache, constipation, a drop in blood pressure upon rising from a seated or prone position, abnormal body movements, hallucinations, and collapse. Breast engorgement and secretion may occur. Antipsychotic drugs make bromocriptine less effective and may cause increased abnormal movements. Oral contraceptives, estrogen, and progestins interfere with the effects of bromocriptine. Levodopa has an additive effect. MAO inhibitors and reserpine (*see both*) may interfere with bromocriptine's benefits. Contraindicated in those who are hypersensitive to ergot derivatives. Should be taken with meals.

BROMODIPHENHYDRAMINE (Rx) • Ambenyl Cough Syrup. Bromo-Benadry. Histabromamine. An antihistamine derived from isopropanol (*see*) and indicated for temporary relief of upper-respiratory symptoms and coughs associated with allergies or the common cold. Has an atropinelike action. May have an additive effect with alcohol.

BROMO-SELTZER • *See* Acetaminophen.

BROMPHEN • *See* Brompheniramine.

BROMPHENIRAMINE (OTC) • Bromphen. Codimal-A. Diamine T.C. Dimetane. Veltane. Combinations: **Dimetane-DC Cough. Dimetapp. Drixoral. Histaject. Nasahist B. ND-Stat. Sinusol-B.** An antihistamine introduced in 1957 as an Rx drug, it was changed to OTC in 1976. Brompheniramine is used for treating allergies such as hay fever, allergic conjunctivitis, hives, and stuffy nose. It is sometimes used to prevent or treat allergic reactions to blood transfusions or X-ray contrast material, and to supplement epinephrine injections in people with acute allergic shock. Potential adverse reactions include drowsiness, blurred vision, dizziness, incoordination, digestive upsets, urinary difficulties, dry mouth, and overstimulation in children. Contraindicated in acute asthmatic attacks. Should be used cautiously in elderly patients, breast-feeding women, and in those with increased eye pressure, overactive thyroid, cardiovascular disease, high blood pressure, kidney disease, bronchial asthma, urine retention, enlarged prostate, bladder-neck obstruction, or peptic ulcers. Brompheniramine will increase the intoxication effect of alcohol. Sedatives may increase the sedative effect of brompheniramine. Anticholinergic drugs are likely to increase the anticholinergic effects of brompheniramine. Monoamine oxidase inhibitors (MAOIs) (*see*) can cause a dangerous rise in blood pressure if taken with brompheniramine. Coffee or tea may reduce drowsiness. Brompheniramine medication should be discontinued four days before taking a skin allergy test, because presence of the drug can lead to inaccurate results.

BRONCHI • The subdivisions of the trachea (*see*), which convey air to and from the lungs. The trachea divides into right and left main bronchi, which, in turn, form lobar, segmental, and subsegmental bronchi.

BRONCHIECTASIS • Dilation of bronchial tubes, usually a result of infection or obstruction by foreign substances.

BRONCHITIS • Inflammation of the linings of the bronchial tubes in the lungs. It leads to excessive mucus and consequent constriction of airways. Can be acute or chronic.

BRONCHITIS FORMULA (H) • Centraria Complex. A homeopathic formula to treat bronchial congestion containing ipecacuanha 4x, sanguisorba 2x, and cetraria islandica 1x. *See* Ipecac, Sanguinaria, and Iceland Moss.

BRONCHO- • Prefix meaning pertaining to the windpipe, as in *bronchial tubes.*

BRONCHOCONSTRICTOR • A substance that causes the airways in the lungs to narrow or constrict. An attack of asthma may be caused by the release of bronchoconstrictor substances such as histamine.

BRONCHODILATOR • Medication that relaxes the smooth muscles lining the airways leading to the lungs, and helps to expand the airways, facilitate normal breathing, and eliminate bronchial spasms. Examples are ephedrine, isoproterenol, and aminophylline (*see all*).

BRONCHOSPASM • Contraction of smooth muscles in the walls of the bronchi and bronchioles causing narrowing of the insides.

BRONDECON (OTC) • *See* Oxtriphylline and Guaifenesin.

BRONITIN • *See* Epinephrine.

BRONKAID TABLETS (OTC) • *See* Ephedrine.

BRONKAID MIST (OTC) • *See* Epinephrine.

BRONKODYL S-R • *See* Theophylline.

BRONKOLIXIR (Rx) • *See* Ephedrine, Phenobarbital, and Theophylline.

BRONKOMETER • *See* Isoetharine.

BRONKOSOL • *See* Isoetharine.

BRONKOTABS (Rx) • *See* Ephedrine, Phenobarbital, Theophylline, and Guaifenesin.

BROOKLIME (H) • *Veronica beccabunga* and *Veronica americana.* **Watercress. Water**

Pimpernel. An herb that grows abundantly in shallow streams, it is believed to have healing properties. It is used to treat boils, ulcers, abscesses, and pimples and is also said to purge the blood of toxins.

BROOM (H) • *Cytisus scoparius. Sarothamnus scoparius.* **Scoparius. Scotch Broom. Spartium. Witch's Broom.** A shrub, it has long been used by herbalists as a diuretic and cathartic. Emetic in large doses. Because of its action on the kidneys, it is contraindicated in acute kidney disease.

BROTANE (OTC) • *See* Brompheniramine.

BRUCELLOSIS • **Malta Fever. Undulant Fever.** An infectious disease transmitted from animals to man, most commonly by contact with cattle or consumption of raw milk products. Symptoms include shifts of body temperature, weakness, fatigability, and excessive sweating.

BRYONIA (H) • **Bryony.** The dried root of *Bryonia alba* or *Bryonia dioica,* native to Europe. It contains glycosides (*see*), stigmasterol, volatile oil, and resin (*see*). It is used in homeopathic medicine for nasal drip, headache, stitching pains, chest pains, and dryness of mucus. It has been used as a cathartic in conventional medicine, but it is toxic.

BRYONY • *See* Bryonia.

B-S-P • *See* Betamethasone.

BSS • Abbreviation for balanced salt solution.

BUCCAL CAVITY • The cavity formed by the cheeks and mouth.

BUCHU (H) • **Hottentot Tea. Zulu Bucu.** The dried leaves of *Barosma betulina* or of *Barosma crenulata,* a citrus shrub grown in South Africa. It is widely used in that country for medicinal purposes. Herbalists use it worldwide to treat diseases of the kidney, urinary tract, and prostate. The leaves contain barosma camphor and essential oil. When given warm, it stimulates sweating. In 1992, the FDA proposed a ban on buchu powdered extract in oral menstrual drug products because it had not been shown to be safe and effective as claimed.

BUCKBEAN (H) • *Menyanthes trifoliata.* **Bog-Bean. Meyanthin. Water Shamrock.** A common plant in bogs, it is used by herbalists as a tonic, to reduce fever, and to treat skin diseases due to rheumatism. Depending on the strength and dosage, its action ranges from that of a bitter tonic and cathartic to a purgative and emetic. In folk medicine, buckbean was used to treat edema, scabies, and fever.

BUCKTHORN (H) • *Rhamnus cathartica.* **Black Adder.** The common shrub contains various glycosides (*see*) in the berries; the bark contains anthraquinone (*see*) derivatives. Herbalists use it as a milk laxative, as a diuretic, and to treat hemorrhoids, colic, and obesity. It is milder than a related compound, cascara (*see*). In 1992, the FDA issued a notice that buckthorn had not been shown to be safe and effective as claimed in OTC digestive-aid products.

BUCLIZINE (Rx) • Vibazine. Acts on the central nervous system to suppress nausea and vomiting. Should not be taken by pregnant women since it causes abnormalities in animal testing. Safety and efficacy for use in children have not been established. This product contains tartrazine, which may cause an allergic-type reaction in those allergic to aspirin. Can be taken without water. Potential adverse reactions include drowsiness, dry mouth, headache, and jitteriness.

BUDESONIDE (Rx) • Rhinocort Nasal Inhaler. A once-daily medication approved in 1994 for the treatment of seasonal and perennial allergic rhinitis in adults and children (ages six and older). It is also approved for nonallergic perennial rhinitis in adults. It has been used in Scandinavia since 1982 and is on the market in thirty-eight other countries. It was reviewed by the FDA for 13.5 months before approval.

BUFF-A COMP (Rx) • A combination of aspirin, butalbital, and caffeine (*see all*), used to treat headache pain.

BUFFERED • Describing a special formulation of a product that minimizes chemical irritation in the stomach.

BUFFERIN (OTC) • *See* Aspirin.

BUFF-OXAL • Used to treat skin eruptions. *See* Benzoyl Peroxide.

BUFOPTO • *See* Atropine Sulfate.

BUGBANE • *See* Black Cohosh.

BUGLE (H) • *Ajuga reptans.* **Carpenter's Herb.** A mint used by homeopaths and herbalists to treat tuberculosis, coughs, and as a mild narcotic. Internally, it has been used in the treatment of internal bleeding, diarrhea, and stomach disorder. No toxicity has been reported, but it does contain cardioactive glycoside and may exert an adverse effect on the heart.

BULIMIA • A disorder characterized by compulsive eating binges followed by some effort to counteract the weight gain that would result from these binges—usually vomiting, but often excessive exercising, fasting, or use of diet pills, laxatives, or diuretics. Overconcern with weight and body shape are also symptoms of bulimia.

BULK-FORMING LAXATIVE • A product that promotes bowel movement by increasing the stool's volume, water, and fiber content, making the stool softer and easier to eliminate. *See* Laxative.

BUMETANIDE (Rx) • Bumex. A strong, fast-acting loop diuretic (*see*) introduced in 1983, it is used to treat fluid retention resulting from heart failure or kidney or liver problems, and to treat high blood pressure. It is useful in people with kidney dysfunction who do not respond to thiazide diuretics (*see*). Bumetanide increases the loss of potassium in the urine, which can cause irregular heartbeat and other problems. Potential adverse effects include ringing in the ears, dizziness, lethargy, cramps, nausea, transient deafness, impaired sexual function, low blood potassium and chloride and other electrolyte imbalances, muscle pain and tenderness, and rash. Nonsteroidal anti-inflammatory drugs (NSAIDs) (*see*) may reduce the effectiveness of bumetanide. Aminoglycoside antibiotics increase the risk of ringing in the ears when taken with bumetanide. Bumetanide may increase the toxicity of lithium if taken together. Contraindicated in absence of urine or states of severe electrolyte depletion. Should be used with caution in patients with liver dysfunction. If you are taking this drug, you should eat foods rich in potassium including citrus fruits, tomatoes, bananas, dates, and apricots. Should be taken in the morning to avoid the need to urinate during the night. May be taken with food.

BUMEX • *See* Bumetanide.

BUPIVACAINE (Rx) • **Marcaine. Sensorcaine.** A long-lasting local anesthetic often used as a nerve block during labor. Onset is four to seventeen minutes, and duration is three to six hours. Potential adverse reactions include skin reactions, swelling, continuous asthma attacks, severe allergic reactions, anxiety, nervousness, seizures followed by drowsiness, unconsciousness, tremors, twitches, shivering, and respiratory arrest. Other potential reactions include blurred vision, ringing in the ears, nausea, and vomiting. Should be used with extreme caution if MAO inhibitors (*see*) or cyclic antidepressants are being taken by the patient.

BUPRENEX • *See* Buprenorphine Hydrochloride.

BUPRENORPHINE HYDROCHLORIDE (Rx) • **Buprenex.** A narcotic analgesic that alters through an unknown mechanism both perception of and emotional response to pain. Used to treat moderate to severe pain. Potential adverse reactions include dizziness, sedation, headache, confusion, nervousness, euphoria, low blood pressure, nausea, vomiting, constipation, itching, sweating, and respiratory depression. Alcohol and central nervous system depressants may add to the effects. Should be used cautiously in head injury and increased pressure on the brain, severe liver and kidney impairment, thyroid irregularities, and prostatic enlargement. May be addictive.

BUPROPION HYDROCHLORIDE (Rx) • **Wellbutrin.** An antidepressant introduced in 1989 that is not a tricyclic antidepressant and does not inhibit MAO inhibitors (*see*), but is a weak inhibitor of the nerve message transmitters norepinephrine, dopamine, and serotonin. Used for the treatment of depression, it was originally approved in 1985, but voluntarily withdrawn to investigate side effects prior to marketing. It is promoted as having few cardiovascular effects, few anticholinergic (*see*) effects, little or no weight gain, little or no daytime drowsiness, and minimal risk of sexual dysfunction. Potential adverse reactions include, as the principal medically important one, seizures. Others include headache, restlessness, anxiety, confusion, decreased libido, delusions, euphoria, hostility, impaired sleep quality, insomnia, sedation, tremor, irregular heartbeat, high or low blood pressure, palpitations, faintness, incoordination, increased appetite, constipation, heartburn, nausea, vomiting, dry mouth, impotence, menstrual problems, urinary frequency, arthritis, chills, fever, sweating, hearing problems, water retention, flulike symptoms, sore mouth, ringing in the ears, and blurred vision. A number of patients lose five pounds or more on the drug. Phenothiazines, phenobarbital, MAO inhibitors, or tricyclic antidepressants (*see*) may cause an increased risk of side effects, including seizures. Should be used cautiously in patients taking L-dopa (*see*). No other medications, including over-the-counter medicine, should be taken without first checking with a physician. Rapid withdrawal of benzodiazepines (*see*) may also cause increased adverse reactions. Contraindicated in patients who are allergic to the drug, patients who have taken MAO inhibitors within two weeks, nursing mothers, and patients with seizure disorders. Should not be used with patients with a history of eating disorders, head trauma, or central nervous system tumors.

BURDOCK (H) • *Arctium lappa.* **Bardane. Beggar's Buttons. Burdock Ointment. Lapp.** The roots, seeds, and leaves of this common roadside plant contain essential oil. The oil contains nearly 45 percent inulin (*see*) and many minerals. Herbalists use it for skin diseases, blood purification, urinary problems, and as a tonic. Chinese burdock is used to eliminate excess nervous energy, and the root is considered to have aphrodisiacal properties. It is sold in drugstores as an ointment to treat minor burns, cuts, or other skin traumas. Traditionally, used by Gypsies to ward off arthritis, in a pouch hung around the neck. Also used to induce sweating in an effort to rid the body of toxins. In modern experiments, burdock root extract has been shown to have antitumor effects, and to produce an increased flow of urine.

BURDOCK OINTMENT • *See* Burdock.

BURNET (H) • *Poterium sanguisorba.* **Burnet Saxifrage. Pimpernel. Pimpinella.** A relative of roses and carrots, used by herbalists to contract small blood vessels and stop bleeding. Revolutionary soldiers in New Jersey reportedly drank it before battles. The ancient Chinese also used it to stop bleeding. Burnet saxifrage has been used internally in the treatment of respiratory problems, gas, and gastric disorders. It is also used in arthritis, kidney disease, and urinary-tract ailments. It has been used for wound healing and to expel bladder stones. It can lead to abortion so should not be used during pregnancy.

BUROW'S SOLUTION • **Star-Optic Ear Solution.** *See* Aluminum Acetate.

BURSA • A sac filled with lubricating fluid, located between opposing surfaces that slide past each other, such as a tendon and a bone. Inflammation of a bursa causes painful bursitis.

BUSPAR • *See* Buspirone.

BUSPIRONE (Rx) • **BuSpar.** An antianxiety drug introduced in 1979, unrelated to Valium or other benzodiazepines. It is less sedating than other antianxiety drugs, but unlike the benzodiazepines is not effective as an anticonvulsant or muscle relaxant. It is also nonaddictive, with no evidence of causing a withdrawal syndrome. Most common potential adverse effects include dizziness, nervousness, nausea, and headache. Other reported adverse effects include drowsiness, insomnia, dry mouth, diarrhea, blurred vision, numbness, rash, and fatigue. It may cause a slow heartbeat, hair loss, changes in sex drive, fever, voice loss, and malaise. Even though it is less sedating than other antianxiety drugs, the manufacturer recommends not driving or operating heavy machinery if you are taking it. If taking buspirone, you should inform your physician about any alcohol, drugs, or medications, prescription or nonprescription, you are now taking or plan to take during treatment. The drug should not be taken with alcohol or other central nervous system depressants. MAO inhibitors (*see*) may elevate blood pressure. Buspirone may take seven days to a month to manifest optimal effects. It should be taken the same way at the same time of day. It is at its highest level in the blood forty to ninety minutes after ingestion. When using buspirone, food seems to take longer to clear from the body, so consult your physician about whether or not to take it with meals.

BUSULFAN (Rx) • **Myleran.** An alkylating agent used in the treatment of certain leukemias. Potential adverse reactions include a drop in white blood count, nausea, vomiting, diarrhea, sore mouth and tongue, wasting, high uric acid, transient discoloration of the skin, enlargement of breasts, loss of hair, and lung damage. Aspirin and anticoagulants should be used cautiously due to possible bleeding.

BUTABARBITAL SODIUM (Rx) • **Barbased. Butalan. Buticaps. Butisol. Sarisol No. 2.** A barbiturate sleeping drug that probably interferes with transmission of impulses from the thalamus to the cortex of the brain. Potential adverse reactions include drowsiness, lethargy, hangover, paradoxical excitement in elderly patients, nausea, vomiting, rash, hives, and swelling. Alcohol or other central nervous system depressants, including narcotic analgesics, may cause central nervous system and respiratory depression. MAO inhibitors (*see*) inhibit metabolism of barbiturates and may cause prolonged central nervous system depression. Aprobarbital may cause a decreased absorption of griseofulvin (*see*) and may make oral blood thinners, estrogens, oral contraceptives, doxycycline, and corticosteroids less effective. Women who use barbital may need to change to other birth control methods. Rifampin may decrease barbiturate levels. Contraindicated in uncontrolled severe pain, respiratory disease, allergy to barbiturates, history of drug abuse, or porphyria. It also must be used with caution in patients with liver or kidney disease. Elderly patients are sensitive to the drug's side effects. Long-term use may lead to dependence.

BUTALAN • *See* Butabarbital Sodium.

BUTALBITAL COMPOUNDS (Rx) • **Amaphen. Bancap. Buff-A Comp. Fioricet. Fiorinal with Codeine. Isocet. Lanorinal. Medigesic. Sedapap-10.** Used in the relief of tension or muscle-contraction headaches and other aches and pains. The active ingredients are aspirin, codeine or acetaminophen, caffeine, and the barbiturate butalbital. The most frequent adverse reactions are drowsiness and dizziness. Less frequent adverse reactions are light-headedness, nausea, vomiting, and gas. May also cause skin reactions. Barbiturates can be habit-forming.

BUTAMBEN (Rx) • **Butesin.** A local anesthetic derived from nitrobenzoic acid and butyl alcohol, it is applied to the skin to relieve the pain of minor burns. One potential adverse reaction is a rash. Should not be applied to large areas.

BUTCHER'S-BROOM (H) • *Ruscus aculeatus.* **Kneeholy. Liliaceae. Pettier. Sweet Broom.** A member of the lily family, this herb contains saponins similar to those in licorice and sarsaparilla, glycosides (*see*), ruscogenins, and neoruscogenins, which are similar to adrenocortical hormones. Herbalists use it to treat inflammation, arthritic pain, and hemorrhoidal swelling. In recent scientific experiments, it has been found to constrict arteries and have anti-inflammatory properties. This may explain why ancient Greek physicians reported curing "swelling" with this herb and why the Roman Pliny said it cured varicose veins.

BUTESIN PICRATE • *See* Butamben.

BUTIBEL (Rx) • *See* Belladonna, Butalbital, and Alcohol.

BUTICAPS • *See* Butabarbital Sodium.

BUTISOL • *See* Butabarbital Sodium.

BUTOCONAZOLE (OTC) • **Femstat.** A drug applied topically to treat vaginal thrush caused by candida. Potential adverse reactions include vaginal itching, soreness, and swelling, and itching of the fingers. Contraindicated during the first three months of pregnancy. Butoconazole may be used with oral contraceptives and antibiotic therapy. Tampons should be avoided during treatment. The patient's sexual partner should wear a condom during intercourse until treatment is complete. Changed from Rx to OTC in 1995. *See* Imidazoles.

BUTORPHANOL (Rx) • **Stadol.** An injectable narcotic analgesic that alters through an unknown mechanism both the perception of and emotional reaction to pain. Used to treat moderate to severe pain. Potential adverse reactions include sedation, headache, dizziness, lethargy, confusion, nervousness, unusual dreams, agitation, euphoria, hallucinations, flushing, palpitations, fluctuations in blood pressure, blurred vision, nausea, vomiting, dry mouth, constipation, rash, hives, cold and clamminess, and respiratory depression. Interacts adversely with alcohol and central nervous system depressants. Contraindicated in narcotic addiction. Should be used cautiously in head injury, increased pressure on the brain, acute heart attack, irregular heartbeat, coronary insufficiency, respiratory disease, and kidney or liver dysfunction. At this writing, the FDA was considering butorphanol in nasal-spray form.

BUTTERCUP • *See* Pilewort.

BUTTERBUR • *Petasites vulgaris.* A plant with broad leaves and purplish flowers, the rhizome or leaves of this herb contain essential oil, mucilage, and tannin (*see all*). It is used for painful menstrual periods, to induce sweating, and reduce fluid retention. The fresh leaves are used for dressing wounds.

BUTTERNUT ROOT BARK (H) • *Juglans cinerea.* White Walnut. During the Revolutionary War, this bark was used as a laxative for the Colonial troops. An early American physician reported experiments in which butternut root bark increased the secretion of bile and also the activity of glands in the walls of the intestinal tract. It is used by herbalists to expel rather than kill worms during the normal course of laxative-induced cleansing. It is used by herbalists to treat cough, asthma, and bronchitis. It is also used to treat skin diseases. It is generally regarded as harmless, but the plant contains ingredients that are toxic to the liver and carcinogenic in animals. Long-term use is hazardous because of cumulative effects. It should not be used as an herbal medicine.

BYCLOMINE • *See* Dicyclomine Hydrochloride.

BYPASS SURGERY • A procedure to bypass the blockage or narrowing of an artery. Blockages can be bypassed using sections of normal artery or vein taken from the patient or by using synthetic tubing.

C

CACHEXIA • A profound and marked state of general ill health and malnutrition.

CAD • Abbreviation for coronary artery disease.

CAFERGOT (Rx) • A combination of ergotamine and caffeine (*see both*).

CAFERGOT P-B (Rx) • A combination of belladonna, ergotamine, caffeine, and pentobarbital (*see all*).

CAFFEDRINE (OTC) • See Caffeine.

CAFFEINE (OTC) • **Anacin Analgesic Coated Caplets. Aspirin Free Excedrin Analgesic. Caffedrine. Dexitac. Excedrin Extra-Strength Analgesic. Histosal. Lanorinal. Maximum Strength Midol Multi-Symptom Menstrual Formula. Medigesic. No Doz. Norgesic Forte. P-A-C Analgesic Tablets. Quick Pep. Rid-A-Pain. Tirend. Vanquish. Vivarin.** A stimulant drug that occurs in coffee, tea, and cola, it is considered the most commonly consumed drug in the United States. Caffeine is added to many analgesic medications and is used to treat breathing problems in newborns. Potential adverse reactions include insomnia, restlessness, nervousness, mild delirium, headache, excitement, agitation, muscle tremors, fast heartbeat, nausea, vomiting, loss of water, and skin sensitivity. Interacts with theophylline and beta-blockers (*see*) to create excessive central nervous system stimulation. Contraindicated in gastric or duodenal ulcer, irregular heartbeat, or those who have had heart attacks. Caffeine-containing beverages should be restricted in patients who have had palpitations. Tolerance or psychological dependence may develop. Americans reportedly consume 2 billion pounds of coffee and 500 million pounds of tea each year. Caffeine content in tea, 40 to 100 mg/180 ml; brewed coffee, 100 to 150 mg/180 ml; and decaffeinated coffee, 1 to 6 mg/180 ml. Caffeine in colas is 17 to 55 mg/180 ml. In nonprescription medication, the caffeine content is: Anacin, 32 mg; Excedrin, 65 mg; aspirin-free Excedrin, 65 mg; Midol, 32 mg; Vanquish, 33 mg; No Doz, 100 mg; Vivarin, 200 mg; Dristan, 16 mg; Dexatrim, 200 mg; and Dietac, 200 mg. Caffeine does not reverse alcohol intoxication or its central nervous system depressant effects. Caffeine may aggravate depression in an already depressed patient. Sudden discontinuation of caffeine may cause headache and irritability. Most health professionals recommend limiting caffeine intake to 200 mg daily. The FDA review panel determined that caffeine is safe and effective as a stimulant in doses of 100 to 200 mg no more often than every three to four hours. In the October 5, 1994, issue of the *Journal of the American Medical Association,* Johns Hopkins researchers reported evidence "suggesting that caffeine exhibits the features of a typical psychoactive substance of dependence," and that would explain why some people feel "compelled to continue caffeine use despite desires and recommendations to the contrary."

CAINE-2 • See Lidocaine.

CAJEPUT • See Cajuput.

CAJUPUT (H) • *Melaleuca leucadendron.* **Cajeput. Tea Tree. White Tea Tree.** The spicy oil contains, among other ingredients, terpenes, limonene, benzaldehyde, valeraldehyde, and dipentene. Native to Australia and Southeast Asia, it is used to treat fungus infections such as athlete's foot, and as a liniment for a wide variety of ailments. Herbalists use it to relieve itchy scalp, arthritic pains, and as an antiseptic for cuts.

CALABAR BEAN (H) (Rx) • **Ordeal Bean.** A climbing, woody plant, *Physostigma venenosum,* native to West Africa and cultivated in some other tropical areas, it has antispasmodic and emetic effects. It is used in homeopathic medicine. It is used in West Africa as an "ordeal poison" to determine a person's guilt. Symptoms of poisoning include excessive sweating, vomiting and diarrhea, tremor, anxiety, severe weakness, decreased heart rate, paralysis of the respiratory muscles, coma, and death. The plant is the source of physostigmine (*see*), now being tested for use in the treatment of Alzheimer's disease. It should be used only under strict medical supervision.

CALADRYL (OTC) • A combination of diphenhydramine and calamine (*see both*).

CALAMINE (OTC) • **Aveeno Anti-Itch Concentrated Lotion. Caladryl. Calamox. Rhulicream. Rhulispray.** A lotion containing zinc oxide and ferric oxide, used to soothe irritated skin. In 1992, the FDA proposed a ban for the use of calamine to treat insect bites and stings and poison ivy, poison oak, and poison sumac because it had not been shown to be safe and effective as claimed in OTC products. The FDA said calamine could be used as "a skin protectant," but not as an "external analgesic."

CALAMOX • *See* Calamine.

CALAMUS (H) • *Acorus calamus.* **Sweet Flag. Sweet Sedge.** The rhizome contains essential oil, mucilage, glycosides, amino acid, and tannins (*see all*). Calamus root is an ancient American Indian and Chinese herbal medicine used to treat acid stomach, irregular heart rhythm, low blood pressure, coughs, and lack of mental focus. Native Americans would chew the root to enable them to run long distances with increased stamina. Massaged on the skin, it was used to induce tranquillity.

CALAN • *See* Verapamil.

CALCAREA CARBONICA • *See* Calc. Carb.

CALCAREA FLURICA • *See* Calc. Fluor.

CALCAREA PHOSPHORICA • *See* Calc. Phos.

CALCAREA SULPHURICA • *See* Calc. Sulph.

CALC. CARB. (H) • **Calcarea Carbonica.** A homeopathic medicine to treat congestion, cold feet, and a hot head. Also used by homeopaths to treat varicose veins and hemorrhoids. It is composed of calcium and carbonate. Calcium is a major mineral in the body and is needed for strong teeth and bones. It also plays a major role in cell metabolism. The combination is used in OTC products as an antacid and calcium supplement. *See* Tissue Salts and Calcium Carbonate.

CALCET (OTC) • A combination of calcium and vitamin D (*see both*). Used to strengthen bones.

CALC. FLUOR. (H) • **Calcarea Flurica.** A homeopathic (*see*) medicine composed of calcium fluoride. Calcium is a major mineral in the body and is needed for strong teeth and bones. It also plays a major role in cell metabolism. Fluoride prevents tooth decay and also strengthens bone. *See* Tissue Salts.

CALCIBIND • *See* Sodium Cellulose Phosphate.

CALCIDRINE SYRUP (Rx) • *See* Codeine and Calcium Iodide.

CALCIFEDIOL (Rx) • **Calderol. 25-HCC.** Vitamin D_3 used in the treatment and management of metabolic bone disease associated with chronic renal failure. Potential adverse reactions include vitamin D intoxication, headache, sleepiness, conjunctivitis, photosensitivity, runny nose, nausea, vomiting, constipation, metallic taste, dry mouth, loss of appetite, diarrhea, frequent urination, weakness, and bone and muscle aches. Cholestyramine may impair absorption. Contraindicated in high blood calcium or vitamin D toxicity. Use cautiously in patients on digitalis because high levels of calcium may precipitate irregular heartbeats. Additional vitamin D should not be taken in prescription or over-the-counter products.

CALCIFEROL • *See* Vitamin D.

CALCIJEX • *See* Calcitriol.

CALCILAC (OTC) • *See* Calcium Carbonate.

CALCIMAR • Approved by the FDA in 1994 for the prevention of osteoporosis. *See* Calcitonin.

CALCIPARINE • *See* Heparin.

CALCITONIN (Rx) • **Calcimar. Miacalcin. Cibacalcin.** A naturally occurring hormone that inhibits bone resorption, secreted by the thyroid gland. Salmon-calcitonin, a synthetic formulation, is used to slow the bone resorption rate in osteoporosis (*see*). Also used to treat Paget's disease (*see*) of the bone and high blood calcium. Potential adverse reactions include nausea, vomiting, facial flushing, high blood sugar, diarrhea, loss of appetite, transient water loss, low blood calcium, tingling, swelling and tenderness of the hand, altered taste, and severe allergic reactions. Contraindicated in allergy to the gelatin used to prepare the drug. Not recommended for breastfeeding mothers, or women who may become pregnant. The drug should not be discontinued suddenly.

CALCITREL (OTC) • A combination of magnesium hydroxide and calcium carbonate (*see both*).

CALCITRIOL (Rx) • **Calcijex. Rocaltrol.** A vitamin D preparation that stimulates calcium absorption from the GI tract and promotes secretion of calcium from bone to blood. Used to treat low blood calcium in patients undergoing chronic dialysis. Potential adverse reactions include nausea, vomiting, headache, sleepiness, red eyes, sensitivity to light, runny nose, loss of appetite, frequent urination, weakness, and bone and muscle pain. Patients should not use magnesium-containing antacids or any over-the-counter drugs without checking with a physician.

CALCIUM (OTC) • **Bugs Bunny Complete. Flintstones Complete. One-A-Day Women's Formula Vitamins and Minerals. Os-Cal.** The adult body contains about three pounds of calcium, 99 percent of which provides hardness for bones and teeth. Approximately 1 percent of calcium is distributed in body fluids, where it is essential for normal cell activity. If the body does not get enough calcium from food, it steals the mineral from bones. Abnormal loss of calcium from bones weakens them and makes them porous or brittle and susceptible to fractures. Calcium deficiencies can result in osteopenia (less bone than normal, a condition preceding osteoporosis) and osteoporosis (a severe decrease in bone mass with diagnosable fractures), which affects 25 percent of postmenopausal women. The percentage of calcium absorption declines progressively with age. The recommended daily allowance (RDA) for calcium is 1,000 mg for adults. There is also some evidence that an intake of about 1,000 mg of calcium may protect against hypertension or high blood pressure. Adverse reactions from intravenous use include tingling sensations and a sense of oppression or heat and, with rapid IV injection, faintness. There may be a mild fall in blood pressure but, with rapid IV injection, dilation of the blood vessels, slowed heartbeat, irregular heartbeat, or cardiac arrest; with oral ingestion, irritation, hemorrhage, and constipation. With IV administration, a chalky taste; with oral calcium chloride, GI hemorrhage, nausea, vomiting, thirst, and abdominal pain. Other reactions to calcium include too much calcium in the blood, frequent urination, and kidney stones. Interaction with cardiac glycosides may increase digitalis toxicity. Calcium is contraindicated in irregular heartbeat, high blood calcium, and kidney stones. Should be used cautiously in patients with sarcoidosis, and kidney or heart disease. Oxalic acid found in rhubarb and spinach, phytic acid in bran and whole cereals, and phosphorus in dairy products may interfere with absorption of calcium and make calcium supplements ineffective. Caffeine and alcoholic beverages may make calcium channel blockers less effective.

CALCIUM ACETATE (OTC) (Rx) • **Brown Acetate of Lime. Phos-Ex. PhosLo.** A white powder used as a source of calcium and to control high phosphate levels in kidney failure. In 1992, the FDA proposed a ban on calcium acetate in astringent (*see*) drug products because it had not been shown to be safe and effective as claimed.

CALCIUM CARBONATE (OTC) • **Alka-Mints. Amitone. Calc. Carb. Calcilac. Calglycine. Cal-Sup. Caltrate. Chooz. Dicarbosil.**

Equilet. Genalac. Glycate. Gustalac. Kanalka. Mallamint. Pama No. 1. Rolaids Calcium Rich. Suplical. Titracid. Titralac. Tums. A calcium salt sold mainly as an antacid. Potential adverse reactions include constipation, gastric distension, gas, rebound hyperacidity, and nausea. Also may cause low phosphate and overload of calcium in the blood if taken with milk or other alkaline products. Effects of allopurinol, antibiotics, corticosteroids, diflunisal, digoxin, iron, isoniazid, penicillamine, phenothiazines, and ranitidine are lessened if used in conjunction. Calcium should not be taken indiscriminately. May cause enteric-coated medications (*see* Enteric Coating) to be released prematurely in the stomach, so doses should be separated by one hour.

CALCIUM CHANNEL BLOCKERS (Rx) •
Drugs that affect the movement of calcium (*see*) into the cells of the heart and blood vessels. As a result, they relax blood vessels and increase the supply of blood and oxygen to the heart, while reducing the work of the organ. Some of the medicines are used to treat high blood pressure. Among calcium channel blockers in use are diltiazem, nicardipine, nifedipine, and verapamil. Potential adverse reactions include breathing difficulty, coughing or wheezing, irregular or fast heartbeat, slow heartbeat, rash, swelling of the ankles, feet, or lower leg, bleeding, tender or swollen gums, chest pain, fainting, and for nifedipine only, eye problems and painful swollen joints. A case-control study reported at the March 10, 1995, meeting of the American Heart Association's 35th Annual Conference on Cardiovascular Disease Epidemiology and Prevention, San Antonio, Texas, suggested that calcium channel blockers may incur a greater risk of heart attack than other blood-pressure-lowering therapies. The study was coordinated by Dr. Bruce Psaty of the University of Washington, Seattle, and funded by the National Heart Institute. Dr. Psaty said the results supported a 1993 study recommending beta-blockers and diuretics be used in preference to calcium channel blockers as first-line antihypertensive agents. *See also* Calcium Messenger System. Grapefruit juice may cause potentially dangerous, increased levels of calcium channel blockers in the blood.

CALCIUM CHLORIDE (Rx) • Cal-Plus.
Used in cardiac resuscitation when epinephrine fails to improve heart contractions, and in cardiac disturbances of high potassium, low calcium, or calcium-channel-blocking-agent toxicity.

CALCIUM CITRATE (OTC) • Citracal.
Used as an adjunct in prevention of postmenopausal osteoporosis, and in prevention and treatment of calcium depletion in the body. *See* Calcium.

CALCIUM DISODIUM EDETATE (Rx) •
Calcium Disodium Ethylenediamine Tetraacetic Acid. Calcium Disodium Versenate. Calcium EDTA. Edetate Calcium Disodium. A chelation (*see*) agent used to treat poisoning from lead and other metals. Potential adverse reactions include nausea, vomiting, loss of appetite, headache, pins-and-needles sensations, numbness, irregular heartbeats, low blood pressure, kidney dysfunction, joint and muscle pains, high blood calcium, and after four to eight hours, sudden fever, chills, fatigue, excessive thirst, sneezing, and nasal congestion. Contraindicated in severe kidney disease.

CALCIUM DISODIUM VERSENATE • *See* Calcium Disodium Edetate.

CALCIUM EDTA • *See* Calcium Disodium Edetate.

CALCIUM GLUBIONATE (OTC) • Neo-Calglucon.
Used as an adjunct in prevention of postmenopausal osteoporosis, and in prevention and treatment of calcium depletion. *See* Calcium.

CALCIUM GLUCONATE (OTC) (Rx) •
Kalcinate. Used in the treatment and prevention of low blood calcium, and of heart disturbances caused by high blood potassium, in cardiac resuscitation when epinephrine fails to increase heart contractions, and in low blood calcium or calcium-channel-blocker toxicity. In 1992, the FDA issued a notice that calcium gluconate had not been shown to be safe and effective as claimed in OTC digestive-aid products.

CALCIUM IODIDE • Calcidrine. Norisodrine. Used in cough medicines to stop coughs and to loosen phlegm. Should not be used by persons sensitive to iodine. Iodide may cause severe and sometimes fatal skin eruptions after prolonged use. Symptoms of adverse effects to iodide include metallic taste, skin lesions, irritation of the mucous membranes, swelling of the salivary glands, and upset stomach.

CALCIUM LACTATE (Rx) • White, almost odorless crystals or powder used as a buffer and, as such, a constituent of baking powders; also used in dentifrices. In medical use it is given for calcium deficiency, but may cause gastrointestinal and cardiac disturbances. In 1992, the FDA proposed a ban on calcium lactate in oral menstrual drug products because it had not been shown to be safe and effective as claimed.

CALCIUM MESSENGER SYSTEM • As calcium increases in the cell, a protein, calmodulin, interacts with other proteins to stimulate responses such as smooth-muscle contraction. The calcium messenger system is believed to play a part in learning, as well as in the functioning of the heart and other vital organs.

CALCIUM PANTOTHENATE (OTC) • Used as a vitamin supplement. Banned as an ingredient in laxatives by the FDA, May 1992 because it had not been shown to be safe and effective as claimed. Its wide use in multivitamins continues.

CALCIUM PHOSPHATE (OTC) • Centrum, Jr. Extra Calcium. Hyland's Teething Tablets. Posture 600. White, odorless powder used to provide a daily source of calcium to help maintain healthy bones or to supplement dietary calcium intake. Also used as an abrasive in toothpaste and tooth powder.

CALCIUM POLYCARBOPHIL (OTC) • Equalactin. Fiberall Tablets. FiberCon. Fiber-Lax. Mitrolan. Used to treat constipation or diarrhea by restoring a more normal moisture level and providing bulk in the intestinal tract. *See* Laxative.

CALCIUM PROPIONATE • Propanoic Acid. Calcium Salt. A mold or rope (slimy strands) inhibitor used as a preservative and as an antifungal medication for the skin.

CALCIUM RICH • *See* Calcium Carbonate.

CALCIUM SALICYLATE (OTC) • In 1992, the FDA proposed a ban on calcium salicylate in internal analgesic products because it had not been shown to be safe and effective as claimed. *See* Salicylates.

CALCIUM UNDECYLENATE (OTC) • Caldesene Medicated Powder. Cruex Antifungal Powder. The calcium salt of undecylenic acid, which occurs in sweat. Used in antifungal and antibacterial skin preparations.

CALC. PHOS. (H) • Calcarea Phosphorica. A homeopathic (*see*) medicine composed of calcium phosphate. Calcium is a major mineral in the body and is needed for strong teeth and bones. It also plays a major role in cell metabolism. Without sufficient phosphate there is abnormal parathyroid-gland function, bone metabolism, intestinal absorption, malnutrition, and kidney malfunction. *See* Tissue Salts.

CALC. SULPH. (H) • Calcarea Sulphurica. A homeopathic medicine (*see*) composed of calcium and sulfate. Calcium is a major mineral in the body and is needed for strong teeth and bones. Sulfate is the salt of sulfuric acid.

CALCULI; RENAL, BLADDER • Stones formed or present in the kidneys or bladder caused by dissolved substances in urine.

CALCULUS • A stone formed in a duct, cyst, or hollow organ of the body, especially the gallbladder and kidney. Most calculi are composed of mineral salts, often with a mixture of organic matter. Stones may cause anything from a few minor symptoms to excruciating pain, depending on whether they pass and where.

CALDEROL • *See* Vitamin D.

CALDESENE (OTC) • *See* Calcium Undecylenate.

CALEN • The abbreviation used in homeopathic medicine for calendula (*see*).

CALENDULA (H) • *Calendula marigold. Calendula officinalis.* **Pot Marigold.** The flower heads contain an essential oil with carotenoids, saponin, resin, and bitter principle. In an oil or ointment, it is used by herbalists and traditional pharmacists to treat minor skin irritations. An infusion is used by herbalists to treat fevers, ulcers, menstrual cramps, and eruptive skin diseases such as measles. They also use it to stop bleeding. Marigold flowers have been reported to lower blood pressure. May be harmful if taken internally by pregnant women.

CALGLYCINE (OTC) • *See* Calcium Carbonate.

CALICYLIC CREME • *See* Salicylic Acid.

CALM-X • *See* Dimenhydrinate.

CALOMEL (OTC) • A mineral containing mercury, which was banned as an ingredient in laxatives by the FDA in May 1992. It is still used as a fungicide and pesticide.

CAL-PLUS (OTC) • *See* Calcium Chloride.

CAL-SUP (OTC) • *See* Calcium Carbonate.

CALTRATE (OTC) • *See* Calcium Carbonate.

CALUMBA (H) • *Jateorhiza palmata.* **Columbo.** A climbing plant native to Mozambique and Madagascar. The root contains alkaloids and glycosides (*see both*) and is used to treat indigestion and to increase the appetite.

CALUSTERONE (Rx) • **Methosarb.** Used in palliation of metastatic breast cancer in which the tumor cells are sensitive to estrogen.

CAMA • *See* Aspirin.

CAMA ARTHRITIS PAIN RELIEVER (OTC) • *See* Aluminum Hydroxide.

CAMALOX (OTC) • A combination of aluminum hydroxide, magnesium hydroxide, and calcium carbonate (*see all*) used as an antacid for stomach upset.

CAMOMILE • *See* Chamomile.

CAMPHO-PHENIQUE (OTC) • *See* Camphor and Phenol.

CAMPHOR (OTC) (H) • *Cinnamomum camphora.* **Camphor Tree. Japanese White Oil. Aurum Analgesic Lotion. Aveeno Anti-Itch Concentrated Lotion. Ben-Gay Ultra Strength Pain Relieving Rub. Caladryl. Campho-Phenique. Feminine Gold Analgesic Relieving Rub. Pazo Hemorrhoid Ointment & Suppositories. Rhulicream. Rhuligel. Rhulispray. Sarna. Theragold Analgesic Lotion. Vicks Vaporub.** Distilled from trees at least fifty years old grown in China, Japan, Taiwan, Brazil, and Sumatra. The camphor tree is used in spice flavorings, in topical applications to give a cool sensation on the skin, and in cold medications and anesthetics. Can cause contact dermatitis. In 1980, the FDA banned camphorated oil as a liniment for colds and sore muscles due to reports of poisonings through skin absorption, and because of accidental ingestion. In 1980, a New Jersey pharmacist had collected case reports and testified before the FDA Advisory Review Panel on Over-the-Counter Drugs. Camphor is readily absorbed through all sites of administration. Ingestion of two grams generally produces dangerous effects in adults. Ingestion by pregnant women has caused fetal deaths. In 1992, the FDA issued a notice that camphor had not been shown to be safe and effective as claimed in OTC products in general, specifically for treating cold sores, fever blisters, insect bites and stings, and in poison ivy, poison oak, and poison sumac drug products. In 1992, the FDA proposed a ban on camphor gum in astringent (*see*) drug products because it had not been shown to be safe and effective as claimed.

CAMPHORATED OPIUM TINCTURE • *See* Paregoric.

CAMPTOSAR • *See* CPT-11.

CANCER • A general term for more than one hundred diseases characterized by abnormal and uncontrolled growth of cells. The resulting mass, or tumor, can invade and destroy surrounding normal tissue.

CANDICIDIN (OTC) • **Vanobid.** An antifungal antibiotic produced by a strain of *Streptomyces griseus*. In 1992, the FDA issued a notice that candicidin had not been shown to be safe and effective as claimed in OTC products.

CANDIDA • A group of yeastlike fungi that may produce infection in the mouth, intestines, vagina, skin and rarely, the whole body.

CANDIDA ALBICANS • A yeastlike fungus that causes a mouth and throat infection called thrush. The fungus also infects the vagina and the intestinal tract.

CANDIDIASIS • A fungal infection, usually of the moist surfaces of the body including the skin, mouth, esophagus, and respiratory tract.

CANKAID (OTC) • *See* Carbamide Peroxide.

CANKER SORES • Ulcers inside the mouth that may be recurrent, but which are not due to herpes (*see*).

CANNABINOIDS (Rx) (H) • Derivatives of marijuana used as anti-emetics (*see*). *See also* Dronabinol and Nabinol.

CANNABIS • *See* Marijuana.

CANNABIS SATIVA • *See* Hemp.

CANTH • Homeopathic abbreviation for *Cantharis vesicatoria* (*see*).

CANTHARIDIN (Rx) • **Cantharone. Verr– Canth.** An antiviral drug used to treat warts. It is applied only by a physician and not dispensed to the patient.

CANTHARIS VESICATORIA (H) • **Caleoptera. Spanish Fly.** An ancient substance from a green beetle found in France and Spain used as an aphrodisiac and to treat edema. It was once used in blistering plasters for arthritis. Homeopaths use it for burns and cystitis. To make the homeopathic medicine, the flies are collected at dawn when they are asleep and are killed by being heated in boiling vinegar steam. They are then crushed and mixed into the remedy. Cantharis is toxic and can cause severe kidney damage.

CANTHARONE • *See* Cantharidin.

CANTHARONE PLUS (Rx) • A combination of cantharidin, podophyllin, and salicylic acid (*see all*) used to treat warts.

CANTIL • *See* Mepenzolate.

CAPASTAT • *See* Capreomycin.

CAPILLARIES • The finest vessels in the body, where nutrient and oxygen exchange occurs. They connect small arteries to small veins.

CAPITAL and CODEINE (Rx) • *See* Acetaminophen and Codeine Phosphate.

CAPITROL • *See* Chloroxine.

CAPLET • A form of medication shaped like a capsule, but solid like a tablet.

CAPOTEN • *See* Captopril.

CAPOZIDE (Rx) • A combination of captopril and hydrochlorothiazide, prescribed for high blood pressure. Hydrochlorothiazide is a diuretic, and captopril is an ACE inhibitor (*see*). Their blood-pressure-lowering effects are greater together than either alone. Potential adverse reactions include kidney dysfunction, liver dysfunction, itching, fever, loss of taste, fatigue, dizziness, headache, stomach upset, chest pain, nausea, vomiting, sweating, flushing, low blood pressure, palpitations, insomnia, cramps, male impotence, swelling, and weakness. Interaction with blood-pressure-lowering drugs may drop the blood pressure too low, and diabetics taking oral antidiabetes drugs may need to have their dosages adjusted. Captopril was relabeled after its introduction to alert doctors and patients that it could dangerously lower the sodium content of the blood. Capozide is contraindicated in people allergic to sulfa drugs, those with kidney dysfunction, asthma, or lupus, or those who take other drugs affecting the white blood cell content. Should be taken on an empty stomach.

CAP-PROFEN (OTC) • *See* Ibuprofen.

CAPREOMYCIN (Rx) • **Capastat.** Used as an adjunctive treatment for tuberculosis (*see* Adjunct). May be toxic to the ears, causing hearing loss, ringing in the ears, and dizziness. May also adversely affect the kidney, liver, and blood. Adversely interacts with many antibiotics and antiarthritic medicines.

CAPRYLIC ACID • A fatty acid that occurs in sweat, fusel oil, in the milk of cows and goats, and in palm and coconut oils. Used as a preservative.

CAPSAICIN (Rx) (OTC) (H) • **Axsain. Zostrix.** A drug derived from cayenne (pepper), it is used for temporary relief of pain after herpes zoster infections, and for relief of postsurgical pain and nerve pains suffered by diabetics. A capsaicin taffy is marketed OTC for pain. Potential adverse reactions include local redness and stinging or burning upon application. Avoid getting drug in the eyes or on broken skin. In 1992, the FDA proposed a ban for the use of capsaicin to treat fever blisters and cold sores because it had not been shown to be safe and effective as claimed in OTC products. Pharmaceutical companies are now studying several capsaicin-based compounds applied to the skin of injured patients for pain relief. *See* Cayenne and Capsicum.

CAPSICUM (H) (OTC) • **Capsaicin. Capsicin.** A member of the nightshade family, it is native to tropical South America. For medicinal purposes, herbalists use capsicum as an internal disinfectant and to protect against infectious disease. Plasters are made for arthritic pains. It increases blood flow to the area of application, and this increased flow results in reduced inflammation of the affected area. In 1992, the FDA issued a notice that capsicum and capsicum fluid extract had not been shown to be safe and effective as claimed in OTC digestive-aid or oral menstrual drug products. The FDA also proposed a ban in 1992 for the use of capsicum oleoresin to treat fever blisters and cold sores because it had not been shown to be safe and effective as claimed in OTC products. *See* Cayenne and Capsaicin.

CAPSICUM FASTIGATUM • *See* Chili.

CAPSULE • A shell of gelatin or other material that can dissolve in the stomach, releasing the capsule's contents. Also, the tough fibrous tissue that encloses an organ or surrounds a joint.

CAPTOPRIL (Rx) • **Capoten.** An ACE inhibitor (*see*) introduced in 1981, this drug reduces the constriction of blood vessels. In 1992, a large study reported at the American College of Cardiology meeting in Dallas, Texas, concluded that, among heart attack victims, this drug could save up to fifteen thousand lives each year. Captopril seems to prevent enlargement of the heart that often follows a heart attack and causes heart failure. The study found that captopril reduced the risk of heart failure by 36 percent, and new heart attacks by 24 percent. The drug must be used with caution in people with kidney disease or immune diseases such as lupus (*see*). Potential adverse reactions include a drop in white blood cells, dizziness, fainting, irregular heartbeat, angina, congestive heart failure, inflammation of the covering of the heart, loss of appetite, loss of taste, kidney dysfunction, skin rash, fever, swelling of the face and extremities, and persistent cough. During the second and third trimesters of pregnancy, ACE inhibitors can cause fetal and neonatal morbidity. Antacids decrease captopril's effect. Captopril may increase concentration of digitalis glycosides in the blood. NSAIDs (*see*) may reduce its blood-pressure-lowering effects. Potassium supplements increase the risk of potassium overload. Used in over-the-counter stimulants, decongestants, and diet pills that raise blood pressure. Aspirin or indomethacin may counteract the benefits of these products. Cimetidine (*see*) increases the risk of adverse effects and reduces the effectiveness of captopril. Captopril should be taken one hour before meals. It should not be discontinued suddenly. As of this writing, captopril is also scheduled for production as a less expensive generic drug.

CARAFATE • *See* Sucralfate.

CARAMIPHEN and PHENYLPROPANO-LAMINE (Rx) • **Tuss-Ornade.** A cough suppressant prepared from caramiphen, a synthetic nonnarcotic cough suppressant, and phenylpropanolamine, a vasoconstrictor with decongestant action on nasal and upper-respiratory-tract mucosal membranes. A final determination has not been made on the effectiveness of this drug in accordance with efficacy requirements of the 1962 amendments to the Food, Drug, and Cosmetic Act. At this writing, attempts were being made to move its classification from Rx to OTC. Potential adverse reactions include nausea, gastrointestinal upset, diarrhea, drowsiness, nervousness, insomnia, palpitations, headache, incoordination, constipation, tremor, difficulty in urinating, painful urination, high blood pressure, low blood pressure, and visual disturbances. Should be used with caution in patients with heart disease, glaucoma, enlarged prostate, thyroid disease, or diabetes. Patients taking this medication should not take other medications containing phenylpropanolamine or amphetamines.

CARAWAY (H) • *Carum carvi.* The use of this herb dates back to ancient Egypt. The plant is a native of southeastern Europe and western Asia. The seeds are used to ease intestinal gas and colic, and to stimulate the appetite. Also used by herbalists to treat bronchitis and laryngitis, and to relieve menstrual-period pains. Has been used to increase the flow of mother's milk.

CARBACEL • *See* Carbachol.

CARBACHOL (Rx) • **Carbacel. Carbamylcholine. Isopto Carbachol. Miostat.** An agent that contracts the pupil of the eye, it is used either in drops or applied topically before or after eye surgery. Also used to treat glaucoma. Potential adverse reactions include abdominal cramps, headache, diarrhea, red eyes, blurred vision, eye and brow pain, sweating, flushing, and asthma.

CARBAMAZEPINE (Rx) • **Epitol. Tegretol.** An anticonvulsant drug introduced in 1962. It limits seizures by controlling the passage of sodium ions across cell membranes in the part of the brain that controls motor-nerve impulses. Used for generalized tonic-clonic and complex-partial seizures, and mixed seizure patterns. Also used to treat trigeminal neuralgia (*see*). Since it may have serious side effects, it is prescribed only after less hazardous drugs have failed. Potential adverse reactions include anemia, dizziness, drowsiness, fatigue, loss of balance, worsening of seizures, congestive heart failure, high or low blood pressure, aggravation of coronary artery disease, conjunctivitis (*see*), dry mouth, blurred vision, double vision, nausea, vomiting, abdominal pain, diarrhea, loss of appetite, sore mouth and tongue, urinary frequency, urine retention, impotence, kidney dysfunction, liver dysfunction, water intoxication, hives, rash, sweating, fever, and chills. Contraindicated in bone-marrow suppression or hypersensitivity to carbamazepine or tricyclic antidepressants (*see*). Should be used cautiously in kidney or liver disease patients and those with increased pressure in the eyes. It may worsen the effects of glaucoma. Children with mixed-seizure disorders given carbamazepine may have increased seizures. Phenytoin, primidone, phenobarbital, and nicotinic acid (*see all*) may make carbamazepine less effective. Phenytoin, warfarin, doxycycline, theophylline, and haloperidol (*see all*) may be less effective when taken with carbamazepine. Propoxyphene, troleandomycin, erythromycin, isoniazid, and verapamil (*see all*) may increase carbamazepine's level in the blood and result in toxicity. MAO inhibitors (*see*) should be discontinued at least two weeks before carbamazepine treatment is initiated. Should be taken at the same time of day, with meals.

CARBAMIDE PEROXIDE (OTC) • Auro Ear Drops. Cankaid. Debrox Drops. Ear Drops by Murine. Gly-Oxide Liquid. Murine Ear Drops. Murine Ear Wax Removal System. Proxigel. Urea Peroxide. A strong oxidizing agent used in drops for softening earwax.

CARBAMYLCHOLINE CHLORIDE • *See* Carbachol.

CARBAPEN • *See* Carbenicillin Disodium.

CARBARYL • Clinicide. Sevin. A pesticide used to kill lice. Potential adverse reactions besides poisoning and death include nausea, vomiting, diarrhea, lung damage, blurred vision, excessive salivation, muscle twitching, convulsions, and eye and skin irritation. It can be absorbed through the skin.

CARBENICILLIN DISODIUM (Rx) • Carbapen. Geocillin. Geopen. Pyopen. A penicillin-type antibiotic introduced in 1964, it is used to treat systemic infections caused by susceptible strains of gram-positive and especially gram-negative (*see both*) organisms, including *Proteus* and *Pseudomonas aeruginosa* (*see both*). It is particularly useful in urinary infections because it concentrates in urine. Potential adverse reactions include bleeding with high doses, a drop in white blood cell and platelet counts, neuromuscular irritability, seizures, nausea, vomiting, low potassium, pain at site of injection, hypersensitivity including potential fatal allergic reactions, and overgrowth of nonsusceptible organisms. Incompatible with aminoglycoside (*see*) antibiotics. Should be taken on an empty stomach.

CARBENOXOLONE (Rx) • A licorice derivative used in the treatment of ulcers. *See* Licorice.

CARBETAPENTANE (Rx) • Germapect. Rynatuss. Sedotussin. Tuclase. Derived from petroleum, it is used to treat coughs. It has antispasmodic properties.

CARBIDOPA-LEVODOPA (Rx) • Lodosyn. Sinemet. Levodopa (*see*) counteracts the depletion in the brain of the neurotransmitter dopamine, while carbidopa inhibits the breakdown of levodopa. The combination is used to treat Parkinson's disease (*see*), and parkinsonism resulting from carbon-monoxide or manganese intoxication. Potential adverse reactions include anemia, involuntary grimacing, awkward or slow movements, jerking, tremor, psychiatric disturbances, memory loss, nervousness, anxiety, bad dreams, euphoria, malaise, fatigue, severe depression, delirium, dementia, hallucinations, a drop in blood pressure upon rising from a seated or prone position, flushing, high blood pressure, phlebitis, spasms of the eyelid, blurred vision, double vision, nasal discharge, nausea, vomiting, loss of appetite, weight loss, stomach pain, hiccups, dry mouth, bitter taste, urinary frequency or retention, incontinence, excessive and inappropriate sexual behavior, priapism (*see*), liver toxicity, hyperventilation, and perspiration. Medications for high blood pressure may cause additive low blood pressure effects. Papaverine, phenothiazines and other antipsychotics, and phenytoin (*see*) may counteract carbidopa-levodopa's beneficial effects. Stimulants may increase the risk of irregular heartbeat.

CARBINOXAMINE (OTC) • An antihistamine used in cough and cold medicines. Should not be taken by patients undergoing an asthma attack or those who are sensitive to it or who have difficulty urinating.

CARBINOXAMINE and PSEUDOEPHEDRINE (Rx) • Rondec. Rondec-DM. Rondec-TR. An antihistamine and decongestant compound used to treat perennial and seasonal allergic rhinitis and other allergic symptoms, including hives. Should be used with caution in patients with high blood pressure, poor circulation, or over sixty years of age. Potential adverse reactions include drowsiness, high blood pressure, dizziness, vomiting, diarrhea, dry mouth, headache, nervousness, loss of appetite, heartburn, weakness, frequent and/or painful urination, irregular heartbeat, respiratory difficulty, convulsions, weakness, and central nervous system stimulation. Antihistamines may enhance the effects of tricyclic antidepressants, barbiturates, alcohol, and other central nervous system depressants. MAO inhibitors (*see*) prolong and intensify the effects of antihistamines. Pseudoephedrine (*see*) may reduce the effectiveness of blood-pressure-lowering drugs.

CARBO BETULA (H) • *See* Birch.

CARBOCAINE • *See* Mepivacaine.

CARBOCHOLINE • *See* Carbachol.

CARBOHYDRATES • Starches and sugars contain a high proportion of carbohydrates. Carbohydrates are chemicals that contain carbon, hydrogen, and oxygen. Gums and mucilages, complex carbohydrates, are ingredients in soothing herbs and medications.

CARBOL-FUCHSIN (Rx) • **Castaderm. Castellani Paint. Magenta Paint.** A topical solution of fuchsin, phenol, resorcinol, acetone, and alcohol used to kill bacterial and fungal skin infections. Potential adverse reactions include bone-marrow depression with use over long periods or at frequent intervals, and skin rash. A stinging sensation usually occurs right after application, followed by the compound's local anesthetic effect.

CARBOLIC ACID • *See* Phenol.

CARBON (OTC) • In 1992, the FDA issued a notice that carbon had not been shown to be safe and effective as claimed in OTC digestive-aid products.

CARBONIC ANHYDRASE INHIBITORS (Rx) • Enzyme inhibitors used to treat glaucoma, seizures, and the effects of mountain (altitude) sickness. Among them: acetazolamide, dichlorphenamide, dorzolamide, and methazolamide (*see all*).

CARBOPLATIN (Rx) • **Paraplatin.** An anticancer drug introduced in 1989, similar to cisplatin (*see*), it is a palliative treatment of ovarian cancer.

Potential adverse reactions include nausea, vomiting, drowsiness, anemia, dizziness, confusion, nerve damage, loss of hair, hypersensitivity, and liver dysfunction. Bone-marrow-depressing drugs and X-ray therapy may increase blood problems. Drugs that affect the kidney may add to carboplatin's kidney effects. Contraindicated in patients with a history of hypersensitivity to platinum-containing compounds.

CARBOPROST (Rx) • **Hemabate. Prostin/15M.** A prostaglandin (*see*) drug introduced in 1979, it produces strong, quick contractions of uterine smooth muscle to abort pregnancy between the thirteenth and twentieth weeks of gestation. Potential adverse reactions include vomiting, diarrhea, nausea, fever, and chills. Contraindicated in pelvic inflammatory disease or active heart, lung, kidney, or liver disease. This drug is administered only in the hospital.

CARBO VEGETABILIS (H) • **Carb-v. Wood Charcoal.** A homeopathic remedy made from charcoal. It is used to treat bad breath, colds, cough, food poisoning, and for people recovering from chest infections.

CARBOXYMETHYLCELLULOSE (OTC) • **Cellufresh Lubricant Ophthalmic Solution. Celluvisc Lubricant Ophthalmic Solution.** An eye lubricant. In eye preparations it is important to avoid contamination and not reuse. If eye pain, changes of vision, continued redness, or irritation of the eye are experienced, or if the condition worsens or persists for more than seventy-two hours, discontinue use and consult a doctor.

CARBUNCLES • Pus-filled cavities that originate at the base of a hair follicle; deep-rooted and often accompanied by extreme pain, fever, and malaise.

CARB-V • Homeopathic abbreviation for carbo vegetabilis (*see*).

CARCINO-, CARCIN- • Prefixes from the Greek *karkinos,* meaning crab, and referring to cancer, as in carcinogen.

CARCINOGEN • Any substance that causes cancer.

CARCINOGENESIS • The origin or production of cancer.

CARCINOID TUMOR • Usually a small, slow-growing tumor covered by mucosa. Such tumors occur anywhere in the lungs and gastrointestinal tract, with approximately 90 percent in the appendix and the rest in the ileum (*see*), but also in the stomach and other parts of the small intestine, colon, and rectum.

CARCINOMA • A malignant growth composed of abnormally multiplying surface tissues such as those of the skin, linings of internal organs, or linings of glands. The most common form of cancer.

CARDAMOM (H) • *Elettaria cardamomum.* **Grains of Paradise.** Grown in India, Ceylon, and Guatemala. The seeds of this aromatic plant contain large amounts of volatile oils that are used by herbalists to stimulate digestion and relieve gas.

CARDEC DM (Rx) • A combination of dextromethorphan, and carbinoxamine and pseudoephedrine (*see both entries*). An antihistamine and decongestant.

CARDENE • *See* Nicardipine.

CARDI-, CARDIO- • Prefixes meaning the heart, as in *cardiovascular.*

CARDIAC GLYCOSIDES • Steroidal compounds affecting the heart. Used in the treatment of congestive heart failure. *See* Glycosides.

CARDIOMYOPATHY • A disease of the heart muscle. It causes reduction in blood circulation to the heart, lungs, and to the rest of the body.

CARDIOQUIN • *See* Quinidine.

CARDIOVASCULAR DISEASE • Disease of the heart and its blood vessels.

CARDIOVASCULAR SYSTEM • Delivers oxygenated blood, nutrients, and hormones to body tissues and removes waste substances such as carbon dioxide and other metabolic products.

CARDIZEM • *See* Diltiazem.

CARDRASE • *See* Ethoxyzolamide.

CARDURA • *See* Doxazosin Mesylate.

CARFIN • *See* Warfarin.

CARISOPRODATE • *See* Carisoprodol.

CARISOPRODOL (Rx) • **Carisoprodate. Rela. Sodol. Soma Compound. Soprodol. Soridol.** A muscle relaxant that reduces transmission of nerve impulses from spinal cord to skeletal muscle. Used to treat painful muscle and bone conditions. Potential adverse reactions include drowsiness, dizziness, loss of balance, tremor, agitation, irritability, headache, depression, insomnia, a drop in blood pressure when rising from a seated or prone position, rapid heartbeat, facial flushing, nausea, vomiting, hiccups, increased bowel movements, heartburn, rash, fever, asthma, tissue swelling, and anaphylaxis. If taken with alcohol, central nervous depression may be increased. Contraindicated in hypersensitivity to the drug or related compounds such as meprobamate and tybamate. Should be used with caution in persons with kidney or liver dysfunction. Should not be discontinued abruptly or mild withdrawal symptoms may occur such as insomnia and headache.

CARLINE THISTLE (H) • *Carlina vulgaris.* The root of this perennial plant contains essential oils, sesquiterpene, and tannin (*see*). Used as a diuretic, to induce sweating, and for healing wounds.

CARMINATIVE • A substance that removes gases from the gastrointestinal tract. Among the herbs used for this purpose are peppermint and aniseed.

CARMOL HC (OTC) • A cream containing hydrocortisone and urea (*see both*).

CARMUSTINE (Rx) • **BCNU. BiCNU.** A drug used in the treatment of tumors of the central nervous system and lymphatic system, the liver, and melanomas, and multiple myeloma. Potential adverse reactions include severe nausea, vomiting, kidney and liver toxicity, bone-marrow depression, high uric acid, facial flushing, intense pain at infusion site, and lung changes. Cimetidine (*see*) may increase carmustine's bone-marrow toxicity.

CARNATION (H) • *Dianthus caryophyllus.* In 1991, researchers at New York University reported an extract from the leaves of the carnation to be effective against the AIDS virus. The extract is also reportedly nontoxic to normal cells and may eventually be used in condoms, vaginal jellies, and toothpastes to minimize the risk of HIV transmission.

CARNITINE (Rx) (OTC) • **Vitamin B$_T$.** A thyroid inhibitor found in muscle, liver, and meat extracts. It stimulates fatty-acid oxidation and manufacture. Muscles, which contain approximately 98 percent of carnitine, must take it up from the blood. When carnitine is deficient, muscles become weak and the person's body becomes intolerant to exercise. *See* Levocarnitine.

CARNITOR • *See* Levocarnitine.

CARNOSINE • A peptide found in the muscle of humans and numerous animals. L-carnosine is being tested as an aid in wound healing.

CAROTENE • A yellow pigment occurring in yellow vegetables, egg yolk, and other foods. The body converts it into vitamin A.

CAROTENOIDS • Found in parsley, carrots, sweet potatoes, and most green, red, and yellow vegetables and fruits, these are vitamin A precursors that are antioxidants and cell-differentiation agents (cancer cells are nondifferentiated). There are hundreds of carotenoids in nature.

CARP- • Prefix meaning the wrist, as in *carpal.*

CARPAL TUNNEL • Space under ligament in the wrist through which the median nerve enters the hand.

CARPHENAZINE (Rx) • A phenothiazine (*see*) antipsychotic drug.

CARPROFEN (Rx) • **Rimadyl.** A nonsteroidal anti-inflammatory drug to treat rheumatoid, gouty, and osteo arthritis. It is effective within one hour and remains so for up to six hours. Potential adverse reactions include nausea, vomiting, drowsiness, headache, dizziness, ringing in ears, rash, heartburn, nervousness, insomnia, depression, confusion, tremor, loss of appetite, fatigue, itching, double or blurred vision, dry or irritated eyes, irregular heartbeat, liver dysfunction, blood disorders, fever, tingling in hands and feet, enlarged breasts, blood in urine, urinary frequency, low blood sugar, kidney damage, asthma, breathing difficulties, fluid retention, and black-and-blue marks. Aspirin and beta-blockers (*see*) make it less effective. Carprofen may increase the side effects of blood-thinning drugs and antidiabetes and antiseizure medications. May be taken with food.

CARRAGEENAN • Banned by the FDA as an ingredient in laxatives, May 1992.

CARROT, WILD (H) • *Daucus carota.* **Bee's Nest. Bird's Nest. Philtron.** A common plant that resembles a bird's nest. It is used by herbalists to treat kidney stones, fluid retention, and bladder problems.

CARTEOLOL (Rx) • **Cartrol.** A beta-blocker (*see*) introduced in 1989 that is used to treat high blood pressure. Potential adverse reactions include weakness, fatigue, sleepiness, heart irregularities, impotence, decreased libido, asthma, and muscle cramps. When used with calcium channel blockers (*see*), blood pressure may drop too low, and heart failure may occur. General anesthetics increase carteolol's blood-pressure-lowering effects. Its use may affect the response to insulin and oral diabetic drugs. Reserpine and other drugs that deplete catecholamine (*see*) may have an additive effect when administered with beta-blockers. Food may slow the rate but not the extent of absorption. The drug should be taken exactly as prescribed and not discontinued suddenly. If shortness of breath, difficulty breathing, unusually fast heartbeat, cough, or fatigue with exertion occur, the prescribing physician should be notified immediately. May be taken with or without meals.

CARTER'S LITTLE PILLS (OTC) • *See* Bisacodyl.

CARTILAGE • **Gristle.** White, elastic connective tissue that forms part of the skeleton and pads the opposing surfaces of joints.

CARTROL • *See* Carteolol.

CARVEDILOL (Rx) • **Coreg.** A beta-blocker (*see*) introduced for high blood pressure. It reduced the risk of death by 67 percent in a large clinical trial of patients with congestive heart failure. Approved by the FDA and available in several countries, it is expected to be on the United States market soon, as of this writing.

CASAMIN (OTC) • Glucosamine, calcium, and vitamin D_3 (*see all*).

CASANTHRANOL (OTC) • **Anticon. Cantralax. Peri-Colace.** A complex mixture derived from Cascara sagrada (*see*) and used as a stimulant laxative. *See also* Laxative.

CASCARA SAGRADA (OTC) (H) • *Rhamnus purshiana.* **Chittembark. Sacred Bark. Nature's Remedy Natural Vegetable Laxative.** Contains anthraquinone glycosides, bitter principle, tannins, and resin. Cascara bark has been called the most widely used cathartic on earth. The bitter principle (*see*) of cascara bark stimulates the entire digestive system. Both herbalists and traditional physicians recommend it as a mild stimulant laxative. In 1992, the FDA issued a notice that cascara sagrada extract had not been shown to be safe and effective as claimed in OTC digestive-aid or menstrual drug products. Cascara should not be used regularly in patients suffering from gastrointestinal irritation or peptic ulcer. It may also cause excessive loss of potassium if used over a long time. *See also* Laxative.

CASODEX • *See* Bicalutamide.

CASTADERM • *See* Carbol-Fuchsin.

CASTELLANI PAINT (OTC) • A mixture of carbol-fuchsin (*see*), phenol, resorcinol, acetone, and alcohol applied locally as an antifungal agent.

CASTOR BEAN (OTC) • *See* Castor Oil.

CASTOR OIL (H) (OTC) • *Ricinus communis.* **Castor Bean. Oleum Ricini. Palma Christi. Alphamul. Emulsoil. Neoloid. Purge Concentrate.** A member of the spurge family, originally native to India, the castor-oil plant is one of the most ancient sources of medicine known. Castor-oil plant seeds have been found in Egyptian tombs thousands of years old. The oil extracted from the bean contains glycerides of ricinoleic, isoricinoleic, and stearic acids. The plant was mentioned by Hippocrates, circa 400 B.C. Both herbalists and medical doctors recommend it as a stimulant laxative. Herbalists also use castor oil to treat food poisoning, as an antihelminthic to aid in expelling worms, and topically to dissolve cysts, growths, and warts. Since the castor bean also contains a highly poisonous substance, only the manufactured products should be used.

CATABOLISM • Metabolism involving the release of energy, resulting from the breakdown of complex material.

CATAPRES • *See* Clonidine.

CATARASE • *See* Chymotrypsin.

CATARRH • Inflammation of a mucous membrane. From the Greek word *katarrhein,* meaning to flow down. Autumnal catarrh is another name for hay fever, nasal catarrh is rhinitis (*see*), and vernal catarrh refers to conjunctivitis (*see*).

CATCHWEED • *See* Cleavers.

CATECHIN (H) • **Catechol. Flavanpentol.** Found primarily in wood such as mahogany and acacia, it is used as an astringent (*see*), particularly to treat diarrhea.

CATECHOLAMINES • A group of chemicals made in the body, such as neurotransmitters and hormones, that can also be made synthetically. Among the major catecholamines are dopamine, norepinephrine, and epinephrine (*see all*). The catecholamines help regulate blood pressure, heart rate, breathing, muscle tone, metabolism, and central nervous system function.

CATECHU • *See* Acacia Gum.

CATHARTIC • A drug that stimulates bowel action to help induce a bowel movement.

CATMINT (H) • *Nepeta cataria.* **Catnep. Catnip.** An aromatic plant of the mint family common to North America and Europe. It was said in folk medicine that the root when chewed made the quietest person fierce and quarrelsome. The leaves contain essential oils and tannin. In modern medicine it is used as a digestive herb, which is prescribed for stomach pains and flatulence. Herbalists use it in a tea as a sedative, for insomnia, fever, colds, and diarrhea. Catmint has been reported effective in treating iron-deficiency anemia, menstrual and uterine disorders, and dyspepsia. In 1992, the FDA issued a notice that catnip had not been shown to be safe and effective as claimed in OTC digestive-aid products.

CATNEP • *See* Catmint.

CATNIP • *See* Catmint.

CAUL • A homeopathic abbreviation for *Caulophyllum thalictroides. See* Blue Cohosh.

CAULOPHYLLUM THALICTROIDES • *See* Blue Cohosh.

CAUSALGIA • Severe pain caused by injury to sensory nerves, especially of the palms and soles.

CAUSTICUM (H) • **Potassium Hydrate.** Homeopathic medicine to treat coughs and sore throat. Causticum was invented by Hahnemann. He made it from burnt or slaked lime (calcium hydroxide), which he mixed with bisulphate of potash. Causticum smells like lye. It has an astringent and burning taste. The caustic characteristic of this compound is one of the major indications for its use as a homeopathic remedy. It is for serious burns that blister. It is also used to treat bed-wetting, constipation, cough, cystitis, indigestion, and joint pain.

CAVACINE • *See* Mepivacaine.

CAYENNE (H) • *Capsicum rutescens.* **Green Pepper. Red Pepper.** Derived from the pungent fruit of the pepper plant, cayenne originated in Central and South America, where it was used by the natives for many diseases, including diarrhea and cramps. It contains capsaicin (*see*), carotenoids, flavonoids, essential oil, and vitamin C. Cayenne is a stimulant, astringent, laxative, and antispasmodic. Cayenne is not irritating when uncooked. Cayenne powder or tincture can be rubbed on toothaches, swellings, and inflammations. Scientists report that cayenne prevents the absorption of cholesterol. It is also reported by herbalists to lower blood pressure and serum cholesterol. Herbalists use it as a rub for inflamed joints, and to stop internal or external bleeding. *See also* Capsicum.

CCK • Abbreviation for cholecystokinin (*see*).

CCNU • *See* Iomutine.

CEBID TIMECELLES • *See* Vitamin C.

CECLOR • *See* Cefaclor.

CEDAX • *See* Cephalosporins.

CEENU • *See* Iomutine.

CEFACLOR (Rx) • **Ceclor.** Introduced in 1979, it is a cephalosporin (*see*) used to treat infections of the respiratory and urinary tracts, skin and soft tissue, and middle ear infections due to *Haemophilus influenzae, Streptococcus pneumoniae, Escherichia coli, Proteus, Klebsiella,* and *Staphylococcus aureus* (*see all*). Potential adverse reactions include anemia, dizziness, headache, sleepiness, nausea, vomiting, diarrhea, loss of appetite, and colitis. May also cause a vaginal superinfection, allergic reactions, fever, and jaundice. Should not be taken with probenecid. Up to 16 percent of those allergic to penicillin will be allergic to cefaclor. May be taken with or without food. As of this writing, cefaclor was soon to become available as a lower-cost generic drug.

CEFADROXIL MONOHYDRATE (Rx) • **Duricef. Ultracef.** A cephalosporin (*see*) antibiotic introduced in 1977, used to treat urinary tract infections caused by *Escherichia coli, Proteus,* and *Klebsiella* (*see all*), infections of skin and soft tissue, and streptococcal sore throat. Reportedly a high cure rate of 90 percent with cefadroxil monohydrate, versus 76 percent for penicillin. Potential adverse effects include anemia, dizziness, headache, malaise, paresthesia (*see*), colitis, nausea, loss of appetite, vomiting, diarrhea, sore throat, heartburn, abdominal cramps, rash, and thrush (*see*). May also cause genital itching, yeast infections, and shortness of breath. Up to 16 percent of those allergic to penicillin will be allergic to cefadroxil. This drug may be taken with food.

CEFADYL • *See* Cephapirin Sodium.

CEFAMANDOLE NAFATE (Rx) • **Mandol.** A cephalosporin (*see*) antibiotic used to treat respiratory and genitourinary tract infections, skin and soft-tissue infections, bone and joint infections, blood poisoning and peritonitis due to *Escherichia coli* (*see*) and other coliform bacteria, *Streptococcus, Klebsiella, Haemophilus influenzae, Proteus,* and *Enterobacter* (*see all*). Potential adverse reactions include anemia, bleeding, headache, malaise, numbness, dizziness, colitis, nausea, loss of appetite, vomiting, diarrhea, sore tongue, heartburn, abdominal cramps, painful spasms of the anal sphincter, genital itching, hives, rashes, pain at injection site, allergic reactions, and shortness of breath. Interacts with alcohol (even several days after discontinuing the medication), and with aspirin and other anticoagulants because it may cause bleeding.

CEFANEX • *See* Cephalexin.

CEFAZOLIN SODIUM (Rx) • **Ancef. Kefzol. Zolicef.** A broad-spectrum cephalosporin (*see*) introduced in 1973, used to treat serious infections of the respiratory and genitourinary tracts, skin and soft-tissue infections, bone and joint infections, blood poisoning, *Haemophilus influenzae, Klebsiella, Proteus, Staphylococcus aureus, Streptococcus pneumoniae,* and bacterial infections of the heart. Potential adverse reactions include anemia, dizziness, headache, malaise, numbness, colitis, nausea, loss of appetite, sore tongue, diarrhea, heartburn, abdominal cramps, itching and/or spasm of the anus, thrush, genital itching, vaginal yeast infections, skin rash, hives, inflammation at the injection site, hypersensitivity, and shortness of breath. Probenecid (*see*) may inhibit excretion and increase blood levels of cefazolin. Given only under close medical supervision.

CEFIXIME (Rx) • **Suprax.** A cephalosporin (*see*) antibiotic introduced in 1989, used to treat urinary-tract infections caused by *Escherichia coli* and *Proteus mirabilis,* ear infections caused by *Haemophilus influenzae, Moraxella,* and *Streptococcus,* and sore throat and tonsillitis caused by *Streptococcus pyrogenes.* Also used to treat bronchitis caused by *Streptococcus pneumoniae.* In one study of 9,600 bronchitis patients, 95 percent were cured or improved by administration of cefixime. Potential adverse reactions include reduction in white blood cells, headaches, dizziness, diarrhea, abdominal pain, nausea, vomiting, dyspepsia, flatulence, colitis, genital itching, vaginitis, genital candidiasis, skin rash, hives, fever, and hypersensitivity reactions. Allergic reactions may occur in up to 10 percent of patients with a history of penicillin allergy. Cefixime may cause a misreading of tests for diabetes. It has the advantage of being administered as a single dose, once a day, or in equally divided doses twice a day. Most effective when taken on an empty stomach, but may be taken with food if stomach upset is a problem.

CEFIZOX • *See* Ceftizoxime Sodium.

CEFLOR • *See* Cefaclor.

CEFMETAZOLE (Rx) • **Zefazone.** A second-generation cephalosporin (*see*) useful on many aerobic and anaerobic bacterial infections.

CEFMETAZOLE SODIUM (Rx) • **Zefazone.** A cephalosporin (*see*) antibiotic used to treat lower-respiratory-tract infections caused by *Streptococcus pneumoniae, Staphylococcus aureus, Escherichia coli,* and *Hemophilus influenzae* (*see all*). Also used to treat urinary tract infections and to prevent infections in patients undergoing colorectal surgery, cesarean sections, and gallbladder surgery. Potential adverse reactions include headache, shock, low blood pressure, nosebleed, lung problems, rash, pain at the site of injection, fever, superinfections, vein blood clots, hypersensitivity, and altered color perception.

CEFOBID • *See* Cefoperazone Sodium.

CEFOL (OTC) • A multivitamin preparation.

CEFONICID SODIUM (Rx) • **Monocid.** A cephalosporin (*see*) antibiotic used to treat serious infections of the lower-respiratory and urinary tracts, skin infections, blood poisoning, and bone and joint bacterial infections. Potential adverse reactions include anemia, dizziness, headache, malaise, numbness, colitis, nausea, loss of appetite, vomiting, diarrhea, sore tongue, heartburn, abdominal cramps, anal pruritus, spasms of the anal sphincter, thrush, genital itching, vaginal yeast infections, rashes, blood clot

in the vein at the site of injection, hypersensitivity, and shortness of breath. Probenecid (*see*) may inhibit excretion and increase blood levels of cefonicid.

CEFOPERAZONE SODIUM (Rx) • **Cefobid.** A cephalosporin (*see*) antibiotic introduced in 1982, used to treat serious bacterial infections of the respiratory tract and the abdomen. Also used to treat gynecological infections, skin infections, and blood poisoning. Potential adverse effects include anemia, bleeding, headache, malaise, numbness, dizziness, colitis, nausea, loss of appetite, vomiting, diarrhea, sore tongue, heartburn, abdominal cramps, spasms of the anal sphincter, itching of the anus and genitalia, thrush, and rashes. May interact with alcohol, even several days after discontinuing the drug. Cefoperazone may also increase the risk of bleeding if aspirin or other anticoagulants are taken, reduce vitamin K so that supplementation may be necessary, and cause false reading of blood sugar tests. Probenecid (*see*) may inhibit excretion and increase blood levels of cefoperazone.

CEFORANIDE (Rx) • **Precef.** A cephalosporin (*see*) antibiotic used to treat blood poisoning and serious infections of the lower-respiratory and urinary tracts, skin, heart, and bones and joints. Potential adverse reactions include a drop in white blood cells, confusion, headache, lethargy, colitis, nausea, loss of appetite, vomiting, diarrhea, sore tongue, heartburn, abdominal cramps, thrush, rash, hives, and pain, clotting, and inflammation at the injection site.

CEFOTAN • *See* Cefotetan Disodium.

CEFOTAXIME SODIUM (Rx) • **Claforan.** A cephalosporin (*see*) antibiotic used to treat some forms of meningitis, blood poisoning, and serious gynecological, lower-respiratory and urinary tract, central nervous system, and skin infections. Potential adverse reactions include anemia, headache, malaise, numbness, dizziness, colitis, nausea, loss of appetite, vomiting, diarrhea, sore tongue, heartburn, abdominal cramps, spasm and itching of the anus, thrush, genital itching, and moniliasis. May also cause hypersensitivity, shortness of breath, and elevated temperature.

CEFOTETAN DISODIUM (Rx) • Cefotan. A cephalosporin (*see*) antibiotic used to treat blood poisoning and serious lower-respiratory and urinary tract, gynecological, skin, abdominal, and bone infections. Potential adverse reactions include anemia, headache, malaise, numbness, dizziness, colitis, nausea, loss of appetite, vomiting, diarrhea, sore tongue, heartburn, abdominal cramps, spasm and itching of the anus, thrush, genital itching, and moniliasis. May also cause hypersensitivity, shortness of breath, and elevated temperature.

CEFOXITIN SODIUM (Rx) • Mefoxin. A cephalosporin (*see*) antibiotic used to treat blood poisoning and serious respiratory and genitourinary tract, skin and soft tissue, bone and joint, and intra-abdominal infections. Potential adverse reactions include anemia, headache, malaise, numbness, dizziness, colitis, nausea, loss of appetite, vomiting, diarrhea, sore tongue, heartburn, abdominal cramps, spasm and itching of the anus, thrush, genital itching, and moniliasis. May also cause hypersensitivity, shortness of breath, and elevated temperature. Probenecid (*see*) may increase blood levels of cefoxitin.

CEFPODOXIME (Rx) • Vantin. A broad-spectrum oral antibiotic, introduced in 1992, for the treatment of mild to moderate infections in adults and children (over six months of age).

CEFPROZIL (Rx) • Cefzil. A broad-spectrum antibiotic introduced in 1991, it is an oral cephalosporin (*see*) used to treat infections, caused by susceptible organisms, of the respiratory tract, ear, skin, bone and joint, and urinary tract; also gynecological infections, sinusitis, and septicemia. It can be prescribed for once-a-day use, an advantage. Penicillin-sensitive patients may also be sensitive to this drug.

CEFTAZIDIME (Rx) • Ceptaz. Magnacef. Tazicef. Tazidime. A cephalosporin (*see*) antibiotic used to treat serious lower-respiratory and urinary tract, gynecological, skin, abdominal, and central nervous system infections. Potential adverse reactions include a drop in white blood cells, headache, malaise, numbness, dizziness, colitis, nausea, loss of appetite, vomiting, diarrhea, bad taste in the mouth, abdominal cramps, spasm and itching of the anus, thrush, genital itching, and moniliasis. May also cause hypersensitivity, shortness of breath, and elevated temperature. Kidney dysfunction has been reported with concomitant use of a cephalosporin and an aminoglycoside antibiotic or potent diuretics. Chloramphenicol is contraindicated for use with this drug.

CEFTIBUTIN (Rx) • Cedax. A once-a-day, broad spectrum oral cephalosporin (*see*) antibiotic, introduced in 1995. It is used for the treatment of acute bacterial worsening of chronic bronchitis (*see*), acute bacterial otitis media, pharyngitis (*see*), and tonsillitis.

**CEFTIN • ** *See* Cefuroxime Axetil and Sodium.

CEFTIZOXIME (Rx) • Cefizox. An antibiotic used to treat infections, caused by susceptible organisms, of the respiratory tract, ear, skin, bone and joint, and urinary tract; also gynecological infections, sinusitis, and blood poisoning. *See* Cephalosporins.

**CEFTIZOXIME SODIUM (Rx) • ** A cephalosporin (*see*) antibiotic used to treat blood poisoning, serious infections of the covering of the brain (meningitis), and lower-respiratory and urinary tract, gynecological, intra-abdominal, and skin infections, and Lyme disease (*see*). Potential adverse reactions include a drop in white blood cells, headache, dizziness, colitis, vomiting, diarrhea, bad taste in the mouth, abdominal cramps, genital itching and moniliasis, rashes, and hives. May cause a reaction at the injection site.

CEFTRIAXONE (Rx) • Rocephin. A cephalosporin (*see*) antibiotic indicated for lower-respiratory and urinary tract, skin, intra-abdominal, and bone and joint infections. It is also used for uncomplicated gonorrhea, pelvic inflammatory disease, and meningitis, and to prevent infections after surgery. Promoted as a once-a-day antibiotic. Potential adverse reactions include pain at the site of injection, hypersensitivity that could be life threatening, a lowering of white blood cells and prolongation of the blood-clotting time, diarrhea, colitis, nausea, vomiting, bad taste in the mouth, kidney and liver dysfunction, headache or dizziness, moniliasis, vaginitis, sweating, and flushing. Contraindicated in patients with known allergy to cephalosporins. Should be used cautiously in patients with a history of gastrointestinal diseases, particularly colitis, and in those sensitive to penicillins in particular, and allergies in general. Ceftriaxone treatment for infections should be continued for at least ten days.

CEFTRIAXONE SODIUM (Rx) • A cephalosporin (*see*) used to treat home-care patients with severe infections, gonorrhea, or chancroid, or who are at high risk of blood poisoning or may have food poisoning such as salmonella (*see*) or shigella, or pneumonia of unknown origin. *See also* Cephalosporins and Shigella Bacillus.

CEFUROXIME AXETIL and SODIUM (Rx) • **Ceftin. Kefurox. Zinacef.** A cephalosporin (*see*) antibiotic introduced in 1976, used for treatment of serious infections of the lower-respiratory and urinary tract, skin infections, blood poisoning, meningitis, and gonorrhea. Potential adverse reactions include anemia, headache, malaise, numbness, dizziness, colitis, nausea, loss of appetite, vomiting, diarrhea, sore tongue, heartburn, abdominal cramps, spasm and itching of the anus, rash, hives, and inflammation at the site of injection. Allergic reactions mild to severe may occur in up to 1 percent of the population; 2.9 percent of those allergic to penicillin will be allergic to cefuroxime. Most effective when taken without food, but may be taken with some food if stomach upset is a problem. *See* Cephalosporins.

CEFZIL • *See* Cefprozil.

CELANDINE (H) • *Chelidonium majus.* **Devil's Milk. Rock Poppy. Swallowwort.** This tall herb contains alkaloids, choline, histamine, tyramine, saponins, chelidoniol, chelidonic acid, carotene, and vitamin C. Herbalists use it for the treatment of hepatitis, jaundice, cancer, psoriasis, eczema, corns, and warts. Used for more than two thousand years to soothe the eyes, it also reputedly detoxifies the liver and relieves muscle spasms and bronchospasms. It is used to treat gallbladder problems. The plant can cause a miscarriage when ingested and therefore should not be used during pregnancy. Sanguinarine found in this plant produces glaucoma in experimental animals and also cancer.

-CELE • Suffix meaning swelling or herniation of a part, such as *cystocele,* prolapse of the bladder.

CELERY SEED (H) • *Apium graveolens.* **Smallage.** One of the first condiments to reach the country of the Gauls and Franks, it was introduced into northern Europe by military men upon returning home from Roman conquests. Celery seed is used by herbalists as a diuretic, blood cleanser, and to treat arthritis. In 1992, scientists reported what herbalists had long known—that celery lowers blood pressure. In Europe, celery seed is a common treatment for gout and rheumatism. Some persons are allergic to celery.

CELESTONE • *See* Betamethasone.

CELIAC SPRUE • **Celiac Disease. Gluten Intolerance. Gluten Sensitive Enteropathy. Nontropical Sprue.** A condition in which gluten (a protein found in wheat, rye, oats, and barley) causes abnormal chemical response in the bowel lining, and malabsorption.

CELL • The smallest living unit that is able to grow and reproduce. A single cell may be a complete organism such as a bacterium or may represent a specialized cell that is part of a large plant or animal.

CELLCEPT • *See* Mycophenolate.

CELLUFRESH LUBRICANT OPHTHALMIC SOLUTION • *See* Carboxymethylcellulose.

CELLULAR IMMUNITY • Produced by B (from bone marrow) and T (from thymus gland) white blood cells that bind to invaders such as germs or cancer cells.

CELLULITIS • An acute, spreading skin infection that extends down to the soft (connective) tissue. It is accompanied by fever, malaise, chills, and extensive spread of a red, hot, swollen lesion that is neither elevated nor has a sharp demarcation.

CELLULOSE • The chief constituent of plant fiber, it is the basic material for cellulose gums used as emulsifiers (*see*). Banned from diet products by the FDA in 1990.

CELLULOSE METHYL ETHER • *See* Methylcellulose.

CELLULOSE SODIUM PHOSPHATE (Rx) • **Calcibind.** A compound used to prevent the formation of calcium-containing kidney stones. Used in patients who absorb too much calcium from their food, it combines with calcium and some minerals in food, thus preventing the calcium from reaching the kidneys where the stones are formed.

CELLUVISC LUBRICANT OPHTHALMIC SOLUTION • *See* Carboxymethylcellulose.

CELONTIN • See Methsuximide.

CEMI-REGROTON (Rx) • A combination of chlorthalidone and reserpine (*see both*).

CENAFED • *See* Pseudoephedrine.

CENA-K • *See* Potassium Chloride.

CENOCORT • *See* Triamcinolone.

CENOLATE • *See* Ascorbic Acid.

CENTAURY (H) • *Erythraea centaureum.* **Red Centaury.** A small, pretty annual native to the United Kingdom, it is a member of the gentian (*see*) family. Used by herbalists for jaundice. A bitter compound gives the herb its strong taste and aids digestion and the flow of gastric juices. It supposedly has a soothing effect on the lining of the intestines. A tisane (*see*) made as a tonic, to stimulate appetite and digestion. A strong antiseptic good for cuts and scratches; also used as a mouthwash.

CENTRAL NERVOUS SYSTEM • CNS. Composed of the brain and the spinal cord with its bundle of nerves running through it.

CENTRAX • *See* Prazepam.

CENTRUM (OTC) • A multivitamin preparation.

CENTURY PLANT • *See* Agave.

CEPACOL DRY THROAT LOZENGES • *See* Benzoyl Peroxide.

CEPASTAT • *See* Phenol.

CEPHAELIS IPECACUANHA • *See* Ipecac.

CEPHAL- • Prefix pertaining to the head, as in *cephalalgia,* head pain.

CEPHALEXIN (Rx) • **Ceporex. Keflet. Keflex. Keftab. Novolexin.** A cephalosporin (*see*) antibiotic introduced in 1969, used to treat respiratory or genitourinary tract, skin and soft-tissue, bone and joint, and middle-ear infections. Potential adverse reactions include anemia, headache, malaise, numbness, dizziness, colitis, nausea, loss of appetite, vomiting, diarrhea, sore tongue, heartburn, abdominal cramps, spasm and itching of the anus, moniliasis vaginitis, rash, hives, shortness of breath, hypersensitivity reactions, and inflammation at the site of injection. Should not be taken with other antibiotics such as erythromycins or tetracyclines (*see both*). Cephalexin may cause a false positive result in a test for sugar in urine. Cephalexin is most effective when taken on an empty stomach, but may be taken with food if stomach upset is a problem.

CEPHALIC • Pertaining to the head.

CEPHALOSPORINS (Rx) • **Anspor. Ceclor. Cefaclor. Cefadroxil. Cefazolin. Cefixime. Cefizox. Cefoperazone. Cefoxitin. Ceftin. Cefuroxime. Cephalexin. Cephalothin. Duricef. Keflex. Keftab. Suprax. Ultracef. Velosef. Cefazolin Sodium. Cefmetazole Sodium. Cefonicid Sodium. Cefoperazone Sodium. Ceforanide. Cefotaxime Sodium. Cefotetan Disodium. Ceftazidime. Ceftizoxime Sodium. Ceftriaxone Sodium. Cefuroxime Axetil. Cephapirin Sodium. Cephradine. Cefpiramide. Moxalactam Disodium.** Broad-spectrum antibiotics of the beta-lactam (*see*) class structurally similar to penicillins. Some people who are allergic to penicillin are also allergic to cephalosporins. The first, cephalosporin A., was isolated in 1948 from a microorganism discovered in the sea near Sardinia. There are now more than twenty. The activity of cephalosporins is due to their ability to inactivate bacterial enzymes involved in cell-wall production, killing the bacteria or interfering with their growth. Cephalosporins are used to treat a number of infections and are sometimes given with other antibiotics. They may be given by injection to prevent infections before, during, and after surgery. The most common side effects are diarrhea, nausea and vomiting, sore mouth or tongue, stomach cramps, and vaginal itching. May less often cause fever, unusual bleeding or bruising, peeling of the skin, convulsions, a decrease in urine, dizziness, joint or muscle pain, loss of appetite, skin rash, shortness of breath, and pain, redness, and swelling at place of injection. One of the most serious but rare side effects is interference with normal blood clotting. Alcohol and alcohol-containing medications may increase cephalosporins' GI disturbances. Blood thinners, carbenicillin, heparin, NSAIDs (*see*), pentoxifylline, plicamycin, sulfinpyrazone, ticarcillin, and valproic acid may increase the chance of bleeding. Probenecid increases cephalosporins' blood levels. Cephalosporins may be taken orally on a full or empty stomach.

CEPHALOTHIN (Rx) • **Ceporacin Seffin. Keflin.** A cephalosporin (*see*) antibiotic. Used in the treatment of susceptible bacterial infections, including those caused by streptococcus. *See* Cephalosporins.

CEPHAPIRIN SODIUM (Rx) • **Cefadyl.** A cephalosporin (*see*) antibiotic used in the treatment of blood poisoning and serious infections of the respiratory, genitourinary, or gastrointestinal tract, skin and soft tissue, bone and joint, and heart. Potential adverse reactions include anemia, headache, malaise, numbness, dizziness, colitis, nausea, loss of appetite, vomiting, kidney dysfunction, diarrhea, sore tongue, heartburn, abdominal cramps, spasm and itching of the anus, moniliasis vaginitis, rash, hives, shortness of breath, hypersensitivity reactions, and inflammation at the site of injection. Use with probenecid (*see*) may increase levels of cephalosporins in the blood. *See* Cephalosporins.

CEPHRADINE (Rx) • **Anspor. Velosef.** A cephalosporin (*see*) antibiotic used in the treatment of blood poisoning and serious infections of the respiratory, genitourinary, or gastrointestinal tract, skin and soft tissue, bone and joint, heart, and middle ear. Potential adverse reactions include a low white blood cell count, headache, malaise, numbness, dizziness, colitis, nausea, loss of appetite, vomiting, kidney dysfunction, diarrhea, sore tongue, heartburn, abdominal cramps, spasm and itching of the anus, oral thrush, rash, hives, shortness of breath, hypersensitivity reactions, and inflammation at the site of injection. Use with probenecid (*see*) may increase levels of cephalosporins in the blood. *See* Cephalosporins.

CEPHULAC • *See* Lactulose.

CEPORACIN • *See* Cephalothin.

CEPOREX • *See* Cephalexin.

CEPTAZ • *See* Ceftazidime.

CEREBRAL PALSY • A general term for disorders of movement and posture resulting from damage to the brain.

CEREBRAL THROMBOSIS • Formation of a blood clot in a vessel leading to the brain.

CEREBROVASCULAR ACCIDENT • A stroke, resulting from the interruption of blood supply to the brain.

CEREBROVASCULAR DISEASE • Disorders of the blood vessels of the brain.

CEREDASE • *See* Alglucerase.

CERESPAN • *See* Papaverine Hydrochloride.

CEREUS • *See* Night-Blooming Cereus.

CEREZYME • *See* Imiglucerase.

CEROSE-DM (OTC) • An expectorant that combines dextromethorphan, phenylephrine, and chlorpheniramine (*see all*). Used for the temporary relief of cough due to minor throat and bronchial irritation as may occur with the common cold or with inhaled irritants. Temporarily relieves nasal congestion and sneezing. May cause marked drowsiness; alcohol may increase the drowsiness effects. Other potential adverse reactions include excitability, especially in children. Unless directed by a physician, contraindicated in people who have heart disease, high blood pressure, thyroid disease, diabetes, asthma, glaucoma, emphysema, chronic lung disease, or difficulty in urination due to enlargement of the prostate gland. The product should not be taken for more than one week.

CERTIFIED • A batch of coal tar or petrochemical color that is certified by the FDA as "harmless and suitable for use." The manufacturer must submit samples of the batch for testing. The lot test number accompanies the colors through all subsequent packaging.

CERUBIDINE • *See* Daunorubicin Hydrochloride.

CERUMENEX • *See* Triethanolamine.

CERVI- • Prefix meaning neck, such as in *cervix,* the "neck" of the womb, or *cervical collar,* a device used in neck injuries.

CERVICAL • Relating to the neck of the uterus.

CERVIX • The narrow outer end of the uterus.

C.E.S. • *See* Estrogen.

CESAMET • *See* Nabilone.

CETACAINE • A combination of benzocaine and tetracaine (*see both*) used as a local anesthetic.

CETACORT • *See* Hydrocortisone.

CETALKONIUM CHLORIDE (OTC) • Derived from ammonia, it is an antibacterial agent. In 1992, the FDA issued a notice that cetalkonium chloride had not been shown to be safe and effective as claimed for poison ivy, poison sumac, and poison oak OTC products.

CETAMIDE • *See* Sulfacetamide.

CETANE (OTC) • *See* Vitamin C.

CETAPRED (Rx) • A combination of prednisolone and sulfacetamide (*see both*) used to treat eye inflammations.

CETIRIZINE (Rx) • **Zyrtec.** An antihistamine approved by the FDA in 1995 for the treatment of seasonal and perennial allergic rhinitis and chronic urticaria (hives) (*see all*). Taken once-a-day, its activity reportedly lasts for 24 hours. Potential adverse effects include drowsiness, fatigue, dry mouth, and dizziness. Alcohol may increase its depressant effect.

CETRARIA ISLANDICA • *See* Iceland Moss.

CETYL ALCOHOL • A waxy, crystalline, and solid substance found in spermaceti (whale oil). It is used as an emollient and emulsion stabilizer in many cosmetic and drug preparations. It has a low toxicity when applied to skin or ingested and is sometimes used as a laxative. It can cause hives.

CETYLPYRIDINIUM CHLORIDE (OTC) • **Cepacol.** A salt of pyridine and cetyl chloride, it is a topical anti-infective and a soothing temporary relief for dry mouth and throat.

CEVALIN (OTC) • *See* Vitamin C.

CEVI-BID (OTC) • *See* Vitamin C.

CEVITA (OTC) • *See* Vitamin C.

CG • Abbreviation for chorionic gonadotropin (*see*).

CHAM • Homeopathic abbreviation for chamomile (*see*).

CHAMAELIRIUM (H) • *See* False Unicorn Root.

CHAMOMILE (OTC) (H) • *Matricaria chamomilla. Anthemis nobilis.* **German Chamomile. Hungarian Chamomile. Roman Chamomile. Hyland's Calms Forte Tablets. Hyland's Colic Tablets. Hyland's Teething Tablets.** A native of Europe, it grows wild in all the temperate parts of the continent. Only the flowers of the herb, a popular plant in herb gardens, are used. It contains flavonoids and glycosides (*see both*) as well as the essential oils chamazulene and bisabolol. In moderate doses, the flowers are used to soothe indigestion, gas, colic, gout, and headaches. A strong infusion acts as an efficient emetic. The oil has stimulant and antispasmodic properties; it is useful in treating gas and is added to purgatives to prevent cramps. The oil is used with crushed poppy heads as a poultice for toothaches and neuralgia as well as for boils and inflammations. Its anti-inflammatory properties have been compared to those of papaverine (*see*). Herbalists claim that chamomile tea prevents nightmares. A chamomile tea is used for relaxation, to aid digestion, to treat coughs, and to increase appetite. If you are allergic to ragweed, chrysanthemums, or asters, you may be allergic to chamomile because it is a member of the same plant family. May cause skin irritation and anaphylaxis (*see*). In 1992, the FDA issued a notice that chamomile had not been shown to be safe and effective as claimed in OTC digestive-aid products.

CHAMOMILE OIL (H) • *See* Matricaria Extract and Oil.

CHANGROLIN (Rx) (H) • An antiarrhythmic (*see*) drug derived from a traditional Chinese antimalarial medication.

CHAPARRAL (H) • *Larrea indentata.* **Creosote Bush. Grease Wood.** The leaf of this dwarf evergreen oak contains antioxidants and is considered an antibiotic by herbalists. It is used for blood purification, cancer and tumors, arthritis, colds, flu, diarrhea, urinary tract infections, and as an antioxidant. Native Americans used it to treat arthritis. A modern Argentine study showed that the primary constituent of chaparral, NDGA (nordihydroguaiaretic acid), an antioxidant, possesses pain-relieving and blood-pressure-lowering properties. Chaparral was removed from the Generally Recognized as Safe (GRAS) list in 1970. Four cases of chaparral-induced toxic hepatitis have been reported by the FDA in the 1990s. One woman required a liver and kidney transplant reportedly due to her self-medication with chaparral to treat her heart disease.

CHARCOAID (OTC) • *See* Charcoal.

CHARCOAL (OTC) (H) • **Actidose-Aqua. Actidose with Sorbitol. Activated Charcoal. Charcoaid. Charcocaps. Liqui-Char.** Activated charcoal is sometimes given to absorb and inactivate poisons or overdosed drugs that have been taken orally. Some activated-charcoal products contain sorbitol, a sweetener that works as a laxative, to eliminate toxins from the body. Activated charcoal without sorbitol may be used to relieve diarrhea and intestinal gas. Potential adverse reactions include nausea, vomiting, and stomach pain. In 1992, the FDA issued a notice that charcoal (wood) had not been shown to be safe and effective as claimed in OTC digestive-aid products.

CHARCOCAPS (OTC) • *See* Charcoal.

CHARDONNA-2 (Rx) • A combination of belladonna and phenobarbital (*see both*).

CHASTE BERRIES (H) • *Vitex agnus-castus.* **Chasteberry. Chaste Tree. Hemp Tree. Monk's Pepper. Vitex.** The fruit contains volatile oil, glycosides, flavonoids, and castine. In ancient times, the berries were used to suppress libido in Greek temple priestesses. The herb is used for premenstrual syndrome (PMS), menopause, and to regulate the menstrual cycle. The plant is claimed to have an inhibiting effect on male sexual desire, hence the common name, monk's pepper.

CHEALAMIDE • *See* Edetate Disodium.

CHECKERBERRY EXTRACT (H) • *See* Wintergreen Oil.

CHECKMATE (OTC) • *See* Sodium Fluoride.

CHELATE • A compound formed when a metallic ion is bound to an organic molecule.

CHELATION • The process by which a compound, such as edetate calcium disodium, binds and precipitates a metal. Such compounds are used to remove lead, iron, and other elements from the body. In experiments by Martin Rubin, Ph.D., professor emeritus of the School of Medicine at Georgetown University, he claims intravenous ethylenediamine can chelate the fat and calcium plaques that block arteries, and the materials are harmlessly excreted in the urine. Chelation for this purpose is controversial.

CHELIDONIUM MAJUS (H) • *See* Celandine.

CHEMET • *See* Succimer.

CHEMOTHERAPY • A cancer treatment that utilizes potent chemicals to kill cancer cells; used alone or in combination depending on the type of disease. A major side effect of many chemotherapeutic drugs is bone marrow (*see*) damage. Other side effects include hair loss and nausea.

CHENIX • *See* Chenodiol.

CHENODEOXYCHOLIC ACID • *See* Chenodiol.

CHENODIOL (Rx) • **Chenodeoxycholic Acid. Chenix.** A digestant that suppresses manufacture by the liver of cholesterol and cholic acid, thus causing gradual dissolution of gallstones. Potential adverse reactions frequently include diarrhea, cramps, heartburn, constipation, nausea, vomiting, loss of appetite, stomach pain, and liver dysfunction. Cholestyramine, colestipol, estrogens, oral contraceptives, and clofibrate decrease chenodiol's effects. Contraindicated in people with liver dysfunction, gallbladder trouble, gallstone pancreatitis, or biliary GI fistula. The drug is particularly effective in breaking up small, floatable gallstones. A low-cholesterol, high-fiber diet is often recommended. Full beneficial effects of this medication may not be evident for up to eighteen months. Chenodiol is most effective when taken on an empty stomach, but may be taken with food if stomach upset is a problem.

CHERACOL (Rx) • A combination of codeine and guaifenesin (*see both*) used to treat coughs.

CHERVIL (H) • *Anthriscus cerefolium.* An herb of the carrot family, native to Europe. Used as a restorative for the elderly, it was called cerefolium, meaning "leaves of the brain," because it was said to be a powerful brain stimulant. It is also a digestive, diuretic, and expectorant. The juice is used for edema, abscesses, eczema, and gout. As a poultice, it is used for arthritic pains. An infusion (*see*) of herbs is made to lower blood pressure.

CHESTNUT (H) • *Castanea vulgaris.* **Horse Chestnut. Spanish Chestnut. Sweet Chestnut.** Nut from a tree of the beech family, used as a remedy for piles, backaches, and for coughs. An astringent, the bark and leaves were used to make a tonic, which was also useful, reportedly, in the treatment of upper-respiratory ailments such as coughs, particularly whooping cough. The bark of Spanish chestnut contains tannins (*see*).

CHIBROXIN • *See* Norfloxacin.

CHICKEN POX • Caused by the varicella-zoster virus of the herpes family, it is an acute but usually benign disease. It causes generalized skin rash of three hundred to five hundred blisters. It is much more serious in adults than in children. The most common complication among adults is pneumonia. After the acute illness, the varicella-zoster virus remains dormant in the infected person's sensory nerve roots for life. Herpes zoster or shingles (*see*) results from reactivation of that virus, usually in adulthood. *See* Varicella Virus Vaccine, Live.

CHICKEN POX VACCINE • *See* Varicella Virus Vaccine, Live.

CHICKEN SOUP • **Jewish Penicillin.** Long used in folk medicine as a cure for the common cold. In the seventies and eighties, researchers found chicken soup contains an amino acid, cysteine, that is similar to a drug, acetylcysteine (*see*), prescribed for people with respiratory infections because it thins the mucus in the lungs.

CHICKWEED (H) • *Stellaria media.* **Herbal Slim. Starweed. Winterweed.** The herb contains saponins, which exert an anti-inflammatory action similar to that of cortisone but, according to herbalists, is much milder and without side effects. Chickweed also is used for weight loss, skin irritation, itches and rashes, and to soothe sore throat and lungs. Excessive doses reportedly can cause temporary paralysis.

CHICORY (H) • *Cichorium intybus.* **Wild Succory.** Related to dandelion, in ancient times it was used as a narcotic, sometimes administered before operations. Used by herbalists to treat liver problems, constipation, and arthritis.

CHIGGERTOX • *See* Benzocaine.

CHILDREN'S IBUPROFEN (Rx) (OTC) • **Children's Advil Suspension.** A reduced dose for children, this anti-inflammatory agent should be used with great care. In clinical studies of adults with rheumatoid arthritis, ibuprofen has analgesic and antifever activities similar to aspirin. Children must be carefully followed for signs and symptoms suggesting liver dysfunction particularly with doses above 30 mg/kg per day, or if abnormal tests have occurred. Children should be carefully followed for signs and symptoms of gastrointestinal ulceration and bleeding. The medication should not be used in cases of kidney failure or dehydration. *See* Ibuprofen.

CHILD-RESISTANT PACKAGING • Packaging designed to prevent young children from opening a medication's container. The resistant packages, however, often prevent older people with arthritis from opening the container. Most pharmacists will provide easier-to-open packages upon request.

CHILI (H) • *Capsicum fastigatum.* Chili is the dried pod of a species of capsicum (*see*), or red pepper. The small pods have been used for dyspepsia (*see*) and dilated blood vessels arising from drunkenness. A capsicum poultice has been used with caution for the relief of aches and pains. Modern herbalists use it in pill and powder form, as a tincture, and as an infusion (*see*) for liniments and gargles. *See* Capsicum.

CHIMPLULA • *See* Pipsisseswa Leaves Extract.

CHIN • Abbreviation for *China officinalis* (*see*).

CHINA OFFICINALIS (H) • **Chin. Cinchona. Loxa Bark. Red Bark.** A homeopathic remedy from the bark of an evergreen tree that is indigenous to tropical forests of South America and cultivated in India. *See* Quinine.

CHINCHONA • *See* Quinine.

CHINESE CUCUMBER • *Trichomatoses kirilowii.* A Chinese herb containing TAP 29 (*see*), which has been reported by researchers at New York University to have potential against the AIDS virus. It is reportedly nontoxic to normal cells and may eventually be used in condoms, vaginal jellies, and toothpastes to minimize the risk of HIV transmission.

CHITIN (OTC) • The principal constituent of the shells of crabs, lobsters, and beetles. It is also found in some fungi, algae, and yeasts. It is used in folk medicine in wound-healing emulsions. *See* Glucosamine.

CHITOSAN • A derivative of chitin (*see*). Mixed with polyethylene oxide, it is being studied as a method of delivery for drugs. Of particular interest to researchers is its use to deliver medication in the stomach to combat *Heliobacter pylori* (*see*), the bacteria now targeted as the culprit in causing many cases of stomach ulcers. Chitosan mixtures allow more of the antibiotics to remain in the stomach and combat the foe.

CHITTEMBARK • *See* Cascara Sagrada.

CHLAMYDIA • A type of microorganism that causes a wide variety of ailments in humans, including "pink eye," prostatitis, urethritis, and epididymitis (an inflammation of a duct leading to the testicle). It is the most common sexually transmitted disease in the United States.

CHLO-AMINE • *See* Chlorpheniramine.

CHLOPHEDIANOL (OTC) • A cough medication closely related to antihistamines. Changed from Rx to OTC.

CHLORACOL • *See* Chloramphenicol.

CHLORAL • *See* Chloral Hydrate.

CHLORAL HYDRATE (Rx) (OTC) • **Trichloroacetaldehyde Monohydrate. Aquachloral Supprettes. Noctec. Somnos.** A short-term sedative and sleeping medication. The mechanism of its effect is unknown. It is rapidly effective and usually does not cause a daytime hangover. It is also used on the skin as an antiseptic. Potential adverse reactions include lung problems, hangover, drowsiness, difficulty swallowing, slow heartbeat, nightmares, dizziness, loss of balance, paradoxical excitement, nausea, vomiting, diarrhea, gas, and hypersensitivity reactions. Alcohol or other central nervous system depressants, including narcotic analgesics, may cause additive central nervous system depression or dilation of the blood vessels. Used with intravenous furosemide (*see*), it may cause sweating, flushing, variable blood pressure, and uneasiness. Oral blood thinners increase the risk of bleeding. Contraindications include liver and kidney impairment, and hypersensitivity to chloral hydrate, stomach disorders, severe heart disease, mental depression, and suicidal tendencies. Abuse may lead to addiction. Should be taken with full glass of fluid. Daytime doses are best taken after meals. In 1992, the FDA proposed a ban for the use of chloral hydrate to treat fever blisters and cold sores, and poison ivy, poison sumac, and poison oak, because it had not been shown to be safe and effective as claimed in OTC products.

CHLORAMBUCIL (Rx) • **Leukeran.** An anticancer drug introduced in 1957 that is used to treat chronic lymphocytic leukemia, lymphomas, Hodgkin's disease, and ovarian cancer. Potential adverse reactions include nausea, vomiting, anemia, bone-marrow suppression, seizures, infertility, high uric acid, liver dysfunction, lung changes, skin problems, and allergic fever reaction. Should be taken with food.

CHLORAMINE • *See* Chlorpheniramine.

CHLORAMPHENICOL (Rx) • **AK-Chlor. Chloromycetin. Chloromycetin Otic. Chloroptic. Econochlor Ophthalmic. I-Chlor. Ophthochlor Ophthalmic. Ophthocort. Sopamycetin.** Introduced in 1947, it is an antibiotic used to treat *Haemophilus influenzae,* salmonella, meningitis, bacteremia, Rocky Mountain spotted fever, lymphogranuloma, psittacosis, and other severe infections caused by *Salmonella* or *Rickettsia,* or various sensitive gram-negative (*see*) organisms. It also is used in topical preparations for eye and ear infections. Given by mouth or injection, it is widely distributed in the body and penetrates the brain as well, making it useful in the treatment of meningitis and brain abscesses. Potential adverse effects include fatal anemia, headache, mild depression, confusion, delirium, nerve damage, sore tongue, blurred vision, nausea, vomiting, diarrhea, colitis, severe allergic reactions, respiratory distress, and death in newborn infants. Instilled in the ear it can cause itching or burning, hives, skin rash, sore throat, and overgrowth of nonsusceptible organisms. Chloramphenicol should be used only to treat infections not responsive to less toxic drugs. It may increase the effect of other drugs including phenytoin, oral antidiabetics, and oral anticoagulants. Phenobarbital, phenytoin, and rifampin may reduce chloramphenicol's effects. Chloramphenicol may inhibit the antibacterial effects of penicillin and erythromycin antibiotics. It may delay the body's response to iron, vitamin B_{12}, or folic acid. Take with a full glass of water on an empty stomach.

CHLORASEPTIC (OTC) • A combination of phenol and menthol (*see both*), it was introduced in 1957 by a dentist for fast relief of dental pain. It is now widely used for sore throat and gum pain. *See also* Benzocaine.

CHLORATE • *See* Chlorpheniramine.

CHLORBUTANOL • A white, crystalline alcohol used as a preservative and as an antioxidant in lotions and oils. It has a camphor odor and taste. Formerly used medicinally as a hypnotic and sedative; today employed as an anesthetic and antiseptic. Potential adverse reactions include central nervous system depression.

CHLORCYCLIZINE (Rx) • **Mantadil Cream.** An antihistamine that blocks the receptor of histamine on the cells that especially affect smooth-muscle contractions and permeability of the skin. It prevents local swelling, is a local anesthetic, and soothes itches.

CHLORDIAZEPOXIDE (Rx) • **A-Poxide. Librax. Libritabs. Librium. Lipoxide. Methaminodiazepoxide. Reposans-10.** A minor tranquilizer introduced in 1960 to treat anxiety and tension, it belongs to the class of benzodiazepines (*see*). It reportedly has a wide margin of safety and few drug interactions. Potential adverse reactions include drowsiness, confusion, depression, lethargy, headache, inactivity, slurred speech, stupor, dizziness, tremor, constipation, dry mouth, nausea, lack

of urinary control, changes in sex drive, irregular menstruation, irregular heartbeat, low blood pressure, fluid retention, blurred or double vision, itching, rash, hiccups, nervousness, insomnia, and liver dysfunction. Contraindicated in those allergic to other benzodiazepines, or with narrow-angle glaucoma. Alcohol and other central nervous system depressants, including antihistamines and sleeping pills, increase chlordiazepoxide central nervous system depressive effects. Smoking may reduce its effectiveness. Cimetidine may prolong its action. Most effective when taken on an empty stomach, but may be taken with food if it causes gastrointestinal problems.

CHLORDIAZEPOXIDE and AMITRIPTYLINE (Rx) • **Limbitrol.** A drug combination used to treat mental depression. *See* Chlordiazepoxide and Amitriptyline, separate listings.

CHLORDIAZEPOXIDE and CLIDINIUM BROMIDE (Rx) • **Librax.** A antianxiety-agent combination used to relax the digestive system and to reduce stomach acid. *See* Chlordiazepoxide and Clidinium Bromide, separate listings.

CHLORESIUM (OTC) • *See* Chlorophyll.

CHLORHEXIDINE GLUCONATE (Rx) • **Hibiclens Antimicrobial Skin Cleanser. Hibistat Germicidal Hand Rinse. Hibistat Towelette.** Derived from methanol, it is a topical anti-infective used to treat sore gums, and as a hand cleanser.

CHLORMEZANONE (Rx) • **Trancopal.** A medication used to relieve nervousness or tension, usually without affecting alertness. The relief of symptoms often occurs within fifteen to thirty minutes and may last up to six hours. Potential adverse reactions include confusion, mental depression, drowsiness, stomach pains, aching muscles and joints, fever and chills, rash, itching, jaundice, swelling of feet or lower legs, and unusual excitement. Chlormezanone will add to the effects of alcohol and other central nervous system depressants, including cold and allergy medications, sedatives, pain medicine, seizure medicine, anesthetics, and muscle relaxants. Doses as low as seven grams have resulted in coma.

CHLOROBUTANOL (Rx) (OTC) • Isopto Pes. Outgro Solution. Colorless to white crystals derived from chloroform and acetone. Used to toughen the skin in ingrown toenails, as an antimicrobial agent, and as an anesthetic in dentistry. In 1992, the FDA proposed a ban on the use of chlorobutanol to treat fever blisters and cold sores, and poison ivy, poison oak, and poison sumac, because it had not been shown to be safe and effective as claimed in OTC products.

CHLOROETHANE • *See* Ethyl Chloride.

CHLOROFAIR • *See* Chloramphenicol.

CHLOROFON-F • *See* Chlorzoxazone.

CHLOROFORM (Rx) (OTC) • A general anesthetic. In 1992, the FDA issued a notice that chloroform had not been shown to be safe and effective as claimed in OTC digestive-aid products.

CHLOROMYCETIN • *See* Chloramphenicol.

CHLOROMYCETIN OTIC • *See* Chloramphenicol.

CHLOR-100 • *See* Chlorpheniramine.

CHLOROPHEN-LA • *See* Oxymetazoline.

CHLOROPHENOTHANE (OTC) • **Dichlorodiphenyltrichloroethane.** In 1992, the FDA proposed a ban on chlorophenothane in lice-killing products because it had not been shown to be safe and effective as claimed.

CHLOROPHYLL (OTC) • Chloresium. Derifil. The green coloring matter of plants, which plays an essential part in photosynthesis. Used topically, it promotes normal healing, relieves pain, inflammation, abrasions, and skin irritation, and reduces malodors in wounds, burns, and surface ulcers. It also is used orally, to control bowel and urinary odors in colostomy (*see*), ileostomy (*see*), and incontinence. Can cause a sensitivity to light.

CHLOROPROCAINE (Rx) • **Nesacaine.** A local anesthetic used to block nerves, and for caudal and epidural anesthesia. Potential adverse reactions include skin reactions, swelling, continuous asthma attacks, severe allergic reactions, anxiety, nervousness, and seizures followed by drowsiness, unconsciousness, tremors, twitches, shivering, and respiratory arrest. Other potential reactions include blurred vision, ringing in the ears, nausea, and vomiting. Contraindicated in patients with hypersensitivity to procaine, tetracaine, or other para-aminobenzoic acid (*see*) derivatives.

CHLOROPTIC • *See* Chloramphenicol.

CHLOROQUIN • *See* Chloroquine Hydrochloride, Phosphate, or Sulfate.

CHLOROQUINE HYDROCHLORIDE, PHOSPHATE, or SULPHATE (Rx) • Aralen HCL. Aralen Phosphate. Chloroquin. Nivaquine. An antimalarial introduced in 1943 to prevent and treat acute attacks of malaria, and some forms of amebic dysentery. Sometimes also used to treat rheumatoid arthritis and related diseases. Potential adverse effects include a drop in white blood cells, anemia, and a drop in blood platelets. May also cause headache, nerve damage, psychic stimulation fatigue, inflammation of the mouth, low blood pressure, visual disturbances, loss of appetite, abdominal cramps, diarrhea, nausea, vomiting, irritability, nightmares, seizures, and dizziness. May be less effective if taken with antacids or kaolin (*see*). Should be taken with food to reduce stomach irritation.

CHLOROTESTOSTERONE • *See* Anabolic Steroids.

CHLOROTHIAZIDE (Rx) • Aldoclor. Azide. Diachlor. Diurigen. Diuril. A thiazide diuretic introduced in 1957 that increases urine excretion of sodium and water and is used to treat edema and high blood pressure. Potential adverse reactions include nausea, loss of appetite, anemia, dehydration, a drop in blood pressure when rising from a seated or prone position, electrolyte imbalance, liver damage, pancreatitis, high blood sugar, impotence, high uric acid, skin rash, photosensitivity, and hypersensitivity reactions such as lung and blood-vessel irritation. Contraindicated in persons allergic to sulfa. Cholestyramine and colestipol make it less effective. Diazoxide increases its blood-pressure-lowering and blood-sugar-raising effects. NSAIDs decrease its effectiveness. Chlorothiazide lowers the potassium level, so the diet should include high-potassium foods such as bananas and apricots, unless a physician has ordered a potassium supplement. In that case, check with the doctor. May be taken after breakfast.

CHLOROTHYMOL (OTC) • A powerful germicide derived from phenol, it is active against *Staphylococcus aureus*. In 1992, the FDA issued a notice that chlorothymol had not been shown to be safe and effective as claimed in OTC products. *See* Staphylococci.

CHLOROTRIANISENE (Rx) • TACE. An estrogen drug used to treat prostate cancer, lack of female hormone in women, menopausal symptoms, and atrophic vaginitis. Potential adverse reactions include nausea, vomiting, depression, high blood pressure, dizziness, migraine, libido changes, water retention, increased risk of stroke, blood clots to the lung, and heart attack. May also worsen nearsightedness, cause intolerance of contact lenses, and lead to loss of appetite, increased appetite, excessive thirst, pancreatitis, bloating, and abdominal cramps. Women may have breakthrough bleeding, altered menstrual flow, painful or absent menstruation, enlargement of benign tumors of the uterus, cervical erosion, abnormal secretions, and vaginal candidiasis. In men there may be enlargement of the breasts, testicular atrophy, and impotence. In both sexes there may be jaundice, high blood sugar, high calcium in the blood, folic-acid deficiency, dark spots appearing on the skin, hives, acne, oily skin, hairiness or loss of hair, leg cramps, and hemorrhages into the skin. Contraindicated in persons with blood-clot disorders, cancer of the breast, reproductive organs, or genitals, in those with undiagnosed abnormal genital bleeding, and in pregnancy. Should be used with caution in high blood pressure, asthma, mental depression, bone disease, blood problems, gallbladder disease, migraine, seizures, diabetes, absences of menstruation, heart failure, liver or kidney dysfunction, and a family history of breast or genital-tract cancer.

CHLOROXINE (OTC) • **Capitrol.** Used in the treatment of dandruff or seborrheic dermatitis of the scalp. Should not be used if blistered, raw, or oozing areas are present on the scalp. Potential adverse reactions include burning of scalp and skin rash. May slightly discolor light hair.

CHLOROXYLENOL (OTC) • **Barri-Care. Care Creme. Concept. Satin Antimicrobial Skin Cleanser. Techni-Care Surgical Scrub.** A skin antiseptic. Active ingredient in germicides, antiseptics, and antifungal preparations. Toxic by ingestion. May be irritating to and absorbed by the skin.

CHLORPACTIN • *See* Oxychlorosene.

CHLORPHED (OTC) • *See* Brompheniramine.

CHLORPHENESIN (Rx) • **Maolate.** A muscle relaxant that reduces the transmission of nerve impulses from the spinal cord to muscles attached to bone. Used as an adjunct in short-term, acute, painful muscle conditions. Potential adverse reactions include a drop in blood platelets and white blood cells, drowsiness, dizziness, confusion, headache, weakness, agitation, insomnia, nervousness, nausea, GI distress, and fatal allergic reaction. Alcohol and central nervous system depressants may increase chlorphenesin's effects. Should be used cautiously in liver or kidney dysfunction, and in patients allergic to aspirin. Should be taken with milk or meals to prevent GI distress. Safe use for more than eight weeks has not been established.

CHLORPHENIRAMINE (OTC) • **Alka-Seltzer Plus Cold Medicine. Aller-Chlor. Allerest. A.R.M. Allergy Relief. BC Cold**

Powder. Cerose-DM. Cheracol. Chloramine. Chlorate. Chlor-100. Chlor-Pro. Chlorspan. Chlortab. Chlor-Trimeton. Comtrex. Contac. Coricidin. Dorcol. Dristan. Fedahist. 4-Way Cold Tablets. Genallerate. Histabid. Histalet. Histamic. Histaspan. Histex. Historal. Histor-D. Histrey. Isoclor. Kloromin. Kronofed. Kronohist. Medi-Flu Caplets. Nasahist. Neotep Granucaps. Nolamine. Novafed A. Novahistine DH. Orthoxicol. PediaCare. Pfeiffer's Allergy. Phenetron. Pyranistan. Pyrroxate. Rhyna. Sinarest Extra Strength. Sine-Off. Singlet. Sinulin. Sinutab Sinus. Sudafed Plus. Telachlor. Teldrin. Theraflu Flu and Cold Medicine. Triaminic. Trymegen. Tussi-Organidin. Tylenol Allergy Sinus. Tylenol Cold & Flu. Vicks Children's NyQuil. Vicks Formula 44. An antihistamine recategorized from Rx to OTC, first in low dosage in 1976, and in stronger strengths in 1981. It is used to treat stuffy nose and other allergy symptoms. Potential adverse effects include stimulation, sedation, drowsiness (in the elderly), excitability (in children), low blood pressure, palpitations, stomach distress, dry mouth, urine retention, rash, hives, and thick bronchial secretions. Central nervous system depressants, including alcohol, increase sedation, and MAO inhibitors may increase blood pressure. Contraindicated in acute asthmatic attacks. Use cautiously in elderly patients, those with glaucoma, overactive thyroid, heart or kidney disease, high blood pressure, bronchial asthma, enlarged prostate, bladder-neck obstruction, and peptic ulcer. Coffee or tea may reduce drowsiness. Medication should be discontinued four days before taking a skin allergy test because it can lead to inaccurate results. In 1992, the FDA issued a notice that chlorpheniramine maleate had not been shown to be safe and effective as claimed in OTC products for poison ivy, poison oak, and poison sumac drug products.

CHLOR-PRO (OTC) • *See* Chlorpheniramine.

CHLORPROMAZINE (Rx) • **Ormazine. Thorazine. Thor-Pram.** An antipsychotic, antinausea medication introduced in the 1950s; also used for intractable hiccups, and mild alcohol withdrawal. Potential adverse reactions include a drop in white blood cells, sedation, parkinsonism-like symptoms, dizziness, a drop in blood pressure when rising from a seated or prone position, vision changes, dry mouth, constipation, urine retention, enlargement of male breasts, inhibited ejaculation, liver dysfunction, weight gain, increased appetite, fever, photosensitivity, irregular heartbeat, and sweating. Tardive dyskinesia (*see*) may occur after prolonged use; and gastritis, nausea, vomiting, dizziness, tremors, sweating, headache, and insomnia may follow abrupt withdrawal. Alcohol and other central nervous system depressants may increase central nervous system depression. Antacids inhibit absorption. Antidepressants and drugs used to treat parkinsonism may increase chlorpromazine's nerve-suppressing activity. Barbiturates and lithium may decrease chlorpromazine's effectiveness. Blood pressure medications that act on the brain may be less effective. Oral blood thinners may be less effective and may also increase blood levels of chlorpromazine. Contraindicated in central nervous system depression, bone-marrow suppression, brain damage, Reye's syndrome, and coma. Also contraindicated with use of spinal or epidural anesthetic, or adrenergic-blocking agents (*see*); in the elderly, patients with liver disease, hardening of the arteries, cardiovascular disease, respiratory disorders, glaucoma, and enlarged prostate, and in acutely ill or dehydrated children. The ingested drug may take effect in thirty to sixty minutes and may last up to three weeks after being discontinued.

CHLORPROPAMIDE (Rx) • **Diabinese. Glucamide.** A member of the sulfonylurea (*see*) family, it is an oral antidiabetes medication prescribed to reduce blood glucose levels by stimulating the pancreas to produce insulin. Adjunct to diet to lower the blood sugar in patients with non-insulin-dependent diabetes. Potential adverse reactions include nausea, vomiting, heartburn, tea-colored urine, sodium loss, low blood sugar, rash, itching, facial flushing, and hypersensitivity reactions. Anabolic steroids (*see*), chloramphenicol, clofibrate, guanethidine, MAO inhibitors (*see*), oral blood thinners, salicylates, and sulfonamides increase blood-sugar-lowering activity.

Beta-blockers (*see*) and clonidine prolong the low blood sugar effect and may mask symptoms of low blood sugar. Corticosteroids, glucagon, rifampin, and thiazide diuretics decrease the blood-sugar-lowering effect. Contraindicated in treating insulin-dependent diabetes, in diabetes adequately controlled by diet, and in type II diabetes complicated by ketosis, acidosis, diabetic coma, Raynaud's disease, gangrene, liver or kidney dysfunction, or thyroid or other endocrine dysfunction. Mild stress such as an infection, minor surgery, or emotional upset can reduce the effectiveness of this drug. The possibility of increased heart deaths is associated with the use of sulfonylureas. Elderly patients may be more sensitive to this drug's adverse reactions.

CHLORPROPHENPYRIDAMINE MALEATE (OTC) • An antihistamine. In 1992, the FDA proposed a ban on chlorprophenpyridamine maleate in oral menstrual drug products because it had not been shown to be safe and effective as claimed. *See* Chlorpheniramine.

CHLORPROTHIXENE (Rx) • Taractan. A phenothiazine (*see*) drug used to treat psychotic disorders, agitation of severe neurosis, and depression. Potential adverse reactions include a drop in white blood cells, tardive dyskinesia (*see*), sedation, pseudoparkinsonism, dizziness, a drop in blood pressure when rising from a seated or prone position, vision changes, dry mouth, constipation, urine retention, menstrual irregularities, enlargement of male breasts, inhibited ejaculation, liver dysfunction, mild photosensitivity, weight gain, increased appetite, fever, irregular heartbeat, and sweating. May lower seizure threshold and cause severe reactions to insulin or electroshock therapy. Abrupt withdrawal may cause gastritis, nausea, vomiting, dizziness, tremors, sweating, headache, and insomnia. Use with alcohol and other central nervous system depressants may increase central nervous system depression. High blood pressure medications that work on the brain may be less effective. Contraindicated in coma, central nervous system depression, bone-marrow suppression, coronary artery or cerebrovascular disorders, brain damage, with use of spinal or epidural anesthetics, or adrenergic-blocking agents (*see*). While taking this drug, a sunscreen should be used to avoid photosensitivity reactions.

CHLORSPAN • *See* Chlorpheniramine.

CHLORTAB • *See* Chlorpheniramine.

CHLORTETRACYCLINE (Rx) • Aureomycin. A tetracycline antibiotic ointment used to treat superficial skin infections. The ointment has a lanolin base and should not be used by persons allergic to wool or lanolin derivatives. Potential adverse reactions include rash and drying of the skin.

CHLORTHALIDONE (Rx) • Combipres. Hygroton. Tenoretic. Thalitone. Uridon. A diuretic introduced in 1960 that acts like a thiazide (*see*) diuretic, increasing excretion of sodium and water. It is used to treat edema, high blood pressure, heart failure, cirrhosis of the liver, kidney dysfunction, and other conditions where fluid retention is a problem. Potential adverse reactions include nausea, loss of appetite, anemia, dehydration, a drop in blood pressure when rising from a seated or prone position, electrolyte imbalance, liver damage, pancreatitis, high blood sugar, high uric acid, skin rash, photosensitivity, and hypersensitivity reactions such as lung and blood-vessel irritation. Cholestyramine and colestipol make it less effective. Diazoxide increases its blood-pressure-lowering and blood-sugar-raising effects. NSAIDs decrease its effectiveness. Contraindicated in absence of urine formation, or in hypersensitivity to thiazides or other sulfonamide-derived drugs. Should be used cautiously in severe kidney disease or impaired liver function. Persons on this diuretic should eat a diet high in potassium that includes citrus fruits, tomatoes, bananas, dates, and apricots. The medication should be taken in the morning after breakfast to avoid having to urinate during the night. A sunscreen should also be worn because this drug can increase sensitivity to the sun.

CHLOR-TRIMETON • *See* Chlorpheniramine.

CHLORZOXAZONE (Rx) • Cetazone. Chlorofon. Lobac. Miflex. Panflex. Paraflex. Parafon Forte. Spasgesic. Strifon Forte. A muscle relaxant introduced in 1958 that reduces transmission of nerve impulses from the spinal cord to skeletal muscles. Used as an adjunct to treat painful muscles. Potential adverse reactions include anemia, drowsiness, dizziness, headache, malaise, excitement, loss of appetite, nausea, vomiting, heartburn, abdominal distress, constipation, diarrhea, urine discoloration, liver dysfunction, hives, redness, itching, pinpoint blood spots on skin, and bruising. A petition has been filed with the FDA by an attorney to take this medication off the market. The attorney, Allen Eaton, contends the original maker of chlorzoxazone hid its toxicity from the agency when the drug was approved for sale in 1959 and fought later FDA attempts to uncover the danger. Eaton said he had uncovered one hundred cases of liver damage linked to the product. Contraindicated in persons with liver dysfunction and/or a history of allergies. Alcohol and central nervous system depressants increase chlorzoxazone central nervous system depressant effects. If taken with AZT or Retrovir, it may increase side effects. May be taken with or without food.

CHLORZOXAZONE WITH APAP (Rx) • *See* Acetaminophen and Chlorzoxazone.

CHOL-, CHOLE- • Prefixes meaning bile as in *cholangitis,* inflammation of the bile ducts.

CHOLAC • *See* Lactulose.

CHOLAGOGUE • Agents that increase the flow of bile into the intestines. Herbs used for this purpose include wild yam root and goldenseal (*see both*).

CHOLECALCIFEROL • *See* Vitamin D.

CHOLECYSTITIS • An inflammation of the gallbladder.

CHOLECYSTOKININ • CCK. A hormone produced by the small intestine during the movement of food from the stomach into the intestine. CCK causes contraction of the gallbladder, thus releasing bile into the small intestine, where enzymes and other components of bile aid digestion. This hormone has also been found in the brain and may help to control overeating. CCK antagonists are in development by several companies.

CHOLEDYL THEOPHYLLINATE • *See* Oxtriphylline.

CHOLERA • An epidemic infectious disease with a high fatality rate, caused by germs transmitted to food and water through bowel discharges of carriers. It is characterized by profuse watery diarrhea, cramps, vomiting, prostration, and suppression of urine.

CHOLERA VACCINE (Rx) • Injection of the gram-negative (*see*) bacillus *Vibrio cholerae,* killed for the purpose of immunization. Potential adverse reactions include malaise, fever, flushing, hives, rapid heartbeat, low blood pressure, diarrhea, headache, severe allergic reaction, and swelling at the injection site.

CHOLESTEROL • A hormonelike chemical present in some foods, notably animal fats, eggs, and dairy products. A high level of cholesterol in the blood is associated with atherosclerosis (*see*) and heart attacks.

CHOLESTOCHECK ONE STEP CHOLESTEROL TEST (OTC) • A kit expected to be approved by the FDA at this writing for both professional use and consumer use at home. It comprises a chemically reactive membrane-based strip, on which a drop of blood is placed. A hand-held electronic meter reads the color reaction of the strip. A system similar to that used by diabetics. The results are available in one minute.

CHOLESTRAK (OTC) • The first nonprescription, home test kit for cholesterol, introduced in 1992. The kit is reportedly as accurate as tests used by doctors and medical laboratories. To perform the test, the user pricks a finger, squeezes blood into a plastic container that holds a test strip, then waits fifteen minutes for results. The strip changes color depending on how much cholesterol is present. The user compares the strip to an accompanying conversion chart to get a cholesterol reading. The test doesn't differentiate between the various types of cholesterol.

CHOLESTYRAMINE (Rx) • Cholybar. Questran. Questran Light. A cholesterol- and fat-lowering medication in the form of a bar or powder, introduced in 1959. The powder should not be taken without fluids. Also used to treat itching and diarrhea due to excess bile acid, it combines with bile acid to form an insoluble compound that is excreted. In the *Annals of Internal Medicine,* September 15, 1994, researchers from University of Texas Southwestern Medical Center reported this drug is safe and effective for lowering cholesterol in patients with adult-onset (type II) diabetes. The drug also had the unexpected benefit of improving diabetes control. Potential adverse reactions include constipation (which is common and may be severe), hemorrhoids, abdominal discomfort, flatulence, nausea, vomiting, rashes, and irritation of the skin, tongue, and perianal area. It may also decrease absorption of vitamins A, D, and K, causing a deficiency. Questran Light contains phenylalanine and should not be used by persons suffering from phenylketonuria. Questran tablets were voluntarily removed from the market because of reports of patients choking and having difficulty swallowing. The powdered form is still widely available. Cholestyramine decreases the absorption of acetaminophen, coumarin anticoagulants, beta-blockers (*see*), corticosteroids, digitalis glycosides, fat-soluble vitamins, iron preparations, thiazide diuretics, and thyroid hormones. Since it binds with other drugs, it is recommended that other drugs be taken at least one hour before or six hours after taking cholestyramine. Contraindicated in patients with complete obstruction of the bile ducts, and in those who have shown hypersensitivity to any of the drug's components. Should not be swallowed as a powder and should be mixed with at least six ounces of fluid. *See also* Bile.

CHOLINE • B complex vitamin found in most animal tissues, either free or in combinations, such as lecithin or acetylcholine. Choline is being actively studied for its effects on brain neurotransmission and memory.

CHOLINE BITARTRATE (OTC) • Geritol Liquid. A white, crystalline powder used as a dietary supplement.

CHOLINE MAGNESIUM TRISALICYLATE (Rx) • Choline Salicylate and Magnesium Salicylate. CMT. Trilisate. A drug similar to aspirin, used in arthritic conditions. It produces analgesia by effecting the hypothalamus in the brain and blocking generation of pain impulses. It exerts an anti-inflammatory effect by inhibiting prostaglandin synthesis. The drug also relieves fever by acting on the hypothalamic heat-regulating center to produce dilation of the blood vessels. This increases peripheral blood supply and promotes sweating, which leads to the loss of heat, and to cooling by evaporation. Potential adverse effects include ringing in the ears, hearing loss, gastrointestinal distress, rash, and rarely, severe allergic reaction. Alcohol, steroids, and other NSAIDs (*see*) increase the risk of adverse GI effects. Ammonium chloride and other urine acidifiers increase blood levels of salicylates and may lead to toxicity. Antacids in high doses and other urine alkalinizers decrease levels of salicylates. Corticosteroids enhance salicylate elimination and may decrease effects. Oral anticoagulants increase risk of bleeding. Should be used cautiously in people with chronic kidney failure, peptic ulcer disease, and gastritis, and in patients with known allergy to salicylates. Causes less GI distress than aspirin. CMT should be taken with food or a full glass of water. Children who have a fever and are dehydrated can develop toxicity rapidly when given CMT.

CHOLINERGIC DRUGS • Medications that affect the action of acetylcholine, a neurotransmitter responsible for transmission of nerve impulses.

CHOLINERGIC SYSTEM • Nerve cells that use acetylcholine (*see*) as their neurotransmitter to send and receive messages.

CHOLINE SALICYLATE (Rx) • Arthropan. A drug similar to aspirin, used in arthritic conditions, and for inflamed gums, minor pain, and fever. Produces analgesia by an ill-defined effect on the hypothalamus, and blocking generation of pain impulses. The peripheral action may involve inhibition of prostaglandin synthesis, by which the drug exerts its anti-inflammatory effect. It relieves fever by acting on the hypothalamic heat-regulating center to produce peripheral vasodilation. This increases peripheral blood supply and promotes sweating, which leads to the loss of heat, and to cooling by evaporation. Potential adverse reactions include ringing in the ears and hearing loss, nausea, vomiting, GI distress, rash and rarely, severe hypersensitivity reaction. Alcohol, steroids, and other NSAIDs (*see*) may increase the risk of adverse GI reactions. Ammonium chloride and other urine acidifiers increase levels of salicylates in the blood. Antacids in high doses and other urine alkalinizers decrease salicylate levels and make them less effective. Corticosteroids enhance salicylate elimination and may make choline salicylate less effective. Choline salicylate should be used cautiously in kidney failure, peptic ulcer disease, gastritis, and in patients with known allergy to salicylates. Because of epidemiologic association with Reye's syndrome, the Center for Disease Control recommends that children or teenagers with chicken pox or influenza-like illness should not be given salicylates. Causes less GI distress than aspirin. Children who are feverish and dehydrated rapidly develop toxicity to salicylates. Unlike aspirin, choline salicylate does not inhibit platelet aggregation.

CHOLINESTERASE • The enzyme that processes the neurotransmitter acetylcholine. There is a great deal of scientific interest in acetylcholine, particularly in the study of Alzheimer's disease, because the enzyme is believed to be involved in poor memory function.

CHOLINE THEOPHYLLINATE • See Oxtriphylline.

CHOLOXIN • *See* Dextrothyroxine Sodium.

CHOLYBAR • *See* Cholestyramine.

CHON-, CHONDRO- • Prefixes meaning cartilage.

CHONDROITIN • A major constituent of cartilage in the body.

CHOOZ • *See* Calcium Carbonate.

CHOREA • A disorder, usually of childhood, characterized by irregular, spasmodic, involuntary movements of the limbs or facial muscles.

CHOREX • *See* Chorionic Gonadotropin.

CHORIONIC GONADOTROPIN (Rx) • Antuitrin. CG. Human Chorionic Gonadotropin. HCG. A.P.L. Chorex. Choron. Corgonject. Follutein. Glukor. Gonic. Pregnyl. Profasi HP. An extract from the urine of pregnant women. A hormone produced by the pituitary gland, it is also made by the tissue of the placenta and is found in urine during pregnancy; also in body fluids of persons having certain tumors. HCG stimulates the Leydig tissue in the male, which results in the secretion of the male hormones, androgens. Used to treat women with infertility problems, to induce ovulation and pregnancy. Given to males with undescended testicles and to men who are deficient in gonadotropic hormones, to increase sperm production. Used occasionally to prevent miscarriage. Potential adverse reactions include headache, fatigue, mood changes, and in women, swollen feet and ankles and abdominal pain. May cause enlarged breasts in men. Alcohol increases the feeling of fatigue.

CHORON • *See* Chorionic Gonadotropin.

CHROMATE • *See* Chromium.

CHROMIUM (OTC) • Chromium Amino Acid Chelate. Chromium Picolinate. Glucose Tolerance Factor. An element occurring in the earth's crust, it plays a vital role in the activities of some enzymes. Chromium is involved in the breakdown of sugar for conversion into energy, and in the manufacture of certain fats. It works together with insulin and is essential to the body's ability to use sugar. Traces of chromium are widely available in food. However, chromium deficiency may frequently occur because the soil in the United States contains low levels. Those who are deficient may show symptoms similar to diabetes, such as fatigue, mental confusion, and numbness or tingling of the hands and feet. Deficiency may worsen preexisting diabetes, depress growth in children, or contribute to the development of narrowing of the arteries. Chromium is poisonous in large amounts. Inhalation of chromium dust can cause irritation and ulceration. Ingestion can result in violent gastrointestinal irritation. Application to the skin may result in allergic reaction. The most serious effect of chromium is lung cancer due to inhalation, which may develop twenty to thirty years after exposure.

CHROMIUM PICOLINATE (H) • In studies of animal cells grown in the laboratory, Dartmouth researchers found chromium picolinate causes considerable damage to chromosomes, which is an indication of a substance's potential to be a human cancer-causing agent. The study, financed by the National Cancer Institute, was a preliminary one. *See* Chromium.

CHROMOGEN CAPSULES • A combination of iron and vitamins B$_{12}$ and C. This iron and vitamin combination is used to treat anemia.

CHRONIC • Long-lasting or frequently recurring conditions.

CHRONIC FATIGUE SYNDROME (CSF) • Formerly called chronic Epstein-Barr virus syndrome, it is a common and frequently debilitating illness, the cause or causes of which are still unknown. At this writing, the diagnosis of this illness is based on clinical observations with the symptoms of persistent or relapsing fatigue with at least 50 percent reduction of activity level for at least six months. May also include mild fever, sore throat, painful glands, muscle weakness and pain, prolonged fatigue after exercise, and headaches.

CHRONIC GRANULOMATOUS DISEASE (CGD) • A congenital defect in the ability of white blood cells to kill bacteria, leaving patients susceptible to severe infections. Nodular lesions, called granulomas, also result and interfere with the function of various organs.

CHRONIC OBSTRUCTIVE PULMONARY DISEASE • COPD. A term that includes chronic bronchitis, emphysema, and asthma. Patients with COPD are susceptible to bacterial infections, which acutely exacerbate their chronic condition.

CHRONULAC • *See* Lactulose.

CHRYSANTHEMUM (H) • **Chrysanthemum. Corn Marigold. Ye Ju.** A large family of perennial herbs thought to originate in Asia. A tea made from this flower is used to treat conjunctivitis and skin diseases. Taken internally, it is used to lower blood pressure. A number of medicines, and the insecticidal pyrethrins (*see*), are derived from this family.

CHYMODIACTIN • *See* Chymopapain.

CHYMOPAPAIN (Rx) • **Chymodiactin. Discase.** An enzyme used to treat herniated disks in the spine. Potential adverse reactions include paralysis, stroke, life-threatening allergic reactions, nausea, headache, dizziness, leg weakness, a feeling of pins and needles, numbness of legs and toes, back pain, stiffness, and back spasm. Contraindicated in patients with a history of allergy to papaya or meat tenderizers, patients who have previously received an injection of chymopapain, and in those with other spinal cord problems. *See* Papaya.

CHYMORAL (Rx) • A combination of trypsin and chymotrypsin (*see both*).

CHYMOTRYPSIN (Rx) • **Avazyme. Catarase. Chymar. Zolyse.** A pancreatic enzyme used in the treatment of cataracts.

CIBACALCIN • *See* Calcitonin.

CIBALITH-S • *See* Lithium Carbonate.

CICLOPIROX (Rx) • **Loprox.** An antifungal drug introduced in 1983, it is prescribed to treat fungal and yeast infections of the skin such as athlete's foot and jock itch. It may also be prescribed to treat less common skin problems such as tinea versicolor (*see*), the symptoms of which are fine scales over the skin, usually on the chest. Ciclopirox may also be given to treat candida (thrush) infections of the vagina or penis. Ciclopirox has a more rapid onset and effect than many other topical antifungal preparations, and fewer adverse reactions. Potential adverse reactions include itching and burning.

CICUTA (H) • A small herb of the family *Umbelliferae*. It has deadly poisonous roots and is used greatly diluted in homeopathic medicines. *See* L.72.

CIDOFOVIR • **Vistide.** An intravenous treatment for cytomegalovirus (CMV) retinitis, an opportunistic infection that afflicts 15 to 40 percent of patients with AIDS and puts them at risk for blindness. The medication was approved by the FDA in June 1996. It is a systemic treatment for CMV retinitis that is delivered by intravenous infusion once a week for two weeks and once every other week thereafter. In contrast, other approved IV treatment for CMV retinitis are given daily or multiple times each day.

CIDOMYCIN • *See* Gentamicin.

CILICANE-VK • *See* Penicillin V.

CILLIUM • *See* Psyllium.

CILOXAN OPHTHALMIC • *See* Ciprofloxacin.

CIMETIDINE (Rx) (OTC) • **Tagamet.** The first histamine H_2 antagonist, it was introduced in 1976 for short-term treatment of active duodenal ulcer, maintenance therapy for duodenal ulcer patients at reduced dosage, and short-term treatment of active benign gastric ulcer, erosive gastroesophageal reflux disease, prevention of upper gastrointestinal bleeding in critically ill patients, and treatment of serious stomach acidity conditions. Potential adverse reactions include rare instances of irregular heartbeat, and a drop in blood pressure. Other potential adverse reactions include diarrhea, dizziness, sleepiness, headache, agitation, psychosis, depression, anxiety, hallucination, a drop in white blood cells, liver or kidney dysfunction, urinary retention, muscle and joint pain, impotence, enlargement of male breasts, enlargement of female breasts with milk production, decreased libido, rash, and rarely, hair loss. Cimetidine may increase toxicity of many drugs including alcohol, antidepressants, blood thinners, and antidiabetes, cancer, and heart drugs. Cimetidine may hide the presence of stomach cancer. Reversible confusion states have been reported, usually in severely ill patients. Cimetidine may increase the effects of warfarin-type blood thinners, phenytoin, propranolol, diazepam, certain tricyclic antidepressants, lidocaine, theophylline, and metronidazole. May have an adverse effect on sperm, but rarely causes impotence. If taken with caffeine-containing drinks such as coffee or cola, or with over-the-counter drugs containing caffeine, stomach irritation may occur, the heart rhythm may become rapid, and blood pressure may rise. This drug should not be discontinued suddenly. Cimetidine should be taken with food and at bedtime to achieve maximum effectiveness. Efforts in 1993 failed to convince the FDA that it was safe for unsupervised use. The FDA's committees twice said there was not sufficient evidence to show that OTC cimetidine was more beneficial for heartburn than a placebo. The committees suggested that the manufacturer, SmithKline Beecham, try again when more data had been collected. In 1995, the company obtained FDA permission to sell the drug over the counter, and the company expects sales to reach $200 to $400 million within two years. Permission was granted on the provision that the label warn users about possible adverse interactions with certain asthma, seizure, and blood-thining medications.

CIMI • Homeopathic abbreviation for cimicifuga. *See* Black Cohosh.

CIMICIFUGA • *See* Black Cohosh.

CIMICIFUGA RACEMOSA • *See* Black Cohosh.

CINA (H) • Used in homoepathic remedies for removing worms. *See* Wormseed.

CINCHONA (H) • *Cinchona ledgeriana.* **Jesuit's Powder. Peruvian Bark.** The extract of the bark of various species of cinchona cultivated in India and South America. The source for quinine (*see*) until that drug was made synthetically, cinchona possesses antiviral, antimalarial, and fever-reducing properties. Cinchona is also used as a tonic, and to stimulate the appetite, as it stimulates digestion. Large amounts of cinchona slow the heart rate. Potential adverse reactions include nausea, dizziness, deafness, and buzzing in the ears.

CINNAMATES (OTC) (H) • Derived from the dried bark of specially cultivated trees, it is used as a sunscreen. May cause sensitivity to light, and allergic reactions.

CINNAMON (OTC) (H) • *Cinnamomum zeylanicum.* Obtained from the dried aromatic bark of cultivated trees of the genus *Cinnamomum,* it is used as a flavoring, and by herbalists to relieve nausea and vomiting and to stop diarrhea. Extracts have been used to break up intestinal gas. However, cinnamon can be irritating to the gastrointestinal system. In 1992, the FDA issued a notice that cinnamon oil had not been shown to be safe and effective as claimed in OTC digestive-aid products.

CINOBAC • *See* Cinoxacin.

CINONIDE • *See* Triamcinolone.

CINOXACIN (Rx) • **Cinobac.** A quinolone (*see*) urinary-tract antiseptic. Potential adverse reactions include dizziness, headache, drowsiness, insomnia, seizure, photosensitivity, ringing in the ears, nausea, vomiting, abdominal pain, diarrhea, rash, and hives. Kidney disease or probenecid (*see*) may increase the side effects of cinoxacin. Those allergic to other quinolones may have a reaction to this drug. Cinoxacin may be taken with food.

CIPRO • *See* Ciprofloxacin.

CIPROFLOXACIN (Rx) • **Cipro.** A broad-spectrum quinolone (*see*) synthetic antibiotic approved in 1989. It is used to treat mild to moderate urinary tract, skin, and sinus infections, and infectious diarrhea. In fact, the British reported in 1995, a single dose of the antibiotic reduces the duration and severity of diarrhea. Potential adverse reactions include headache, restlessness, tremor, light-headedness, confusion, hallucinations, seizures, crystals in urine, rash, and inflammation at the site of IV administration. May also cause allergic reactions; those allergic to other quinolones should not be given cipro. Prolonged use of cipro may cause an overgrowth of bacteria resistant to it. Antacids containing magnesium hydroxide or aluminum hydroxide decrease cipro's effectiveness. Probenecid (*see*) may elevate its level in the blood. Cipro also may interact with and increase theophylline's (*see*) level in the blood, causing serious and even fatal side effects, particularly in older patients. Caffeine may also have cumulative effects if ingested while taking this drug. Cipro may be taken with or without food.

CIRRHOSIS • A chronic liver disease in which liver cells are damaged and replaced by scar tissue.

CISAPRIDE (Rx) • **Propulsid.** A medication to treat heartburn and gastroesophageal reflux disease (*see*). Potential adverse effects include headache, diarrhea, abdominal pain, nausea, constipation, gas, and heartburn. Physicians were notified by the FDA in 1995 that use in combination with the oral antifungal ketoconazole (*see*) or other oral anti-infectives, itraconazole and miconazole, and troleandomycin, is contraindicated because of the possibility of cardiac side effects. Cisapride may also increase the sedative effects of alcohol and certain tranquilizers. Cisapride should be taken fifteen minutes before meals.

CISPLATIN (Rx) • **Platinol.** An anticancer drug introduced in 1970 as an adjunctive therapy in testicular and ovarian cancers that have spread, and for treatment of advanced bladder cancer. It is an alkylating agent (*see*). Potential adverse reactions include nausea, vomiting, mild bone-marrow suppression, anemia, nerve damage, loss of taste, seizures, ringing in the ears, hearing loss, diarrhea, metallic taste, kidney toxicity, and life-threatening allergic reactions. Aminoglycoside (*see*) antibiotics add to cisplatin's kidney toxicity.

CITRACAL (OTC) • *See* Calcium Citrate.

CITRA FORTE (OTC) • A combination of vitamin C, hydrocodone, and pheniramine (*see all*) used to treat colds.

CITRATES (Rx) • **Potassium Citrate. Sodium Citrate. Bictria. Oracit. Polycitra-K. Urocit-K.** The salts of citric acid (*see*) are used to make urine less acidic. This helps prevent certain kinds of kidney stones. Citrates are sometimes used with other medicines to help treat kidney stones that may occur with gout. They also are used to make the blood more alkaline in certain conditions.

CITRIC ACID (OTC) • **Alka-Seltzer Effervescent Antacid. Maintenance Solution. Oracit. Ricelyte Rice-Based Oral Electrolyte. Shohl's Solution.** One of the most widely used acids in cosmetics and foods, it is derived from citrus fruit by fermentation of crude sugars. Employed as a preservative, sequestering agent, and to adjust acid-alkali balance. The clear, crystalline, water-absorbing chemical is used to prevent scurvy, a deficiency disease, and as a refreshing drink with water and sugar added.

CITROBACTER • A gram-negative bacteria (*see*) found in feces, soil, water, sewage, and urine. Some may inhabit normal intestines, but can cause meningitis, and infections of the stomach, gallbladder, urinary tract, and wounds.

CITROCARBONATE (OTC) • A combination of sodium bicarbonate and sodium citrate (*see both*).

CITROMA • *See* Magnesium Citrate.

CITRO-NESIA • *See* Magnesium Citrate.

CITROVORUM FACTOR • *See* Leucovorin.

CITRUCEL • *See* Methylcellulose.

CITRUS PECTIN • In 1992, the FDA issued a notice that citrus pectin had not been shown to be safe and effective as claimed in OTC digestive-aid products.

CLA • *See* Clarithromycin.

CLAFORAN • *See* Cefotaxime Sodium.

CLARITHROMYCIN (Rx) • **Biaxin. CLA.** A macrolide (*see*) antibiotic introduced in 1991. It is indicated for the treatment of moderate infections, including pharyngitis, tonsillitis, pneumonia, sinusitis, chronic bronchitis, and skin infections and abscesses usually requiring surgical drainage. Promoted as causing less gastrointestinal upset than erythromycin. Contraindicated in people allergic to erythromycin, or any of the macrolide antibiotics. The most common adverse effects are diarrhea, nausea, abnormal taste, heartburn, abdominal pain, and headache. Rarely, macrolide antibiotics have been associated with irregular heartbeat and liver dysfunction. Biaxin may make theophylline (*see*) levels toxic and increase the levels of carbamazepine in the blood (*see*). Can be taken without regard to meals.

CLARITIN (Rx) • *See* Loratadine.

CLARITIN-D (RX) • *See* Loratadine and Pseudoephedrine.

CLAUDICATION • Cramping in one or both legs, which develops while walking. In intermittent claudication, the pain lessens after a short rest. The condition is usually caused by blockage or narrowing of fat-clogged arteries.

CLAVULANATE • **Augmentin Tablets.** An oral antibacterial combination consisting of the semisynthetic antibiotic amoxicillin and an enzyme inhibitor, clavulanate potassium. The clavulanate extends the effectiveness of amoxicillin to other bacteria that would not be affected by it alone. May cause serious hypersensitive reaction as far as the penicillin component. Colitis has also been reported. Among other potential adverse reactions are anemia, agitation, and insomnia. *See* Amoxicillin.

CLEARASIL (OTC) • *See* Benzoyl Peroxide.

CLEAR BLUE EASY (OTC) • A diagnostic test for pregnancy.

CLEAR BY DESIGN (OTC) • *See* Benzoyl Peroxide.

CLEAR EYES (OTC) • *See* Naphazoline.

CLEARPLAN EASY (OTC) • A diagnostic test for ovulation.

CLEAVERS (H) • *Galium aparine.* **Burweed. Catchweed. Clivers. Goosegrass. Love Man. Scratch Weed.** A native of Europe, Asia, and North America. The Greeks called it *philantropon* because they considered its trait of clinging to walls showed a love of mankind. In rural medicine it was used for jaundice, scarlet fever, and measles. The crushed herb was folded into a cloth and applied hot in cases of earache and toothache. A cooling drink was given every spring as a tonic. It was also used by dieters to keep them lean and lank. In homeopathic medicine it is used for skin diseases such as psoriasis and scurvy and as a diuretic and astringent. The whole herb is used by herbalists to treat kidney and bladder problems and gallstones. Has diuretic properties. Contraindicated in patients with diabetes because of the strong diuretic effect of the plant.

CLEMASTINE (OTC) • **Tavist. Tavist-D. Tavist-1.** An antihistamine changed from Rx to OTC in 1992, it is used to treat stuffy nose and allergy symptoms. Potential adverse reactions include anemia, a drop in blood platelets, sedation and drowsiness (especially in elderly patients), low blood pressure, palpitations, rapid heartbeat, stomach distress, loss of appetite, nausea, vomiting, constipation, dry mouth, urine retention, rash, hives, and thick bronchial secretions. Central nervous system depressants, including alcohol, increase sedation. Coffee or tea may reduce drowsiness. MAO inhibitors may shoot up blood pressure. Should be used cautiously in elderly patients, those with glaucoma, overactive thyroids, heart or kidney disease, high blood pressure, bronchial asthma, enlarged prostate, bladder-neck obstruction, and peptic ulcer. Medication should be discontinued four days before taking a skin allergy test because it can lead to inaccurate results. Clemastine is most effective when taken on an empty stomach, but may be taken with food if stomach upset is a problem.

CLEOCIN • *See* Clindamycin.

CLERZ • *See* Hydroxyethylcellulose.

C-LEXIN • *See* Cephalexin.

CLIDINIUM BROMIDE (Rx) • **Librax. Quarzan.** An antispasmodic drug used in irritable-bowel syndrome, and as an adjunctive therapy for peptic ulcers. Potential adverse reactions include headache, insomnia, drowsiness, dizziness, confusion, excitement, nervousness, weakness, palpitation, rapid heartbeat, blurred vision, increased eye pressure, sensitivity to light, impotence, dry mouth, difficulty swallowing, loss of taste, nausea, vomiting, paralytic ileus, constipation, urinary retention, hives, decreased sweating, fever, and allergic reactions. Contraindicated in glaucoma, particularly in patients over forty years of age, obstructions of the urinary or GI tracts, severe ulcerative colitis, myasthenia gravis, hypersensitivity to anticholinergics, heart problems, nerve damage, overactive thyroid, coronary artery disease, high blood pressure, hiatal hernia, and liver or kidney disease. Should be taken before bedtime and thirty minutes to one hour before meals.

CLIMARA (Rx) • A transdermal (through the skin) method approved in 1995 for delivering estradiol (*see*).

CLINDAMYCIN (Rx); –HYDROCHLO-RIDE, –PALMITATE, –PHOSPHATE (Rx) • **Cleocin. Cleocin T Topical Gel, Lotion, Solu-**

tion. **Dalacin C.** Introduced in the early 1970s, it is used to treat infections caused by staphylococci, streptococci, pneumococci, and other aerobic and anaerobic organisms. Because it penetrates bone and joints, it is prescribed for bone and joint infections, including osteomyelitis. In topical solutions, lotions, or gel, it is used to treat infections of the oil glands in the skin. It is one of the few oral drugs effective against anaerobic (*see*) infections. Potential adverse effects include blood problems, nausea, vomiting, abdominal pain, diarrhea, potentially fatal colitis, esophagitis, gas, loss of appetite, bloody stools, trouble swallowing, rash, hives, bad taste in the mouth, and fatal allergic reactions. Erythromycin (*see*) makes it ineffective. Kaolin decreases absorption of oral clindamycin. Makes medicines for myasthenia gravis, such as neostigmine, less effective. When using skin preparations, avoid abrasive or medicated soaps and cleansers, as well as acne preparations, or any containing a peeling agent (benzoyl peroxide, salicylic acid, sulfur, resorcinol, tretinoin). Also to be avoided are alcohol-containing products such as aftershave, perfumed toiletries, shaving creams or lotions, and cosmetics. Soaps or cosmetics with strong drying effects, isotretinoin, and medicated cosmetics or "cover-ups" may cause cumulative drying or irritation resulting in excessive skin irritation. Take oral clindamycin with a full glass of water or food to prevent stomach irritation and throat pain.

CLINISTIX (OTC) • A diagnostic test for sugar in urine.

CLINITEST (OTC) • A diagnostic test for sugar in urine.

CLINORIL • *See* Sulindac.

CLIOQUINOL (Rx) (OTC) • **HCV Cream. Iodo. Mity-Ouin. Torofor. Vioform.** A topical anti-infective medication to treat skin infections. Available without prescription. When combined with hydrocortisone (*see*), however, it is only available Rx. Potential adverse reactions include itching, rash, redness, swelling, and blistering, or other signs of irritation.

CLIVERS (H) • *See* Cleavers.

CLOBETASOL (Rx) • **Dermovate. Temovate.** A potent corticosteroid ointment or cream used to treat skin inflammations. Potential adverse reactions include burning, itching, irritation, dryness, inflammation of the hair follicles, acne, rash around the mouth, spots of pigment loss, hairiness, allergic contact dermatitis, and if covered with a dressing, secondary infection, atrophy, streaks, and blisters. Should be used cautiously in skin problems caused by viruses such as herpes, and in fungal or bacterial skin infections. Should not be used for more than two weeks due to potential absorption into the system, consequently affecting the hypothalamus, and pituitary and adrenal glands. Should not be applied near eyes or mucous membranes, under the arms, on the face, groin, or under the breast, unless medically specified.

CLOCORTOLONE (Rx) • **Cloderm.** A corticosteroid ointment or cream used to treat skin inflammation. Potential adverse reactions include burning, itching, irritation, dryness, inflammation of the hair follicles, acne, rash around the mouth, spots of pigment loss, hairiness, allergic contact dermatitis, and if covered with a dressing, secondary infection, atrophy, streaks, and blisters. Should be used cautiously in skin problems caused by viruses such as herpes, and in fungal or bacterial skin infections. Should not be used for more than two weeks due to potential absorption into the system, consequently affecting the hypothalamus, and pituitary and adrenal glands. Should not be applied near eyes or mucous membranes, under the arms, on the face, groin, or under the breast, unless medically specified.

CLOCREAM • *See* Vitamin A and Vitamin D.

CLODERM • *See* Clocortolone.

CLOFAZIMINE (Rx) • **Lamprene.** Inhibits the growth of the bacteria that cause leprosy and reduces inflammation. May cause eye irritation, stomach pain, diarrhea, nausea, vomiting, bowel obstruction, GI bleeding, pigmentation of the skin, dryness, and rash.

CLOFIBRATE (Rx) • **Atromid-S.** Used to lower blood fats and to reduce fat plaques. Potential adverse reactions include a low white blood cell count, fatigue, weakness, irregular heartbeat, nausea, diarrhea, vomiting, heartburn, gas, gallstones, rashes, hives, dry skin and hair, muscle pain, joint pain, weight gain, fever, decreased sex drive, and impotence. May pose an increased risk of gallstones, heart disease, and cancer. Contraindicated in severe kidney or liver disease. Clofibrate may potentiate the blood-thinning effects of warfarin or dicoumarol. Oral contraceptives and rifampin (*see*) may decrease clofibrate's effects. Clofibrate may increase the clinical effect of furosemide and sulfonylureas (*see both*). Probenecid and alcohol may increase clofibrate's effects to toxic levels. Clofibrate may be taken with food or milk.

CLOMID • *See* Clomiphene Citrate.

CLOMIPHENE CITRATE (Rx) • **Clomid. Milophene. Serophene.** A drug introduced in 1967, it induces ovulation by stimulating the release of pituitary hormones that stimulate the ovaries. Potential adverse reactions include nausea, vomiting, bloating, high blood pressure, blurred vision, headache, restlessness, insomnia, dizziness, depression, fatigue, tension, sensitivity to light, double vision, blurred vision, increased appetite, weight gain, urinary frequency, ovarian enlargement and cyst formation, high blood sugar, hives, rash, hot flashes, hair loss, and breast discomfort. The possibility of multiple births exists with this drug. Prolonged use of clomiphene during infertility treatment has been associated with an increased risk of ovarian tumors in a study published in the *New England Journal of Medicine* (September 22, 1994). Although the findings do not prove that the infertility drugs cause ovarian cancer, they do add to the data supporting such a link. Contraindicated in undiagnosed abnormal genital bleeding, ovarian cyst, liver disease, or in patients with a history of blood clots. The drug should be stopped as soon as pregnancy is suspected.

CLOMIPRAMINE HYDROCHLORIDE (Rx) • **Anafranil.** A tricyclic antidepressant introduced in 1970 to treat obsessions and compulsions. It is believed to have an effect on serotonin, a brain chemical that has been reported to be above normal in these patients. The drug should not be given within fourteen days before or after treatment with monoamine oxidase inhibitors (MAOIs) (*see*). Contraindicated in patients who have recently suffered a heart attack or are hypersensitive to anafranil or other tricyclic antidepressants. Potential adverse reactions include dry mouth, sleepiness, tremor, dizziness, constipation, low blood pressure and irregular heartbeat, seizures, muscle pain, liver changes, anemia, increased body heat, sexual dysfunction, weight gain, and neuropsychiatric symptoms, including delusions, hallucinations, and psychotic episodes. Tobacco smoking lowers the concentrations of clomipramine, while coadministration of haloperidol (*see*) increases its concentration in the blood. Coadministration with phenobarbital increases blood concentration of phenobarbital. Use with MAO inhibitors may lead to a fever crisis, seizures, coma, and death. Alcohol, barbiturates, and other central nervous system depressants may cause an exaggerated response. May be taken with or without food.

CLONAZEPAM (Rx) • **Clonopin. Klonopin. Rivotril.** A benzodiazepine (*see*) anticonvulsant introduced in 1977 that seems to work in the brain to control seizures. Used to treat Lennox-Gastaut syndrome and atypical absence seizures, akinetic status epilepticus, and myoclonic seizures. Potential adverse reactions include a drop in white blood cells, drowsiness, loss of balance, slurred speech, tremor, confusion, increased salivation, double vision, abnormal eye movements, constipation, gastritis, change in appetite, nausea, great thirst, sore gums, painful urination, urinary retention, bed-wetting, skin rash, and respiratory depression, and behavioral disturbances, especially in children. Elderly people are more sensitive to clonazepam. It should not be withdrawn suddenly. Alcohol and central nervous system depressants increase its central nervous system depression. Contraindicated in glaucoma, liver and kidney disease, and in those sensitive to chlordiazepoxide, diazepam, or other benzodiazepines. Phenobarbital and phenytoin may reduce clonazepam's effectiveness. Clonazepam is most effective when taken on an empty stomach, but may be taken with a small amount of food if stomach upset is a problem.

CLONE • A genetically identical cell or organism.

CLONIDINE (Rx) • **Catapres. Catapres-TTS.** Introduced in 1969 in tablet form and later as a transdermal patch, clonidine inhibits the center in the brain that controls signals to the autonomic nervous system, which regulates the beating of the heart. It causes dilation of certain blood vessels, thereby decreasing blood pressure. It is also used to suppress symptoms during narcotics withdrawal, and as a prophylactic treatment for migraine and for menopausal flushing. Potential adverse effects include drowsiness, dizziness, fatigue, sedation, nervousness, headache, vivid dreams, low blood pressure, dry mouth, constipation, urine retention, impotence, rash, severe rebound high blood pressure, and transient glucose intolerance after large doses. Clonidine increases the action of central nervous system depressants. Propranolol and other beta-blockers cause a paradoxical hypertensive response when taken with clonidine. Tricyclic antidepressants and MAO inhibitors (*see*) may decrease clonidine's effectiveness. Persons taking the drug should rise from a sitting or lying position slowly. The last dose should be taken just before retiring. Most effective when taken on an empty stomach, but may be taken with a small amount of food if stomach upset is a problem.

CLONOPIN • *See* Clonazepam.

CLOPRA • *See* Metoclopramide.

CLORAZECAPS • *See* Clorazepate Dipotassium.

CLORAZEPATE DIPOTASSIUM (Rx) • **Gen-XENE. Tranxene.** A benzodiazepine (*see*) antianxiety drug introduced in 1968 that depresses the central nervous system limbic and subcortical levels of the brain. The drug is not meant for everyday stress. As an anticonvulsant it suppresses the spread of seizure activity in the brain. Potential adverse reactions include drowsiness, lethargy, hangover, fainting, dry mouth, transient high blood pressure, nausea, vomiting, and abdominal discomfort. Should not be used with alcohol or other central nervous system depressants. Use with cimetidine increases sedation. Contraindicated in glaucoma, depression, psychosis, and in children under eighteen years of age. Must be used with caution when liver or renal damage is present. The drug should not be discontinued suddenly. It is best taken on an empty stomach, but may be taken with a small amount of food if stomach upset is a problem.

CLOSTEBOL • *See* Anabolic Steroids.

CLOSTRIDIUM DIFFICILE • The leading cause of nosocomial intestinal infections, which can manifest as uncomplicated diarrhea and colitis. The disease occurs when antibiotics or other factors disrupt the resistance of normal colonic flora. Most antibiotics share the risk of further perturbing the protective normal flora in the colon and making the patient more susceptible to *C. difficile*. The incidence may range from 5 percent to 21 percent of hospitalized patients, and mortality may occur from complications such as toxic megacolon or intestinal perforation.

CLOTRIMAZOLE (OTC) • **Gyne-Lotrimin. Lotrimin. Lotrisone. Mycelex.** An antifungal and antiyeast medication in the form of lozenges, cream, topical lotion or solution, and vaginal cream or tablets. It is used to treat tinea pedis, tinea cruris, tinea corporis, tinea versicolor, and candidiasis (*see all*). It was reclassified OTC from RX in 1989 and 1990. Potential adverse reactions include nausea and vomiting (with lozenges), mild vaginal burning and irritation (with vaginal preparations), blistering, redness, swelling, itching, burning, stinging, peeling, hives, skin fissures, and general irritation. In treatment of a vaginal infection, the sexual partner should wear condoms until the treatment is finished.

CLOVE (H) • *Eugenia aromatica.* An evergreen tree, the clove is native to the Moluccas, the "Spice Islands," and is cultivated in Ceylon, Zanzibar, Java, and other tropical areas. The oldest medical use was in China, where it was taken for various ailments as early as 240 B.C. Medicinally, herbalists use cloves to treat flatulence and diarrhea, and for liver, stomach, and bowel ailments. It is also used as a stimulant for nerves. Clove oil is still sold in modern drugstores as a treatment for toothaches. Clove tea with mace is used in a tea for nausea. In 1992, the FDA proposed a ban on clove oil in astringent (*see*) drug products, because it had not been shown to be safe and effective as claimed.

CLOVER, RED (H) • *Trifolium pratense.* A perennial common throughout Europe, it is used in medicine as a tea and sometimes is combined with other herbs, as a tonic. Red clover also is given as a cure for indigestion, bronchitis, and whooping cough and is reputedly good for the nerves due to its sedative properties. A salve is made to heal fresh wounds, ulcers, and sores. Used by some herbalists to help cancer patients.

CLOXACILLIN SODIUM (Rx) • **Alclox. Apo-Cloxi. Austrastaph. Bactopen. Cloxapen. Novocloxin. Orbenin. Orbenin Injection. Tegopen.** A penicillin antibiotic introduced in 1962 for systemic infections caused by penicillinase-producing staphylococci (*see*). May cause lung problems (eosinophilia), nausea, vomiting, gastric distress, diarrhea, liver problems, overgrowth of nonsusceptible organisms, and hypersensitivity, including potentially fatal allergic reaction. Cloxacillin is most effective if taken on an empty stomach with a full glass of water.

CLOXAPEN • *See* Cloxacillin Sodium.

CLOZAPINE (Rx) • **Clozaril.** An antipsychotic drug introduced in 1990 for the treatment of schizophrenia in severely ill patients unresponsive to other therapies. It reportedly caused improvement in 30 percent of the cases that had not responded to other medications. Clozapine has to be carefully monitored. Potential adverse reactions include a drop in white blood cells, drowsiness, sedation, seizures, dizziness, fainting, headache, tremor, disturbed sleep or nightmares, restlessness, confusion, fatigue, insomnia, loss of balance, slurred speech, irregular heartbeat, low or high blood pressure, chest pain, constipation, nausea, vomiting, dry mouth, salivation, urinary problems, abnormal ejaculation, fever, muscle pain or spasm, muscle weakness, a drop in blood pressure when rising from a seated or prone position, weight gain, and rash. Blood pressure drugs may drop pressure too low when used with clozapine. Anticholinergics (*see*) may potentiate the muscle-relaxing effects of clozapine. Bone marrow suppressant drugs may increase bone marrow toxicity. Central nervous system–active drugs may have possible additive effects. Increased serum levels of warfarin, digoxin, and other highly protein-bound drugs may occur. Contraindicated in patients with adverse reactions to clozapine, or with severe central nervous system depression, coma, or enlarged prostate. Patients on clozapine should check with a physician before taking over-the-counter drugs. May be taken with or without food.

CLOZARIL • *See* Clozapine.

CL-719 • *See* Gemfibrozil.

CLUB MOSS (H) • *Lycopodium clavatum.* American Indians sprinkled a powder made from this herb on wounds to stop bleeding. The powder is used today for minor skin wounds. Both the spores and the whole herb are considered by herbalists as diuretic and antispasmodic, and decoctions were used in rheumatism and diseases of the lungs and kidneys.

CLUSAMIN (OTC) • A combination of glucosamine, calcium citrate, and vitamin D_3 (*see all*).

CLUSIVOL (OTC) • A multivitamin preparation.

CLYSODRAST • *See* Bisacodyl.

CMV • Abbreviation for cytomegalovirus (*see*).

CNICUS BENEDICTUS • *See* Blessed Thistle.

CNS • Abbreviation for central nervous system (*see*).

COAKUM • *See* Pokeweed.

COAL TAR (OTC) (H) • **Denorex Medicated Shampoo. Fototar. L.C.D. MG Psoriasis Ointment and Lotion. Neutrogena T/Gel. Oxipor. P & S Plus Tar Gel. Sebutone Cream Shampoo. Tarpaste. Tegrin. X-Sebt.** A thick liquid or semisolid tar obtained from bituminous coal, it contains many constituents, including benzene, xylenes, naphthalene, pyridine, quinoline, phenol, and creosol. The main concern about coal tar derivatives is that they not only cause cancer in animals, but are frequent sources of allergic reactions, particularly skin rashes, and hives. Coal tar is included in many topical preparations for the treatment of psoriasis and dandruff. In 1992, the FDA ruled that coal tar over-the-counter products for dandruff, seborrheic dermatitis, and psoriasis must have stated on their packaging the concentrations of coal tar contained in any solution, or the derivative or fraction of coal tar used in the source of the product. In 1992, the FDA also issued a notice that coal tar had not been shown to be safe and effective as claimed in OTC products.

COBIOTIC (Rx) • *See* Neomycin, Polymyxin B, and Hydrocortisone.

COCA • *See* Cocaine.

COCAINE • *Erythroxylon coca.* **Coca. Coke. Crack. Nose Candy. Snow.** Derived from the leaves of the coca plant, cultivated widely in South America. Once widely used as a local anesthetic, it is still sometimes given for topical anesthesia in the mouth, throat, and nose before surgery or other procedures. Because of its side effects and potential for abuse, it has been replaced in medicine, for the most part, by safer local anesthetics. Cocaine is a central nervous system stimulant. It can increase blood pressure and thus can counteract medications for high blood pressure. It also can cause a dangerous rise in blood pressure if taken concurrently

with MAO inhibitors (*see*). Cocaine also can increase adverse effects on the blood vessels and heart when taken with certain general anesthetics. Heavy regular use of cocaine can cause restlessness, anxiety, excitability, nausea, insomnia, and weight loss. Continued use may lead to increasing paranoia and psychosis. Repeated sniffing damages the lining of the nose and may eventually lead to the destruction of the structure separating the nostrils. Use of cocaine by people with heart disease, high blood pressure, and/or an overactive thyroid can result in a high risk of heart problems.

COCC • Homeopathic abbreviation for cocculus (*see*).

COCC-C • Homeopathic abbreviation for coccus cacti (*see*).

COCCI • Spherical bacterial cells; cocci may exist singly, in pairs (diplococci), chains (streptococci), or clusters (staphylococci).

COCCULUS (H) • *Anamirta cocculus.* **Fishberry.** A climbing plant. Cocculus preparations are used only in great dilutions in homeopathic medicine to treat heart conditions. Externally, it has been used to destroy lice. The plant is highly toxic.

COCCUS CACTI (H) • **Cocc-C.** A homeopathic remedy made from cochineal (*see*). It is used to treat coughs.

COCHINEAL CARMINE • A crimson pigment derived from a Mexican beetle and cacti.

COCHLEARIA OFFICINALIS • *See* Scurvy Grass Extract.

COCKLEBUR • *See* Agrimony.

COCOA BUTTER (OTC) (H) • **Theobroma Oil. Nupercainal Suppositories. Preparation H Hemorrhoidal Suppositories. Wyanoids Relief Factor Hemorrhoidal Suppositories.** A solid fat expressed from the roasted seeds of the cocoa plant, cocoa butter softens and lubricates the skin.

In 1992, the FDA proposed a ban on cocoa butter in diaper-rash drug products because it had not been shown to be safe and effective as claimed.

COCONUT OIL (OTC) (H) • pHisoDerm Cleansing Bar. The white, semisolid, highly saturated fat expressed from the kernels of the coconut. Used in cleansing preparations. May cause allergic skin rashes. In 1992, the FDA proposed a ban on coconut oil soap (aqueous) in lice-killing products because it had not been shown to be safe and effective as claimed.

CODEINE PHOSPHATE and SULFATE (Rx) • Capital and Codeine. Fiorinal with Codeine. Guaituss AC. Methyl Morphine. Naldecon CX. Nucofed. Ryna-C. Tussi-Organidin. Tylenol with Codeine. An analgesic that alters both the perception of and emotional response to pain, through an unknown mechanism, and the cough reflex. Used to treat mild to moderate pain. Potential adverse reactions include sedation, euphoria, dizziness, lack of alertness, seizures, low blood pressure, irregular heartbeat, nausea, vomiting, constipation, dry mouth, urine retention, itching, flushing, and respiratory depression. Alcohol and central nervous system depressants add to its effects. It should be used with extreme caution in head injury, increased pressure on the brain, liver or renal disease, low thyroid conditions, Addison's disease, acute alcoholism, seizures, severe central nervous system depression, breathing problems, shock, and in elderly or debilitated patients. May be addictive. Codeine should be taken with food to reduce gastrointestinal symptoms. In 1992, the FDA proposed a ban on codeine, codeine phosphate, and codeine sulfate in internal analgesic products, because they had not been shown to be safe and effective as claimed. Codeine was also on the ban list for menstrual drug products.

CODESOL • *See* Prednisolone.

CODICLEAR (Rx) • *See* Hydrocodone and Potassium Guaiacolsulfonate.

CODIMAL-A • *See* Brompheniramine.

CODIMAL LA (OTC) • *See* Chlorpheniramine and Pseudoephedrine.

COD LIVER OIL (OTC) • Desitin Ointment. The fixed, pale yellow, fishy-smelling oil expressed from fresh codfish liver, which is rich in vitamins A and D. These vitamins promote healing of wounds and abscesses.

CODOXY (Rx) • *See* Oxycodone Hydrochloride, Pectin, and Aspirin.

CODROXOMIN • *See* Vitamin B_{12}.

COENZYME Q_{10} (OTC) • Ubiquinone. A naturally occurring antioxidant nutrient and a cofactor in the energy production of the cell. Chemically similar to vitamins E and K. Its use in medicine to aid muscle function in diseases such as multiple sclerosis and heart failure is still being studied. It is also being tested in Denmark as an adjunctive treatment for breast cancer.

COFFEE (OTC) (H) • The most common psychoactive drug used, *Coffea arabica* is an evergreen shrub cultivated in many tropical regions. Its roasted seeds contain 1 to 3 percent caffeine and small amounts of theobromine and theophylline. It is used as a brain stimulant, diuretic, and heart stimulant by the general public in the form of a beverage. In some people, even a low dose of coffee may cause nervousness, restlessness, excitement, and even insomnia. Since coffee increases secretion of stomach acid, excessive use may contribute to hyperacidity. Contraindicated in individuals with peptic ulcers, hyperacidity, high blood pressure, heart and blood-vessel disorders, or those suffering from nervous excitement and anxiety.

COGENTIN • *See* Benztropine.

CO-GESIC (Rx) • *See* Acetaminophen and Hydrocodone.

COGNEX • *See* Tacrine.

COLA • *See* Kola Nut.

COLACE (OTC) • *See* Docusate.

COLASPASE • *See* Asparaginase.

COLBENEMID • *See* Probenecid and Colchicine.

COLBENL-MOR • *See* Probenecid.

COLCH • Homeopathic abbreviation for *Colchicum autumnale. See* Meadow Saffron.

COLCHICINE (Rx) (H) • Colabid. Colbenemide Tablets. Colsalide. Novocolchicine. A drug introduced in 1763 prepared from roots of the meadow saffron (*see*). It is specific in relieving gout, but why it works is unclear. Potential adverse reactions include nausea, vomiting, abdominal pain, anemia, diarrhea, hives, skin rash, and hair loss. Alcohol and diuretics may make it less effective. Colchicine impairs the absorption of vitamin B$_{12}$. Phenylbutazone may increase its adverse effects on white blood cells. Should be used cautiously in persons with liver dysfunction, heart disease, blood problems, kidney disease, GI disorders, and in elderly or debilitated patients. The following drugs decrease colchicine's effectiveness: anticancer drugs, butenamide, diazoxide, thiazide diuretics, ethacrynic acid, furosemide, mecamylamine, pyrazinamide, and triamterene. Colchicine can be taken with or without food.

COLCHICUM AUTUMNALE • *See* Meadow Saffron.

COLD SORE • Common term for herpes of the lip or vagina.

COLESTID • *See* Colestipol Hydrochloride.

COLESTIPOL HYDROCHLORIDE (Rx) • **Colestid.** A lipid-lowering drug introduced in 1974, it combines with bile acid to form an insoluble compound that is excreted. Potential adverse reactions include headache, dizziness, constipation, fecal impaction, hemorrhoids, abdominal discomfort, flatulence, nausea, vomiting, rashes, and irritation of the skin, tongue, and perianal area. May cause a deficiency of vitamins A, D, and K from decreased absorption. Contraindicated in persons sensitive to it or cholestyramine (*see*). Oral antidiabetic drugs may antagonize the response to colestipol. Colestipol may decrease the absorption of any orally administered drugs. All other medications, therefore, should be administered at least one hour before or four to six hours after taking colestipol. Take colestipol before meals. It may be mixed with juices or water.

COLIC • Abdominal cramps and, often, increased gas, usually in infants.

COLIC ROOT • *See* True Unicorn Root.

COLISTIN SULFATE (Rx) • **Coly-Mycin S. Coly-Mycin S Otic. Polymixin E.** Introduced in 1962, the sulfate form is used to treat diarrhea in infants and children caused by susceptible organisms, especially *E. coli* and *Shigella.* Combined with neomycin and hydrocortisone (*see both*) it is also used to treat superficial infections of the external ear canal and mastoid infections. It rarely causes adverse reactions, although itching, redness, and rash may occur, most often due to other ingredients in the preparations.

COLITIS • Inflammation of the colon (large intestine) causing diarrhea, usually with blood and mucus, and sometimes with abdominal pain and fever. Colitis may be due to a variety of causes, including infection by a virus, amoeba, or bacterium that produces toxins that irritate the intestinal lining. Antibiotic therapy for more than two weeks may result in a form of colitis caused by the bacterium.

COLLAGEN • An insoluble protein found in connective tissue, including skin, bone, ligaments, and cartilage. Collagen represents about 30 percent of total body protein.

COLLAGENASE (Rx) • **Biozyme-C. Santyl.** An enzyme to promote sloughing of dead tissue in skin ulcers and severe burns.

COLLINSONIA (H) • *Collinsonia canadensis.* **Horse Balm. Knob Root. Richweed. Stoneroot.** The root from a plant grown in North America. Contains saponin, alkaloid, tannin, and resin. It is used by herbalists to treat hemorrhoids. It also is used for varicose veins and diarrhea. In 1992, the FDA proposed a ban on collinsonia in oral menstrual drug products because it had not been shown to be safe and effective as claimed.

COLLODION (OTC) • A solution of nitrocellulose (plant material) in a solvent such as alcohol. The solution dries to form a sticky film and is used to protect broken skin.

COLLOIDAL OATMEAL (OTC) (H) • **Aveeno Bath Products.** Meal obtained by grinding oats. Soothing to the skin. In 1992, the FDA proposed a ban on colloidal oatmeal in astringent (*see*) drug products because it had not been shown to be safe and effective as claimed.

COLLYRIUM • *See* Boric Acid.

COLLYRIUM 2 (OTC) • *See* Tetrahydrozoline Hydrochloride, Glycerin, and Sodium Borate.

COLOC • Homeopathic abbreviation for colocynthis (*see*).

COLOCYNTH (OTC) • A cathartic prepared from a vine related to watermelon. Banned as an ingredient in laxatives by the FDA, May 1992.

COLOCYNTHIS • **Coloc.** From the family of Cucurbitaceae, colocynthis is a trailing plant that grows in sandy places. Homeopaths mix the powdered dried fruit with alcohol and allow the compound to sit for a week. This is one of the main colic remedies used by homeopaths. *See* Colocynth.

COLOGEL • *See* Methylcellulose.

COLONY STIMULATING FACTORS (Rx) • **CFSs.** Proteins that control the production of white blood cells. Cancer chemotherapy and inherited disorders are among the causes of low white blood cell counts, which lower resistance to infection. CSFs can stimulate the production of white blood cells.

COLORINGS • Many of the colorings used in pharmaceuticals are manufactured, frequently from coal tar (*see*) colors. The coal tar derivatives need to be certified, which means that batches of the dyes are chemically tested and approved by the FDA. *See also* FD&C Colors, D&C, and individual colors.

COLOSCREEN (OTC) • A diagnostic test for blood in feces.

COLOSTOMY • From the Greek words *kolon,* for colon, and *stoma,* for mouth, it refers to the establishment of an artificial opening into the colon.

COLREX EXPECTORANT (OTC) • A combination of acetaminophen, codeine, phenylephrine, and chlorpheniramine (*see all*) used to treat coughs. *See* Guaifenesin.

COLSALIDE • *See* Colchicine.

COLTSFOOT (H) • *Tussilago farfara.* **Coughwart. Horsehoof.** The Latin name means "the plant that stops coughing." It contains large quantities of vitamin C, calcium, and potassium. Used in a tea for upper-respiratory infections. Also used to soothe inflammation, and as an astringent. The plant is toxic to the liver and potentially carcinogenic in humans. In the 1990s, a case was reported of an infant born with severe liver damage blamed on the mother's drinking of coltsfoot tea during pregnancy. The child died after five weeks. There is a movement to ban the use of this plant in herbal remedies.

COLUMBINE (H) • **Crowfoot.** A slender perennial native to Europe and Asia and cultivated as an ornamental plant. Its seeds contain cyanogenic glycosides, tannins, resin, and alkaloids. Its seeds have been used by herbalists to treat skin diseases and jaundice. Extracts from the columbine herb have been used in homeopathic medicine to treat menopause and nervous disorders. Externally, seed decoctions have been used to treat sore throats and eczema. Severe injury and even fatalities have been reported in children who ate excessive amounts of the seeds.

COLY-MYCIN M • *See* Colistin.

COLY-MYCIN S • *See* Colistin.

COLY-MYCIN S OTIC (Rx) • A combination of colistin and hydrocortisone (*see both*), used to treat ear inflammation and infection.

COLYTE (OTC) • A drug used for clearing the bowel. *See* Polyethylene Glycol and Laxative.

COMBANTRIN • *See* Pyrantel.

COMBIPRES (Rx) • A combination of clonidine and chlorthalidone (*see both*), it reduces blood pressure by dilating blood vessels and reducing excess fluid. Potential adverse reactions include nausea, vomiting, weight gain, loss of hair, breast enlargement, heart problems, dry or burning eyes, sexual impotence, tingling in the limbs, sensitivity to sunlight, breathing difficulties, muscle spasms, fatigue, and blurred vision. Combipres may interact with digitalis to cause irregular heartbeat. If administered while taking lithium, it may increase lithium's toxicity. Central nervous system depressants such as alcohol, barbiturates, sedatives, and tranquilizers should be avoided while taking this drug. Combipres may be taken with or without food.

COMBISTIX (OTC) • A diagnostic test for sugar in the urine.

COMEDO • **Blackhead.** A blocked skin pore.

COMFREY (H) • *Symphytum officinale.* **Blackwort. Healing Herb. Knitbone.** The leaf and root contain allantoin, mucilage, tannins, starch, inulin (*see*), steroidal saponins, and pyrrolizidine alkaloids. It has been reported to be toxic when taken internally and to cause liver damage. Herbalists recommend comfrey for rapid wound and bone healing and use a decoction for diarrhea, hemorrhage, and bleeding. Potential adverse reactions include liver dysfunction. Pyrrolizidine alkaloids have been found to cause cancer in laboratory rats. Comfrey was formerly regarded as safe, but reports of toxic effects surfaced when its use became popular. Symptoms of poisoning appear after a few months of use. It is a strong liver toxin. Comfrey was banned in Canada in 1989.

COMHIST LA (OTC) • A cold-relief preparation containing chlorpheniramine, phenylephrine, atropine sulfate, and phenyltoloxamine (*see all*).

COMMON CENTAURY • *See* Centaury.

COMMON IVY • *See* Ivy.

COMPAL (Rx) • A combination of acetaminophen, caffeine, and dihydrocodeine (*see all*) used as an analgesic.

COMPAZINE • *See* Prochlorperazine.

COMPETE (OTC) • A multivitamin preparation with iron and zinc (see both).

COMPLEMENT • A complex series of blood proteins whose action "complements" the work of antibodies. Complement destroys bacteria, produces inflammation, and regulates immune reactions.

COMPOUND E • *See* Cortisone.

COMPOUND F • *See* Hydrocortisone.

COMPOUND S • *See* Zidovudine.

COMPOUND W (OTC) • A combination of salicylic acid, menthol, acetic acid, and camphor (*see all*).

COMPOZ (OTC) • Approved by the FDA as a sleep aid. *See* Diphenhydramine.

COMPULSION • An insistent, repetitive, and unwanted urge to perform an act as a means of relieving anxiety. However, the ritualistic behavior, such as repeated hand washing, is not realistically related to what the person is trying to avoid.

COMTREX (OTC) • A multisymptom cold-relief preparation. The "day" version contains acetaminophen, pseudoephedrine, and dextromethorphan (*see all*). The "night" version has the added antihistamine chlorpheniramine. Comtrex products should not be taken by persons with asthma, glaucoma, emphysema, chronic pulmonary disease, high blood pressure, heart disease, thyroid disease, diabetes, shortness of breath, or difficulty in urination due to prostate gland enlargement, unless directed by a doctor. Alcoholic beverages, sedatives, or tranquilizers can add to sedation. Should not be taken if a prescription for high blood pressure or depression is being taken, without first consulting a physician.

CON • Homeopathic abbreviation for conium (*see*).

CONACETOL • *See* Acetaminophen.

CONAR-A (OTC) • A cough medication containing acetaminophen, phenylephrine, guaifenesin, and noscapine (*see all*).

CONCEPTROL (OTC) • *See* Nonoxynol-9.

CONDURANGO (H) • *Marsdenia condurango.* The dried bark contains glycosides, resin, tannin (*see all*), and oils. A bitter-tasting herb, it is used to treat digestive and stomach problems, stimulate appetite, and relax nerves.

CONDYLOMA • Warty growths on the skin around the anus and external sex organs.

CONDYLOX • *See* Podofilox.

CONGENITAL • Refers to a condition present at birth.

CONGESPIRIN • *See* Dextromethorphan.

CONGESTIVE HEART FAILURE • Reduction of the pumping action of the heart caused by prolonged high blood pressure, damage from heart attack, or other disease of the heart muscle.

CONGRESS (Rx) • A cough medication containing pseudoephedrine and guaifenesin (*see both*).

CONIUM (H) • *Conium maculatum.* The dried, unripe fruit of the hemlock, it is used in homeopathic medications as a sedative, antispasmodic, and anodyne (*see*). Highly toxic. *See also* Hemlock.

CONJUGATED ESTROGENS (Rx) • **Premarin. Progens.** A mixture of estrogens (female hormones) obtained from natural sources such as pregnant mare's urine. Conjugated estrogens are used to relieve the symptoms of menopause such as hot flashes and sweating, and to treat underdeveloped ovaries and bleeding from the womb due to hormone imbalance. They also are used to treat and prevent osteoporosis (*see*), which may occur after menopause. Potential adverse reactions include nausea, vomiting, depression, high blood pressure, reduced sex drive, chest pain, vaginal bleeding, and breast swelling and tenderness. Tobacco smoking increases the risk of serious side effects. There is a risk of uterine cancer after menopause when conjugated estrogens are used without a progestin (*see*).

CONJUNCTIVA • The mucous membrane that lines the eyelids and covers the white portion of the eyes.

CONJUNCTIVITIS • **Pink Eye.** An infection of the membrane that lines the eyelids and covers the white portion of the eye.

CONSTANT-T • *See* Theophylline.

CONSTILAC • *See* Lactulose.

CONSTIPATION • Inadequate, infrequent, or difficult bowel movements.

CONSTULOSE • *See* Lactulose.

CONTAC (OTC) • A cold-relief medicine containing chlorpheniramine and phenylpropanolamine (*see both*).

CONTACT DERMATITIS • Skin eruption, redness, and inflammation, resulting from contact with substances that touch the skin.

CONTRAINDICATED • Means that a medication may hold a risk for an individual because of heredity, other medications being taken, kidney or liver problems, or other reasons that may lead to an adverse reaction.

CONTRAST MEDIUM • A substance, such as barium, that is relatively opaque to X rays and is given to patients to enhance the visualization of certain organs on X-ray examination.

CONTROL • *See* Phenylpropanolamine.

CONTUSS (OTC) • A combination of guaifenesin, phenylpropanolamine, and phenylephrine (*see all*) used to treat coughs.

COPAXONE • *See* Copolymer 1.

COPD • Abbreviation for chronic obstructive pulmonary disease (*see*).

COPHENE-B • *See* Brompheniramine.

COPHENE PL (OTC) • A combination of chlorpheniramine, phenylephrine, and phenylpropanolamine (*see all*) used to treat stuffy nose and symptoms of allergy.

COPOLYMER 1 (Rx) • **Copaxone.** A drug being developed in Israel and being tested in the United States for the treatment of relapsing-remitting multiple sclerosis, in which unpredictable attacks leave the victims increasingly disabled. U.S. multiple sclerosis researchers have said the results, thus far, have been "encouraging."

COPPER (Rx) (OTC) • **Copper Chloride Dihydrate. Copper Gluconate. Copper Sulfate. Cupric Chloride.** One of the earliest-known metals. An essential nutrient for all mammals. Naturally occurring or experimentally produced copper deficiency in animals leads to a variety of abnormalities including anemia, skeletal defects, and muscle degeneration. Copper deficiency is extremely rare in humans. The body of an adult contains from 75 to 150 mg of copper. Copper is an essential constituent of several proteins and enzymes. It plays an important role in the development of red blood cells, helps form the dark pigment that colors hair and skin, and helps the body to use vitamin C. It is essential for the formation of collagen and elastin (*see both*) and the proper formation and maintenance of bones. It is also required for central nervous system activity. Concentrations are highest in the brain, liver, and heart. A copper intake of 2 mg per day appears to maintain a balance in adults. An ordinary diet provides 2 to 5 mg daily. Copper is nontoxic, but soluble copper salts, notably copper sulfate, are highly irritating to the skin and mucous membranes and, when ingested, can cause serious vomiting. In 1992, the FDA proposed a ban on copper oleate in lice-killing products because it had not been shown to be safe and effective as claimed.

COPPER CHLORIDE DIHYDRATE • *See* Copper.

COPPER GLUCONATE • *See* Copper.

COPPER SULFATE • *See* Copper.

CORALONE • *See* Prednisolone.

CORDARONE • *See* Amiodarone.

CORDILATE • *See* Erythrityl Tetranitrate.

CORDILOX • *See* Verapamil.

COREG • *See* Carvedilol.

CORDRAN • *See* Flurandrenolide.

CORGARD • *See* Nadolol.

CORIANDER OIL (H) • *Coriandrum sativum.* The colorless or pale yellow, volatile oil from the dried ripe fruit of a plant grown in Asia and Europe. The name means "buglike odor." The ancient Egyptians used it for headaches. In the seventeenth century it was used to dispel "wind." It still is used today as a laxative and to aid digestion. Coriander is used (up to one gram) to break up intestinal gas. It is also employed as a flavoring agent in dentifrices. Can cause allergic reactions, particularly of the skin.

CORICIDIN (OTC) • A combination of aspirin and chlorpheniramine (*see both*).

CORICIDIN NASAL MIST (OTC) • *See* Oxymetazoline.

CORNEA • The outer "clear window" of the eye that allows light in.

CORN OIL • **Maize Oil. Lipomul Oral.** Edible oil used as a vehicle for injections.

CORN SILK (H) • *Stigmata maydis. Zea mays.* **Yumix.** The herb contains a large number of substances, including fatty acids, menthol, glycosides, thymol, saponins, sucrose, steroids, and vitamins C and K (*see all*). In Europe and the United States, corn silk is used in over-the-counter diuretics to reduce fluid retention. Herbalists maintain that corn silk reduces the painful symptoms and swelling due to cystitis, pyelitis, hepatitis, and all fluid-retention conditions. In 1992, the FDA proposed a ban on corn silk in oral menstrual drug products because it had not been shown to be safe and effective as claimed.

CORNSTARCH • Many containers are powdered with cornstarch to prevent sticking. The dietetic grade is marketed as Maizena and Mondamin. It is an absorbent dusting powder and a demulcent for irritated colons. May cause allergic reactions, including skin rashes and asthma.

CORONARY ARTERIES • Arteries that supply blood and oxygen to the tissues of the heart.

CORONARY ARTERY DISEASE • **CAD.** A progressive condition in which the heart muscle eventually receives inadequate blood supply via the coronary arteries (*see*).

CORRECTOL (OTC) • *See* Docusate and Phenolphthalein.

CORTAID (OTC) • *See* Hydrocortisone.

CORTALONE • *See* Prednisolone.

CORTAN • *See* Prednisone.

CORTATRIGEN (Rx) • *See* Neomycin, Polymyxin B, and Hydrocortisone.

CORT-DOME • *See* Hydrocortisone.

CORTEF • *See* Hydrocortisone.

CORTENEMA • *See* Hydrocortisone.

CORTEX • The external layer of gray matter covering the hemispheres of the cerebrum and cerebellum.

CORTICAINE (Rx) • *See* Dibucaine and Hydrocortisone.

CORTICOSTEROIDS (Rx) (OTC) • A class of compounds comprising natural steroid hormones, which are secreted by the adrenal cortex, and synthetic analogs. In pharmacologic doses introduced in 1948, corticosteroids were used primarily for their anti-inflammatory and/or immunosuppressive effects. Topical corticosteroids, such as betamethasone (*see*), are effective in the treatment of corticosteroid-responsive skin problems primarily because of their anti-inflammatory, anti-itching, and vasoconstrictive (*see*) actions. The absorption through the skin of topical corticosteroids involves many factors, including the vehicle, skin condition, and the use of covering dressings. Topical corticosteroids can be absorbed from normal, intact skin. The adverse effects of long-term use of corticosteroids include osteoporosis, cataracts, poor wound healing, gastrointestinal bleeding, high blood sugar, high blood pressure, and increased risk of infection. Some of these effects, such as gastrointestinal bleeding and osteoporosis, may be more severe in the elderly.

CORTICOTROPIN (Rx) • Adrenocorticotropic Hormone. ACTH. Acthar. Cortigel. Cortopic-Gel. Cortrophin G. Cortrophin Zinc. H.P. Acthar Gel. A hormone released from the pituitary gland. Used to treat acute exacerbations of multiple sclerosis, as a diagnostic aid in adrenocortical insufficiency, and to treat severe muscle weakness in myasthenia gravis (*see*). Potential adverse reactions include nausea, vomiting, euphoria, seizures, dizziness, pressure in the eyes, headache, insomnia, mood swings, personality changes, depression, psychosis, cataracts, glaucoma, peptic ulcer, hemorrhage, pancreatitis, abdominal distension, ulcers in the esophagus, menstrual irregularities, sodium and fluid retention, calcium and potassium loss, negative nitrogen balance, impaired wound healing, thin, fragile skin, bleeding into the skin, facial redness, increased sweating, acne, brown spots on the skin, hairiness, allergic skin reactions, muscle weakness, muscle damage, osteoporosis, compression fractures of the spine, cushingoid state (*see* Cushing's syndrome), suppression of growth in children, activation of latent diabetes, a progressive increase in antibodies, loss of ACTH stimulatory effect, and hypersensitivity. Contraindicated in scleroderma (*see*), osteoporosis, fungal infections, herpes, infection of the eyes, recent surgery, peptic ulcer, congestive heart failure, high blood pressure, sensitivity to pork and pork products, overactive adrenal gland or insufficiency of the gland, or Cushing's syndrome. Should be used with caution in pregnant women, breast-feeding mothers, and women of childbearing age, and in low thyroid, cirrhosis, infection, acute gouty arthritis, emotional instability, diabetes, kidney dysfunction, and myasthenia gravis. ACTH may mask signs of chronic disease and decrease resistance to infections.

CORTICOTROPIN-RELEASING FACTOR (CRF) • A neurotransmitter involved in appetite and stress reactions.

CORTIFOAM • *See* Hydrocortisone.

CORTIGEL • *See* Corticotropin.

CORTINAL • *See* Hydrocortisone.

CORTISOL • *See* Hydrocortisone.

CORTISONE (Rx) (OTC) • Cortone Acetate. A hormone secreted by the adrenal gland that affects carbohydrate and protein metabolism. Used as an anti-inflammatory drug in the treatment of acute arthritis, Addison's disease (*see*), allergic reactions, and inflammations of the eyes and skin. Most adverse reactions to cortisone result from dosage or length of time of administration. Potential adverse reactions include euphoria, insomnia, psychotic behavior, high blood pressure, swelling, cataracts, glaucoma, peptic ulcer, GI irritation, increased appetite, high blood sugar, growth suppression in children, delayed wound healing, acne, skin eruptions, muscle weakness, pancreatitis, hairiness, decreased immunity, and acute adrenal gland insufficiency. When withdrawn, there may be rebound inflammation, fatigue, weakness, joint pain, fever, dizziness, lethargy, depression, fainting, a drop in blood pressure upon rising from a seated or prone position, shortness of breath, loss of appetite, and high blood sugar. Sudden withdrawal of cortisone can be fatal. Contraindicated in systemic fungal infections. Should be used cautiously in patients with GI ulceration or kidney disease, high blood pressure, diabetes, chicken pox, osteoporosis, Cushing's syndrome (*see*), blood-clotting disorders, seizures, myasthenia gravis (*see*), congestive heart failure, tuberculosis, herpes, and emotional instability. When taking the drug, patients may need low-sodium diets and potassium supplements. Barbiturates, phenytoin, and rifampin (*see all*) increase its effects. Indomethacin and aspirin may increase the risk of GI distress and bleeding. Should be taken with food or milk to reduce GI irritation. *See also* Corticosteroids.

CORTISPORIN CREAM (Rx) • A combination of bacitracin, hydrocortisone, neomycin, and polymyxin B (*see all*), used to treat skin inflammations and infections.

CORTISPORIN OTIC (Rx) • A combination of hydrocortisone and neomycin (*see both*).

CORTONE ACETATE • *See* Cortisone.

CORTRIL • *See* Hydrocortisone.

CORTROPHIN G • *See* Corticotropin.

CORTROPHIN ZINC • *See* Corticotropin.

CORTROSYN • *See* Cosyntropin.

CORYBAN-D (OTC) • A combination of chlorpheniramine, phenylpropanolamine, and caffeine (*see all*).

CORYNEBACTERIUM PARVUM (Rx) • A drug derived from bacteria that stimulates the immune response, used in the treatment of certain cancers.

CORZIDE • *See* Nadolol and Bendroflumethiazide.

COSMEGEN • *See* Dactinomycin.

COSTMARY (H) • *Chrysanthemum majus.* A fragrant perennial grown in ancient Egypt, Greece, and Rome. It is said to be dedicated to Mary Magdalene, the patron saint of fallen women, because it was an infusion of costmary that she used to wash Jesus' feet. Physicians in the Middle Ages used costmary to treat indigestion, dysentery, ague, and weight loss. The bruised leaves were rubbed on insect bites and stings, and a lotion was made to remove head lice. As an herbal tea, it is used for catarrh (*see*).

COSTO-, -COSTAL • Prefix and suffix meaning pertaining to the ribs.

COSYNTROPIN (Rx) • **Cortrosyn. Synacthen. Tetracosactide.** An injectable synthetic replacement for the biologically active part of the ACTH molecule (*see* Corticotropin), cosyntropin stimulates the adrenal gland to secrete its entire spectrum of hormones. Used to diagnose adrenocortical function. Potential side effects include itching, flushing, and hypersensitivity reactions. Should be used cautiously in patients with hypersensitivity to natural corticotropin but, reportedly, is less likely to produce an allergic reaction than the natural product.

COTAZYM • *See* Pancrelipase.

COTRIM • *See* Co-Trimoxazole.

CO-TRIMOXAZOLE (Rx) • **Bactrim. Bethaprim. Comoxol. Cotrim. Septra. SMZ-TMP. Sulfamethoprim. Sulfatrim. Sulfoxaprim. Sulmeprim. TMP-SMZ. Trisulfam. Uroplus.** A combination of sulfamethoxazole and trimethoprim (*see both*), it is an inexpensive antibiotic used in the oral treatment of urinary tract infections, acute otitis media in children, acute exacerbations of chronic bronchitis in adults, prophylaxis and treatment in typhoid fever, shigellosis, and other infections. It has been found to be useful in treating *Pneumocystis carinii* pneumonia (PCP), the most common life-threatening opportunistic infection affecting those with AIDS. Potential adverse reactions include nausea, vomiting, allergic reactions, blood disorders, arthritislike pains, abdominal pain, diarrhea, headache, tingling in the arms or legs, depression, convulsions, hallucinations, ringing in the ears, dizziness, insomnia, malaise, weakness, kidney dysfunction, sensitivity to light, and nervousness. Contraindicated if a folic-acid deficiency is present or allergy exists to any of the ingredients. Septra may prolong the effects of blood thinners such as warfarin and antidiabetic oral drugs. Take each dose with a full glass of water and continue to drink fluids throughout the day to decrease chances of kidney problems.

COTTON (H) • *Gossypium hebaceum.* An erect annual or perennial native to India and extensively cultivated worldwide for commercial purposes. Its seeds and root bark are used by herbalists to induce abortion, to bring on menstruation, and as a contraceptive in males. Both bark and seeds are highly toxic.

COTYLENOL (OTC) • A combination of acetaminophen, chlorpheniramine, and pseudoephedrine (*see all*) used to treat headache and other discomforts due to colds and allergies.

COUCH GRASS (H) • *Agropyrum repens.* **Dog Grass. Quack Grass. Twitch Grass.** A weed that herbalists use to cool fevers and soothe and treat internal irritation or inflammation. Dogs and cats, when they have upset stomachs, will seek out and eat this plant. The roots possess both diuretic and demulcent properties and have been used by herbalists for centuries to treat bladder problems in humans. Couch grass contains a high concentration of soft mucilage, which gives the plant its soothing effect on mucous membranes. The plant also is reported to have antibiotic activity. In 1992, the FDA proposed a ban on couch grass in oral menstrual drug products because it had not been shown to be safe and effective as claimed.

COUGH SUPPRESSANT • **Antitussive.** A medication that suppresses or inhibits coughing. Most suppressants act directly to inhibit the brain's cough-control center.

COUGHWART • *See* Coltsfoot.

COUMADIN • *See* Warfarin.

COUMARIN (H) • **Curmarin. Tonka Bean.** A fragrant ingredient of tonka beans, sweet woodruff, cramp bark, and many other plants. Made synthetically as well. Has anti-blood-clotting effects, and anticlotting agents are derived from it. Coumarin is prohibited in foods by the FDA because it is carcinogenic and toxic by ingestion.

COUNTERIRRITANT • A substance applied directly to the skin to stimulate nerve endings to feel warmth, coolness, or substitute milder pain.

COVERA-HS (Rx) • A so-called "smart drug" that is a version of verapamil formulated in a way that allows its concentration in the blood to peak at around 6 A.M., when blood pressure and heart rate

naturally fall. It is believed that such "timing" will make the drug more effective because it will be present in high concentration when needed.

COVERT • *See* Ibutilide Fumarate.

COWBERRY (H) • **Red Whortleberry.** A small evergreen shrub, *Vaccinium vitis-idaea,* native to Europe, North America, and Asia. The leaves are used by herbalists as a diuretic, astringent, and urinary disinfectant. The leaves contain arbutin (*see*). Potential adverse effects include vomiting, spasms, anemia, stomach irritation, and constipation.

COWSLIP (H) • *Primula veris.* A primrose prevalent in Britain, it is an old folk remedy, used in a tea for migraine or insomnia. Contains saponins, glycosides, essential oils, and flavonoids (*see all*). Used as a sedative, and to treat colds, chills, and coughs.

COZAAR (Rx) • *See* Losarton Potassium.

CPK • Abbreviation for creatinine phosphokinase (*see*).

CPM • Abbreviation for cyclophosphamide (*see*).

CPT-11 (Rx) • **Camptosar.** The first major anticancer drug in a long time, it was developed by a Japanese yogurt company. The medication is from a Chinese tree. It was approved by the FDA in 1996 for the treatment of advanced colorectal cancer that has metastasized, or spread beyond the original site. In tests, between 40 and 60 percent of patients who had tumors growing at distant sites, such as the liver and the lung, had their tumors stabilized for a prolonged period of time.

CRAMP BARK (H) • *Vigurnum opulus.* **Guelder Rose. Snowball Tree.** The bark contains hydroquinones, arbutin, coumarins, tannins, and catechins (*see all*). Used to treat the cramps and discomfort of menstruation. Also has been used to prevent miscarriage and to treat the symptoms of menopause. A decoction is recommended by herbalists for asthma, and as a sedative. Contraindicated if anticoagulant drugs are being used.

CRANESBILL ROOT (H) • *Geranium maculatum.* **Alumroot. Storksbill. Spotted Geranium. Wild geranium.** The root contains tannic and gallic acids, starch, pectin, and gum. Used by early American Indians to treat dysentery, leukorrhea, and hemorrhoids, among other conditions. These people passed on the knowledge of the herb to early settlers. Used by herbalists today to treat diarrhea and dysentery, colitis, bleeding, and vaginal discharge. It is being studied by researchers at universities and the National Cancer Institute as a potential cancer remedy.

CRANIO- • Prefix meaning skull, as in *craniotomy,* a brain operation.

CREAMALIN • *See* Dextromethorphan.

CREATININE • A waste product of protein breakdown, reflecting renal function.

CREATININE PHOSPHOKINASE • **CPK or CK.** The most important cardiac enzymes. Levels are monitored to discern the extent of myocardial damage following a heart attack.

CREMACOAT 2 (OTC) • *See* Guaifenesin.

CREON • *See* Pancrelipase.

CREOSOTE (OTC) • Obtained from wood tar. Used locally as an antiseptic and internally as an expectorant. Large doses taken internally may cause stomach irritation, heart problems, and death. Also used as a mild insect repellent. In 1992, the FDA issued a notice that creosote (beechwood) had not been shown to be safe and effective as claimed in OTC products, including those to treat poison ivy, poison sumac, and poison oak.

CRESOL (OTC) • Obtained from coal tar and wood, cresols are antiseptic and disinfectant. Chronic poisoning may occur from oral ingestion or absorption through the skin. Cresols may also produce digestive disturbances and nervous disorders, with fainting, dizziness, mental changes, skin eruptions, jaundice, uremia, and lack of urine. In 1992, the FDA proposed a ban on cresol in astringent (*see*) drug products because it had not been shown to be safe and effective as claimed.

CRIXIVAN (Rx) • An experimental AIDS drug that is a protease inhibitor (*see*). In combination therapy with other AIDS drugs, participants had greatly reduced levels of virus in their blood after four months.

CROHN'S DISEASE • *See* Inflammatory Bowel Diseases.

CROMOGLICIC ACID • *See* Cromolyn Sodium.

CROMOLYN SODIUM (Rx) • **Gastrocrom. Intal Inhaler. Nalcrom. Nasalcrom. Opticrom. Rynacrom.** An allergy medication that reportedly is 70 to 75 percent effective in long-term prevention of asthma attacks. A *New England Journal of Medicine* review article, September 19, 1991, described cromolyn as having the fewest adverse effects of any antiallergic medication. However, it is poorly absorbed. It is used in eyedrops to treat and prevent allergic eye disorders. Potential adverse reactions to eyedrops include temporary stinging or burning upon instillation. The preparation contains benzalkonium chloride (*see*) as a preservative, so soft contact lenses should not be worn during the treatment period. Relief of symptoms may take several days to a week. In capsules, aerosols, or sprays, it is used to treat severe bronchial asthma, food allergy, exercise-induced asthma, and inflammatory bowel disease. Potential adverse reactions include nausea, dizziness, headache, throat irritation, cough, nasal congestion, wheezing, painful or frequent urination, rash, hives, joint swelling and pain, tearing, swollen glands, and pneumonia. Contraindicated in acute asthma and continuous asthma attacks. It is useful only in preventing attacks. Must be used cautiously in patients with coronary artery disease or irregular heartbeat. A candidate for OTC status.

CROSS-REACTION • *See* Cross-Reactivity.

CROSS-REACTIVITY • A phenomenon where cells or microorganisms resistant to a certain drug tend to be resistant to all other chemically related drugs.

CROTALINE ANTIVENIN POLYVALENT (Rx) • An antivenin used to treat rattlesnake bites. Potential adverse reactions include severe allergic reactions, nerve damage, and serum sickness. Antihistamines increase the toxicity of rattlesnake venoms.

CROTAMITON (Rx) • **Eurax.** A cream applied topically, used to treat scabies (*see*). May cause skin irritation. Contraindicated when skin is raw or inflamed. Should not be applied to face, eyes, or mucous membranes.

CROTON (H) • *Croton tiglium.* A small shrub or tree, the seeds of which are used in Chinese and homeopathic medicines as a strong cathartic, rubefacient, and vesicant. It is toxic and a potential cancer promoter.

CROWN VETCH (H) • *Coronilla varia.* A leafy perennial native to Europe and cultivated in North America. The herb and seeds contain cardiac glycosides and tannins. Homeopathics use it as a diuretic, emetic, laxative, and cardiotonic. The plant is toxic, particularly the seeds. In excessive amounts, it can cause heart failure.

CRUCIFEROUS VEGETABLES • A family of plants characterized by flowers and fruits that bear a cross. The genus is being studied intensively for anticancer properties. Among the vegetables are brussels sprouts, cauliflower, and broccoli.

CRUEX (OTC) • *See* Calcium Undecylenate.

CRY-, CRYO- • Prefixes meaning icy cold.

CRYPTOCOCCAL MENINGITIS • A fungal infection that affects the three membranes surrounding the brain and spinal cord. Symptoms include severe headache, dizziness, nausea, loss of appetite, sight disorders, and mental degeneration.

CRYSTAL VIOLET • *See* Gentian Violet.

CRYSTAMINE • *See* Vitamin B_{12}.

CRYSTAPEN • *See* Penicillin G.

CRYSTICILLIN A.S. • *See* Penicillin G and Procaine.

CRYSTODIGIN • *See* Digitoxin.

C-SOLVE 2 • *See* Erythromycin.

C-SPAN (OTC) • *See* Vitamin C.

CS-T (OTC) • A diagnostic test for blood in feces.

CUBEB BERRIES (H) • *Piper cubeba.* **Java Pepper. Tailed Pepper.** The dried unripe fruit of a perennial vine native to the East Indies, Java pepper was formerly used to stimulate healing of mucous membranes. The fruit has been used as a stimulant and diuretic and is sometimes smoked in cigarettes. The oil is used for chronic bladder troubles and is reputed to increase the flow of urine. Contraindicated in cases of inflammatory disease of the intestinal tract.

CUCUMBER (H) • *Cucumis sativus.* The juice of the cucumber was reputedly used by Cleopatra to preserve her skin. The juice is soothing to the skin and imparts a cool feeling. Herbalists believe it to be a good diuretic and to prevent constipation by ingestion. Researchers are now studying its effect on cholesterol.

CUDWEED (H) • *Gnaphalium ulginosum.* Used by herbalists to treat upper-respiratory inflammation, including laryngitis, tonsillitis, and bronchitis. Grown widely in North America.

CULVER'S ROOT (H) • *Leptandra virginica. Veronica virginica.* **Black Root. Physic Root.** The root of this perennial, which may be seen in borders and along roadsides, contains volatile oil, saponins, mannitol, dextrose, tannins, and other constituents. It induces sweating. American Indians used it as a laxative. It is an old American folk medicine for liver congestion and constipation. The plant is hazardous and should not be used.

CUMIN (H) • *Cuminum cyminum.* A fragile dwarf plant cultivated in Asia and the Middle East, it contains cuminic aldehyde, which may have some antiviral properties, and cumene, which is narcotic in high doses and potentially toxic by ingestion. The seed was used medically in ancient times as a stimulant and a remedy for stomach ailments. Used by herbalists to treat sore eyes.

CUPR • Homeopathic abbreviation for cupric metallicum. *See* Copper.

CUPRIC CHLORIDE • *See* Copper.

CUPRIC METALLICUM (H) • **Cupr.** Homeopaths use it to treat restlessness, colic, convulsions, and cough. *See* Copper.

CUPRIC SULFATE (OTC) • **Blue Vitriol Copper Sulfate.** Occurs in nature as hydrocyamite. Used as an agricultural fungicide, an herbicide, in the preparation of azo dyes (*see*), and as a skin fungicide. Irritating if ingested. In 1992, the FDA proposed a ban on cupric sulfate in astringent (*see*) drug products because it had not been shown to be safe and effective as claimed.

CUPRID • *See* Trientine.

CUPRIMINE • *See* Penicillamine.

CURARE (Rx) (H) • *Chondodendron tomentosum.* **Pareira.** A woody vine native to South America. The root and stem extract were made famous by B movies about arrow poisons and hard-to-solve murders. It was formerly used in folk medicine to treat kidney and bladder inflammations, jaundice, and arthritis. Curare is a source of d-tubocurarine, which is used to induce muscle relaxation during surgery. Curare is one of the most poisonous plants known.

CURCUMA (H) • Family of herbs that includes turmeric, licorice root, and flaxseed, all of which are being studied for their anticancer properties.

CURLED DOCK • *See* Sour Dock.

CURRANTS (H) • **Ribes.** A variety of small raisins grown in Greece. Red and white currants are antiseptic and, according to herbalists, are effective against many blood disorders as well as jaundice and other liver disorders. Herbalists maintain that currant jelly is served with game or roast mutton to counteract any potential bacterial illnesses caused by the meat. Black currants are used to treat infant thrush. Persons with bladder problems and pain caused by urinary retention may find relief in drinking an infusion made from freshly gathered black currant.

CURRETAB • *See* Medroxyprogesterone.

CUSHING'S SYNDROME • A disease caused by excessive steroid hormones in the blood, either from production by the adrenal gland lying above the kidney or by ingestion of steroids.

CUTANEOUS • Pertaining to the skin.

CYA • *See* Cyclosporine.

CYAN-, CYANO- • Prefixes meaning blue, as in *cyanosis,* blue coloring due to lack of oxygen to the tissues.

CYANOCOBALAMIN • *See* Vitamin B_{12}.

CYANO-GEL • *See* Vitamin B_{12}.

CYANOJECT • *See* Vitamin B_{12}.

CYANOSIS • Bluish discoloration of the skin, lips, and nail beds due to an inadequate level of oxygen in the blood.

CYCLAN • *See* Cyclandelate.

CYCLANDELATE (Rx) • **Cyclan. Cyclospasmol.** A drug that directly relaxes smooth muscle. Used in the treatment of cerebrovascular and peripheral disorders, including Raynaud's phenomenon and nocturnal leg cramps. Potential adverse reactions include headache, sweating, tingling of the extremities, dizziness, flushing, irregular heartbeat, belching, and heartburn. Should be used with caution in people with severe heart and blood-vessel disease because circulation may be compromised by the blood-vessel-expanding actions of the drug. Should be taken with food or antacids to lessen stomach upset.

CYCLIZINE (Rx) (OTC) • **Antivert. Antrizine. Dizmiss. Marazine. Meclizine. Meni-D. Ru-Vert-M.** Used in the prevention and treatment of nausea, vomiting, and dizziness of motion sickness. It reduces the sensitivity of the inner-ear apparatus and acts on the nerve pathways to the vomiting center in the brain. Potential adverse reactions include drowsiness, sensitivity, dry mouth, rash, hives, loss of appetite, diarrhea, urinary frequency, urinary retention, low blood pressure, palpitations, rapid heartbeat, and dry nose.

CYCLOBENZAPRINE (Rx) • **Flexeril.** A drug that reduces transmission of impulses from the spinal cord to skeletal muscles, used in the short-term treatment of muscle spasms. Potential adverse reactions include drowsiness, euphoria, weakness, headache, insomnia, nightmares, numbness, tingling, dizziness, depression, visual disturbances, and seizures. May also cause irregular heartbeat, rash, hives, itching, and urine retention. Cyclobenzaprine interferes with the blood-pressure-lowering effects of guanethidine (*see*). The drug is usually used for a short term only, but should not be discontinued abruptly or withdrawal symptoms such as nausea, headache, and malaise may result. Should be given with food or antacids to lessen stomach irritation. A candidate for OTC status.

CYCLOCORT • *See* Amcinonide.

CYCLOFLEX • *See* Cyclobenzaprine.

CYCLOGYL • *See* Cyclopentolate.

CYCLOMYDRIL OPHTHALMIC (Rx) • *See* Phenylephrine and Cyclopentolate. Used to treat eye inflammations.

CYCLOPAR • *See* Tetracycline Hydrochloride.

CYCLOPENTOLATE (Rx) • **AK-Pentolate. Cyclogyl Ocu-Pentolate.** A potent eye solution to dilate the pupil for diagnostic procedures. Potential adverse reactions include a burning sensation on instillation, blurred vision, eye dryness, eye redness, sensitivity to light, flushing, rapid heartbeat, urine retention, confusion, dry skin, fever, irritability, hallucinations, seizures, and behavioral disturbances in children.

CYCLOPHOSPHAMIDE (Rx) • **Cytoxan. Neosar.** An anticancer drug introduced in 1959 for breast, head, neck, lung, and ovarian cancer, Hodgkin's disease, chronic lymphocytic leukemia, chronic myelocytic leukemia, acute lymphoblastic leukemia, neuroblastoma, retinoblastoma, non-Hodgkin's lymphoma, multiple myeloma, mycosis fungoides, and sarcomas. Potential adverse reactions include nausea, vomiting, anemia, heart toxicity, loss of appetite, sore mouth, gonadal suppression, hemorrhagic cystitis, bladder fibrosis, kidney toxicity, high uric acid, reversible hair loss in 50 percent of the patients, especially with high doses, secondary malignancies, and lung fibrosis. Barbiturates increase the drug's effects and toxicity. Drugs toxic to the heart increase adverse cardiac effects. Corticosteroids and chloramphenicol (*see both*) reduce its effectiveness. Succinylcholine may cause breathing problems. While taking this medicine, it is important to drink a lot of fluids.

CYCLOSERINE (Rx) • **Seromycin.** An antibiotic used to treat tuberculosis, it may cause drowsiness, headache, tremor, dizziness, confusion, loss of memory, and psychotic symptoms. May also cause allergic skin rashes and should not be taken with alcohol or ethionamide. People with seizures, kidney problems, or emotional disorders are poor risks for this drug.

CYCLOSPASMOL • *See* Cyclandelate.

CYCLOSPORINE (Rx) • **CYA. Cyclosporine A. Sandimmune.** An immunosuppressive agent introduced in 1983, widely used in the field of transplantation since the 1970s, and at this writing, in trials for rheumatoid arthritis, psoriasis, and other autoimmune diseases. It is extracted from a culture of the fungus *Tolypocladium inflatum* GAMS. Potential adverse reactions include nausea, abdominal pain, heartburn, vomiting, diarrhea, hairiness, numbness, headache, tremor, flushing, gum disorders, kidney dysfunction, liver dysfunction, high blood pressure, and possibly lymphomas. The vast majority of drugs that interact with cyclosporine generally cause either an increase or decrease of its levels in the blood, thereby exposing the patient to the increased risk of developing renal dysfunction. Cyclosporine reduces the clearance of prednisolone (*see*), and conversely, high-dose methylprednisolone can increase blood concentrations. Cyclosporine may enhance the potential of lovastatin and colchicine (*see both*) to induce muscular toxicity. Aminoglycosides, amphotericin B, co-trimoxazole, and NSAIDs (*see all*) increase risk of kidney damage. Azathioprine, corticosteroids, cyclophosamide, and verapamil increase immunosuppression. Carbamazepine, isoniazid, phenobarbital, phenytoin, and rifampin may decrease immunosuppression. Ketoconazole, amphotericin B, cimetidine, diltiazem, erythromycin, n-cilastatin, metoclopramide, and prednisolone may increase levels of cyclosporine in the blood. Most effective when taken on an empty stomach, but may be taken with food if gastric distress is a problem.

CYCLOTHIAZIDE • *See* Thiazide Diuretics.

CYCRIN • *See* Medroxyprogesterone.

CYLERT • *See* Pemoline.

CYMEVENE • See Ganciclovir.

CYPERUS (H) • *Cyperus rotundus.* **Sedge Root.** A common wayside weed, it is closely related to the Egyptian papyrus plant. The root contains essential oils (*see*), including pinene and sesquiterpenes. It is used by herbalists to treat stomach cramps, colds, flu, menstrual irregularities, and depression.

CYPROHEPTADINE HYDROCHLORIDE (Rx) • **Periactin.** An antihistamine that is also used to stimulate appetite and treat allergy symptoms and itching. Potential adverse reactions include drowsiness (especially in elderly patients), dizziness, headache, fatigue, nausea, vomiting, stomach pain, dry mouth, urine retention, rash, and weight gain. Central nervous system depressants, including alcohol, increase sedation. MAO inhibitors may rapidly raise blood pressure. Use cautiously in elderly patients, and those with glaucoma, overactive thyroid, heart or kidney disease, high blood pressure, bronchial asthma, enlarged prostate, bladder-neck obstruction, and peptic ulcer. Coffee or tea may reduce drowsiness. Medication should be discontinued four days before taking a skin allergy test, as it can lead to inaccurate results. The elderly are more sensitive to this drug. It can be taken with or without food.

CYRONINE • *See* Liothyronine.

CYST- • Prefix meaning pertaining to a bladder or sac.

CYSTAGON • *See* Cysteamine Bitartrate.

CYSTEAMINE BITARTRATE (Rx) • **Cystagon.** An oral medication for the management of a rare disease, cystinosis, in children and adults, introduced in 1994. Cystinosis is an inherited metabolic disorder. The drug was reviewed and approved in nineteen months under a priority status. This medication replaces two drugs no longer available—cysteamine hydrochloride and phosphocysteamine—for the management of nephropathic cystinosis, which affects about four hundred persons in the United States.

CYSTEINE (OTC) • A nonessential amino acid. In 1992, the FDA proposed a ban on cysteine hydrochloride in diaper-rash drug products because it had not been shown to be safe and effective as claimed.

CYSTIC FIBROSIS • A genetic disorder causing abnormal mucous secretion that obstructs glands and ducts in various organs.

CYSTINE (OTC) • A product of cysteine (*see*) produced by oxidation and sometimes found in urine. Used to treat brittle nails.

CYSTITIS, INTERSTITIAL • *See* Interstitial Cystitis.

CYSTOSPAZ • *See* Hyoscyamine.

CYTADREN • *See* Aminoglutethimide.

CYTARABINE (Rx) • **Arabino-sylcytosine. Ara-C. Cytosar-U. Cytosine Arabinoside.** An antimetabolite (*see*) medication derived from chemicals found in a Caribbean sponge, *Tethya crypta*, used to treat some kinds of cancer, particularly leukemia. Cytarabine interferes with the growth of cancer cells, which are eventually destroyed. Normal body cells are also affected by cytarabine, and some of the side effects may be serious. This medicine causes temporary loss of hair; after the treatment has stopped, the hair grows back. Potential adverse reactions include black, tarry stools, cough or hoarseness, fever or chills, lower-back pain, side pain, painful urination, unusual bleeding or bruising, sores in the mouth and on the lips, joint pain, numbness or tingling in the fingers, toes, or face, swelling of the limbs, fatigue, bone pain, red eyes, shortness of breath, rash, weakness, ulcers, liver damage, high uric acid, loss of appetite, nausea, vomiting, dizziness, diarrhea, headache, itching, skin freckling, and flulike symptoms.

-CYT-, -CYTE, CYTO- • Signifying cell such as leukocytes (*see*), white blood cells.

CYTISUS SCOPARIUS • *See* Broom.

CYTOKINES • Naturally occurring proteins that regulate or modify the growth of specific cells. They act as immune-system hormones or messengers. *See* GM-CSF.

CYTOMEGALOVIRUS • **CMV.** An opportunistic infection that can cause blindness and be fatal to AIDS patients.

CYTOMEL • *See* Liothyronine.

CYTOPENIA • An abnormally low number of blood cells.

CYTOSAR-U • *See* Cytarabine.

CYTOSINE ARABINOSIDE • *See* Cytarabine.

CYTOTEC • *See* Misoprostol.

CYTOTOXICS • Drugs that destroy rapidly dividing cells; usually used to treat cancer and, more recently, autoimmune diseases. This drug group includes methotrexate, azathioprine, chlorambucil, and cyclophosphamide. Rapidly dividing cells include lymph cells found in the synovial fluid of joints and, unfortunately, in bone marrow, where all blood cells originate, and mucosal tissue. Because of their toxicity, these drugs are generally used in severe rheumatoid arthritis only after other agents have failed.

CYTOVENE • *See* Ganciclovir.

CYTOXAN • *See* Cyclophosphamide.

D

DACARBAZINE (Rx) • **DIC. DTIC-Dome.** An anticancer alkylating agent (*see*) used in the treatment of the skin cancer, melanoma, and Hodgkin's disease. Potential adverse reactions include severe nausea and vomiting beginning one to three hours after administration in 90 percent of patients and lasting up to twelve hours; also loss of appetite, a drop in white blood cells, phototoxicity, flulike symptoms, muscle pain beginning a week after treatment has stopped and possibly lasting up to two weeks, loss of hair, severe allergic reaction, and rarely, liver dysfunction.

DACODYL • *See* Bisacodyl.

DACTINOMYCIN (Rx) • **Actinomycin D. Cosmegen.** A cytotoxic (*see*), antibiotic anticancer drug used to treat melanomas, sarcomas, uterine tumors, testicular cancer, Wilms's tumor, rhabdomyosarcoma, and Ewing's sarcoma (*see all*). Potential adverse reactions include nausea, vomiting, loss of appetite, anemia, abdominal pain, diarrhea, sore mouth, reddened skin, dark spots on the skin, acnelike eruptions, blood clots in the injected vein, reversible hair loss, and liver toxicity.

DA HUANG • *See* Rhubarb, Chinese.

DAILY REFERENCE VALUES • **DRVs.** Introduced in 1994 by the FDA, these values are for nutrients for which no set of standards previously existed, such as fat, cholesterol, carbohydrates, proteins, and fibers. DRVs for these energy-producing nutrients are based on the number of calories consumed per day. For labeling purposes, two thousand calories has been established as the reference for calculating percent daily values. This level was chosen, in part, because many health experts say it approximates the maintenance calories requirements of the group most often targeted for weight reduction: postmenopausal women. *See* Reference Daily Intakes.

DAILY VALUES • **DV.** Two sets of references for nutrients. *See* Daily Reference Values and Reference Daily Intakes.

DAINITE KL • *See* Aminophylline.

DAIRY EASE (OTC) • *See* Lactase.

DAISY (H) • *Bellis perenis.* The fresh or dried flowers of this plant, which is cultivated or grows wild all over North America, are used in an infusion or tincture. The flowers contain saponins, tannin, essential oil, flavones, bitter principle, and mucilage (*see all*). Daisy is used for coughs and inflammations of the mucous lining. It reputedly also helps arthritis, as well as liver and kidney problems.

DAISY 2 (OTC) • A diagnostic test for pregnancy.

DALACIN C • *See* Clindamycin.

DALALONE L.A. and DALALONE D.P. • *See* Dexamethasone.

DALCAINE • *See* Lidocaine.

DALICOTE • *See* Dexamethasone.

DALIDYNE • *See* Dexamethasone.

DALMANE • *See* Flurazepam.

DALPRO ACID • *See* Valproic Acid.

DALTEPARIN SODIUM • **Fragmin.** A low-molecular-weight heparin (*see*) that is injected once daily for the prevention of deep-vein blood clots and blood clots in the lungs of patients undergoing abdominal surgery who are at risk for such clotting complications. It was introduced in 1994 after a review of nearly two years by the FDA. It is used in fifteen countries including Germany, which introduced the compound in 1985.

DAMASON-P • *See* Hydrocodone and Aspirin.

DAMIANA (H) • *Turnera diffusa. Turnera aphrodisiaca.* **Pastorata.** From the leaves of a tropical plant that contain volatile oil, hydrocyanic glycoside, bitter principle, tannin, and resin. The drug is used by herbalists as a mild aphrodisiac for both sexes. Reputed to be the safest of plant aphrodisiacs. Also is believed to counteract depression and coughs. Contraindicated in severe urinary-tract disease because it can worsen existing conditions.

D-AMP • *See* Ampicillin.

DANAZOL (Rx) • **Cyclomen. Danocrine.** A drug introduced in 1976 that inhibits the effects of estrogen by suppressing hormones from the front of the pituitary gland. Used to treat endometriosis, fibrocystic breast disease, and to prevent hereditary angioedema (*see all*). Potential adverse reactions in women include acne, water retention, weight gain, hairiness, hoarseness, clitoral enlargement, decrease in breast size, changes in libido, male pattern baldness, oiliness of the skin or hair, a drop in blood platelets, dizziness, headache, sleep disorders, fatigue, tremor, irritability, excitation, lethargy, mental depression, high blood pressure, visual disturbances, gastric irritation, nausea, vomiting, diarrhea, constipation, change in appetite, blood in urine, jaundice, flushing, sweating, vaginitis, emotional mood swings, nervousness, menstrual irregularities, and muscle cramps and spasms. Contraindicated in undiagnosed abnormal genital bleeding, and kidney, heart, or liver dysfunction. Must be used cautiously in epileptics or those with migraine headaches. Washing after intercourse and the wearing of cotton underwear is usually suggested to decrease the risk of vaginal inflammation.

DANDELION (H) • *Taraxacum officinale.* **Blow Ball. Clock. Gowans Milk. Priest's Crown. Pu Gong Ging. Wiggers.** Native to Europe and eastern Asia, it is believed to have derived its name from the Norman *dent de leon,* "lion's tooth," referring to its sharply toothed leaves. The milky juice, called "devil's milk," was used to treat pimples and warts. It was so effective as a diuretic, it was nicknamed "piss-a-bed" in the United States and Britain. In Chinese medicine, it is used to treat problems of the liver (including hepatitis) and pancreas. The reputa-

tion of the plant as a remedy against swooning and passion gave it the name heart-fever grass in Ireland. Used in an herbal tea as a tonic and blood purifier by herbalists. Rich in beta-carotene (*see*) and lecithin and contains several choleretic compounds, which stimulate the liver. Among the substances within dandelion and the related chicory (*see*) root are tannin, inulin (*see both*), and sugars. In 1992, the FDA proposed a ban on *Taraxacum officinale* in oral menstrual drug products because it had not been shown to be safe and effective as claimed.

DANDRUFF • An FDA regulation issued in 1991 lists the following as safe and effective: coal tar preparations and salicylic acid for dandruff, seborrheic dermatitis (*see*), and psoriasis (*see*); pyrithione zinc and selenium sulfide for dandruff and seborrheic dermatitis; sulfur for dandruff; and a combination of salicylic acid and sulfur for dandruff.

DANG SHEN • *See* Salvia.

DANOCRINE • *See* Danazol.

DANTHRON • A stimulant laxative banned by the FDA. *See* Laxative.

DANTRIUM • *See* Dantrolene.

DANTROLENE (Rx) • **Dantrium.** A muscle relaxant introduced in 1974 that acts directly on skeletal muscle to interfere with the movement of calcium in the cells. Used to treat spasticity and other muscle disorders due to chronic conditions such as cerebral palsy, multiple sclerosis, and spinal cord injury. Also used to prevent recurrence of malignant high temperature. Potential adverse reactions include muscle weakness, drowsiness, dizziness, malaise, headache, confusion, nervousness, insomnia, seizures, rapid heartbeat, excessive tearing, visual disturbances, urinary frequency, incontinence, constipation, cramping, loss of appetite, difficulty swallowing, metallic taste, severe diarrhea, impotence, hepatitis, skin rash, itching, hives, photosensitivity, hairiness, drooling, sweating, chills, fever, and muscle pain.

Alcohol and central nervous system depressants increase dantrolene's central nervous system effects. Use with verapamil (*see*) may cause heart stoppage. Contraindicated in rheumatic disorders and in breast-feeding women. Used with caution in patients with severely impaired heart, lung, or liver function and in patients over thirty-five years of age. Should be taken with meals or milk to prevent GI distress.

DAPA (OTC) • *See* Acetaminophen.

DAPEX • *See* Phentermine.

DAPIPROZOLE (Rx) • **Rev-Eyes.** Introduced in 1990, it is an alpha-blocking agent (*see* Alpha Blockers) that acts by blocking the receptors in smooth muscle and affects the dilator muscles of the iris in the eye. It is used to treat dilation of the pupil of the eye.

DAPSONE (Rx) • **Avlosulfon. Dapsone 100. DDS.** Introduced in 1957 to treat all forms of leprosy (Hansen's disease), it may cause anemia and other blood problems, psychosis, headache, dizziness, lethargy, numbness, ringing in the ears, stuffy nose, loss of appetite, abdominal pain, nausea, and vomiting. Also may adversely affect the liver and cause allergic skin rash. Interacts with probenecid (*see*), causing dapsone's levels to increase in the body. May have to be taken from three years to life.

DARANIDE • *See* Dichlorphenamide.

DARAPRIM • *See* Pyrimethamine.

DARVOCET-N (Rx) • **Dolene-AP 65. DOXA-PAP-N. Genagesic. Lorcet. Propacet N. Prox/APAP. Wygesic.** A combination of propoxyphene and acetaminophen (*see both*), used to relieve mild to moderate pain. Propoxyphene is a derivative of methadone, a stronger pain reliever than codeine (*see both*). Contains FD&C Yellow No. 6 (*see*). Potential adverse reactions include nausea, vomiting, constipation, rash, abdominal pain, light-headedness, weakness, headache, euphoria, and allergic reactions. Long-term use may cause anemia. Alcohol, tranquilizers, sedatives, sleeping pills, or antihistamines may increase the side effects of darvocet. Should be taken with a full glass of water or with food to reduce gastrointestinal disturbances.

DARVON • *See* Propoxyphene.

DARVON COMPOUND 65 (Rx) • *See* Aspirin, Propoxyphene, and Caffeine.

DARVON N (Rx) • *See* Butylparaben and Propoxyphene Napsylate.

DATRIL (OTC) • *See* Acetaminophen.

DA T'SAO • *See* Jujube Date.

DATURA STRAMONIUM • *See* Jimsonweed.

DAUNOMYCIN • *See* Daunorubicin Hydrochloride.

DAUNORUBICIN HYDROCHLORIDE (Rx) • **DNR. Cerubidine. Daunomycin. Rubidomycin.** A cytotoxic antibiotic used to treat leukemia. Potential adverse reactions include nausea, vomiting, bone marrow suppression, sore throat, loss of appetite, diarrhea, irreversible heart injury, kidney toxicity, liver toxicity, rash, pigmentation of fingernails and toenails, sloughing tissue at injection site, fever, chills, and generalized, usually reversible, loss of hair. Urine may be red for one or two days, but not due to bleeding. Persons taking this drug are usually advised to drink fluids liberally.

DAYPRO • *See* Oxaprozin.

DAZAMIDE • *See* Acetazolamide.

D&C • Abbreviation for colors approved by the United States Food and Drug Administration (USFDA) for use only in drugs and cosmetics, and not in food. *See* FD&C Colors.

D&C BLUE NO. 1 ALUMINUM LAKE • **Brilliant Blue Lake.** Insoluble pigment prepared from FD&C Blue No. 1 (*see*). A coal tar derivative, this brilliant blue is used as a coloring in cosmetics and drugs. May cause allergic reactions. It will produce malignant tumors in rats at the site of injection. On the FDA permanent list of color additives. Rated 1A for toxicology by the World Health Organization, meaning it is completely acceptable for use in foods, drugs, and cosmetics. *See also* FD&C Colors.

D&C BLUE NO. 2 ALUMINUM LAKE • **Acid Blue 74. Indigetine 1A. Indigo Carmine.** An indigo dye (*see*). *See also* FD&C Colors.

D&C BLUE NO. 4 • Acid Blue 9 (Ammonium Salt). Bright greenish blue. A coal tar color permanently listed by the FDA, January 3, 1977. *See also* FD&C Colors.

D&C BLUE NO. 6 • Indigo. An indigo (*see*) dye. *See also* FD&C Colors.

D&C BROWN NO. 1 • Resorcin Brown. Acid Orange 24. Light orange brown. A diazo dye (*see*) made with resorcinol (*see*), which can be irritating to the skin and mucous membranes. Absorption can cause depletion of oxygen in the body, and death. Also used as an antiseptic and fungicide. Permanently listed in 1976 for external use only. *See also* FD&C Colors.

D&C GREEN NO. 3 ALUMINUM LAKE • **Food Green 3.** The aluminum salt of FD&C Green No. 3. A brilliant but not colorfast dye. *See* Aniline and FD&C Colors.

D&C GREEN NO. 5 • Acid Green 25. Dullish blue green. Classed chemically as an anthraquinone color (*see* Colorings). Used in suntan oils, toothpastes, and soaps. Low skin toxicity, but may cause skin irritation and sensitivity. Permanently listed by the FDA in 1982. *See also* FD&C Colors.

D&C GREEN NO. 6 • Solvent Green 3. Dull blue green. Classified chemically as an anthraquinone (*see*) color. Permanently listed by the FDA in 1982. *See also* FD&C Colors.

D&C GREEN NO. 8 • Solvent Green 7. Transparent orange classed chemically as a monoazo color (*see*). Permanently listed by the FDA in 1976. *See also* FD&C Colors.

D&C ORANGE NO. 4 • Acid Orange 7. Bright orange. Transparent orange used in lipsticks and face powders. Classed chemically as a monoazo color (*see*). Permanently listed by the FDA in 1977. *See also* FD&C Colors.

D&C ORANGE NO. 4 ALUMINUM LAKE • Persian Orange. An insoluble pigment prepared from D&C Orange No. 4 (*see*). *See also* Colorings, Lakes, Color, and FD&C Colors.

D&C ORANGE NO. 5 • Acid Orange 11. Solvent Red 72. Dibromofluorescein. Reddish orange. Permanently listed by the FDA in 1982 for use in lipsticks, mouthwashes, and dentifrices. Permanently listed in 1984 for externally applied drugs and cosmetics. *See also* Dibromofluorescein and FD&C Colors.

D&C ORANGE NO. 5 ALUMINUM LAKE • Dawn Orange. Manchu Orange. Insoluble pigment prepared from D&C Orange No. 5 (*see*). *See also* Colorings and Lakes, Color.

D&C ORANGE NO. 5 ZIRCONIUM LAKE • Petite Orange. Dawn Orange. Acid Red 26. Ponceau R. A monoazo color (*see*). *See also* FD&C Colors, Lakes, Color.

D&C ORANGE NO. 10 • Solvent 73. Diiodofluorescein. Reddish orange. Classed chemically as a fluoran (*see*) color. *See also* FD&C Colors.

D&C ORANGE NO. 10 ALUMINUM LAKE • Solvent Red 73. Erythrosine G. A xanthene color (*see*). *See also* FD&C Colors.

D&C ORANGE NO. 11 • Clear red. Classed chemically as a xanthene color (*see*). It is the conversion product of D&C Orange No. 10 (*see*) to the sodium or potassium salt. *See also* FD&C Colors.

D&C ORANGE NO. 17 • Permanent Orange. Pigment Orange 5. Bright orange. Classed chemically as a monoazo color (*see*). The FDA permanently listed D&C Orange No. 17, but its ruling was reversed in 1987 by the United States Court of Appeals for the District of Columbia, which said the FDA lacked legal authority to approve the coloring since it was found to induce cancer. The court's ruling was in response to a lawsuit by the Public Citizen Health Research Group, a consumer advocacy group. *See also* FD&C Colors.

D&C ORANGE NO. 17 LAKE • Permanent Orange. Solvent Red 23. Sudan III. A diazo dye (*see*). *See also* FD&C Colors.

D&C RED NO. 2 ALUMINUM LAKE • An insoluble pigment prepared from FD&C Red No. 2 (*see*). *See also* FD&C Colors.

D&C RED NO. 3 ALUMINUM LAKE • An insoluble pigment prepared from FD&C Red No. 2 (*see*) and aluminum. *See also* FD&C Colors.

D&C RED NO. 4 ALUMINUM LAKE • Food Red 1. A monoazo color (*see*). *See also* FD&C Colors.

D&C RED NO. 6 • Lithol Rubine B. Medium red. Classed chemically as a monoazo color (*see*). It is the calcium salt of D&C Red No. 7 (*see*). Lithol is a topical antiseptic. Permanently listed by the FDA in 1983. *See also* FD&C Colors.

D&C RED NO. 6 ALUMINUM LAKE • Pigment Red 57. Lithol Rubine. A monoazo color (*see*). *See also* FD&C Colors.

D&C RED NO. 6 BARIUM LAKE • Pigment Red 57. Rubine Lake. Lithol Rubine B. A monoazo color (*see*). An insoluble pigment prepared from D&C Red No. 6 (*see*) and barium. *See also* FD&C Colors.

D&C RED NO. 6 POTASSIUM LAKE • An insoluble pigment composed of the potassium salt of D&C Red No. 6 (*see*). *See also* FD&C Colors.

D&C RED NO. 7 • Lithol Rubine B Ca. Bluish red. Classed chemically as a monoazo color (*see*). Also used as a topical antiseptic. Permanently listed by the FDA in 1987. *See also* FD&C Colors.

D&C RED NO. 7 ALUMINUM LAKE • Pigment Red 57. *See* Azo Dyes, Lakes, Color, and FD&C Colors.

D&C RED NO. 7 BARIUM LAKE • An insoluble pigment prepared from D&C Red No. 7 (*see*). *See also* Lakes, Color, and FD&C Colors.

D&C RED NO. 7 CALCIUM LAKE • Pigment Red 57. Lithol Rubine B. A monoazo color (*see*). An insoluble pigment prepared from D&C Red No. 7 (*see*) and calcium. *See also* Lakes, Color, and FD&C Colors.

D&C RED NO. 7 ZIRCONIUM LAKE • Pigment Red 57. Lithol Rubine B. A monoazo color (*see*). Carcinogenic in animals. Ruling postponed. *See also* Lakes, Color, and FD&C Colors.

D&C RED NO. 8 • Lake Red C. Pigment Red 53. Orange. Classed chemically as a monoazo color (*see*). Carcinogenic in animals. Permanently listed in 1987 by the FDA. This permanent listing of D&C Red No. 8 has been challenged in a lawsuit by the Public Citizen Health Research Group, a consumer advocacy group. *See also* Lakes, Color, and FD&C Colors.

D&C RED NO. 8 BARIUM LAKE • Acid Red 88. Fast Red A. A monoazo color (*see*). *See* Azo Dyes, FD&C Colors, and Lakes, Color.

D&C RED NO. 8 SODIUM LAKE • An insoluble pigment prepared from D&C Red No. 8 (*see*). *See also* FD&C Colors and Lakes, Color.

D&C RED NO. 9 • Lake Red C Ba. Scarlet coloring. The barium salt of D&C Red No. 8 (*see*). Permanently listed in 1987 by the FDA. The permanent listing of this color, which has shown to be carcinogenic in animals, was challenged in 1988 by the Public Citizen Health Research

Group, a consumer advocacy organization. *See also* Lakes, Color, and FD&C Colors.

D&C RED NO. 9 BARIUM LAKE • An insoluble pigment prepared from D&C Red No. 9 and barium (*see both*). *See also* FD&C Colors.

D&C RED NO. 9 ZIRCONIUM STRONTIUM LAKE • Similar to D&C Red No. 8 (*see*). *See also* FD&C Colors.

D&C RED NO. 10 • **Litho Red.** Yellowish red. *See* FD&C Colors.

D&C RED NO. 17 • **Toney Red.** Classed chemically as a diazo (*see*) color. Carcinogenic in animals. No longer used much in lipsticks. The FDA permanently listed Red No. 17 in 1988, but its ruling was later reversed by the United States Court of Appeals for the District of Columbia, which said the FDA lacked legal authority to approve Red No. 17 since it was found to induce cancer. The court's ruling was in response to a lawsuit by the Public Citizen Health Research Group, a consumer advocacy group. *See also* FD&C Colors.

D&C RED NO. 19 • **Rhodamine B.** Magenta. Classed chemically as a xanthene (*see*) color. Its greenish crystals or yellow powder turns violet in solution. The FDA permanently listed D&C Red No. 19 in 1988, but its ruling was reversed by the United States Court of Appeals for the District of Columbia, which said the FDA lacked legal authority to approve Red No. 19 since it was found to induce cancer. The court's ruling was in response to a lawsuit by the Public Citizen Health Research Group, a consumer advocacy group. *See also* FD&C Colors.

D&C RED NO. 19 BARIUM LAKE • **Rhodamine B.** Magenta. Violet in solution. A xanthene (*see*) dye. *See also* FD&C Colors.

D&C RED NO. 19 ZIRCONIUM LAKE • **Vat Red 1. Thioindigo Pink R.** A thioindigoid dye. *See* FD&C Colors and Indigo.

D&C RED NO. 21 • **Solvent Red 43. Tetrabromofluorescein.** Classed chemically as a fluoran (*see*) color. Permanently listed by the FDA in 1982. *See also* FD&C Colors.

D&C RED NO. 21 ALUMINUM LAKE • An insoluble pigment prepared from D&C Red No. 21 (*see*) and aluminum. *See* FD&C Colors.

D&C RED NO. 21 ZIRCONIUM LAKE • **Solvent Red 43. Merry Pink.** A xanthene (*see*) dye. *See also* FD&C Colors.

D&C RED NO. 22 • **Eosine YS.** Yellowish pink. Classed chemically as a xanthene (*see*) color. Brownish red powder, or red crystals with a bluish tinge. Lethal dose in animals is quite small. Permanently listed in 1982 by the FDA. *See also* FD&C Colors.

D&C RED NO. 27 • **Solvent Red 48. Philoxine B. Veri Pink.** A xanthene (*see*) dye. Classed chemically as a fluoran (*see*) color. A deep bluish red stain. Permanently listed in 1982 by the FDA. *See also* FD&C Colors.

D&C RED NO. 27 ALUMINUM LAKE • **Terabromo Terachloro Fluorescein Lake.** An insoluble pigment prepared from D&C Red No. 27 (*see*) and aluminum. *See also* FD&C Colors.

D&C RED NO. 27 BARIUM LAKE • **Solvent Red 48. Petite Pink.** A xanthene (*see*) dye. *See also* FD&C Colors.

D&C RED NO. 27 ZIRCONIUM LAKE • **Solvent Red 48.** A xanthene (*see*) dye, deep bluish red. *See also* FD&C Colors.

D&C RED NO. 28 • **Acid Red 92. Phloxine B.** Classed chemically as a xanthene (*see*) color. The conversion product of D&C Red No. 27 (*see*) to the sodium salt. Permanently listed in 1982 by the FDA. *See also* FD&C Colors.

D&C RED NO. 30 • **Helindone Pink CN. Vat Red 1.** Bluish pink. Classed chemically as an indigoid (*see* Indigo) color. *See* FD&C Colors.

D&C RED NO. 30 ALUMINUM LAKE • **Vat Red 1. Thioindigo Pink R.** A thioindigo color. A red vat dye made from indigo and sulfur (*see both*). *See also* FD&C Colors.

D&C RED NO. 30 CALCIUM LAKE • **Vat Red 1. Thioindigo Pink R. Permanent Pink.** A thioindigo dye. *See also* FD&C Colors and Indigo.

D&C RED NO. 30 LAKE • An insoluble pigment prepared from D&C Red No. 30 (*see*) with an approved metal. *See* FD&C Colors.

D&C RED NO. 31 • **Brilliant Lake Red R.** Classed chemically as a monoazo color (*see*). *See also* FD&C Colors.

D&C RED NO. 31 CALCIUM LAKE • **Brilliant Lake Red R.** A monoazo color (*see*). *See also* FD&C Colors.

D&C RED NO. 33 • **Acid Red 33.** Dull bluish red. Classed chemically as a monoazo color (*see*). Was to be permanently listed in 1988, but the ruling has been postponed to allow the FDA "additional time to study complex scientific and legal questions about it." *See also* FD&C Colors.

D&C RED NO. 34 • **Deep Maroon. Fanchon Maroon.** Classed chemically as a monoazo color (*see*). *See also* FD&C Colors.

D&C RED NO. 34 CALCIUM LAKE • An insoluble pigment prepared from D&C Red No. 34 (*see*). *See also* FD&C Colors.

D&C RED NO. 36 • **Pigment Red 4. Tiger Orange.** A monoazo color (*see*). Bright orange. Was to be permanently listed in 1988, but the ruling has been postponed to allow the FDA "additional time to study complex scientific and legal questions about it." *See also* FD&C Colors.

D&C RED NO. 36 BARIUM LAKE • **Pigment Red 4. Permanent Red 12.** Orange hue. A monoazo color (*see*). *See also* FD&C Colors.

D&C RED NO. 36 LAKE • **Chlorinated Para Lake. Tang Orange.** An insoluble pigment prepared from D&C RED No. 36 (*see*). *See also* FD&C Colors.

D&C RED NO. 36 ZIRCONIUM LAKE • **Pigment Red 4.** *See* D&C Red No. 36 Barium Lake and FD&C Colors.

D&C RED NO. 39 • An azo dye (*see*) containing benzoic acid (*see*). Used for coloring quaternary-ammonium-compound (*see*) germicidal solutions for external applications only. Must not exceed 0.1 percent by weight of the finished product. Must be certified (*see*). *See also* FD&C Colors.

D&C RED NO. 40 • Bluish pink. Classed chemically as a xanthene (*see*) color. Used in soaps. *See also* FD&C Colors.

D&C VIOLET NO. 2 • **Alizurol Purple SS. Solvent Violet 13.** Classed chemically as an anthraquinone (*see*) color. Dull bluish violet. *See also* FD&C Colors.

D&C YELLOW NO. 5 ALUMINUM LAKE • Greenish yellow. An insoluble pigment prepared from FD&C Yellow No. 5 (*see*) and aluminum. *See also* FD&C Colors.

D&C YELLOW NO. 5 ZIRCONIUM LAKE • An insoluble pigment prepared from FD&C Yellow No. 5 (*see*) and zirconium. *See also* FD&C Colors.

D&C YELLOW NO. 6 ALUMINUM LAKE • An insoluble pigment prepared from FD&C Yellow No. 6 (*see*) and aluminum. *See also* FD&C Colors.

D&C YELLOW NO. 7 • **Acid Yellow 73. Fluorescein.** Classed chemically as a fluoran (*see*) color. A water-absorbing, yellowish red powder, freely soluble in water. The fluorescence disappears when the solution is made acid and reappears when it is made neutral. *See also* FD&C Colors.

D&C YELLOW NO. 8 • **Naphthol Yellow S. Sodium Fluorescein. Uranine.** Classed chemically as a xanthene (*see*) color. The sodium salt of D&C Yellow No. 7 (*see*). Light yellow or orange-yellow powder soluble in water. *See also* FD&C Colors.

D&C YELLOW NO. 10 • **Acid Yellow 3. Quinoline Yellow.** One of the quinolines (*see*). A bright greenish yellow used in toothpastes, soaps, and shampoos. A potential allergen. It is present in yellow Irish Spring, Pink Dove, and Caress Bath Soap. May cross-react with other quinoline colors used in drugs. *See also* FD&C Colors.

D&C YELLOW NO. 10 ALUMINUM LAKE • An insoluble pigment prepared from D&C Yellow No. 10 (*see*) and aluminum. *See also* FD&C Colors.

D&C YELLOW NO. 11 • **Solvent Yellow 33.** Classed chemically as a quinoline (*see*) color. A bright greenish yellow used in soaps, shampoos, suntan oils. *See also* FD&C Colors.

DCF • *See* Pentostatin.

DDAVP • *See* Desmopressin.

DDC • *See* Zalcitabine.

DDI • *See* Didanosine.

DDS • *See* Dapsone.

DEADLY NIGHTSHADE (H) • *See* Belladonna.

DEAD SEA MINERAL BATH SALTS (OTC) (H) • Concentrated mineral water used to treat psoriasis (*see*). Many psoriasis sufferers visit the Dead Sea in Israel each year to soak in it.

DEBRISAN (OTC) • *See* Dextranomer.

DEBROX (OTC) • *See* Carbamide Peroxide.

DECABID (Rx) • *See* Indecainide.

DECADERM (Rx) • *See* Dexamethasone.

DECADRON (Rx) • *See* Dexamethasone.

DECA-DURABOLIN (Rx) • *See* Nandrolone.

DECAJECT • *See* Dexamethasone.

DECASPRAY • *See* Dexamethasone.

DECHOLIN • *See* Dehydrocholic Acid.

DECLOMYCIN • *See* Demeclocycline.

DECOCTION • Made by simmering an herb in water in a covered container for ten to twenty minutes.

DECOFED (OTC) • *See* Pseudoephedrine.

DECOLONE • *See* Nandrolone.

DECONADE (OTC) • *See* Chlorpheniramine and Phenylpropanolamine.

DECONAMINE SR (OTC) • *See* Chlorpheniramine and Pseudoephedrine.

DECONGESTANT • Congestion in the nose, sinuses, and chest is due to swollen, expanded, or dilated blood vessels in the membranes of the nose and air passages. Oral or topical decongestants cause constriction or tightening of the blood vessels in those membranes, which then forces much of the blood out of the membranes so that they shrink and the air passages open up again. Decongestants are chemically related to adrenaline, the natural decongestant, which is also a type of stimulant. Therefore, the side effects of these medications include nervousness, insomnia, and elevated blood pressure and pulse rate. Decongestants should not be used by people with irregular heart rhythm, high blood pressure, or heart disease. Also should not be used by patients with glaucoma or problems in urinating.

DECONSAL • *See* Phenylephrine.

DECONSAL II (Rx) • Indicated for the relief of nasal congestion and cough associated with respiratory-tract infections and related conditions such as sinusitis, pharyngitis, bronchitis, and asthma, it is a combination of pseudoephedrine (*see*) and guaifenesin (*see*) in a sustained-release formulation. Although both ingredients are in many over-the-counter products, the combination in this form contains higher dosages that are slowly released. It is claimed to be especially effective in dry, nonproductive cough, which tends to injure the mucous membranes of the air passages. It should be used cautiously by people who have hypersensitivity to any of the ingredients, which may be manifested by insomnia, dizziness, weakness, tremor, or irregular heartbeat. Pseudoephedrine is contraindicated in patients with high blood pressure, ischemic heart disease, diabetes, increased pressure in the eye, overactive thyroid, or enlarged prostate. It is not recommended for use in children under two years. The elderly may be more likely to have adverse reactions to the medication. An overdose in this age group may cause hallucinations, convulsions, CNS depression, and death.

DEER ANTLER (H) • *Cervus nippon.* **Lu Rong.** The antler of the sika, a red deer of northern China, is one of the most precious of Chinese tonics. Usually administered by itself in an alcoholic extract, it is taken through the cold winter months by people over forty years of age. It is reputedly a powerful aphrodisiac for both men and women.

DEFEROXAMINE (Rx) • **Desferal.** A chelating (*see*) agent used in iron poisoning. Potential adverse reactions include pain at injection site, redness, hives, low blood pressure, shock, and with long-term use, hypersensitivity reactions, leg cramps, fever, rapid heartbeat, pain when urinating, diarrhea, abdominal discomfort, blurred vision, and cataracts. Contraindicated in severe kidney disease. Should not be used with vitamin C, which may increase the toxicity of deferoxamine.

DEFICOL (OTC) • *See* Bisacodyl.

DEGEST 2 (OTC) • *See* Naphazoline.

DEHIST • *See* Brompheniramine.

DEHYDRATION • A loss of water from the body, often due to severe vomiting or diarrhea.

DEHYDROCHOLIC ACID (Rx) • **Atrocholin. Decholin.** A laxative derived from cholic acid in bile (*see*). It has a stimulating effect upon the secretion of bile by the liver and improves the absorption of essential food materials. *See also* Laxative.

DEHYDROEPIANDROSTERONE • Full name for DHEA (*see*).

DEKASOL • *See* Dexamethasone.

DELADUMONE • *See* Estradiol and Testosterone.

DELALUTIN • *See* Hydroxyprogesterone.

DELATEST • *See* Testosterone.

DELATESTRYL • *See* Testosterone.

DELAXIN • *See* Methocarbamol.

DELAYED HYPERSENSITIVITY • Manifested primarily as contact dermatitis due to parabens (*see*), a common preservative in topical medications, or to drugs such as neomycin (*see*). Certain multiple allergic reactions to drugs such as penicillin, nitrofurantoin, and hydantoins may also fall into this category.

DELESTROGEN • *See* Estradiol.

DELFEN (OTC) • A spermicidal foam containing nonoxynol-9 (*see*).

DELIRIUM TREMENS • A group of symptoms that may occur if an alcoholic abstains from drinking. Symptoms range from shaking to hallucinations and convulsions.

DELSYM (OTC) • *See* Dextromethorphan.

DELTA-CORTEF • *See* Prednisolone.

DELTACORTISONE • *See* Prednisone.

DELTA-D • *See* Vitamin D.

DELTADEHYDROCORTISONE • *See* Prednisolone.

DELTASONE • *See* Prednisone.

DEMAZIN (OTC) • *See* Chlorpheniramine and Phenylpropanolamine.

DEMECARIUM BROMIDE (Rx) • **Humorsol.** A drug to contract the pupil, used in the treatment of glaucoma. Potential adverse reactions include aching brow, unusual fatigue or weakness, headache, slow or irregular heartbeat, eye pain, retinal detachment, iris cysts, lens opacities, a paradoxical increase in eye pressure, tearing, obstruction of the tear ducts, burning, redness, stinging, irritation, twitching of the eyelids, blurred vision, nausea, vomiting, diarrhea, stomach cramps, and loss of bladder control. Anticholinergics and other cholinesterase inhibitors increase the possibility of toxicity. Inhalation or skin absorption of carbamate or organophosphate-type insecticides, local anesthetics, and ophthalmic tetracaine increase the risk of whole-body toxicity. Demecarium increases the toxicity risk of cocaine. Contraindicated in patients with bronchial asthma, slow heartbeat or low blood pressure, Down's syndrome, epilepsy, spastic GI disturbances, Parkinson's disease, heart diseases, or a history of retinal detachment (*see*). Toxicity is cumulative; symptoms may not appear for weeks or months after start of therapy.

DEMECLOCYCLINE (Rx) • **Declomycin. Ledermycin.** A tetracycline (*see*) antibiotic introduced in 1959 to treat infections caused by gram-negative and gram-positive (*see*) organisms, trachoma, and rickettsiae. Potential adverse side effects include a drop in white blood count, inflammation of the heart, trouble swallowing, sore tongue, loss of appetite, nausea, vomiting, diarrhea, colitis, and inflammation around the anus. May also cause rashes, photosensitivity, increased pigmentation, and hives and other allergic reactions. Demeclocycline should not be taken with food, milk or other dairy products, or antacids and laxatives containing aluminum, magnesium, or calcium, because they decrease its absorption, making it ineffective. Iron and zinc also make it less potent. Oral contraceptives may be less effective. It should also be used with extreme caution in patients with impaired liver or kidneys.

DEMENTIA • A disorder in which there is loss or impairment of mental powers, due to physical disease, severe enough to interfere with work or social functioning. Memory disturbance is the most prominent symptom. Other symptoms include personality change and impairment of abstract thinking, judgment, and control of impulses.

DEMEROL • *See* Meperidine.

DEMETHYCHLORTETRACYCLINE • *See* Demeclocycline.

DEMI-REGROTON • *See* Chlorthalidone and Reserpine.

DEMSER • *See* Metyrosine.

DEMULCENT • A soothing, usually thick, oily or creamy substance used to relieve pain in inflamed or irritated mucous surfaces. Gum acacia or oatmeal, for instance, are used as demulcents.

DEMULEN • *See* Ethinyl Estradiol, Ethynodiol, and Oral Contraceptives.

DENDRITES • Spiderlike projections from the cell body, which receive and send messages between nerve cells.

DENOREX (OTC) • *See* Coal Tar.

DENQUEL SENSITIVE TEETH • *See* Potassium Nitrate.

DENT-, DENTO- • Prefixes meaning pertaining to a tooth or teeth.

DENTAPAIN GEL (OTC) • *See* Benzocaine.

DEOXYACYCLOVIR (Rx) • A derivative of acyclovir (*see*).

DEOXYCOFORMYCIN (Rx) • *See* Pentostatin.

DEOXYDOXORUBICIN • *See* Doxorubicin.

DEOXYSPERGUALIN (Rx) • **Gusperimus.** A Japanese-developed drug to treat multiple sclerosis that has shown beneficial effects in a clinical study and is expected at this writing to be on the German market soon. Bristol-Meyers Squibb, is developing it for the U.S. and Canadian markets.

DEPA • *See* Valproic Acid.

DEPAKENE • *See* Valproic Acid.

DEPAKOTE • *See* Valproic Acid.

DEPANDROGYN (Rx) • *See* Estradiol and Testosterone.

DEPEN (Rx) • *See* Penicillamine.

DEPGYNOGEN (Rx) • *See* Estradiol.

DEPMEDALONE (Rx) • *See* Methylprednisolone.

DEPO-ESTRADIOL (Rx) • *See* Estradiol.

DEPO-ESTRONE (Rx) • *See* Estrone.

DEPOGEN (Rx) • *See* Estradiol.

DEPO-MEDROL (Rx) • *See* Methylprednisolone.

DEPONIT (Rx) • *See* Nitroglycerin.

DEPOPRED (Rx) • *See* Methylprednisolone.

DEPO-PROVERA (Rx) • The FDA recommended the approval of depo-provera, a long-acting injectable contraceptive, in June 1992. An earlier FDA advisory committee had recommended approval of the drug in the mid-1970s as a general contraceptive, but a congressional report raised questions about the drug's possible link to cervical cancer. Worries about the risk of breast cancer, particularly in women under the age of thirty-four, and osteoporosis continued to delay the drug's approval. Depo-provera has been on the market for more than twenty years to ease the effects of cancer of the uterine lining. World Health Organization studies seemed to show that it might increase breast cancer, but the FDA considered the statistics as not significant. Those in favor of depo-provera maintain that there might be 5.6 cases of breast cancer for every 100,000 women taking the drug, but that it seems to prevent an estimated 19.2 cases of uterine cancer. As of this writing, there are still many questions about the safety of depo-provera. *See* Medroxyprogesterone.

DEPOTEST • *See* Testosterone.

DEPO-TESTADIOL (Rx) • *See* Estradiol and Testosterone.

DEPOTESTOGEN (Rx) • *See* Estradiol and Testosterone.

DEPO-TESTOSTERONE • *See* Testosterone.

DEPRENYL • *See* Selegiline Hydrochloride.

DEPRESSION • When used to describe a mood, depression refers to what may be normal feelings of sadness, despair, and discouragement. More serious depression may be a symptom of a variety of physical and mental disorders. The disorder known as major depression is characterized by slow thinking, decreased purposeful physical activity, sleep and appetite disturbances, low self-esteem, loss of sex drive, and feelings of guilt and hopelessness.

DEPROL (Rx) • *See* Meprobamate and Benactyzine.

DERIFIL (OTC) • *See* Chlorophyll.

-DERM, DERMA- • Suffix and prefix meaning pertaining to skin.

DERMABET • *See* Betamethasone.

DERMACOMB (Rx) • *See* Nystatin and Triamcinolone.

DERMACORT (OTC) • *See* Hydrocortisone.

DERMATOHELIOSIS • See Photoaging.

DERMOLATE (OTC) • *See* Hydrocortisone.

DERMOPLAST (OTC) • *See* Benzocaine.

DERMOVATE (Rx) • *See* Clobetasol.

DES • *See* Diethylstilbestrol.

DESENEX (OTC) • *See* Undecylenic Acid.

DESENEX FOOT & SNEAKER DEODORANT SPRAY (OTC) • *See* Aluminum Chlorohydrate.

DESENUISANA PLUS • *See* Undecylenic Acid.

DESERPIDINE (Rx) • **Enduronyl. Harmonyl.** An antihypertensive drug that acts by inhibiting the release of the natural nerve stimulant norepinephrine and depletes the norepinephrine stores in the adrenal gland's nerve endings. Potential adverse effects include mental confusion, depression, drowsiness, nervousness, paradoxical anxiety, nightmares, sedation, irregular heartbeat, dry mouth, nasal stuffiness, hypersecretion of gastric acid, nausea, vomiting, gastrointestinal bleeding, rash, impotence, and weight gain. If used with MAO inhibitors (*see*), it may cause excitability and a rise in blood pressure.

DESFERAL • *See* Deferoxamine.

DESFLURANE (Rx) • **Suprane.** A fast-acting inhalation anesthetic for inpatient and outpatient surgery in adults, and for maintenance of anesthesia in infants and children. Introduced in 1992.

DESIPRAMINE (Rx) • **Norpramin. Pertofrane.** A tricyclic antidepressant introduced in 1964 that increases the amount of the neurotransmitters norepinephrine or serotonin, or both, in the central nervous system. Potential adverse reactions include drowsiness, dizziness, excitation, tremors, weakness, confusion, headache, nervousness, a drop in blood pressure upon rising from a sitting or prone position, changes in libido, impotence, painful male orgasm, swelling of testicles, female breast enlargement with milk production, irregular heartbeat, high blood pressure, blurred vision, ringing in the ears, dry mouth, constipation, nausea, vomiting, loss of appetite, intestinal paralysis, urine retention, rash, hives, sweating, and allergy. Sudden discontinuation may cause nausea, headache, and malaise. Barbiturates decrease levels of desipramine in the blood. Cimetidine may increase levels of desipramine in the blood and cause increased adverse reactions. Epinephrine and norepinephrine increase effects on blood pressure. MAO inhibitors may cause severe excitation, high fever, or seizures. Methylphenidate increases desipramine's effect. Contraindicated soon after a heart attack, in patients with a history of seizures, and in men with enlarged prostates. Should be used cautiously in patients with heart disease, urine retention, glaucoma, thyroid disease, blood problems, liver dysfunction, or who are suicide risks. The drug takes effect in about two weeks. No other drugs, including over-the-counter medication, should be taken without first checking with a physician. Desipramine is most effective when taken on an empty stomach, but may be taken with food.

DESITIN (OTC) • *See* Zinc Oxide, Cod Liver Oil, and Talc.

DESLANOSIDE (Rx) • **Cedilanid-D.** A cardiac glycoside (*see*), it is used to treat congestive heart failure, irregular heartbeat, and flutter. Potential adverse reactions include fatigue, generalized muscle weakness, agitation, hallucinations, loss of appetite, nausea, vomiting, headache, dizziness, stupor, numbness, and increased severity of congestive heart failure, which may be life threatening. Should not be used with amphotericin B, carbenicillin, ticarcillin, corticosteroids, or diuretics because it may predispose patients to low blood potassium and digitalis toxicity.

DESMETHYLIMIPRAMINE • *See* Desipramine.

DESMOPRESSIN (Rx) • **DDAVP. Stimate.** A nasal solution of a pituitary hormone, vasopressin, used for the long-term treatment of diabetes insipidus and for controlling bleeding in certain types of hemophilia. Also sometimes used for nighttime bed-wetting. Potential adverse reactions include headache, confusion, convulsions, rapid weight gain, a slight rise in blood pressure at high dosage, stuffy nose, nausea, vaginal pain, and flushing. Should be used with caution in coronary artery disease or high blood pressure.

DESOGEN (Rx) • An oral contraceptive for women, introduced in 1992 in the United States. It combines a new-generation progestin with desogestrel (*see*) and ethinyl estradiol (*see* Estrogen). Introduced in Germany in 1982 and now used in fifty-six countries, it is reportedly the most prescribed birth control pill worldwide. Both desogestrel and ethinyl estradiol are derived from the root of the Mexican plant *Dioscorea mexicana,* a type of wild yam. *See* Discorea and Wild Yam Root.

DESOGESTREL (Rx) (H) • Derived from the plant *Dioscorea mexicana*—a type of wild yam—it is a natural chemical that is converted into a progestin. It is used in the most widely prescribed birth control pill worldwide (*see* Desogen and Discorea).

DESONIDE (Rx) • **DesOwen. Tridesilon.** A corticosteroid (*see*) ointment or cream used to treat skin inflammations. Potential adverse reactions include burning, itching, irritation, dryness, inflammation of the hair follicles, acne, rash around the mouth, spots of pigment loss, hairiness, allergic contact dermatitis, and if covered with a dressing,

secondary infection, atrophy, streaks, and blisters. Should be used cautiously in skin problems caused by viruses such as herpes, and in fungal or bacterial skin infections. Should not be used for more than two weeks due to potential absorption into the system, consequently causing an effect on the hypothalamus, and pituitary and adrenal glands. Should not be applied near eyes or mucous membranes, under the arms, on the face, groin, or under the breast unless medically specified.

DESOWEN • *See* Desonide.

DESOXIMETASONE (Rx) • **Topicort.** A corticosteroid (*see*) ointment or cream introduced in 1958 to treat skin inflammation. Potential adverse reactions include burning, itching, irritation, dryness, inflammation of the hair follicles, acne, rash around the mouth, spots of pigment loss, hairiness, allergic contact dermatitis, and if covered with a dressing, secondary infection, atrophy, streaks, and blisters. Should be used cautiously in skin problems caused by viruses such as herpes, and in fungal or bacterial skin infections. Should not be used for more than two weeks due to potential absorption into the system, consequently causing an effect on the hypothalamus, and pituitary and adrenal glands. Should not be applied near eyes or mucous membranes, under the arms, on the face, groin, or under the breast unless medically specified.

DESOXYEPHEDRINE (OTC) • **Vicks Inhaler.** A blood-vessel constrictor, obtained from laudanosine or papaverine, both derived from the poppy. Used for the relief of stuffy nose due to the common cold, hay fever, upper-respiratory allergies, and sinusitis. The recommended dosage should not be exceeded because burning, stinging, sneezing, or increase of nasal discharge may occur. The inhaler is effective for a minimum of three months after first use. However, it should be used by one person only, and not for more than a week.

DESOXYN • *See* Methamphetamine.

DESOXYPHENOBARBITAL • *See* Primidone.

DESYREL • *See* Trazodone Hydrochloride.

DEVIL'S APPLE • *See* Jimsonweed.

DEVIL'S CLAW (H) • *Harpagophytum procumbens.* **Devil's Craw Root. Grapple Plant.** A perennial herb introduced into North America relatively recently. It has been used in South Africa for more than 250 years by the natives as a tonic for arthritis.

DEVIL'S DUNG • *See* Asafetida.

DEVROM (OTC) • *See* Bismuth.

DEXACIDIN • *See* Dexamethasone, Neomycin, and Polymyxin B.

DEX-A-DIET (OTC) • *See* Phenylpropanolamine.

DEXAIR • *See* Dexamethasone.

DEXAMETHASONE (Rx) • **Aeroseb-Dex. Ak-Dex. Dalalone. Decaderm. Decadrol. Decadron. Decadron Phosphate Turbinaire. Decaject-LA. Decameth LA. Decaspray. Deronil. Dexacen LA. Dexameth. Dexasone-LA. Dexone. Gammacorten. Hexadrol. Infectrol. Maxidex Ophthalmic Suspension. Maxitrol. Mymethasone. NeoDecadron. Solurex-LA.** A synthetic cortisol (*see*) introduced in 1958, it decreases inflammation, suppresses the immune system, stimulates bone marrow, and influences protein, fat, and carbohydrate metabolism. Used to treat brain swelling, inflammation, irregular menstruation, allergic reactions, and abnormal growths. In eye ointments and solutions it is used to treat inflammations of the eyes and eyelids, chemical or heat injury to the cornea, penetration of foreign bodies, and allergic conjunctivitis. In nose sprays, it is used to treat allergic or inflammatory conditions and nasal polyps. Also used in an ointment or cream to treat skin inflammations. Most adverse reactions are the result of dosage or length of time between dosages when taken orally. Dexamethasone may activate latent diabetes, glaucoma, peptic ulcer disease, and tuberculosis. Potential adverse reactions include euphoria, insomnia, psychotic behavior, high blood pressure, swelling, cataracts, glaucoma, peptic ulcer, GI irritation, increased appetite, high blood sugar, growth suppression in children, delayed wound healing, acne, skin eruptions, muscle weakness, pancreatitis, hairiness, decreased immunity, and acute adrenal gland insufficiency. When withdrawn, there may be rebound inflammation, fatigue, weakness, joint pain, fever, dizziness, lethargy, depression, fainting, a drop in blood pressure upon rising from a seated or prone position, shortness of breath, loss of appetite, and high blood sugar. Sudden withdrawal may be fatal. Eye preparations may cause the following adverse reactions: increased pressure within the eye, thinning of the cornea, interference with wound healing, increased susceptibility to viral or fungal infections of the eye, corneal ulcers, and with excessive or long-term use, cataracts, worsening of glaucoma, eye-nerve damage, mild blurred vision, burning, stinging, redness, and watery eyes. In nose sprays, potential adverse reactions may include nasal irritation, dryness, rebound nasal congestion, hypersensitivity reactions, depression of pituitary and adrenal glands, congestive heart failure, high blood pressure, low potassium, headaches, convulsions, peptic ulcer, blood spots in the skin, and masking of infection. In skin ointment or cream, potential adverse reactions include burning, itching, irritation, dryness, inflammation of the hair follicles, acne, rash around the mouth, spots of pigment loss, hairiness, allergic contact dermatitis, and if covered with a dressing, secondary infection, atrophy, streaks, and blisters. Should be used cautiously in skin problems caused by viruses such as herpes, and in fungal or bacterial skin infections. Contraindicated in systemic fungal or viral infections. Should be used cautiously in patients with GI ulceration or kidney disease, high blood pressure, diabetes, chicken pox, osteoporosis, Cushing's syndrome, blood-clotting disorders, seizures, myasthenia gravis, congestive heart failure, tuberculosis, herpes, and emotional instability. The nasal spray is contraindicated in tuberculosis of the skin, and fungal and herpes lesions. Dexamethasone may interfere with insulin and oral antidiabetes medication. Phenobarbital, ephedrine, and phenytoin may make dexamethasone less effective. Interactions with diuretics may cause loss of potassium. When taking the drug, patients may need low-sodium diets and potassium supplements. Barbiturates, phenytoin, and rifampin (*see all*) increase its effects. Indomethacin (*see*) and aspirin may increase the risks of GI distress and bleeding. May worsen ulcers. Skin preparations should not be used for more than two weeks due to potential absorption into the system, consequently causing an effect on the hypothalamus, and pituitary and adrenal glands. Mothers should not breast-feed, as systemic absorption can occur. Should not be applied near eyes or mucous membranes, under the arms, on the face, groin, or under the breast unless medically specified. Oral doses may be taken with food to avoid stomach upset.

DEXASONE-LA • *See* Dexamethasone.

DEXASPORIN (Rx) • *See* Neomycin, Polymixin B, and Dexamethasone.

DEXATRIM (OTC) • Contains 200 mg of caffeine. *See* Phenylpropanolamine and Caffeine.

DEXBROMPHENIRAMINE (OTC) • **Disophrol. Drixoral.** An antihistamine that provides relief of sneezing, watery, itchy eyes, and runny nose due to hay fever and other upper-respiratory allergies. Reclassified from Rx to OTC in varying strengths in 1982, 1985, and 1987. Contraindicated in those taking a medication for high blood pressure.

DEXCHLORPHENIRAMINE (OTC) (Rx) • **Dexchlor. Poladex. Polaramine. Polargen.** Both a prescription and nonprescription antihistamine, used to treat stuffy nose, allergy symptoms, contact dermatitis, and itching. Potential adverse reactions (especially in the elderly) include drowsiness, dizziness, stimulation, nausea, dry mouth, frequent or painful urination, and urinary retention. Central nervous system depressants, including alcohol, increase sedation. MAO inhibitors (*see*) may quickly raise blood pressure.

Use cautiously in elderly patients, those with glaucoma, overactive thyroid, heart or kidney disease, high blood pressure, bronchial asthma, enlarged prostate, bladder-neck obstruction, and peptic ulcer. Coffee or tea may reduce drowsiness. Medication should be discontinued four days before taking a skin allergy test because it can lead to inaccurate results.

DEXEDRINE • *See* Dextroamphetamine.

DEXFENFLURAMINE (Rx) • **Redux.** An appetite suppressant available in Europe for seven years. Fenfluramine (*see*), its parent compound, has been used for weight loss for more than twenty years with reportedly no users developing neurological disease. Dexfenfluramine is marketed in more than sixty countries. It was approved by the FDA in 1996.

DEX-IDE (Rx) • *See* Neomycin, Polymixin B, and Dexamethasone.

DEXITAC • *See* Caffeine.

DEXONE • *See* Dexamethasone.

DEXPANTHENOL (Rx) • **Ilopan.** A drug related to panthenol (*see*), used to relieve flatulence and, topically, for various skin conditions such as burns and eczema. Also used to prevent or minimize paralyzed intestines and for treatment of postoperative distension. In 1992, the FDA issued a notice that dexpanthenol had not been shown to be safe and effective as claimed in OTC poison ivy, poison oak, and poison sumac products.

DEXTRAN (Rx) (OTC) • **Dextran 40. Dextran 70. Feronim. Gentran 40. Hydextran. Hyskon. LMD. Macrodex. Promit. Rheomacrodex.** In eye preparations, it provides artificial tears. The container must be handled carefully to avoid contamination. In injectable form, it expands blood plasma and provides fluid replacement and prevents blood clots in the veins. Potential adverse reactions include a decreased level of red blood cells, nausea, vomiting, liver dysfunction, hives, and serious allergic reactions. Contraindicated in certain blood problems, fluid in the lungs, kidney disease, or extreme dehydration.

DEXTRANOMER (Rx) • A compound that absorbs moisture and small molecules from wounds. Potential adverse reactions include allergic skin reactions.

DEXTROAMPHETAMINE (Rx) • **Adderall. Dexampex. Dexedrine. Ferndex. Obetrol. Oxydess II. Robese. Span Cap No. 1.** An amphetamine brain stimulant, it is used to treat narcolepsy (*see*), obesity (a use prohibited in some states), and attention deficit disorders with hyperactivity. Potential adverse reactions include restlessness, tremor, hyperactivity, talkativeness, insomnia, irritability, dizziness, headache, chills, overstimulation, palpitations, irregular heartbeat, low blood pressure, high blood pressure, nausea, vomiting, cramps, dry mouth, diarrhea, constipation, metallic taste, loss of appetite, weight loss, hives, impotence, and altered libido. Ammonium chloride, phenothiazine, haloperidol, and vitamin C make it less effective. Antacids, sodium bicarbonate, and acetazolamide may increase its effectiveness. Caffeine may increase its effects. MAO inhibitors (*see*) may cause a severe rise in blood pressure. Must be taken at least six hours before bedtime to avoid insomnia. May alter insulin needs. Contraindicated in overactive thyroid, severe high blood pressure, angina or other severe cardiovascular disease, glaucoma, and a history of drug abuse. May be taken with food.

DEXTROMETHORPHAN (OTC) • **Alka-Seltzer Plus Cold & Cough Medicine. Benylin DM. Cerose-DM. Cheracol D and Plus. Comtrex Cough Formula. Congespirin. Contac Cough and Chest Cold. Creamcoat. Delsym. Dimacol. Dimetapp-DM. DM Cough. Dorcol Children's Cough Syrup. Dristan Cold and Flu. Hold. Medi-Flu. Mediquell. Naldecon. Novahistine DX. PediaCare 1. Pertussin 8 Hour Cough Formula. St. Joseph for Children. Sucrets Cough Control Formula.** Commonly available in combination: **Contac Cough and Sore Throat Formula. Contac Nighttime Cold Medicine. Guaituss DM. Novahistine DMX Liquid. Phenergan with Dextromethorphan. Robitussin-DM. Rondec-DM. Triaminicol Multi-Symptom Cold. Trind-DM Liquid. Tussi-Organidin DM. Vicks Formula 44.** A synthetic morphine derivative used as a cough medication, it works directly on the cough center in the brain. It has no central depressant or analgesic action. Is not believed to be addictive. Potential adverse reactions include drowsiness, chest pain, rapid or irregular heartbeat, stomach pain, dizziness, and nausea. May cause an increase in blood cholesterol. Contraindicated in patients who are taking or have taken within two weeks MAO inhibitors (*see*). Dextromethorphan may alter the effectiveness of blood-thinning medications and cholesterol-lowering drugs. All drugs that have a sedative action may increase the sedative properties of dextromethorphan.

DEXTROPROPOXYPHENE HYDROCHLORIDE (Rx) • *See* Propoxyphene and Propoxyphene Napsylate.

DEXTROSE (Rx) (OTC) • **Emetrol. Glutose.** A sugar used to treat insulin-induced low blood sugar or to relieve nausea by local action on the wall of the hyperactive GI tract. Reduces smooth muscle contraction in proportion to the amount used. Works rapidly. Patient should not take more than five doses in one hour.

DEXTROSTIX (OTC) • A diagnostic test for sugar in the blood.

DEXTROTHYROXINE SODIUM (Rx) • **Choloxin. D-Thyroxine Sodium.** A lipid-lowering drug that accelerates the liver's processing of cholesterol and increases bile secretion to lower cholesterol levels. Potential adverse effects include palpitations, angina pectoris, irregular heartbeat, a decrease of blood to the heart, heart attack, visual disturbances, drooping eyelid, nausea, vomiting, diarrhea, constipation, decreased appetite, insomnia, weight loss, sweating, flushing, increased body temperature, hair loss, and menstrual irregularities. Dextrothyroxine may increase blood sugar levels in diabetics, and also the need for insulin, diet therapy, or oral antidiabetes drugs. It may enhance the clinical effects of digitalis and the anticoagulants warfarin or dicumarol. Also may precipitate irregular heartbeat or coronary insufficiency in patients with cardiac disease. Contraindicated in hepatic or renal disease. Patients with a history of heart disease, including irregular heartbeat, high blood pressure, or angina, should receive small doses. May be taken with food.

DEY-DOSE ATROPINE • *See* Atropine.

DEY-DOSE ISOETHARINE • *See* Isoetharine.

DEY-DOSE ISOPROTERENOL • *See* Isoproterenol.

DEY-DOSE METAPROTERENOL • *See* Metaproterenol.

DEY-DROPS OPHTHALMIC SOLUTION • *See* Silver Nitrate.

DEY-LUBE (OTC) • An eye lubricant. *See* Artificial Tears.

DEY-LUTE • *See* Isoetharine.

DEZOCINE (Rx) • **Dalgan.** An injectable synthetic opioid narcotic with postoperative pain-killing properties similar to morphine's. Potential adverse effects include oxygen in the blood, sedation, dizziness, anxiety, mood disorders, sleep disturbances, headache, slurred speech, water retention, low or high blood pressure, irregular heartbeat, chest pain, nausea, vomiting, dry mouth, constipation, diarrhea, abdominal distress, skin rash, itching, sweating, chills, flushing, and blood clots. Alcohol or other central nervous system depressants may cause additive central nervous system depression. Should be used with caution in elderly patients.

d-FENCHONE (OTC) • A synthetic flavoring occurring naturally in common fennel (*see*). An oily liquid with a camphor smell. Practically insoluble in water. Used as a counterirritant (*see*).

DFMO • *See* Eflornithine.

DFP • *See* Isoflurophate.

DHAD • *See* Mitoxantrone.

D.H.E. 45 (Rx) • *See* Ergotamine Tartrale.

DHEA (Rx) (OTC) • Dehydroepiandrosterone. An adrenal hormone that is converted by the body into a variety of hormones that decline with age, including those governing sexual and immune functions. A version made from yams is sold over the counter. A prescription version is made by compounding pharmacists or imported from overseas. The over-the-counter is sold as a means to improve immunity and strength. It is being studied under grants from the National Institute on Aging to determine its part in aging since it is one of the hormones that declines significantly with age.

DHPG SODIUM • *See* Ganciclovir.

DHS TAR (OTC) • *See* Coal Tar.

DHS ZINC • *See* Zinc Pyrithione.

DHT • *See* Dihydrotachysterol.

DIA- • Prefix meaning through.

DIABETA (Rx) • *See* Glyburide.

DIABINESE (Rx) • *See* Chlorpropamide.

DIACETYLMORPHINE (Rx) • *See* Heroin.

DIACHLOR (Rx) • *See* Chlorothiazide.

DIA-GESIC • *See* Hydrocodone.

DIALOSE • *See* Docusate.

DIALUME ALUMINUM • *See* Hydroxide.

DIAMINE TC • *See* Brompheniramine.

DIAMINODIPHENYLSULFONE • *See* Dapsone.

DIAMOX • *See* Acetazolamide.

DIAPARENE (OTC) • A combination of methylbenzethonium chloride, cornstarch, and magnesium carbonate (*see all*), used to treat diaper rash.

DIAPER RASH • **Ammonia Dermatitis.** Skin irritation caused by urine and feces; also by soap or detergents left in diapers if they are not thoroughly rinsed. The skin becomes red, spotty, sore, and moist.

DIAPER RASH DRUG PRODUCTS • In 1992, the FDA issued a notice that no OTC products with ingredients labeled for use in treating or preventing diaper rash have been shown to be safe and effective as claimed.

DIAPHORESIS • Perspiration.

DIAPHORETIC • An agent that increases perspiration.

DIAR-AID (OTC) • *See* Attapulgite.

DIASORB (OTC) • *See* Attapulgite.

DIASTASE (OTC) • In 1992, the FDA issued a notice that diastase and diastase malt aluminum hydroxide have not been shown to be safe and effective as claimed in OTC digestive-aid products.

DIASTIX (OTC) • A diagnostic test for glucose in urine.

DIASTOLIC BLOOD PRESSURE • Blood pressure when the heart is relaxing.

DIAZEPAM (Rx) • **Diazepam Intensol. Q-Pam. Valium. Valrelease. Vazepam. Zetran.** An antianxiety agent introduced in 1963 that depresses the central nervous system at the area controlling emotions. Should not be used for everyday stress. As an anticonvulsant, it suppresses the spread of seizure activity produced by epilepsy. It also is used to treat skeletal muscle spasm. Potential adverse reactions include drowsiness, lethargy, hangover, loss of balance, fainting, slurred speech, tremor, transient low blood pressure, slow heartbeat, cardiovascular collapse, double vision, blurred vision, uncontrolled movement of the eyes, nausea, vomiting, abdominal discomfort, rash, hives, and respiratory depression. Contraindicated in shock, coma, acute alcohol intoxication, glaucoma, psychoses, myasthenia gravis, and in children under six months. Should be used with caution in persons with blood problems, liver, lung, or kidney damage, depression, glaucoma, and in the elderly and debilitated. Should not be used with alcohol or other central nervous system depressants. Cimetidine (*see*) increases sedation. Use of diazepam with phenobarbital (*see*) increases the effects of both drugs. Diazepam may be addicting. Should not be discontinued suddenly. May be taken with or without food.

DIAZO • A compound containing two nitrogen atoms, such as diazepam (*see*).

DI-AZO • *See* Phenazopyridine Hydrochloride.

DIAZO DYES (Rx) • Coloring agents that contain two linked nitrogen atoms united with an aromatic group and an acid radical.

DIAZOXIDE (Rx) • **Hyperstat. Proglycem.** A sulfa drug that is used to treat low blood sugar and high blood pressure. It relaxes the smooth muscle walls of arteries. It works by preventing release of insulin from the pancreas. Potential adverse reactions include headache, dizziness, lightheadedness, euphoria, sodium and water retention, a drop in blood pressure upon standing, sweating, flushing, warmth, angina, a reduction in blood to the heart, hairiness, irregular heartbeat, nausea, vomiting, abdominal discomfort, high blood sugar, high uric acid, and inflammation. Hydralazine (*see*) may interact and cause severe low blood pressure. Thiazide diuretics (*see*) may increase the effects of diazoxide.

DIBENT • *See* Dicyclomin.

DIBENZYLINE • *See* Phenoxybenzamine.

DIBROMOFLUORESCEIN • A coloring made by heating resorcinol and phthalic anhydride (*see both*) to produce fluorescent orange-red crystals. Ingestion can cause gastrointestinal symptoms. Skin application can cause skin sensitivity to light, inflamed eyes, skin rash, and even respiratory symptoms.

DIBUCAINE (OTC) • **Nupercainal Hemorrhoidal and Pain Relief Cream.** A local synthetic anesthetic used for temporary relief of pain, itching, and burning due to hemorrhoids or other anorectal disorders. Also may be used topically for temporary relief of pain and itching associated with sunburn, minor burns, cuts, scrapes, insect bites, or minor skin irritation. Toxic if swallowed. Should not be used if the condition worsens or does not improve within a week. Potential adverse reactions include allergy, irritation, swelling, pain, and bleeding.

DIC • *See* Dacarbazine.

DICAL D (OTC) • A combination of calcium and vitamin D (*see both*).

DICARBOSIL • *See* Calcium Carbonate.

DICHLORALPHENAZONE (Rx) • **Atarin. Isocom. Midrin.** A white, crystalline powder with a bitter taste, used as a mild sedative to reduce emotional reaction to the pain of both vascular and tension headaches. Potential adverse reactions include dizziness and skin rash in hypersensitive patients.

DICHLOROPHEN (OTC) • A fungicide and bactericide used in cosmetic products and dentifrices. A potent allergen closely related to hexachlorophene (*see*). In 1992, the FDA issued a notice that dichlorophen had not been shown to be safe and effective as claimed in OTC products.

DICHLORPHENAMIDE (Rx) • **Daranide.** A drug to treat glaucoma that decreases the secretion of the fluid in the eye, thereby lowering pressure within the eye. Potential adverse reactions include nausea, vomiting, drowsiness, a feeling of pins and needles in the limbs, transient nearsightedness, loss of appetite, kidney stones, low blood potassium, rash, acidosis caused by high chloride in the blood, and anemia. Contraindicated in liver dysfunction, kidney failure, inadequate hormone production by the adrenal gland, high levels of chloride in the blood, low levels of sodium or potassium, severe lung obstruction, or Addison's disease (*see*).

DICLOFENAC POTASSIUM (Rx) • **Cataflam.** A nonsteroidal anti-inflammatory medication that has an enteric-coated (*see*) delayed release formulation. It is indicated for the relief of painful menstruation. It is contraindicated in patients hypersensitive to aspirin, other NSAIDs, or diclofenac. As with other NSAIDs, the most common side effects relate to the gastrointestinal tract. In patients treated over a period of time with NSAID therapy, serious gastrointestinal toxicity such as bleeding, ulceration, and perforation can occur. May also affect the liver. *See* Diclofenac Sodium.

DICLOFENAC SODIUM AND POTASSIUM (Rx) • **Voltaren. Cataflam.** An antiarthritis drug introduced in 1989. Enteric-coated tablets or suppositories produce anti-inflammatory, analgesic, and fever-reducing effects, possibly through inhibition of prostaglandin (*see*) synthesis. Also used to relieve menstrual cramps. Promoted as causing less stomach upset. Also administered in eyedrops and as an emulgel, a cross between a cream and an ointment. People allergic to aspirin or other nonsteroidal anti-inflammatory drugs (*see* NSAIDs) may also be allergic to diclofenac. Potential adverse reactions include gastrointestinal bleeding and peptic ulceration as well as anxiety, depression, drowsiness, insomnia, irritability, headache, congestive heart failure, high blood pressure, abdominal pain or cramps, constipation, diarrhea, indigestion, nausea, abdominal distension, flatulence, colitis, appetite change, uremia, acute renal failure, excessive urination, impotence, memory loss, ringing in the ears, excessive sweating, swelling of the throat, lips, and tongue, fluid retention, liver damage, asthma, rash, hives, eczema, loss of hair, sensitivity to light, and potentially fatal allergic reactions. When used with anticoagulants, increased bleeding may result. Should not be used with aspirin. Cyclosporine, digoxin, lithium, and methotrexate may rise to toxic levels in the blood when used with diclofenac. The drug may decrease the effectiveness of diuretics. Diclofenac may produce a need for adjustment in diabetes medications. Also may enhance potassium retention, resulting in a possible potassium overload. Contraindicated in patients allergic to diclofenac, aspirin, or other NSAIDs. Should be used cautiously in patients with peptic ulcer diseases. Should be taken with meals or milk to minimize GI distress. As of this writing, slated to be produced in a lower-cost, generic form.

DICLOFENAMIDE • *See* Dichlorphenamide.

DICLOXACILLIN SODIUM (Rx) • **Dicloxacil. Dycill. Dynapen. Pathocil.** A penicillin antibiotic used to treat systemic infections caused by penicillinase-producing staphylococci (*see*) and other bacterial infections. May cause lung problems (eosinophilia), neuromuscular irritability, seizures, nausea, vomiting, gastric distress, flatulence, diarrhea, hypersensitivity including possibly fatal allergic reaction, and overgrowth of nonsusceptible organisms. Its effectiveness is reduced by other antibiotics. Should be taken on an empty stomach.

DICUMAROL (Rx) • **Bishydroxycoumarin.** An anticoagulant that inhibits vitamin K–dependent activation of clotting factors that are formed in the liver. Used to treat blood clots to the lungs, for prevention and treatment of deep-vein blood clots, heart attack, rheumatic fever with heart-valve damage, and irregular heartbeat. Potential adverse reactions include hemorrhage, a drop in white blood cells, loss of appetite, nausea, vomiting, cramps, diarrhea, mouth ulcers, blood in the urine, fever, rash, hives, and hair loss. Fever and rash signal possible severe adverse reactions. Acetaminophen increases bleeding if taken over a long period. Allopurinol, amiodarone, chloramphenicol, clofibrate, diflunisal, thyroid drugs, heparin, anabolic steroids, cimetidine, disulfiram, glucagon, inhalation anesthetics, metronidazole, quinidine, ethacrynic acid, indomethacin, mefenamic acid, oxyphenbutazone, salicylates, influenza vaccines, sulindac, sulfinpyrazone, sulfonamides, and tricyclic antidepressants (*see all*) increase the possibility of bleeding. Cholestyramine, griseofulvin, haloperidol, ethchlorvynol, carbamazepine, and rifampin (*see all*) decrease the effectiveness of dicumarol. Contraindicated in hemophilia, leukemia, open wounds or ulcers, impaired liver or kidney function, severe high blood pressure, and infection of the heart. Those taking this drug should shave with an electric razor and use a soft toothbrush to avoid causing bleeding.

DICYCLOMINE (Rx) • **Antispas. Bemote. Bentyl. Byclomine. Dibent. DiCyclonex. Dicycloverine Hydrochloride. Dilomine. Di-Spaz. Neoquess. OR-TYL. Spasmoject.** An anticholinergic, atropinelike antispasmodic drug introduced in 1952. Used to treat GI disorders such as irritable bowel syndrome and infant colic, and as an adjunctive therapy for peptic ulcers. Potential adverse reactions include headache, insomnia, drowsiness, dizziness, palpitations, rapid heartbeat, nausea, constipation, vomiting, paralytic ileus (*see*), urinary retention, impotence, hives, decreased sweating, fever, and allergic reactions. Contraindicated in obstructive urinary-tract and GI-tract diseases, severe ulcerative colitis, myasthenia gravis (*see*), hypersensitivity to anticholinergics, paralytic ileus, intestinal flaccidity, unstable cardiovascular state, or toxic megacolon. Should be used cautiously in glaucoma, overactive thyroid, coronary artery disease, irregular heartbeat, congestive heart failure, high blood pressure, hiatus hernia (*see*), liver or kidney dysfunction, and ulcerative colitis. Should be taken thirty minutes to one hour before meals and at bedtime.

DICYCLOVERINE HYDROCHLORIDE • *See* Dicyclomine.

DIDANOSINE (Rx) • **DDI. Videx.** Introduced in 1991, it is used for the treatment of adult and pediatric patients (over six months of age) with advanced HIV infections. Used for patients who are intolerant of zidovudine (*see*).

DIDREX • *See* Benzphetamine.

DIDRONEL • *See* Etidronate.

DIENESTROL (Rx) • **DV. Ortho Dienestrol.** A vaginal estrogen cream used to treat inflammation of the vagina in postmenopausal women. Potential adverse reactions include vaginal discharge, increased discomfort, burning sensation, breast tenderness, and with excessive use, uterine bleeding. Contraindicated in pregnancy, and in persons with blood-clot disorders, cancer of the breast, reproductive organs, or genitals, and in those with undiagnosed abnormal genital bleeding. Should be used with caution in menstrual irregularities or endometriosis. Systemic reactions are possible with normal intravaginal use. Prolonged therapy with estrogen-containing products is contraindicated.

DIET GUM • *See* Phenylpropanolamine.

DIETHYLCARBAMAZINE (Rx) • **Hetrazam. Notezine.** A treatment to rid the body of worms. Potential adverse reactions include itching and swelling of the face, fever, swollen glands, rash, loss of vision, night blindness, tunnel vision, dizziness, headache, joint pain, fatigue, nausea, and vomiting. Should be taken immediately after meals.

DIETHYLPROPION (Rx) • **Depletite. Ten-Tab. Tenuate. Tepanil.** An appetite suppressant that releases stored norepinephrine (*see*) from nerves in the brain. It is not an amphetamine but produces the same potential adverse reactions including headache, nervousness, dizziness, irregular heartbeat, palpitations, a rise in blood pressure, blurred vision, nausea, abdominal cramps, dry mouth, diarrhea, constipation, hives, impotence, altered libido, and menstrual changes. If taken with MAO inhibitors (*see*), high blood pressure may shoot up to dangerous levels. Contraindicated in overactive thyroid, high blood pressure, angina, severe cardiovascular disease, glaucoma, or a history of drug abuse. Should be used with caution in epilepsy, diabetes, and hyperexcitability. May alter the need for insulin dosage. Dependence may occur. Caffeinated drinks should be avoided. The medication should not be used for more than three months. Should be taken at least six hours before bedtime to avoid interference with sleep.

DIETHYLSTILBESTROL (Rx) • **DES. Stilbestrol. Stilphostrol.** A synthetic compound possessing estrogenlike actions. Used in women with inactive or absent ovaries, in menopausal women, as a postcoital contraceptive, and in postpartum breast engorgement in women who are not breastfeeding. Used in men to palliate prostatic cancer. Potential adverse reactions include nausea, vomiting, dizziness, high blood pressure, headache, depression, lethargy, blood clots, swelling, increased risk of stroke, blood clot to the lung, heart attack, worsening of nearsightedness, intolerance to contact lenses, abdominal cramps, bloating, diarrhea, constipation, loss of appetite, weight changes, increased appetite, excessive thirst, pancreatitis, jaundice, high blood sugar, high calcium, folic-acid deficiency, brown spots on the skin, hives, acne, oily skin, hairiness or loss of hair, leg cramps, and breast tenderness or enlargement. In women potential adverse reactions include breakthrough bleeding, altered menstrual flow, painful or absent menstruation, cervical erosion, enlargement of benign tumors of the uterus, vaginal candidiasis, and loss of libido; in men, breast enlargement, atrophy of testicles, and impotence. Contraindicated in pregnancy, and in persons with blood-clot disorders, cancer of the breast, reproductive organs, or genitals, and in those with undiagnosed abnormal genital bleeding. Should be used with caution in high blood pressure, asthma, mental depression, bone disease, blood problems, gallbladder disease, migraine, seizures, diabetes, absence of menstruation, heart failure, liver or kidney dysfunction, and a family history of breast or genital-tract cancer. Can be harmful to the fetus, so women should stop medication if they suspect pregnancy has occurred. Concurrent use of estrogen is associated with increased risk of endometrial cancer and possibly breast cancer. Diethylstilbestrol may be taken with or without food.

DIFENOXIN (Rx) • Motofen. An antidiarrheal that exerts a direct effect on the intestinal wall to slow movement. Used as an adjunct in acute non-specific diarrhea and acute worsening of chronic diarrhea. Potential adverse reactions include dizziness, drowsiness, headache, fatigue, nervousness, insomnia, confusion, burning eyes, blurred vision, nausea, vomiting, dry mouth, stomach pain, and constipation. Alcohol, central nervous system depressants, tranquilizers, narcotics, and barbiturates increase difenoxin's central nervous system effects. MAO inhibitors (*see*) may cause severe high blood pressure. Contraindicated in patients with hypersensitivity to difenoxin or atropine, with diarrhea from colitis associated with antibiotics, and in children under two years of age. Also contraindicated in patients with jaundice, or diarrhea from organisms that may penetrate the intestinal mucosa, including *Escherichia coli, Salmonella,* and *Shigella.* Alcohol and other central nervous system depressants including antihistamines and sleeping medications will increase the sedative effects of difenoxin.

DIFLORASONE (Rx) • Florone. Flutone. Maxiflor. Psorcon. A corticosteroid ointment or cream used to treat skin inflammations. Potential adverse reactions include burning, itching, irritation, dryness, inflammation of the hair follicles, acne, rash around the mouth, spots of pigment loss, hairiness, allergic contact dermatitis, and if covered with a dressing, secondary infection, atrophy, streaks, and blisters. Should be used cautiously in skin problems caused by viruses such as herpes, and in fungal or bacterial skin infections. Should not be used for more than two weeks due to potential absorption into the system, consequently causing an effect on the hypothalamus, and pituitary and adrenal glands. Should not be applied near eyes or mucous membranes, under the arms, on the face, groin, or under the breast unless medically specified.

DIFLUCAN • *See* Fluconazole.

DIFLUNISAL (Rx) • Dolobid. A nonsteroidal anti-inflammatory drug introduced in 1977 to treat mild to moderate pain and osteoarthritis. The mechanism of the drug's action is unknown, but it is thought to inhibit prostaglandin synthesis. Potential adverse effects include dizziness, sleepiness, insomnia, headache, fatigue, ringing in the ears, visual disturbances, nausea, heartburn, gastrointestinal pain, diarrhea, vomiting, constipation, flatulence, rash, sweating, dry mucous membranes, and sore mouth. Aspirin and antacids decrease levels of diflunisal in the blood. Oral anticoagulants and anti-blood-clotting agents may be enhanced by diflunisal. Diflunisal decreases the effects of sulindac (*see*). Contraindicated for patients in whom acute asthmatic attacks, hives, or stuffy nose are precipitated by aspirin or other nonsteroidal anti-inflammatory drugs. Should be used cautiously in patients with active GI bleeding, history of peptic ulcer disease, renal impairment, liver disease, compromised heart function, or those taking anticoagulants. Diflunisal does not have an effect on blood platelets. Use of diflunisal in children and teenagers with viral illnesses and flu should be avoided due to possible association with Reye's syndrome. May be taken with food, milk, or water. It is a candidate for OTC status, as of this writing.

DI-GEL (OTC) • *See* Simethicone.

DIGITALIS (Rx) • Ouabain. A drug that is a powerful stimulant of heart-muscle contractions, derived from the foxglove plant (*see*). The plant contains a number of active agents that are isolated pharmaceutically, such as digitoxin (*see*).

Digitalization is the procedure of administering digitalis until a desired concentration of the drug is built up in the patient's body. The toxic effect of digitalis is close to the therapeutic effect, thus expert medical supervision is necessary. Should not be taken with prune juice, bran cereals, or foods high in fiber because they may undermine the effectiveness of digitalis.

DIGITALIS PURPUREA • *See* Foxglove.

DIGITOXIN (Rx) • **Crystodigin. Purodigin.** The main ingredient in digitalis (*see*), digitoxin is found in the leaves of the foxglove plant (*see*). Used to treat congestive heart failure, and irregular heartbeat and flutter. It strengthens the force of the heart's contractions and regulates abnormal heart rhythms, especially fast, irregular heartbeat. To be effective, the dose must be close to toxic and thus has to be monitored carefully. Potential adverse reactions include fatigue, generalized muscle weakness, agitation, hallucinations, headache, malaise, dizziness, stupor, numbness, and potentially lethal increased severity of congestive heart failure and irregular heartbeat. Diuretics can lower levels of potassium in the body, which increases the adverse effects with digitoxin. Quinidine and verapamil increase the amount of digitoxin in the blood, thus increasing the risk of adverse effects. Drugs that increase heartbeat, such as epinephrine and isoproterenol, may increase risk of abnormal heart rhythms if taken with digitoxin. Phenobarbital decreases digitoxin's effectiveness. Digitoxin should be taken with breakfast and should not be discontinued suddenly.

DIGOXIN (Rx) • **Lanoxicaps. Lanoxin.** Digoxin is the most widely used form of digitalis (*see*), a drug extracted from the leaves of the foxglove plant (*see*) and introduced in 1934. Used to treat congestive heart failure, and irregular heartbeat and flutter. Also helps to control water retention and fatigue. Digoxin has a narrow margin of safety; treatment dose is 60 percent of toxic dose. Potential adverse reactions include fatigue, generalized muscle weakness, agitation, hallucinations, headache, malaise, dizziness, stupor, numbness, and potentially lethal increased severity of congestive heart failure and irregular heartbeat. Many drugs interact with digoxin. Diuretics may increase the risk of adverse effects. Amiloride may make it less effective. Amphotericin B, carbenicillin, ticarcillin, and corticosteroids may cause low blood potassium, predisposing patients to digitalis toxicity. Antacids and kaolin-pectin decrease absorption from digoxin. Anticholinergics may increase digoxin absorption from oral tablets. Cholestyramine, colestipol, and metoclopramide decrease its effectiveness. Injectable calcium, quinidine, diltiazem, amiodarone, nifedipine, and verapamil may increase digoxin's toxicity. High-fiber foods decrease the drug's absorption. Digoxin should be taken after breakfast.

DIGOXIN IMMUNE FAB (Rx) • **Digibind.** A drug that counteracts digoxin and digitoxin (*see both*) that is used to treat potentially fatal digoxin or digitoxin intoxication. Potential adverse reactions include rapid heartbeat, congestive heart failure, low blood potassium, and hypersensitivity.

DIHYDROCODEINE (Rx) • A narcotic analgesic. *See* Codeine.

DIHYDROERGOTAMINE (Rx) • **DHE-45.** An injectable drug used to treat migraine headaches and cluster headaches. Most effective if used at first indication of a migraine, it inhibits the effects of epinephrine and norepinephrine (*see both*). It reportedly relieves migraine attacks within thirty minutes and is useful in all stages of the headache. Reportedly unlike narcotics and analgesics that simply alleviate headache pain, DHE-45 acts directly upon the headache mechanism to eradicate headache at its sources. It binds to the serotonin receptors in the brain that regulate the release of this brain chemical that plays a part in dilating blood vessels and increasing inflammation. A nasal spray is reportedly being tested. Contraindicated in pregnancy and in high blood pressure, liver or kidney dysfunction, blood poisoning, or blood-vessel and heart disease. Potential side effects include numbness and tingling in fingers and toes, transient rapid heartbeat or slow heartbeat, chest pain, increase in blood pressure, nausea, vomiting, itching, weakness in legs, muscle pains, and swelling. Prolonged exposure to cold weather may increase adverse reactions. Propranolol and other beta-blockers may cause excessive constriction of blood vessels.

DIHYDROERGOTOXINE • *See* Ergoloid Mesylates.

DIHYDROHYDROXYCODEINONE • *See* Oxycodone Hydrochloride.

DIHYDROMORPHINONE • *See* Hydromorphone.

DIHYDROTACHYSTEROL (Rx) • **DHT. Hytakerol.** A vitamin D preparation that stimulates calcium absorption from the GI tract and promotes secretion of calcium from bone to blood. Used to treat low blood calcium associated with an underactive parathyroid gland (*see*), calcium loss due to chronic kidney dysfunction, and to prevent low calcium following thyroid surgery. Potential adverse reactions include nausea, vomiting, headache, sleepiness, red eyes, sensitivity to light, runny nose, loss of appetite, frequent urination, weakness, and bone and muscle pain. Thiazide diuretics may cause too high a level of calcium in patients with underactive parathyroid glands. Adequate dietary calcium is recommended. Contraindicated in high or low blood calcium associated with kidney dysfunction and high phosphate in the blood, renal stone, hypersensitivity to vitamin D, and in breast-feeding mothers.

DIHYDROXYALUMINUM SODIUM CARBONATE (OTC) • **Rolaids.** An aluminum antacid that provides rapid neutralization of stomach acid. Used for the relief of heartburn and sour stomach, or acid indigestion. Potential adverse reactions include loss of appetite, constipation, and intestinal obstruction. Allopurinol, antibiotics, corticosteroids, diflunisal, digoxin, iron, isoniazid, penicillamine, phenothiazines, and ranitidine may be less effective because absorption may be impaired. Use cautiously in the elderly, especially those with slow digestion, and

those receiving antidiarrheals, antispasmodics, or anticholinergics; also in persons who are dehydrated, have chronic kidney disease, or suspected intestinal obstruction. Plain Rolaids has a high sodium content and should not be taken by persons with kidney dysfunction or who are on a low-salt diet. (Rolaids Sodium Free, which has calcium carbonate, may be taken by those who have to watch salt intake.) Rolaids or any other antacid should not be taken indiscriminately. May cause enteric-coated drugs to be released prematurely in the stomach, so doses should be separated by one hour.

DIHYDROXYANTHRACENEDIONE • *See* Mitoxantrone Hydrochloride.

DIIODOHYDROXYQUIN • *See* Iodoquinol.

DIISOPROPYL FLUOROPHOSPHATE • *See* Isofluorophate.

DILACOR • *See* Diltiazem.

DILANTIN • *See* Phenytoin.

DILANTIN WITH PHENOBARBITAL • *See* Phenobarbital and Phenytoin.

DILAR • *See* Pentaerythritol Tetranitrate.

DILATRATE-SR • *See* Isosorbide Dinitrate.

DILAUDID • *See* Hydromorphone.

DILL (H) • *Anethum graveolens.* A hardy herb native to southern Europe and western Asia as well as the Americas, it was said by the ancient Greek physician Galen that it "procureth sleep." The name *dill* is derived from a Saxon word meaning to lull. Used by herbalists to treat symptoms of colic in children and insomnia in adults caused by indigestion. Chewing dill seeds supposedly cures bad breath, and drinking dill tea calms upset stomach and hiccups. Dill contains volatile oils that include carvone, which is used by herbalists to break up intestinal gas, and limonene, used in foods as a flavoring. Dill in hot milk is recommended by herbalists as a drink that calms the nerves. Herbalists say that taken by nursing mothers, it increases milk production. Limonene can be a skin irritant and sensitizer.

DILOCAINE • *See* Lidocaine.

DILOMINE • *See* Dicyclomine.

DILOR • *See* Dyphylline.

DILTIAZEM (Rx) • **Cardizem. Cardizem SR. Dilacor. Dilacor XR (once-a-day). Tiazac.** Introduced in 1984, Diltiazem belongs to the family of calcium channel blockers (*see*). These interfere with the conduction of signals in the muscles of the heart and blood vessels. Diltiazem is used to treat angina and high blood pressure. It reduces the frequency of angina attacks but does not work quickly enough to reduce the pain. It is particularly useful for asthmatics because it does not adversely affect breathing as some other angina drugs do. Diltiazem XR is a newer version that need be taken only once a day. Diltiazem is contraindicated in patients with sick sinus syndrome or heart blocks, except if a pacemaker has been inserted. Also contraindicated in patients with low blood pressure and those hypersensitive to the drug or who have had recent heart attacks and lung congestion. May worsen heart problems and liver dysfunction. Potential side effects include headache, loss of appetite, nausea, weight gain, double vision, thirst, rash, photosensitivity, constipation, tiredness, dry mouth, leg and ankle swelling, dizziness, and rash. May also cause abnormal dreams, amnesia, depression, gait abnormality, hallucinations, insomnia, nervousness, numbness, personality change, sleepiness, ringing in the ears, and tremor. May increase the effects of high blood pressure medications. It may interact with digoxin (*see*) causing increased adverse effects. Diltiazem should be taken with *extreme caution with any drug that affects heart contractions*. Diltiazem should be taken on an empty stomach. As of this writing, Diltiazem was slated to become available in a lower-cost, generic drug. Grapefruit juice may cause potentially dangerous, increased levels of this medication in the blood.

DIMACOL • *See* Dextromethorphan.

DIMENHYDRINATE (OTC) • **Dramamine. Calm X. Dimentabs. Dinate. Dommanate. Dramanate. Dramilin. Dramocen. Dramoject. Dymenate. Gravol. Hydrate. Marmine. Motion-Aid. Nico-Vert. Nidryl. Reidamine. Tega-Vert. Triptone Caplets. Wehamine.** Introduced in 1949, it is an antihistamine used to prevent nausea and vomiting, especially when occurring with vertigo. Also used to relieve the symptoms of inner-ear disorders such as Ménière's disease, and to prevent and treat motion sickness. Also may counteract the effects of radiation, drug-induced nausea and vomiting, and the morning sickness of pregnancy. Potential adverse effects include drowsiness, dry mouth, palpitations, ringing in the ears, and blurred vision. Should not be taken with sedatives, which may increase the effects of dimenhydrinate. Abuse of the drug by teenagers in Canada has been reported. Should be used cautiously in patients with glaucoma, GI obstruction, and in elderly males with possibly enlarged prostate. May mask the ear toxicity of aminoglycoside (*see*) antibiotics and serious conditions such as brain tumor or intestinal obstruction. May be taken with food or milk.

DIMERCAPROL (Rx) • **BAL in Oil.** A chelating (*see*) agent used to treat metal poisoning. Potential adverse reactions include pain or tightness in throat, chest, or hands, headache, a pins-and-needles sensation, muscle pain or weakness, high blood pressure, twitching of the eyelid, conjunctivitis, tearing, runny nose, excessive salivation, bad breath, nausea, vomiting, a burning sensation in the lips, mouth, and throat, abdominal pain, painful urination, kidney damage, fever, sweating, and tooth pain. Contraindicated in liver and kidney dysfunction and used cautiously in persons with high blood pressure.

DIMENTABS (OTC) • *See* Dimenhydrinate.

DIMETANE-DC COUGH SYRUP (OTC) • *See* Brompheniramine.

DIMETANE DECONGESTANT (OTC) • *See* Brompheniramine.

DIMETANE ELIXIR (OTC) • *See* Brompheniramine.

DIMETANE EXTENTABS (OTC) • *See* Brompheniramine.

DIMETANE TABLETS (OTC) • *See* Brompheniramine.

DIMETAPP (OTC) • A combination of the antihistamine brompheniramine and the nasal decongestant phenylpropanolamine (*see both*). For use when a cough is present, Dimetapp-DM contains dextromethorphan (*see*).

DIMETHICONE (OTC) • **Moisturel.** A water-repellent silicone oil used as a topical drug vehicle and skin protectant.

DIMETHISOQUIN (OTC) • A local anesthetic derived from quinoline (*see*).

DIMETHYL SULFOXIDE (Rx) • **DMSO. Rimso-50.** A drug administered into the bladder to treat interstitial cystitis (*see*). It has not been approved for any other indication. Potential adverse reactions include a garliclike taste within a few minutes after instillation and moderately severe discomfort on administration. The discomforts reportedly become less severe upon repeated instillations.

DIMETHYL TUBOCURARINE • *See* Metocurine.

DINOPROST (Rx) • **Prostin F$_2$ Alpha.** A prostaglandin (*see*) drug used to stimulate contractions of the uterus. Used to cause abortion during the second trimester of pregnancy. Has many adverse reactions and must be administered only under a physician's supervision.

DINOPROSTONE (Rx) • **Prostin E$_2$. PGE$_2$.** A prostaglandin (*see*) drug used to stimulate contractions of the uterus to abort second-trimester pregnancies and to evacuate the uterus in cases of missed abortion, intrauterine fetal deaths up to twenty-eight weeks of gestation, or benign hydatidiform mole, the end stage of a degenerating pregnancy. In a study by Johns Hopkins obstetricians reported in 1991, prostaglandin E$_2$ shortened the time of labor and made it easier. The substance, according to the Johns Hopkins researchers, reduced the numbers of cesarean sections. Potential adverse reactions include nausea, vomiting, diarrhea, low blood pressure, vaginal pain and inflammation, fever, shivering, chills, joint inflammation, nighttime leg cramps, and bronchospasm.

DIOS • Homeopathic abbreviation for dioscorea (*see*).

DIOSCOREA (H) • **Devil's-Bones. Wild Yam.** A perennial creeper or vine that grows wild. The homeopathic remedy is made from the plant's long, knotted root. It is used for colic. It is also the basis for ancient and modern birth control preparations. *See* Wild Yam Root.

DIOCTO-C • *See* Docusate.

DIODOQUIN • *See* Iodoquinol.

DIOEZE • *See* Docusate.

DIONEX • *See* Docusate.

DIOSUCCIN • *See* Docusate.

DIOTHRON • *See* Docusate and Casanthranol.

DIOVAL • *See* Estradiol.

DIPENTUM • *See* Olsalazine Sodium.

DIPERODON (OTC) • **Bactine. Campho-Phenique Triple Antibiotic.** Obtained by condensing a piperidine and glycerol chlorohydrin with an alkali. Used as an anesthetic in solution to ease itching and minor skin irritations. For external use only. Not recommended to be used for more than seven days. Should be kept away from the eyes. In 1992, the FDA issued a notice that diperodon had not been shown to be safe and effective as claimed in OTC poison ivy, poison oak, and poison sumac products.

DIPHENATOL • *See* Difenoxin.

DIPHEN COUGH (OTC) • *See* Diphenhydramine.

DIPHENHYDRAMINE (Rx) (OTC) • **Aller May. Beldin. Belex. Bena-D. Benadryl. Benahist. Ben-Allergen. Benaphen. Bendylate. Benylin. Caladryl. Cold Control +. Dihydrex. Diphehist. Diphenacen-50. Diphen Cough. Dormarex. Extra-Strength Doan's P.M. Fenylhist. Hydramine. Hydramyn. Hydril. Insomnal. Nervine Nighttime Sleep Aid. Noradryl. Nytol. Sleep-Eze. Sominex. Tusstat. Twilite. Valdrene. Wehdryl. Ziradryl.** Introduced in 1945, diphenhydramine is one of the oldest and most common over-the-counter antihistamines. Used to treat allergies, including life-threatening allergic reactions and hypersensitivity reactions to foods, drugs, or insect stings. Because it has anticholinergic properties, it is used to treat parkinsonism and movement disorders caused by antipsychotic drugs. From 1982 to 1987, strong versions of the drug to treat coughs, insomnia, and vomiting were reclassified from Rx to OTC. One of the most sedating of antihistamines, it is used in over-the-counter sleep aids. In 1995, diphenhydramine became indicated for coughs in certain combination OTC cough/cold medications. Potential side effects include drowsiness, dry mouth, nausea, abdominal pain, blurred vision, urinary difficulties, hives, rash, excessive perspiration, fast heartbeat, palpitations, anemia, incoordination, epigastric distress, loss of appetite, urinary frequency, urinary retention, thickening of bronchial secretions, wheezing, nasal stuffiness, insomnia, and disorientation. Used with sedatives, it may increase central nervous system depression. Monoamine oxidase inhibitors (MAOIs) (*see*) used with this drug may increase blood pressure to dangerous levels. Other anticholinergic drugs (*see*) may increase the slowing of heart rhythms and gastrointestinal movements caused

by diphenhydramine. Contraindicated in acute asthmatic attacks. Should be used cautiously in elderly patients, people with glaucoma, overactive thyroid, heart or kidney disease, high blood pressure, bronchial asthma, enlarged prostate, bladder-neck obstruction, and peptic ulcer. Coffee or tea may reduce drowsiness. May cause photosensitivity, so sunscreens and sunglasses should be worn. In 1992, the FDA proposed a ban on diphenhydramine hydrochloride in poison ivy, poison oak, and poison sumac drug products because it had not been shown to be safe and effective as claimed. Medication should be discontinued four days before taking a skin allergy test because it can lead to inaccurate results. May be taken with food.

DIPHENIDOL (Rx) • **Vontrol.** A drug to counteract nausea and vomiting, and to treat Ménière's disease and other middle-ear problems. Potential adverse reactions include drowsiness, dizziness, sleep disturbance, confusion, and auditory and visual hallucinations and disorientation that may occur within three days of starting the drug and subside within three days after discontinuing it. Also may cause temporary low blood pressure, dry mouth, nausea, indigestion, heartburn, blurred vision, and hives. May mask more serious illnesses such as intestinal obstruction and brain tumor. Contraindicated in patients with urinary retention. Should be used cautiously in patients with glaucoma, GI obstruction, and in elderly males with possibly enlarged prostate. May be taken with food or a glass of water or milk to lessen stomach irritation. However, if vomiting has already occurred, it should be taken with a small amount of water on an empty stomach.

DIPHENOXYLATE (Rx) • **Diphenatol. Lofene. Logen. Lomotil. Lonox. Lo-Trol. Low-Quel. Nor-Mil.** Introduced in 1960, it is a narcotic antidiarrheal drug related to opiate analgesics. Reduces bowel contractions and decreases secretions. Available as tablets and liquid, it is not suitable for diarrhea caused by infection, antibiotics, or poisons because it may delay recovery by slowing the expulsion of harmful substances from the bowels. Potentially dangerous in ulcerative colitis. Especially dangerous for young children. Should not be used to treat acute diarrhea for more than two days. Not likely to be effective if there is no response within forty-eight hours. Potential adverse effects include drowsiness, restlessness, headache, blurred vision, rash, urine retention, hives, respiratory depression, bowel paralysis, constipation, nausea, and abdominal swelling and pain. Should not be taken by anyone with impaired liver function, severe abdominal pain, bloody diarrhea, glaucoma, or urinary difficulties. Also may interact adversely with antibiotics, MAO inhibitors (*see*), and many other medications. Alcohol may increase its depressant action on the brain. Diphenoxylate may be taken with or without food.

DIPHENYLHYDANTOIN • *See* Phenytoin.

DIPHENYLPYRALINE (Rx) • **Hispril.** An antihistamine prepared from piperidine, which occurs naturally in black pepper, and xylene, a hydrocarbon used often as a solvent.

DIPHTHERIA • An acute contagious disease once fatal to many children, but no longer a problem due to vaccination.

DIPHTHERIA ANTITOXIN, EQUINE (Rx) • An injection that neutralizes and binds toxin. Used to prevent and treat diphtheria. Potential adverse reactions include severe allergic reactions and serum sickness, which may occur in seven to twelve days.

DIPIVALYL EPINEPHRINE • *See* Dipivefrin.

DIPIVEFRIN (Rx) • **Propine.** A drug related to epinephrine, it is used to reduce pressure inside the eye in the treatment of glaucoma. Potential adverse reactions include rapid heartbeat, high blood pressure, and burning and stinging upon instillation. Digitalis, inhalation hydrocarbon anesthetics, and tricyclic antidepressants increase the risk of heart side effects if systemic absorption occurs.

DIPLOPIA • Double vision, due usually to weakness or paralysis of some of the eye muscles.

DIPRIVAN • *See* Propofol.

DIPROLENE • *See* Betamethasone.

DIPROSONE • *See* Betamethasone.

DIPYRIDAMOLE (Rx) • **Dipridacot. Persantine. Pyridamole.** Introduced in the late 1970s as an antiangina medication, it is now used as an antiplatelet drug. Usually given with aspirin to thin the blood of recent heart attack and stroke victims, or of those who have undergone coronary artery surgery. Also used to reduce the frequency of temporary shutoffs of blood to the brain (transient ischemic attacks). Its action reduces platelet stickiness, preventing blood-clotting within arteries. Potential side effects include nausea, headache, flushing, dizziness, and rash. Should not be taken with anticoagulants because it may cause uncontrolled bleeding. Should be taken before meals.

DIRITHROMYCIN (Rx) • **Dynabac.** An oral, once-a-day antibiotic, introduced in 1995, for the treatment of certain bacteria that cause lower-respiratory tract infections, pharyngitis (*see*), tonsillitis, community-acquired pneumonia, and skin infections in patients twelve years and older. Should not be used with terfenadine, theophylline, antacids, triazolam, anticoagulants, ergotamine and has reported to also interact with concomitant administration of erythromycin and cyclopsprins. Potential adverse reactions include abdominal pain, headache, nausea, diarrhea, and it may also increase platelet count and potassium. Should be taken with food.

DISALCID • *See* Salsalate.

DISC • The cartilage cushion found between the vertebrae of the spinal column. It may bulge beyond the vertebrae and compress nearby nerve roots, causing pain (slipped disc).

DISCASE • *See* Chymopapain.

DISIPAL • *See* Orphenadrine.

DISODIUM CROMOGLYCATE • *See* Cromolyn Sodium.

DISODIUM EDTA • *See* Edetate Disodium.

DISODIUM PHOSPHATE (OTC) • **Afrin Saline Mist.** Provides soothing moisture to dry, inflamed nasal membranes due to colds, allergies, low humidity, and other minor nasal irritation. It is innocuous and may be used with other cold, allergy, and sinus medications.

DISOPHROL • *See* Pseudoephedrine and Dexbrompheniramine.

DISOPYRAMIDE (Rx) • **Napamide. Norpace. Norpace CR.** An antiarrhythmic drug introduced in 1978, used for ventricular and supraventricular arrhythmias. Narrow margin of safety. Potential side effects include dizziness, agitation, depression, fatigue, muscle weakness, fainting, low blood pressure, coronary heart failure, weight gain, water retention, blurred vision, dry eyes, nose, or mouth, nausea, vomiting, loss of appetite, abdominal pain, constipation, impotence, jaundice, low blood sugar, and rash. Because it reduces the force of the heartbeat, it can worsen existing heart failure and low blood pressure. Interacts with antiarrhythmics, which may increase or decrease its effects. Phenytoin and rifampin (*see both*) make it less effective. Most effective on an empty stomach, but may be taken with food if stomach upset is a problem. *See also* Arrhythmia.

DI-SOSUL • *See* Docusate.

DISOTATE • *See* Edetate Disodium.

DI-SPAZ • *See* Dicyclomine Hydrochloride.

DISULFIRAM (Rx) • **Antabuse. Cronetal. Ro-Sulfiram 500.** Introduced in 1948, it is used to help alcoholics maintain abstinence. If alcohol is ingested, the drug produces nausea and vomiting, flushing, throbbing headache, breathlessness, depression, thirst, palpitations, dizziness, and fainting. Such reactions may last from thirty minutes to several hours, leaving the person feeling drowsy. Other potential adverse reactions include garlic taste, temporary impotence, and blurred vision. In severe reactions, unconsciousness and death may result. Should not be taken within twelve hours of alcohol ingestion, in psychoses, heart attack, or patients receiving metronidazole, paraldehyde, or alcohol-containing preparations, including over-the-counter medications. Contraindicated in pregnancy, diabetes, low thyroidism, epilepsy, brain damage, nerve inflammation, liver cirrhosis or insufficiency, abnormal brain waves, or multiple-drug dependence. Should not be taken with phenytoin, anticoagulants, or isoniazid because these may increase adverse effects. May be taken with food to reduce stomach upset.

DISULFIRAMLIKE REACTION • The interaction of any drug with alcohol that produces effects, such as the nausea, vomiting, and other symptoms, similar to those caused by disulfiram (*see*) and alcohol.

DITHIOGLYCEROL • *See* Dimercaprol.

DITI CREAM • *See* Diethylstilbestrol.

DITROPAN • *See* Oxybutynin.

DIUCARDIN • *See* Hydroflumethiazide.

DIUCHLOR • *See* Hydrochlorothiazide.

DIUPRES • *See* Chlorothiazide and Reserpine.

DIURETIC • A drug used to remove excess fluids from the body by increasing the flow of urine. Diuretics should not be taken with foods containing the additive monosodium glutamate (MSG) or potassium- or sodium-rich foods because these may cause tightness in the chest or flushing of the face. Among herbs that are considered diuretics are cleavers, celery seed, and yarrow (*see all*). Rx diuretics include bumetanide, furosemide, and chlorothiazide (*see all*). *See also* Loop Diuretics.

DIURIGEN • *See* Chlorothiazide.

DIURIL • *See* Chlorothiazide.

DIUTENSIN-R • *See* Methyclothiazide and Reserpine.

DIVERTICULITIS • *See* Diverticulosis.

DIVERTICULOSIS • The presence of little sacs (diverticula) in the walls of the intestines and gallbladder. A common condition in older people. Diverticulitis involves inflamed diverticula.

DIZMISS (OTC) • *See* Meclizine.

DIZYMES • *See* Pancreatin.

DMSO • *See* Dimethyl Sulfoxide.

DNA • Abbreviation for deoxyribonucleic acid. A chain of molecules that contains the genetic code (blueprint) of cells.

DNR • *See* Daunorubicin Hydrochloride.

DOAK (OTC) • *See* Coal Tar.

DOBUTAMINE (Rx) • **Dobutrex.** A drug used to treat heart failure and occasionally shock. It directly stimulates receptors of the heart to increase its pumping action. Potential adverse reactions include headache, increased heart rate, high blood pressure, premature heartbeats, angina, chest pain, nausea, vomiting, and shortness of breath. Beta-blockers (*see*) may make it less effective. General anesthetics may increase incidence of irregular heartbeat.

DOCUSATE (OTC) • **Afko-Lube. Anticon. Colace. Coloxyl Enema. Correctol. Dialose. Diocto. Diocto-K. Dioeze. Diosuccin. DioSul. Disonate. Di-Sosul. DOK Liquid. DOK-250. Doss 300. Doxinate. D-S-S. Duosol. Feen-A-Mint. Ferro-Sequels. Genasoft. Geriplex-FS. Hemaspan FA. Kasof. Laxinate 100. Modane Soft. Phillips LaxCaps. Pro-**

Cal-Sof. Regulax SS. Regutol. Stulex Surfak. A laxative with detergent activity that promotes softening of stools. Potential adverse reactions include throat irritation, bitter taste, mild abdominal cramping, diarrhea, and laxative dependence after long-term or excessive use. Should not be taken with mineral oil as it may increase the oil's absorption, causing a type of pneumonia. Should be used only occasionally and not for more than one week. In 1992, the FDA proposed a ban on docusate sodium in lice-killing products because it had not been shown to be safe and effective as claimed.

DODEX • *See* Vitamin B_{12}.

DOGBANE • *See* Dog Grass.

DOG GRASS (OTC) (H) • *Agropyron repens.* **Triticum.** In 1992, the FDA issued a notice that dog grass had not been shown to be safe and effective as claimed in OTC digestive-aid products or oral menstrual drugs. *See* Couch Grass.

DOGTOOTH VIOLET • *See* Adder's-Tongue.

DOGWOOD (H) • *Cornus florida* or *fanguinea.* **Boxwood. Green Ozier.** *Piscidia erythrina.* A small tree found in many areas of the United States. The bark possesses astringent, stimulant, and tonic properties and was used by herbalists for malaria, especially when cinchona (*see*) bark was unavailable.

DOKTORS DURATION • *See* Phenylephrine.

DOLACET (Rx) • A combination of acetaminophen and hydrocodone (*see both*) used to treat coughs.

DOLANEX • *See* Acetaminophen.

DOLENE • *See* Propoxyphene and Propoxyphene Napsylate.

DOLOBID • *See* Diflunisal.

DOLOPHINE • *See* Methadone.

DOMEBORO ASTRINGENT (OTC) • *See* Aluminum Acetate.

DOMEBORO OTIC (OTC) • *See* Acetic Acid.

DOME-PASTE (OTC) • *See* Zinc.

DOMPERIDONE (Rx) • **Motilium.** A drug expected to be approved to treat diabetes.

DONATUSSIN (OTC) • *See* Chlorpheniramine.

DONG QUAI (H) • *Angelica sinensis.* **Tang Kwei.** The root of the herb, which contains safrole and coumarin (*see both*), is used for the treatment of female gynecological ailments, particularly menstrual cramps, irregularity, and malaise during the menstrual period. Also used to relieve the symptoms of menopause. Dong quai is used by herbalists as an antispasmodic for treating insomnia, high blood pressure, allergies, and cramps. It is reputedly useful in treating anemia and constipation. Excessive doses may cause contractions of the uterus and should not be used during pregnancy. Because of the presence of safrole, it may be carcinogenic in humans. *See also* Angelica.

DONNAGEL (OTC) • **Liquid and Tablets.** Used to relieve diarrhea, the liquid contains attapulgite (*see*) plus 1.4 percent alcohol, magnesium aluminum silicate, sorbitol, FD&C Blue No. 1 (*see*), and a number of other ingredients. The tablets contain D&C Yellow No. 10 Aluminum Lake, FD&C Blue No. 1 Aluminum Lake, mannitol, saccharin, sorbitol (*see all*), and other inactive ingredients. Should not be used for more than two days, or in the presence of fever, or by children under three years.

DONNAGEL-PG (Rx) • Contains powdered opium, kaolin, pectin, hyoscyamine, atropine, scopolamine, sodium benzoate, 5 percent alcohol, citric acid, D&C Yellow No. 10, carboxymethylcellulose (*see all*), and sugars. Contraindicated in glaucoma, advanced liver or kidney disease, or hypersensitivity to any of the ingredients. Should be used cautiously in patients with enlarged prostate or urinary-bladder-neck obstruction. Potential adverse reactions include diarrhea, blurred vision, dry mouth, difficulty in urinating, and dryness of the skin. Should not be used for more than two days.

DONNAPECTOLIN-PG (Rx) • A combination of hyoscyamine, atropine, kaolin, pectin, and opium (*see all*), used in the treatment of diarrhea.

DONNATAL (Rx) • **Barbidonna. Barophen. Bellastal. Donnamor. Donnapine. Donphen Tablets. Haponal. Hybephen. Hyosophen. Malatal. Myphentol. Relaxadon. Seds. Spaslin. Spasmolin. Spasmophen. Spasquid. Susano.** A combination of hyoscyamine, atropine, scopolamine, and phenobarbital, it is used to relieve stomach spasms and other cramps, and motion sickness. Potential adverse reactions include blurred vision, dry mouth, difficulty in urinating, flushing, dry skin, irregular heartbeat, sensitivity to light, loss of taste, headache, nervousness, tiredness, fever, stuffy nose, heartburn, loss of sex drive, decreased sweating, constipation, bloated feeling, and allergic reactions. Alcohol, antihistamines, tranquilizers, sleeping pills, and narcotics may increase central nervous system depression. Should be taken an hour before meals.

DONNAZYME (Rx) • A combination of belladonna, phenobarbital, and pepsin (*see all*), used to treat upset stomach due to anxiety.

DON SEN (H) • *Codonopsis pilosula.* **Tang Shen.** The root is used as a tonic. It is similar to ginseng, but is less expensive and can be taken on a daily basis. The action is milder and can be used for longer treatment. Don sen reputedly strengthens the function of the spleen and pancreas. Used for treating infection, inflammation, diabetes, and to aid digestion.

DOPAMINE • A natural neurotransmitter (*see*) involved in movement and mood. A precursor of norepinephrine and epinephrine (*see both*).

DOPAMINE HYDROCHLORIDE (Rx) • **Intropin.** A drug that stimulates the release of dopamine. Used to treat shock, increase blood flow to the heart, correct low blood pressure, and treat kidney failure. Potential adverse reactions include headache, irregular heartbeat, angina, palpitations, low blood pressure, slow heartbeat, constriction of the blood vessels, nausea, vomiting, and shortness of breath. Beta-blockers (*see*) may make it less effective. Use with ergot alkaloids or MAO inhibitors (*see*) may quickly raise blood pressure to dangerous levels. Phenytoin may lower blood pressure too much. Contraindicated in several forms of heart disease, cold injuries, in pregnancy, and in those taking MAO inhibitors. *See also* Alkaloids.

DOPAR • *See* Levodopa.

DOPASTAT • *See* Dopamine.

DOPRAM • *See* Doxapram.

DORAL • *See* Quazepam.

DORAPHEN • *See* Propoxyphene and Propoxyphene Napsylate.

DORCOL CHILDREN'S COUGH SYRUP (OTC) • Contains pseudoephedrine, guaifenesin, dextromethorphan, benzoic acid, edetate disodium, glycerin, propylene glycol, sodium hydroxide, sucrose, and tartaric acid (*see all*). Should not be given to a child who has high blood pressure or is taking an antidepressant drug containing monoamine oxidase, unless it is under a physician's supervision.

DORCOL CHILDREN'S DECONGESTANT LIQUID (OTC) • Contains pseudoephedrine (*see*). Other ingredients include benzoic acid, edetate disodium, sodium hydroxide, sorbitol, and sucrose (*see all*).

DORCOL CHILDREN'S LIQUID COLD FORMULA (OTC) • A combination of pseudoephedrine hydrochloride and chlorpheniramine (*see both*). Other ingredients include benzoic acid, sorbitol, sucrose, and sodium hydroxide (*see all*). Potential adverse reactions that may occur at high

doses include nervousness, dizziness, and sleeplessness. *See also* Chlorpheniramine.

DORIDEN (Rx) • A medicine to treat insomnia. Effective for short-term use only. Potential adverse reactions that may occur at high doses include nervousness, dizziness, and sleeplessness. May interact with alcohol. *See* Glutethimide.

DORIGLUTE • *See* Glutethimide.

DORMALIN • *See* Quazepam.

DORNASE (Rx) • **Dnase. Pulmozyme.** A drug introduced in 1994 used for the treatment of cystic fibrosis (*see*). It is the first new therapeutic approach to be developed for cystic fibrosis in more than thirty years. It is not a cure or a replacement for current therapies, but acts on the accumulation and reduction of the viscosity of mucous secretions. This leads to an improvement in lung function and a reduction in infection risks. Now approved in eighteen countries, Dornase reduces respiratory infections and improves breathing in cystic fibrosis patients. It is also being tested as a treatment for other respiratory ailments.

DORYX • *See* Doxycycline.

DORZOLAMIDE (Rx) • **Trusopt.** An opthalmic solution—the first topical carbonic anhydrase inhibitor—for the treatment of elevated pressure inside the eye in patients with ocular high blood pressure or open-angle glaucoma. Dorzolamide can be used in combination with other topical glaucoma agents such as timolol maleate (*see*). Dorzolamide reportedly has the potential to reduce the systemic side effects, such as gastrointestinal disturbances and drowsiness, of carbonic anhydrase inhibitors (*see*) taken orally.

DOSS • *See* Docusate.

DOTHIEPIN (Rx) • **Prothiaden.** An antidepressant expected to be approved.

DOUBLE-BLIND • A trial in which patients receive either a placebo or a drug, and neither patients nor persons administering these know which product is being administered.

DOU FU-TOFU • *See* Bean Curd.

DOVALPROEX SODIUM • *See* Valproic Acid.

DOW-ISONIAZID • *See* Isoniazid.

DOXAPHENE • *See* Propoxyphene and Propoxyphene Napsylate.

DOXAPRAM (Rx) • A respiratory stimulant used after surgery to stimulate breathing in drug-induced central nervous system depression, and chronic lung disease. Potential adverse reactions include nausea, vomiting, diarrhea, seizures, headache, dizziness, apprehension, disorientation, flushing, sweating, numbness, chest pain and tightness, high blood pressure, irregular heartbeat, urine retention or incontinence, wheezing, coughing, throat and lung spasms, hiccups, rebound slow breathing, and itching. MAO inhibitors and sympathomimetics (*see both*) may potentiate adverse effects on the heart. Contraindicated in seizure disorders, head injury, heart disease, overactive thyroidism, and muscle disorders.

DOXAZOSIN MESYLATE (Rx) • **Cardura.** An antihypertensive drug introduced in 1986 that blocks the nerve signals that trigger constriction of blood vessels. Reportedly does not have an adverse effect on blood sugar as some blood-pressure-lowering drugs do. Potential adverse reactions include dizziness, headache, sleepiness, fatigue, fainting, numbness, a drop in blood pressure when standing, water retention, palpitations, irregular heartbeat, and reduction in blood supply to the heart. Also may cause rash, joint and muscle aches, weakness, and stuffy nose. Because it may cause drowsiness at first, driving a car or working with machinery should be postponed until adjustments are made to the effects of the drug. Should be taken at bedtime to avoid a drop in blood pressure when rising from a seated or prone position. May be taken with or without food.

DOXEPIN (Rx) • **Adapin. Sinequan.** Introduced in 1969, doxepin belongs to a family of antidepressants known as the tricyclics (*see*). Used in the treatment of major depressions including manic depression, it elevates mood, increases physical activity, improves appetite, and renews interest in everyday activities. Since it has more sedative effects than many other antidepressants, it is used for patients who suffer from sleep problems and anxiety. Potential side effects include drowsiness, sweating, flushing, dry mouth, blurred vision, dizziness, female breast enlargement with milk production, swelling of the testicles, fainting, rash, urinary difficulties, and palpitations. Doxepin interacts with sedatives, increasing central nervous system depression. It also interacts with high blood pressure drugs, counteracting their effectiveness. When used with monoamine oxidase inhibitors (*see*), seizures and delirium may occur. Heavy smoking may reduce the antidepressant effect of doxepin. Most effective when taken on an empty stomach, but may be taken with a small amount of food.

DOXIDAN (OTC) • *See* Danthron and Docusate.

DOXINATE • *See* Docusate.

DOXORUBICIN (Rx) • **ADR. Adriamycin. Deoxydoxorubicin. DOX-SL. Rubex.** One of the most effective of anticancer drugs, it was introduced in 1974 and is often used in conjunction with other drugs. Doxorubicin is an effective treatment for acute leukemia, cancer of the lymph nodes (Hodgkin's disease), and lung, breast, bladder, stomach, thyroid, and reproductive-organ cancers. Potential adverse reactions include vomiting, nausea, hair loss, diarrhea, mouth ulcers, sore throat, pigmentation of the skin, and palpitations. The most serious adverse reactions include bleeding, anemia, infections, and heart problems. Medications for gout may have to be increased because doxorubicin increases levels of uric acid in the blood. Streptozocin (*see*) may make it more toxic. *See* DOX-SL.

DOX-SL (Rx) • A formulation of doxorubicin that achieved accelerated approval by the FDA for the treatment of Kaposi's sarcoma (*see*). An FDA committee recommended DOX-SL for use in the treatment of the AIDS-related cancer in patients who had failed prior systemic combination chemotherapy. *See* Doxorubicin.

DOXY-CAPS • *See* Doxycycline.

DOXYCHEL • *See* Doxycycline.

DOXYCYCLINE (Rx) • **AK-Ramycin. AK-Ratabs. Doxy-Caps. Doxychel. Doxy-Lemmon. Doxylin. Doxy-100. Doxy-Tabs. Doxy-200. Vibramycin. Vibra-Tabs. Vivox.** A long-acting tetracycline (*see*) antibiotic introduced in 1967 used to treat infections caused by gram-negative and gram-positive (*see both*) organisms, trachoma, rickettsiae, mycoplasma, chlamydia, and Lyme disease (*see all*). May also be used in gonorrhea patients allergic to penicillin. Potential adverse reactions include a drop in white blood cells, pressure on the brain, inflammation of the heart, sore throat, sore tongue, trouble swallowing, loss of appetite, nausea, vomiting, colitis, anogenital inflammation, skin rash, photosensitivity, increased pigmentation, and hives and other hypersensitivity reactions. Blood clots at the site of injection may occur. Less toxic to the kidney than some other tetracyclines, it is less likely to cause diarrhea. Usually not prescribed for children up to age eight because it has been shown to discolor permanent teeth. It may also retard growth. Antacids including sodium bicarbonate, and laxatives containing aluminum, magnesium, or calcium, may make the drug less effective. Iron, zinc, and phenobarbital also decrease its effect. Oral contraceptives and penicillin may be ineffective while taking doxycycline. Oral blood thinners increase the anticoagulant action of this drug. Barbiturates, carbamazepine, and phenytoin reduce the effectiveness of doxycycline. May be taken with food or milk. Cases of damage to the esophagus caused by this drug have been reported since 1970. To help prevent such damage when taking doxycycline, patients are recommended to take the capsules or tablets while in an upright position, along with at least eight ounces of water, several hours before bedtime.

DOXY-II • *See* Doxycycline.

DOXYLAMINE (Rx) (OTC) • **Mereprine. Unisom. Vicks NyQuil Nighttime Cold/Flu.** An antihistamine used to induce sleep, it was reclassified from Rx to OTC in 1978, and in stronger doses in 1987. A coal tar derivative, it shows a high level of sedation. In some studies, it was chosen as the antihistamine, based on dosage, causing the earliest onset of sleep. Should be taken only at bedtime. Contraindicated for asthma, glaucoma, and enlargement of the prostate gland. Should not be taken if alcohol is being consumed, or by patients taking other drugs, without consulting a physician. Should not be taken for longer than two weeks.

DOXY-LEMMON • *See* Doxycycline.

DOXY-TABS • *See* Doxycycline.

DPE • *See* Dipivefrin.

D-PENICILLAMINE (Rx) • *See* Penicillamine.

DPH • *See* Phenytoin.

DPT (Rx) • **Diphtheria and Tetanus Toxoids and Pertussis Vaccine. Tri-Immunol.** A vaccine combining immunization against diphtheria, pertussis, and tetanus, administered in a single injection. The primary injection is usually given to children six weeks to six years. Potential adverse reactions include slight fever, chills, malaise, seizures, brain swelling, severe allergic reaction, loss of appetite, vomiting, and soreness and redness at site of injection. In rare instances, sudden infant death syndrome has been suspected. Should not be given if the child has a fever, is taking corticosteroids, or is immunosuppressed.

DRAGON WORT • *See* Bistort.

DRAMAMINE (OTC) • *See* Dimenhydrinate.

DRAMILIN (OTC) • *See* Dimenhydrinate.

DRENISON • *See* Flurandrenolide.

DRI/EAR • *See* Boric Acid.

DRISDOL • *See* Vitamin D.

DRISTAN COLD AND FLU (OTC) • A lemon-flavored hot-drink mix containing acetaminophen, pseudoephedrine, chlorpheniramine, and dextromethorphan (*see all*).

DRISTAN 12-HOUR NASAL SPRAY (OTC) • *See* Oxymetazoline.

DRITHOCREME • *See* Anthralin.

DRITHO-SCALP • *See* Anthralin and Salicylic Acid.

DRIXINE NASAL • *See* Oxymetazoline.

DRIXORAL (OTC) • **Bromfed. Brompheril. Disobrom. Disophrol/Chronotabs.** A combination of brompheniramine and pseudoephedrine (*see both*). An antihistamine-decongestant used to relieve the symptoms of common colds, allergies, and other upper-respiratory conditions. Potential adverse reactions include anxiety, drowsiness, palpitations, restlessness, tremor, weakness, insomnia, sweating, loss of appetite, nausea, vomiting, dizziness, and constipation. Alcoholic beverages, sedatives, tranquilizers, antihistamines, and sleeping pills may cause excessive drowsiness. Over-the-counter drugs for the relief of cold symptoms may increase the side effects of Drixoral, including high blood pressure, heart disease, diabetes, and thyroid disease. Do not take Drixoral if you are taking or have taken an MAO inhibitor (*see*) within two weeks. Severe high blood pressure may result. Drixoral may be taken with food.

DROMOSTANOLONE (Rx) • An androgenic drug sometimes used in the treatment of breast cancer. *See* Androgens.

DRONABINOL (Rx) • **Marinol. Tetrahydrocannabinol. THE.** A drug derived from marijuana. Used primarily to treat nausea and vomiting induced by anticancer drugs. It is also approved as a treatment for appetite loss associated with AIDS. Potential adverse reactions include dizziness, loss of balance, disorientation, hallucinations, headache, paranoia, memory lapses, irritability, rapid heartbeat, a drop in blood pressure when rising from a seated or prone position, dry mouth, and visual disturbances. Alcohol, central nervous system depressants, and sedatives cause additive effects. Contraindicated for nausea and vomiting from any cause other than cancer therapy; contraindicated also in patients hypersensitive to sesame oil. Should be used cautiously in elderly patients and those with high blood pressure, heart disease, or psychiatric illness.

DRONCIT • *See* Praziquantel.

DROPERIDOL (Rx) • **Inapsine. Innovar.** A drug given as premedication or as an anesthetic during surgery, and to suppress vomiting and dizziness associated with Ménière's disease. Potential adverse reactions include a drop in white blood cells, movement disorders, seizures, low blood pressure, rapid heartbeat, and spasms of the throat and lungs. Should be used cautiously in elderly or debilitated patients, those with low blood pressure, impaired kidneys or liver, and Parkinson's disease.

DROS • Homeopathic abbreviation for drosera (*see*).

DROSERA (H) • **Dew Plant. Red Rot. Youth Wort.** A small, perennial carnivorous plant that grows close to the ground on mossy, marshy ground throughout Britain, northern Europe, Asia, and North America. A homeopathic medicine to treat coughs. *See* Sundew.

DROTIC (Rx) • A combination of neomycin, polymyxin B, and hydrocortisone (*see all*).

DROXOMIN (OTC) • *See* Vitamin B_{12}.

DRUG DELIVERY SYSTEMS • The following are methods of administering drugs to the body.

Physically Controlled Drugs. These are the familiar capsules, tablets, and solutions.

Chemically Modified Drugs. These include prodrugs (*see*) and soft drugs that must be transformed by chemicals in the body before eliciting an effect. Prodrugs are inactive drugs that can be converted to the active form by the body's chemistry. For example, since tumors tend to lack oxygen compared with normal tissue, prodrugs may be activated in areas of oxygen deprivation. Scientists are also working on developing soft drugs that fall apart to nontoxic compounds after performing their therapeutic tasks. Both types of drugs are expected to cause fewer undesirable side effects than the highly toxic agents now in use.

Osmotically Controlled Drugs. These are the preparations that use pressure exerted by water moving across a membrane to release a steady flow of drug from a reservoir.

Diffusion Controlled Drugs. These include hydrogels (gelatins that melt and release drugs), matrix systems, and transdermal delivery systems in which a drug moves steadily from areas of high concentration to areas of low concentration. Matrix systems are synthetic molecules that uniformly distribute a drug through a synthetic polymer (bead). As water enters the matrix, the drug dissolves and escapes into the body. Matrix systems containing insulin also release the hormone at a steady rate. Transdermal delivery systems release a steady flow of drug, reducing side effects. They are being widely used to treat the chest pain of angina, for high blood pressure, and to administer estrogen in postmenopausal women.

Mechanically Controlled Infusion Pumps. These pumps are used by people with insulin-dependent diabetes to deliver a constant flow of insulin. A sophisticated model now in the developmental stage will release the drug as needed. Mechanically controlled systems also are used to deliver cancer-fighting drugs to malignant cells.

Targeted Drug Delivery Monoclonal Antibodies and Liposomes. Each monoclonal antibody is a genetically uniform and highly specific immune-system protein that can be produced through biotechnology. A monoclonal antibody moves like an arrow to a specific target. It hits only that target. Scientists are experimenting with ways of combining monoclonals with anticancer drugs such as chemotherapeutic agents, toxins, and radioactive isotopes to help detect, target, and destroy malignant cells while leaving healthy cells alone. Liposome carriers deliver medications. Liposomes containing antifungal and antibacterial agents have proven to be effective long-acting agents against certain diseases.

In the future, patients may wear a watch containing drugs to be released automatically at just the right time through the skin or from a reservoir under the skin.

DRUG FEVER • An elevated body temperature, a side effect caused by a drug, usually due to an allergy. Among the drugs commonly known to sometimes cause drug fever are allopurinol, antihistamines, atropinelike drugs, barbiturates, coumarin anticoagulants, hydralazine, iodides, isoniazid, methyldopa, nadolol, novobiocin, para-aminosalicylic acid, penicillin, pentazocine, phenytoin, procainamide, propylthiouracil, quinidine, rifampin, and sulfonamides.

DRUG INTERACTION • The modification of the effect of one drug by another in a way that diminishes, negates, or enhances the effectiveness or safety of one or both drugs.

DRY AND CLEAR (OTC) • *See* Benzoyl Peroxide.

DRYSOL (OTC) • An antiperspirant preparation containing aluminum chloride (*see*).

DTO (Rx) • An opium (*see*) tincture.

DUCK'S FOOT • *See* Mayapple.

DULC • Homeopathic abbreviation for dulcamara (*see*).

DULCAMARA (H) • **Bittersweet Night-shade.** An extract of the dried stems of *Solanum dulcamara,* belonging to the family of the night-shades. It is used as a preservative food additive. The ripe berries are used for pies and jams. A homeopathic medicine to treat coughs and congestion. It is also used by herbalists as an ointment to treat skin cancers and burns. It induces sweating. Dulcamara's unripened berries are deadly. *See also* Horse Nettle.

DULCOLAX (OTC) • *See* Bisacodyl.

DULL-C • *See* Vitamin C.

DUO-CYP (Rx) • *See* Estradiol and Testosterone.

DUODENAL ULCER • An open sore in the lining of the duodenum, the top portion of the small intestine.

DUODENUM • The portion of the small intestine directly connected to the stomach. The duodenum receives digestive enzymes and bile from the pancreas and gallbladder. ·

DUOFILM • *See* Salicylic Acid.

DUOLUBE (OTC) • An emollient eye preparation containing white petrolatum and mineral oil.

DUO-MEDIHALER (Rx) • *See* Isoproterenol, Phenylephrine, and Pyrilamine.

DUOSOL • *See* Docusate.

DUOTRATE • *See* Pentaerythritol Tetranitrate.

DUPHALAC • *See* Lactulose.

DUPHRENE (OTC) • A combination of chlorpheniramine, phenylephrine, and pyrilamine (*see all*), used to treat allergy symptoms.

DUPLEX (OTC) • *See* Coal Tar.

DURABOLIN • *See* Nandrolone.

DURACILLIN • *See* Penicillin G.

DURADYNE (OTC) • A combination of acetaminophen, aspirin, and caffeine (*see all*), used as a painkiller.

DURA-ESTRIN • *See* Estradiol.

DURAGEN • *See* Estradiol.

DURAGESIC (Rx) • A transdermal patch for severe pain. *See* Fentanyl and Transdermal.

DURALUTIN • *See* Hydroxyprogesterone.

DURAMIST PLUS • *See* Oxymetazoline.

DURAMORPH • *See* Morphine Sulfate or Hydrochloride.

DURANEST • *See* Etidocaine.

DURAPAM • *See* Flurazepam.

DURAPHYL • *See* Theophylline.

DURAPRED • *See* Prednisolone.

DURAQUIN • *See* Quinidine.

DURATEARS (OTC) • *See* Artificial Tears.

DURATEST • *See* Testosterone.

DURATESTRIN • *See* Estradiol and Testosterone.

DURATHESIA • *See* Procaine.

DURATION 4-WAY LONG LASTING NASAL (OTC) • *See* Oxymetazoline.

DURICEF • *See* Cefadroxil Monohydrate.

DURRAX • *See* Hydroxyzine.

DUSTY MILLER (H) • *Senecio cineraria.* The sterilized juice of this herb is used to treat eye problems. It is sold by homeopathic pharmacies to treat cataracts and to brighten vision. Contains pyrrolizidine alkaloids and should not be used internally.

DUVOID • *See* Bethanechol.

DV CREAM • *See* Dienestrol.

DWARF ELDER • *See* Elder.

DWARFISM • A condition of being markedly undersized. *See* Somatomedin C.

D-XYLOSE (Rx) (H) • **Wood Sugar. Xylo-Pfan.** A sugar used for evaluating intestinal absorption and diagnosing malabsorptive states.

DYAZIDE (Rx) • **Maxzide.** A diuretic, a combination of hydrochlorothiazide and triamterene. Used to treat high blood pressure and other conditions where fluid retention is a problem. Dyazide helps the body retain potassium while producing a diuretic effect. This balances the potassium loss due to hydrochlorothiazide. Potential adverse reactions include loss of appetite, drowsiness, lethargy, headache, gastrointestinal upset, cramps and diarrhea, confusion, rash, fever, malaise, impotence, red and/or burning tongue, tingling in limbs, restlessness, anemia, sensitivity to sunlight, a drop in blood pressure when rising from a prone or seated position, muscle spasms, gout, weakness, and blurred vision. Contraindicated in people with severe kidney dysfunction, those with an allergy to sulfa drugs, or with bronchial asthma. Potassium supplements or foods high in potassium should not be taken unless directed by a physician. Dyazide increases the effect of other blood-pressure-lowering drugs. May alter the dose needed for antidiabetes drugs and cause lithium to become more toxic. Over-the-counter cough, cold, and allergy remedies may counteract its effects. May be taken with food.

DYCILL • *See* Dicloxacillin Sodium.

DYCLONE • *See* Dyclonine.

DYCLONINE (OTC) • **Sucrets.** A topical anesthetic that relieves minor sore-throat pain and mouth irritations. Was reclassified from RX to OTC in 1982. Potential adverse reactions due to large overdosage are systemic and involve the central nervous system and cardiovascular system. Central nervous system reactions are characterized by excitation and/or depression. Nervousness, dizziness, blurred vision, or tremors may occur. Also may cause low blood pressure and slowed heartbeat.

DYMELOR • *See* Acetohexamide.

DYNABAC (Rx) • *See* Dirithromycin.

DYNACIRC • *See* Isradipine.

DYNAPEN • *See* Dicloxacillin.

DYPHYLLINE (Rx) • **Brophylline. Dilin. Dilor. Dyflex. Dylline. Emfabid. Lufyllin. Neothylline.** A xanthine (*see*) bronchodilator used for the relief of acute and chronic bronchial asthma and bronchospasm associated with chronic bronchitis and emphysema. Potential adverse reactions include restlessness, dizziness, headache, insomnia, light-headedness, seizures, muscle twitching, palpitations, rapid heartbeat, flushing, low blood pressure, increased respiratory rate, nausea, vomiting, loss of appetite, bitter taste in mouth, heartburn, stomach discomfort, and hives. Barbiturates, phenytoin, and rifampin make it less effective. Beta-blockers (*see*) may cause bronchospasm when used with dyphylline. Flu vaccine, oral contraceptives, troleandomycin, erythromycin, and cimetidine may increase the toxic effects of dyphylline. Contraindicated in people hypersensitive to xanthine compounds such as caffeine and theobromine, and in patients with heart irregularities. Should be used cautiously in young children, in elderly patients with congestive heart failure, and in circulatory, kidney, or liver dysfunction. Also in those with peptic ulcer, overactive thyroid, or diabetes. Should be taken after meals.

DYRENIUM • *See* Triamterene.

DYREXAN • *See* Phendimetrazine.

DYS-, DIS- • Prefixes meaning bad or difficult, as in *dyscrasia,* usually meaning bad blood.

DYSENTERY • Inflammation of the colon with severe diarrhea, abdominal cramps, and painful and ineffectual rectal straining. Stools may contain blood and mucus.

DYSESTHESIA • A condition in which a disagreeable sensation is produced by ordinary touch, temperature, or movement.

DYSGEUSIA • Distorted taste.

DYSLEXIA • Difficulty in reading and/or understanding written material. For reasons not fully understood, the brain misinterprets what the eye sees.

DYSMENORRHEA • Painful menstruation.

DYSMETRIA • A movement disorder in which the subject is unable to arrest muscular movement at the desired point.

DYSOSMIA • Distorted smell.

DYSPEPSIA • Disturbed digestion. Also known as acid indigestion and sour stomach.

DYSPHAGIA • Difficulty in swallowing.

DYSPHASIA • Difficulty in speaking or understanding language due to a brain lesion, and without mental impairment, either by failure to find words or to express them.

DYSPLASIA • Abnormal growth of cells. Often a premalignant condition.

DYSPNEA • Difficulty in breathing.

DYSTROPHY • Degeneration, wasting, abnormal development.

DYSURIA • Difficult or painful urination.

E

EAR-DRI (OTC) • *See* Boric Acid.

EARLY BIRD • *See* Pyrantel, Embolate, and Pamoate.

EARLY DETECTOR (OTC) • A diagnostic test for blood in feces.

EAROCOL • *See* Auralgan.

EASPRIN • *See* Aspirin.

EASTER ROSE • *See* Primrose.

EBV • Abbreviation for Epstein-Barr virus (*see*).

ECCHYMOSIS • Bleeding into and discoloration of the skin.

ECHINACEA (H) • *Echinacea angustifolia.* **Coneflower. Snakeroot. Serpentary. Stoneflower.** The roots and leaves of this herb served as a medicine for the Plains Indians. Said by herbalists to be a natural antibiotic and immune enhancer. Contains an antiseptic volatile oil, glycosides (*see*), and phenol, which is also an antiseptic. It was widely used by Dr. Wooster Beach, who in the mid-1800s founded Eclectic medicine, a blending of homeopathic and North American herbalism. Echinacea has been found to increase the ability of white blood cells to fight, destroy, and digest toxic organisms that invade the body. It is taken to combat colds, infections, and inflammations. The herb produces a numbing sensation when held in the mouth for a few minutes.

ECHOTHIOPHATE (Rx) • **Ecothiophate Iodide.** An eye solution used in the treatment of glaucoma. Potential adverse reactions include aching brow, unusual fatigue or weakness, headache, slow or irregular heartbeat, eye pain, retinal detachment, iris cysts, lens opacities, a paradoxical increase in eye pressure, tearing, obstruction of the tear ducts, burning, redness, stinging, irritation, twitching of the eyelids, blurred vision, nausea, vomiting, diarrhea, stomach cramps, and loss of bladder control. Anticholinergics and other cholinesterase inhibitors increase the possibility of toxicity. Inhalation or skin absorption of carbamate or organophosphate-type insecticides, local anesthetics, and ophthalmic tetracaine increase the risk of whole-body toxicity. Echothiophate increases the toxic risk of cocaine. Contraindicated in patients with bronchial asthma, slow heartbeat or low blood pressure, Down's syndrome, epilepsy, spastic GI disturbances, Parkinson's disease, heart diseases, or a history of retinal detachment (*see*). Toxicity is cumulative; symptoms may not appear for weeks or months after start of therapy.

ECLAMPSIA • Convulsions. A serious form occurs in late pregnancy, or even during or after delivery. An extreme manifestation of toxemia of pregnancy, often associated with kidney disorders.

EC-NAPROSYN • Enteric-coated (*see*) naproxen (*see*).

ESCHERICHIA COLI • A type of bacteria normally found in the gut of most animals, including humans. Much of the work scientists have done using recombinant DNA (*see*) techniques has used *E. coli* as a carrier because it is well understood.

ECONAZOLE (Rx) • **Ecostatin. Spectazole.** An antifungal cream used to treat athlete's foot, jock itch, ringworm, and candidiasis (yeast infection). Potential adverse effects include local burning, itching, stinging, redness, and possibly, liver toxicity if used in large amounts over a long period. If condition does not improve within two weeks, check with your physician. Topical corticosteroids (*see*) may inhibit antifungal effect. *See also* Imidazoles. A candidate for OTC status.

ECONOCHLOR OPHTHALMIC • *See* Chloramphenicol.

ECONOPRED • *See* Prednisolone.

ECOSTATIN • *See* Econazole.

ECOSTIGMINE IODIDE • *See* Echothiophate.

ECOTRIN (OTC) • Enteric-coated aspirin. *See* Enteric Coating.

ECTASULE • *See* Ephedrine.

-ECTOMY • Suffix meaning surgical removal, as in *lumpectomy,* the removal of a breast lump.

E-CYPIONATE • *See* Estradiol.

ECZEMA • An inflammation of the skin.

EDATHAMIL DISODIUM • *See* Edetate Disodium.

EDECRIN • *See* Ethacrynate Sodium.

EDEMA • An excessive accumulation of watery fluid in body cavities.

EDETATE CALCIUM DISODIUM • *See* Calcium Disodium Edetate.

EDETATE DISODIUM (Rx) • **Disodium EDTA. Disotate. Endrate Sodium Versenate.** A chelation agent (*see*) used to reduce calcium levels in the blood and to control certain types of irregular heartbeats. Potential adverse reactions include nausea, vomiting, diarrhea, a drop in blood pressure upon rising from a seated or prone position, sensation of pins and needles, numbness, headache, malaise, fatigue, muscle pain or weakness, high blood pressure, blood clots in the veins, kidney damage, severe low calcium level in the blood, decreased magnesium, and redness, pain, and rash at the site of injection. Contraindicated in patients with kidney disease, brain lesions, hardening of the arteries, or a history of seizures. Should be used carefully in patients with poor heart function or diabetes.

EDROPHONIUM (Rx) • **Reversolo. Tensilon.** A drug that inhibits the destruction of acetylcholine (*see*) and stimulates muscles. Used to diagnose myasthenia gravis (*see*) and to treat rapid beating of the heart. Potential adverse reac-

tions include seizures, weakness, trouble swallowing, respiratory paralysis, sweating, low blood pressure, slow heartbeat, heart block, excessive tearing, double vision, nausea, vomiting, diarrhea, abdominal cramps, excessive salivation, urinary frequency, increased bronchial secretions, bronchospasm, and muscle cramps and twitches. Contraindicated in intestinal or urinary obstructions, slow heartbeat, and low blood pressure. Should be used with caution in persons with overactive thyroid, heart disease, peptic ulcer, or bronchial asthma. Digitalis (*see*) may increase the action of edrophonium. Procainamide and quinidine (*see both*) may reduce its effectiveness.

EDTA • *See* Edetate Disodium.

EES • *See* Erythromycin.

EFEDRON • *See* Ephedrine.

EFEDRON NASAL JELLY (OTC) • *See* Ephedrine.

EFFECTIVENESS • The ability of a medication to do what it claims to do.

EFFER-K. (OTC) • *See* Potassium Bicarbonate and Potassium Citrate.

EFFER-SYLLIUM (OTC) • *See* Psyllium.

EFFEXOR • *See* Venlafaxine.

EFIDAC/24 (OTC) • Introduced in 1993, it is the first twenty-four-hour time-released cold remedy. The technology uses a controlled-release system that provides a continuous dose of nasal decongestant. Its active ingredient is pseudoephedrine (*see*), which is discharged in a three-part delivery system through osmosis over a twenty-four-hour period. The amount of pseudoephedrine is 250 mg, and if you have high blood pressure, difficulty urinating, anxiety or insomnia, you are cautioned, as with other products of this type, not to take it. If you do have an adverse reaction, you will have a day's worth of waiting until the medication gets out of your system.

EFLORNITHINE (Rx) • **DFMO. Ornidyl.** Inhibits the enzyme ornithine decarboxylase and stops cell differentiation and division. Used in the treatment of brain swelling and irritation due to sleeping sickness (*Trypanosoma brucei gambiense* or *Trypanosoma brucei rhodesiense*). May cause anemia and other blood problems, seizures, hearing impairment, dizziness, headache, and numbness. Diarrhea, vomiting, abdominal pain, loss of appetite, swelling of the face, and hair loss may also occur.

EFODINE (OTC) • *See* Povidone-Iodine.

EFUDEX • *See* Fluorouracil.

EHDP • *See* Etidronate.

8-MOP • *See* Methoxsalen.

ELASE • *See* Fibrinolysin.

ELASTIN • A protein in connective tissue.

ELATERIN RESIN • An ingredient in laxatives, banned by the FDA in 1992.

ELAVIL • *See* Amitriptyline.

ELDEPRYL • *See* Selegiline.

ELDER (H) • *Sambucus nigra. Sambucus canadensis. Sambucus ebulus.* **Black Elder. Bourtree. Judas Tree. Sambucus.** An herbal additive to a Chinese tea, it contains essential oil, terpenes, glycosides (*see*), rutin, quercetin (*see*), mucilage, and tannin (*see*). The fruits are high in vitamin C. The elder flower is used to treat colds and flu, and in salves to treat burns, rashes, and minor skin ailments and to diminish wrinkles. Was used by herbalists to soothe the nerves. Hippocrates mentioned its use as a purgative. The inner bark and the young leaf buds, as well as the juice root, are all considered cathartics. The berries induce sweating and act as a diuretic. Only

the black elder is safe to use internally. Red elder and dwarf elder are toxic.

ELDOPAQUE • *See* Hydroquinone.

ELDOQUIN • *See* Hydroquinone.

ELECAMPANE (OTC) (H) • *Inula helenium.* **Elf-Dock. Hose-Heal. Scabwort.** A perennial of the daisy family, elecampane is native to China, Korea, and many parts of Europe. Has been used in folk medicine for thousands of years. The plant contains inulin, an antiseptic and bactericide that is used by herbalists in surgical dressings. Also contains bitter principle (*see*). Used in an herbal tea for coughs, and to relieve hay fever and asthma. It has also been reputed to help digestion and promote menstruation. In 1992, the FDA issued a notice that elecampane had not been shown to be safe and effective as claimed in OTC digestive-aid products.

ELECTROCARDIOGRAM • A graphic tracing of the electric current produced when the heart muscle contracts.

ELECTROLYTES • Dissolved salts or ions in body fluids that conduct electric current. They participate in many chemical processes of life.

ELEUTHERO (H) • *Eleutherococcus senticosus.* A relative of ginseng, the roots and leaves are considered by the Chinese to be the best medicine for treating insomnia. Also widely used to treat bronchitis and chronic lung ailments. Employed in the treatment and prevention of heart disease, to lower blood pressure, and to reduce cholesterol levels. Has also been used to treat arthritis, low hemoglobin, impotence, and stress.

ELIMITE • *See* Permethrin.

ELIXICON • *See* Theophylline.

ELIXIR • A sweetened liquid, generally containing alcohol, that forms a base for many medications, such as those to treat coughs.

ELIXOPHYLLIN • *See* Theophylline.

ELLAGIC ACID • A polyphenol (*see*) of great scientific interest today. It is in various fruits and nuts and has been found to inhibit the induction of tumors of the esophagus and those caused by aflatoxin from molds and by hydrocarbons such as cigarette smoke.

ELOCON • *See* Mometasone Furoate.

ELSPAR • *See* Asparaginase.

EMBOLEX • *See* Heparin.

EMBOLISM • Sudden blockage of a blood vessel by an embolus (*see*).

EMBOLUS • A blood clot or other material such as a fragment of fat carried along in the bloodstream.

EMCYT • *See* Estramustine.

EMESIS • Vomiting.

EMETE-CON • *See* Benzquinamide.

EMETIC • A substance that induces vomiting, such as ipecac (*see*). Used in the treatment of certain types of poisonings.

EMETINE HYDROCHLORIDE (Rx) • A drug used for sympathetic relief of amebic dysentery (*see*). Also used for amebic hepatitis and abscess. Side effects include dizziness, headache, central nerve function changes, aching and/or stiff muscles, and tremor. Acute toxicity can occur at any dose, causing low blood pressure, heartbeat irregularities, shortness of breath, and heart failure. Other side effects include nausea, vomiting, diarrhea, cramps, loss of the sense of taste, rash, and fluid retention.

EMINASE (Rx) • **Anistreplase. APSAC.** Thrombolytic agent; derivative of an enzyme that breaks up blood clots. Eminase has been reported to significantly reduce incidences of death from a heart attack caused by blood clot, if given within the first six hours of the onset of symptoms. Because this medication thins the blood, it is contraindicated in persons with active internal bleeding, a history of stroke or head trauma, severe, uncontrolled high blood pressure, brain tumors, and blood-vessel malformation. Patients who have had an allergic reaction to eminase or to streptokinase (*see*) should not be given the drug.

EMITRIP • *See* Amitriptyline.

EMKO (Rx) • A spermicidal vaginal foam containing nonoxynol-9.

EMLA (Rx) • **Eutectic Mixture of Local Anesthetics.** A combination of the anesthetics lidocaine (*see*) and prilocaine in an oil and water emulsion used in a cream that can take the pain out of getting injections. The cream is applied to the skin and covered with an airtight bandage for at least sixty minutes. The skin is then anesthetized for up to two hours after the bandage is removed. Introduced in 1993 in the United States, it has been available for more than ten years in seventeen other countries.

EMMENAGOGUE • An agent that induces or increases menstrual flow. Among the herbs used for this purpose are motherwort, cramp bark, and fenugreek (*see all*).

EMOLLIENT • Preparations that help the skin feel softer and smoother and reduce roughness, cracking, and irritation of the skin. Among the herbs used for this purpose are balm of Gilead and mallow (*see both*).

EMPHYSEMA • A condition in which lung tissue becomes less elastic and accumulates too much air, making it difficult to exhale.

EMPIRIN (OTC) • *See* Aspirin and Codeine.

EMULSIFIERS • Agents used to assist in the production of an emulsion (*see*). Among common emulsifiers: potassium and sodium stearates and cholesterol.

EMULSION • What is formed when two or more nonmixable liquids are shaken so thoroughly together that the mixture sustains a homogenized appearance. Most oils form emulsions with water.

E-MYCIN • *See* Erythromycin.

ENALAPRIL (Rx) • **Enalaprilat. Vaseretic. Vasotec.** An ACE inhibitor (*see*) that inhibits an enzyme in the blood and dilates blood vessels and rapidly lowers blood pressure. Introduced in 1981, it is effective in controlling mild to severe high blood pressure. Has been found to improve cardiac performance and prolong life in acute congestive heart failure. In 1995, French researchers reported that enalapril slows progression of kidney disease in patients with high blood pressure and chronic kidney failure. Potential adverse reactions include a drop in white blood cells, headache, dizziness, fatigue, insomnia, low blood pressure, diarrhea, nausea, kidney dysfunction, rash, cough, and swelling. May increase the toxicity of lithium. NSAIDs (*see*) may reduce its antihypertensive effects. If combined with other blood-pressure-lowering drugs, extreme caution must be used because a dangerous drop in blood pressure may result. If potassium supplements are taken, they may cause an overload of potassium in the blood. Over-the-counter drugs such as diet pills, decongestants, and stimulants may counteract its effects. Enalapril should not be discontinued suddenly. Most effective when taken on an empty stomach at the same time each day.

ENALAPRILAT • *See* Enalapril.

ENANTHATE • *See* Fluphenazine.

ENARAX • *See* Hydroxyzine and Oxyphencyclimine.

ENCAINIDE (Rx) • **Enkaid.** The sale of this antiarrhythmic drug to treat life-threatening irregular heartbeat was discontinued in 1992 because it was found that encainide worsened heartbeat irregularities in certain patients and increased mortality rates. The manufacturer continues to make it available to patients with special needs, within specific guidelines.

ENCAPRIN • *See* Aspirin.

ENCARE (OTC) • Spermicidal vaginal suppositories containing nonoxynol-9 (*see*).

ENCEPHALITIS • An inflammation of the brain caused most often by viruses.

ENDEP • *See* Amitriptyline.

ENDO- • Prefix from the Greek word *endon,* meaning within. Used in medicine to indicate "within," "inner," "absorbing," or "containing."

ENDOCRINE GLAND • A gland that furnishes an internal secretion, usually having an effect on another organ.

ENDOCRINOPATHY • Any disease due to abnormality of quantity or quality in one or more of the internal glandular secretions.

ENDOGENOUS • Arising from within the body.

ENDOMETRIAL • Relating to the lining of the uterus (endometrium).

ENDOMETRIOSIS • Presence of abnormal fragments of the membrane that lines the cavity of the uterus. The rogue tissue "menstruates" in place and tends to cause pain and inflammation and to form cysts.

ENDORPHINS • Tranquilizers and painkillers manufactured by the body. Each endorphin is composed of a chain of amino acids and acts on the nervous system to reduce pain.

ENDOTHELIUM • A layer of flat cells that lines the inside of the arteries, veins, and capillaries.

ENDRATE • *See* Edetate Disodium.

ENDURON • *See* Methyclothiazide.

ENDURONYL • *See* Methyclothiazide and Deserpidine.

ENFLURANE (Rx) • An inhalation anesthetic that is fast-acting and allows a fast recovery. It is used to relieve the pain of childbirth. Can cause low blood pressure and must be used with caution in persons with kidney dysfunction.

ENISYL • *See* Lysine Hydrochloride.

ENKAID • *See* Encainide.

ENKEPHALINS • The body's self-made painkillers, to which endorphins (*see*) belong.

ENLON • *See* Edrophonium.

ENOVID (Rx) • *See* Mestranol and Norethynodrel.

ENOVIL • *See* Amitriptyline.

ENOXACIN (Rx) • **Penetrex.** A drug introduced in 1991, used to treat urinary tract infections caused by bacteria and gonorrhea.

ENOXAPARIN (Rx) • **Lovenox.** An anti-blood-clot medication introduced in 1993 to prevent deep-vein thrombosis (DVT), which may lead to pulmonary embolism (PE), a potentially fatal blood clot in the lung following hip-replacement surgery. In 1992, the American College of Chest Physicians Consensus Conference concluded that fatal PE may be the most common preventable cause of hospital deaths. On the market in Europe since 1987, enoxaparin was given a priority review by the FDA. The first of a new class of anti-blood-clotting agents known as low-molecular-weight heparins (LMWHs), the medication reportedly causes fewer bleeding complications than standard heparin (*see*) and has fewer drug interactions than low-dose warfarin (*see*). It does not require, according to its manufacturer, monitoring of coagulation times—an uncomfortable and costly procedure. It is approved for the prevention of deep-vein blood clots. Hip and knee replacements are two of the highest-risk surgeries with respect to deep-vein blood clots, with a 45 to 70 percent incidence without the use of prophylaxis.

EN-tabs • *See* Sulfasalazine.

ENTACEF • *See* Cephalexin.

-ENTER-, ENTERO- • Combination forms meaning pertaining to the intestines, as in *gastroenteritis,* inflammation of the intestines and stomach.

ENTERIC • Pertaining to the small intestine.

ENTERIC COATING • Coating on a medicine allowing it to bypass the stomach and dissolve in the intestine, thereby helping to lessen stomach upset and irritation.

ENTEROBACTER • Gram-negative (*see*) bacteria that occur in the feces of humans and other animals, and in sewage, soil, water, and dairy products. They are sometimes found in urine, pus, and other germ-filled materials from animals.

ENTERODOPHILUS (OTC) • *See* Acidophilus.

ENTEX LA (OTC) • **Dura-Vent. UTEX-S.R.** A combination of phenylpropanolamine and guaifenesin (*see both*), used as a decongestant and expectorant for treating symptoms of allergies and colds. Potential adverse reactions include nausea, vomiting, high blood pressure, weakness, irritability, loss of appetite, difficulty in urinating, breathing difficulties, rapid heartbeat, anxiety, and insomnia. Should not be taken with MAO inhibitors (*see*), and should be used with caution with any other stimulant, including other cold and allergy medications. The phenylpropanolamine in this compound may interfere with the effects of blood-pressure-lowering medications. Phenylpropanolamine can also aggravate diabetes, heart disease, hyperthyroid disease, high blood pressure, a prostate condition, stomach ulcers, and urinary blockage.

ENTOLASE-HP • *See* Pancrelipase.

ENTOZYME (Rx) • A combination of pancre-atin, pepsin, and bile salts (*see all*), used to aid digestion impaired by an enzyme deficiency.

ENTUSS (Rx) • *See* Pseudoephedrine, Guaifen-esin, and Hydrocodone.

ENUCLENE (OTC) • An artificial-tear (*see*) preparation containing benzalkonium chloride and tyloxapol.

ENULOSE • *See* Lactulose.

ENZYMES • Substances in the body necessary for accomplishing chemical changes such as pro-cessing sugar to create energy, or breaking down food in the intestines for digestion.

EOSINOPHILIA • A lung condition in which infiltrates are accompanied by blood. Often symp-tomless, in most cases it is due to worm infiltra-tion. It may also be a side effect of drugs such as dicloxacillin sodium (*see*).

EPAZOTE (H) • *Chenopodium ambrosioides.* **American Wormseed. Mexican Wormseed.** The herb contains geraniol, cymene, terpene, methyl salicylate (*see*), butyric acid, and terpenes. The seeds have long been used by herbalists to treat hookworms, pinworms, and tapeworms. Southwesterners use a pinch of the leaves when cooking pinto beans, to reduce flatulence. The oil is highly toxic. It is contraindicated in persons with heart disease, kidney or liver dysfunction, or gastrointestinal inflammations. A one-year-old baby died when given a dose of only four drops of pure oil three times daily for two days.

EPEG • *See* Etoposide.

EPHED • *See* Ephedrine.

EPHEDRA (H) • *Ephedra equisetina.* *Ephedra gerardiana.* **E. helvetica. E. sinica. E. trifurca. Ma Huang. Mormon Tea.** About forty species of this herb are mentioned in ancient scriptures of India. Used by the Chinese for more than five thousand years. The stems contain alka-loids (*see*), including ephedrine (*see*). Herbalists use the herb to treat arthritis, asthma, emphy-sema, bronchitis, hay fever, and hives. This herb taken with other stimulants or combined with them in a compound can cause severe adverse re-actions including death. The FDA issued a warn-ing in 1995 that the agency had received more than one hundred reports of adverse reactions ranging from heart attacks to hepatitis and several deaths. Among the stimulants that can add to the adverse reactions is caffeine, contained in colas and coffee.

EPHEDRINE (OTC) • **Adrenaline Chloride. Bronkaid. Bronkolixir. Bronkotabs. Dey-Pak. Efedron Nasal Jelly. Ephed. Ephedsol. Kie. Marax. Pazo Hemorrhoid Ointment & Suppositories. Primatene. Rynatuss. Va-tro-nol Nose Drops. Vicks Vatronol Nose Drops.** The alkaloid ephedrine is derived from *Ephedra equi-setina* and other members of the forty species of the genus *Ephedra* (*see*), or produced synthetically. Ephedra has been used for more than five thousand years in Chinese medicine and has become more and more popular in Western medicine. It acts like epinephrine (*see*) and is used as a bronchodilator, a nasal decongestant, to raise blood pressure, and topically to constrict blood vessels. In nasal jelly or drops, it is used to treat stuffy noses. Also pre-scribed for bed-wetting in children, stress inconti-nence of the bladder in adults, and delayed ejaculation. Potential side effects include insom-nia, nervousness, dizziness, headache, muscle weakness, sweating, euphoria, confusion, delirium, palpitations, rapid heartbeat, high blood pressure, dry throat and nose, nausea, vomiting, loss of ap-petite, urine retention, and painful urination. ACE inhibitors and beta-blockers (*see both*) may cause a drop in blood pressure when used with ephedrine. High blood pressure medications and methyldopa make it less effective. Digitalis, levodopa, and gen-eral anesthetics increase the risk of irregular heart-beat. Ergot, guanadrel, and guanethidine (*see all*) may increase its blood-vessel-constricting and blood-pressure-raising effects. MAO inhibitors and tricyclic antidepressants (*see both*) may cause severe high blood pressure. Contraindicated in porphyria (*see*), severe coronary artery diseases, irregular heartbeat, glaucoma, and in neurotic patients, and those on MAO inhibitors. Should be used with caution in the elderly and those with high blood pressure, enlarged prostate, heart disease, or anxiety. To prevent insomnia, it should be taken more than two hours before bedtime. Tolerance develops to the drug after two to three weeks. The Ohio State Board of Pharmacy has restricted the sale of single-ingredient ephedrine products because they are being abused. Other states restricting the sale of such products include Arizona, New Mexico, Washington, and Oregon. However, those states have exempted those ephedrine-containing products considered to have a high threshold of abuse.

EPHEDSOL • *See* Ephedrine.

EPI- • Prefix from the Greek word *epi,* meaning on, at, besides, following, or subsequent to.

EPIDEMIOLOGICAL STUDY • A study that measures the incidence of disease in large population groups and looks for associations with various genetic or environmental factors.

EPIDERMIS • Four to five layers of cells covering the skin (dermis).

EPIDERMOID CANCER • Malignancy of the outermost layer of tissue, either the epidermis or resembling the epidermis (*see*).

EPIDURAL • Space upon or over the dura, a membrane surrounding the brain and spinal cord.

EPIFOAM • *See* Hydrocortisone and Pramoxine Hydrochloride.

EPIFRIN • *See* Epinephrine.

EPIGASTRIC • Refers to the epigastrium (*see*), the upper region of the abdomen.

EPIGASTRIUM • Upon the stomach; the upper-middle portion of the abdomen.

E-PILO • *See* Epinephrine and Pilocarpine.

EPIMEDIUM (H) • *Epimedium grandiflorum.* **Lusty Goatherb.** An herb widely used in Chinese medicine, it contains benzene, sterols, tannin, palmitic acid, linolenic acid, oleic acid, and vitamin E. Used to treat kidney dysfunction, lower-back pain, impotence, high blood pressure, arthritis, chronic bronchitis, and asthma.

EPINAL • *See* Epinephryl Borate.

EPINEPHRINE (RX) (OTC) • **Adrenaline Chloride. Asthma-Haler Mist. Bronitin Mist. Bronkaid Mist. Epifrin. Epinal. EpiPen. Epitrate. Eppy/N. Glaucon. Medihaler-Epi. Micronefrin. Mytrate. Primatene Mist. Sus-Phrine. Vaponefrin.** The major hormone of the adrenal gland, epinephrine increases heart rate and contraction, vasoconstriction, vasodilation, relaxation of the muscles in the lungs and smooth muscles in the intestines, and the processing of sugar and fat. Epinephrine is the hormone that readies us for "fight or flight" in stressful situations. It was introduced as a medication in 1900 to treat bronchospasm, hypersensitivity reactions, and anaphylaxis, a life-threatening allergic reaction. Also used to restore heart rhythm in cardiac arrest. In eye solutions, it is used to dilate the pupil in the treatment of glaucoma and during surgery. In nose drops, it is used to relieve stuffy nose and local superficial bleeding. Potential adverse reactions include nervousness, tremor, euphoria, anxiety, coldness, vertigo, headache, sweating, disorientation, agitation, and in patients with Parkinson's disease, increased rigidity and tremor. Other adverse reactions include palpitations, high blood pressure, rapid heartbeat, irregular heartbeat, stroke, angina, high blood sugar, fluid in the lungs, shortness of breath, and pallor. In eye medications, it may cause redness, fluid retention, rash, severe stinging, burning, and tearing upon instillation, aching brow, palpitations, and rapid heartbeat. ACE inhibitors (*see*) may cause a drop in blood pressure. Beta-blockers (*see*) may cause increased constriction of the blood vessels and slowing of the heart. Digitalis, levodopa, and general anesthetics may increase the risk of irregular heartbeat. Doxapram, mazindol, methylphenidate, ergot, and guanadrel (*see*) may increase epinephrine's blood-pressure-raising effects. MAO inhibitors (*see*) may cause severe high blood pressure. Tricyclic antidepressants (*see*), antihistamines, and thyroid hormones when given with epinephrine may cause severe adverse heart effects. Contraindicated in glaucoma, shock, organic brain damage, heart problems, during general anesthesia with halogenated hydrocarbons or cyclopropane, and in labor. Should be used with extreme caution in chronic bronchial asthma and emphysema, in elderly patients, and those with overactive thyroid, angina, high blood pressure, neurosis, and diabetes. Frequent use of this drug at short intervals can make it ineffective.

EPINEPHRYL BORATE (Rx) • An epinephrinelike drug. *See* Epinephrine.

EPIPEN • *See* Epinephrine.

EPIPHYSES • Ends of the long bones, which in children are separated from the bone shafts by a layer of cartilage. As growth progresses, this cartilage layer disappears, the epiphyses are said to have "closed," and the bones do not grow longer. When this process is complete, ultimate height has been attained.

EPITHELIAL • Refers to those cells that form the outer layer of the skin and line all the portions of the body that have contact with external air, and those that are specialized for secretion.

EPITHELIOMAS • Skin tumors of varying malignancy.

EPITHELIUM • The cellular covering of internal and external body surfaces, including the lining of vessels and small cavities. The epithelium consists of cells joined by small amounts of cementing substances and is classified according to the number of layers and the shape of the cells.

EPITOL • *See* Carbamazepine.

EPITRATE • *See* Epinephrine.

EPIVIR (Rx) • *See* Lamivudine.

E.P. MYCIN • *See* Oxytetracycline.

EPO • *See* Erythropoietin.

EPOETIN ALFA • *See* Erythropoietin.

EPOGEN • *See* Erythropoietin.

EPOPROSTENOL (Rx) • **Flolan.** A medication, introduced in 1995, that is delivered by continous infusion. It is indicated for the long-term intravenous treatment of primary pulmonary hyptertension. It is an orphan drug (*see*).

EPPY/N (Rx) • **Epinephryl Borate.** An ophthalmic solution. *See* Epinephrine.

EPROLIN • *See* Vitamin E.

EPSOM SALTS • *See* Magnesium Sulfate.

EPSTEIN-BARR VIRUS • **EBV.** One of five members of the human herpes family. Causes infectious mononucleosis and possibly chronic fatigue syndrome (*see*).

e.p.t. (OTC) • A diagnostic test for pregnancy.

EPT • *See* Teniposide.

EQUAGESIC (Rx) • **Epronate-M. Equazine-M. Meprogesic-Q. Micrainin.** A combination of aspirin and meprobamate (*see both*), used to relieve the pain of muscle spasms. Potential adverse reactions include nausea, vomiting, stomach upset, dizziness, drowsiness, allergic reactions, rash, fever, fluid in the arms and/or legs, faintness, and breathing difficulties. Meprobamate may cause drowsiness and interact with other central nervous system depressants, including alcohol and sleeping pills. The aspirin in the medication may cause excessive bleeding if taken with blood-thinning drugs.

EQUALACTIN (OTC) • *See* Calcium Polycarbophil.

EQUANIL • *See* Meprobamate.

EQUILET (OTC) • *See* Calcium Carbonate.

EQUISETUM HYEMALE (H) • *See* Scouring Rush and Horsetail.

ERCY • *See* Erythromycin.

ERG- • Prefix from the Greek word *ergon,* meaning work.

ERGAMISOL • **Viosterol.** *See* Levamisole.

ERGOCALCIFEROL • *See* Vitamin D.

ERGOLOID MESYLATES (Rx) • **Dihydroergotoxine. Deapril-ST. Gerimal. Hydergine. Hydro-Ergoloid. Niloric. Uni-Gine.** As ergot (*see*) alkaloids, mesylates are used to treat some changes in mood, memory, behavior, or dizziness, and other problems that may be due to poor blood circulation to the brain. They are sometimes prescribed in primary progressive dementia, Alzheimer's dementia, and senility at onset. Mesylates differ from other ergot alkaloids such as ergotamine in that they do not relieve migraine headaches. The way they act on the body is unknown. Potential adverse reactions include dizziness, rash, slow pulse, soreness under the tongue, flushing, fainting, headache, nausea, vomiting, stomach cramps, loss of appetite, and stuffy nose. Must be used with caution in persons with liver disease, low blood pressure, emotional problems, and slow heartbeat. Under-the-tongue tablets should be dissolved slowly and not chewed or swallowed. Eating, drinking, or smoking should be avoided while the tablet is dissolving.

ERGOMAR • *See* Ergotamine Tartrate.

ERGOMETRINE MALEATE • *See* Ergonovine.

ERGONOVINE (Rx) • **Ergometrine Maleate. Ergotrate Maleate.** A drug derived from ergot (*see*), introduced in 1935 to prevent or treat postpartum and postabortion hemorrhage due to uterine problems. Potential adverse reactions include nausea, vomiting, dizziness, headache, ringing in the ears, uterine cramping, high blood pressure, sweating, shortness of breath, and hypersensitivity. Contraindicated for induction or augmentation of labor, before delivery of placenta, in threatened spontaneous abortion, and in patients with allergy or sensitivity to ergot preparations. Should be used with caution in persons with kidney or liver disease, high blood pressure, Raynaud's disease (*see*), and angina or other heart problems or blood-vessel disease. *See also* Ergot.

ERGOSTAT • *See* Ergotamine Tartrate.

ERGOT (Rx) (OTC) (H) • *Claviceps purpurea.* **Ergot of Rye. Hornseed. Smut of Rye.** A fungus found most frequently growing on rye. In the Middle Ages, epidemics of ergotism from eating contaminated rye flour produced gangrene and convulsions. The principal uses of ergot are as a uterine stimulant and vasoconstrictor. Also used to check excessive menstrual bleeding. Ergot alkaloids are widely used today in the treatment of migraine, and to stimulate the heart and other involuntary muscles. Ergot is known to contain a number of complex and potent alkaloids, some of which are similar to lysergic acid (LSD). The two major alkaloids are ergonovine (*see*), which acts primarily to contract uterine muscles and constrict blood vessels of the endometrium of the uterus, and ergotamine tartrate (*see*), which acts primarily on the blood vessels of the brain. Long-term use of ergot may cause constriction of the blood vessels of the extremities, which may result in gangrene. In 1992, the FDA proposed a ban for the use of Ergot Fluidextract to treat insect bites and stings because it had not been shown to be safe and effective as claimed in OTC products.

ERGOTAMINE TARTRATE (Rx) • **Bellergal-S. Ergomar. Ergostat. Medihaler Ergotamine. Migergot. Wigraine. Wigrettes.** Introduced in 1926, it inhibits the effects of epinephrine and norepinephrine (*see both*) and also has an antiserotonin effect (*see*). Combined with caffeine to enhance absorption. Used in the treatment of migraine, vascular, and histamine headaches. In combination with belladonna (*see*), used to treat premenstrual and menopausal symptoms. Potential side effects include numbness and tingling in fingers and toes, transient rapid heartbeat or slow heartbeat, chest pain, increased blood pressure, nausea, vomiting, itching, weakness in legs, muscle pains, and swelling. May also cause abortion, gangrene of the fingers, toes, or intestines, and may aggravate coronary artery disease. Contraindicated in pregnancy and in high blood pressure, liver or kidney dysfunction, blood poisoning, and blood-vessel and heart disease. Most effective for migraine if used at first indication. Prolonged exposure to cold weather may increase adverse reactions. Propranolol and other beta-blockers (*see*) may cause excessive constriction of blood vessels. Excessive use of ergotamine can actually cause migraines. *See also* Ergot and Serotonin.

ERGOTRATE MALEATE • *See* Ergonovine.

ERIDIUM • *See* Phenazopyridine Hydrochloride.

ERIGERON (OTC) (H) • **Fleabane Oil. Horseweed.** Oil derived from the leaves and tops of *Erigeron canadensis,* a plant grown in the northern and central United States. In 1992, the FDA proposed a ban on oil of erigeron in oral menstrual drug products because it had not been shown to be safe and effective as claimed.

ERT • Abbreviation for estrogen replacement therapy (*see*).

ERYC • *See* Erythromycin.

ERYCETTE • *See* Erythromycin.

ERYDERM • *See* Erythromycin.

ERYMAX • *See* Erythromycin.

ERYPAR • *See* Erythromycin.

ERYSIPELAS • A type of cellulitis (*see*) of the skin in which the dermis and lymphatic systems become involved. Characterized by a painful, bright red lesion, swelling, "orange-peel" skin texture, and fever. Often affects the lower extremities.

ERY-TAB • *See* Erythromycin.

ERYTH-, ERYTHRO- • Prefixes meaning redness, as in *erythema,* flushed skin.

ERYTHRAEA CENTAUREUM • *See* Centaury.

ERYTHROCIN • *See* Erythromycin.

ERYTHROCYTES • Red blood cells; elastic, jellylike disks containing hemoglobin, the oxygen-carrying cells.

ERYTHROMYCIN (Rx) • **Akne-mycin. A/T/S. C-Solve 2. E-Base. E-Mycin. ERYC. Erycette. EryDerm. Erygel. Erymax. Erypar. EryPed. Ery-Sol. Ery-Tab. Erythrocin. ETS-2%. GTS. Ilosone. Ilotycin. Ilotycin Ophthalmic. PCE. Pediamycin. Robimycin. RP Mycin. Staticin. T-Stat. Wyamycin S.** An antibacterial introduced in 1952, it is obtained from strains of *Streptomyces erythraeus* found in soil. Used to treat a wide range of bacterial infections, including acute pelvic inflammatory disease, Legionnaires' disease, conjunctivitis, intestinal amebiasis, mild to moderately severe respiratory-tract infections, and skin and soft-tissue infections, caused by bacteria such as *Streptococcus, Mycoplasma, Legionella pneumophila, Diplococcus pneumoniae, Bordetella pertussis,* and *Listeria.* Gram-positive bacteria are usually more susceptible to its actions than are gram-negative (*see both*) bacteria. Erythromycin is used to prevent heart infections due to dental procedures and in eye ointments to treat acute and chronic conjunctivitis, trachoma, and other eye infections. Also put on the eyes of newborns shortly after birth to prevent infection. A useful alternative for those allergic to penicillins and tetracycline. In ointments or other topical formulations, it is used to treat acne and superficial skin infections due to susceptible organisms. Potential adverse effects include hearing loss with high IV doses, abdominal pain and cramping, nausea, vomiting, diarrhea, jaundice, hives, rashes, vein irritation and clotting (IV), overgrowth of nonsusceptible bacteria or fungi, fever, and severe allergic reactions. Liver problems are most common with erythromycin estolate. In eye ointments it can slow wound healing, cause blurred vision, and an overgrowth of resistant organisms with long-term use. In skin preparations it may cause minor skin irritation, possible sensitivity to light, and allergic rashes. Increases the effects of blood thinners. Clindamycin and lincomycin make it less effective. Erythromycin may increase blood levels of digoxin and of carbamazepine (*see both*). Theophylline decreases erythromycin's effectiveness, increases its own, and may increase the risk of side effects. Warfarin (*see*) increases the risk of bleeding when taken with erythromycin. Erythromycin should be used cautiously in patients who have had an unusual reaction to it, in those on a low-sodium, low-sugar, or other special diet, or who are allergic to any foods, sulfites, or other preservatives or dyes that may also be in the erythromycin-based drug. Also in those who have had liver disease or hearing loss. Erythromycin should be taken with a full glass of water one or two hours before meals. If it causes nausea or cramping, it may be taken with meals to reduce those side effects. E-Mycin, E-Base, and Ery-Tab are enteric coated (*see*). Should not be taken with acidic fruits or juices, carbonated beverages, wines, or syrups because these may decrease the effectiveness of the antibiotic. It is a candidate for OTC status as of this writing.

ERYTHROPOIETIN (Rx) • EPO. Epogen. Epoetin Alfa. Procrit. Introduced in 1989, it is a hormone whose deficiency in kidney disease results in anemia, a deficiency in red blood cell production. EPO, made by genetic engineering, can add more red blood cells to correct chronic anemias. Research is in progress to use EPO for other types of anemia, including those resulting from arthritis and the side effects of the AIDS drug AZT. Potential adverse reactions include nausea, vomiting, diarrhea, iron deficiency, elevated platelet count, headache, seizures, high blood pressure, rash, and increased clotting of vein grafts. Contraindicated in patients with uncontrolled high blood pressure.

ERYZOLE • *See* Erythromycin and Sulfisoxazole.

ESCHERICHIA COLI • A gram-negative (*see*) bacterium commonly found in fecal matter and in the human intestines. Certain strains may cause intestinal and urinary-tract infections.

ESERINE SALICYLATE • *See* Physostigmine.

ESGIC (Rx) • A combination of acetaminophen, butalbital, and caffeine (*see all*) used to treat pain.

ESIDRIX • *See* Hydrochlorothiazide.

ESIMIL • *See* Hydrochlorothiazide.

ESKALITH • *See* Lithium Carbonate.

ESMOLOL HYDROCHLORIDE (Rx) • Brevibloc. An antiarrhythmic drug, short acting; a beta-blocker (*see*) used for emergency control of irregular heartbeat. Potential adverse reactions include dizziness, sleepiness, headache, agitation, fatigue, low blood pressure, nausea, vomiting, local inflammation at infusion site, and bronchospasm (asthmalike lung problem). Causes an increase of digoxin in the blood if used with that drug. Morphine raises esmolol levels. Reserpine and other catecholamine-depleting drugs may cause increased irregular rhythms and low blood pressure.

E-SOLVE 2 • *See* Erythromycin.

ESOPHAGEAL VARICES • Dilated, weakened veins in the walls of the lower part of the esophagus that can rupture and cause acute bleeding.

ESOPHAGITIS • Inflammation of the esophagus, usually caused by the backup of acid contents of the stomach.

ESOPHAGUS • That portion of the digestive canal between the throat and the stomach.

ESSENTIAL HYPERTENSION • High blood pressure that has no apparent cause.

ESSENTIAL OILS • The oily liquids obtained from plants through a variety of processes. The essential oils are called volatile because most of them are easily vaporized. They are called essential because the oils were believed to be (1) essential to life, and (2) the "essence" of the plant. The use of essential oils as preservatives is ancient. A large number of oils have antiseptic, germicidal, and preservative action. A teaspoonful may cause illness in an adult and less than an ounce may kill.

ESTAR (OTC) • A coal tar gel. *See* Coal Tar.

ESTAZOLAM (Rx) • **ProSom.** A sleeping medication that acts on the limbic system and thalamus of the brain by binding to specific benzodiazepine receptors. Potential adverse reactions include fatigue, dizziness, daytime drowsiness, and headache. Use with alcohol, central nervous system depressants, including antihistamines, opiate painkillers, and other benzodiazepines increases central nervous system depression. Cimetidine, oral contraceptives, disulfiram, and isoniazid may impair the metabolism and clearance of benzodiazepines and prolong their stay in the body. Rifampin and cigarette smoking may make estazolam less effective. Estazolam may make theophylline less effective. Contraindicated in patients who are allergic to benzodiazepines, pregnant, or have sleep apnea (*see*).

ESTER • A compound formed from an alcohol and an acid by elimination of water, as is ethyl acetate (*see*). Usually, esters are fragrant liquids used for artifical scents and flavors. Esterification can also reduce the allergy-causing properties of a chemical. Toxicity varies with the ester.

ESTINYL • **Feminone.** *See* Estradiol.

ESTIVIN • *See* Naphazoline.

ESTRACE • *See* Estradiol.

ESTRADERM (Rx) • A transdermal (*see*) preparation of estradiol (*see*), used to treat menopausal symptoms and/or to prevent osteo-porosis (*see*). The Estraderm system releases through the skin small amounts of estradiol, a female hormone made by the ovaries. Potential adverse reactions include nausea, retention of fluid, breast tenderness, breakthrough bleeding, vomiting, bloating, cramps, gallbladder disease, abnormal blood clotting, migraine, elevated calcium, growth of benign fibroid tumors in the uterus, jaundice, darkening of the skin, defects in the fetus, and liver tumors. Redness, irritation, or rash may occur at the site of Estraderm application. The risk of cancer of the uterine lining, the endometrium, is greater in estrogen users than in nonusers. In certain animals treated with estrogen, cancer of the cervix, vagina, and liver occurred more frequently. Although reported in some studies, an increase in breast cancer due to estrogen use has not been confirmed. Contraindicated in pregnancy, in cancer of the breast or uterus, unusual vaginal bleeding, endometriosis, or abnormal blood clotting. Should be used cautiously in patients with high blood pressure, heart or kidney dysfunction, asthma, skin allergy, epilepsy, migraine, diabetes, and depression. *See also* Estrogen.

ESTRADIOL (Rx) • **Delestrogen. depGynogen. Depo-Estradiol. Dioval. Dura-Estrin. Duragen-10. E-Cypionate. Ertrogel. Estinyl. Estrace. Estraderm. Estradrol-LA. Estra-O. Estraval. Estro-Cyp. Estrofem. Estroject-LA. Genora. Gynogen LA. Halodrin. Levlen. Loestrin. Menaval. Nordette. Oestradiol. Progynon. Triphasil. Valergen-40.** An estrogen drug given by skin patch, tablets, injection, or vaginal cream, used to treat menopausal symptoms, the effects of a hysterectomy, primary ovarian failure, atrophic vaginitis, postpartum breast engorgement, and inoperable prostate cancer. The drug has also been approved for the prevention of osteoporosis. Potential adverse reactions include nausea, vomiting, depression, high blood pressure, dizziness, migraine, libido changes, blood clots, water retention, increased risk of stroke, blood clots to the lung, and heart attack. May also worsen nearsightedness, cause intolerance to contact lenses, and lead to loss of appetite, increased appetite, excessive thirst, pancreatitis, bloating, and abdominal cramps. Women may have breakthrough bleeding, altered menstrual flow, painful or absent menstruation, enlargement of benign tumors of the uterus, cervical erosion, abnormal secretions, and vaginal candidiasis. In men there may be enlargement of the breasts, testicular atrophy, and impotence. In both sexes there may be jaundice, high blood sugar, high calcium in the blood, folic-acid deficiency, dark spots appearing on the skin, hives, acne, oily skin, hairiness or loss of hair, leg cramps, and hemorrhaging into the skin. Contraindicated in persons with blood-clotting disorders, cancer of the breast, reproductive organs, or genitals, in those with undiagnosed abnormal genital bleeding, and in pregnancy. Should be used with caution in high blood pressure, asthma, mental depression, bone disease, blood problems, gallbladder disease, migraine, seizures, diabetes, absence of menstruation, heart failure, liver or kidney dysfunction, and a family history of breast or genital tract cancer. *See* Estrogen.

ESTRADURIN • *See* Polyestradiol.

ESTRA-L • *See* Estradiol.

ESTRAMUSTINE (Rx) • **Emcyt.** A combination of estrogen and an alkylating agent (*see*), it is an anticancer drug used as a palliative treatment of metastatic or progressive cancer of the prostate. Potential adverse reactions include nausea, vomiting, diarrhea, a drop in white blood cells, heart attack, fluid retention, blood clots to the lung or in the veins, high blood pressure, rash, itching, painful swelling of the breasts, thinning of the hair, and high blood sugar. Calcium-rich foods such as milk and dairy products cause malabsorption of estramustine. Contraindicated in patients hypersensitive to estradiol and nitrogen mustard (*see* Mechlorethamine). Also contraindicated in active blood-clot disorders, except when the actual tumor mass is the cause of the blood clots.

ESTRATAB • *See* Estrogens, Esterified.

ESTRATEST (Rx) • A combination of esterified estrogens and methyltestosterone (*see both*).

ESTROGEL • *See* Estradiol.

ESTROGEN (Rx) (OTC) • A hormone produced by the ovaries, it is mainly responsible for female sexual characteristics. Estrogen influences bone mass by slowing or halting bone loss, improving retention of calcium by the kidneys, and improving the absorption of dietary calcium by the intestines. Estrogen is given to relieve menopausal symptoms, prevent or relieve aging changes in the vagina and urethra, and to help prevent osteoporosis (*see*). Potential adverse reactions include increased risk of uterine cancer, increased frequency of gallstones, accelerated growth of preexisting fibroid tumors of the uterus, fluid retention, nausea, rash, hives, itching, headache, nervous tension, irritability, accentuation of migraine, bloating, diarrhea, pigmentation of the face, postmenopausal bleeding, deep-vein blood clots (less likely with conjugated estrogens), increased blood pressure, and decreased sugar tolerance. May cause swelling and tenderness of breasts, milk production, and increased vaginal secretions. When taking estrogens, it is recommended that salt be used sparingly if fluid retention is a problem. Smoking cigarettes may increase the side effects of estrogen.

ESTROGEN REPLACEMENT THERAPY (Rx) • **ERT.** A treatment that restores estrogen lost when natural estrogen production in the ovaries is dramatically reduced due to the onset of menopause. Physicians question the risk of ERT replacement causing breast cancer, especially for women who have a family history of breast cancer. *See* Estrogen.

ESTROGENS AND PROGESTINS • *See* Oral Contraceptives.

ESTROGENS, CONJUGATED (Rx) • **Premarin. Progens.** A mixture of estrogens obtained from natural sources. Used to prevent postmenopausal osteoporosis (*see*); reportedly reduces hip and wrist fractures by as much as 62 percent. Also used to prevent moderate to severe hot flashes. There is no evidence that estrogens are effective for the nervous symptoms or depression that may occur during menopause, but there is new research that shows estrogen may protect the brain against Alzheimer's disease. Vaginal estrogen cream is also used in the treatment of age-related changes in the vagina. The drug has been approved by the FDA for osteoporosis. Contraindicated in pregnancy, known or suspected cancer of the breast, with some exceptions, known or suspected estrogen-dependent growths, undiagnosed abnormal genital bleeding, active blood-clot disorders, and those hypersensitive to the ingredients. Some studies suggest a possible increased incidence of breast cancer in women taking higher doses of estrogen for prolonged periods. Endometrial cancer risk among estrogen users has been reported to be about four times greater than in nonusers and appears dependent on treatment duration and dosage. The use of progestin (see) with estrogen has reportedly significantly lowered the risk of endometrial cancer. Large doses of estrogens, such as those used to treat prostate and breast cancer, have been shown to increase the risk of nonfatal heart attacks, and blood clots to the lungs and veins have been shown in men. Researchers cannot say definitely if the risk is the same in women. Among the potential adverse reactions known to exist are vaginal bleeding, increase in size of fibroid tumors in the uterus, vaginal candidiasis, change in the amount of cervical secretion, enlargement or tenderness of the breasts, nausea, vomiting, abdominal cramps, bloating, jaundice, brown spots on the skin, rash, loss of scalp hair, hairiness, intolerance to contact lenses, headache, migraine, dizziness, mental depression, increase or decrease in weight, reduced carbohydrate tolerance, swelling, and changes in libido. Estrogens should not be discontinued abruptly.

ESTROGENS, ESTERIFIED (Rx) • **Estratab. Menest.** A mixture of the sodium salts of sulfate esters of estrogens. Used for oral therapy. *See* Estrogen.

ESTRONE (Rx) • **Theelin.** An estrogen (*see*) used to treat atrophic vaginal inflammation, primary failure of the ovaries, symptoms of menopause, cancer of the prostate, and to prevent osteoporosis.

ESTROPIPATE (Rx) • **Ogen.** *See* Estrogen.

ETHACRYNATE SODIUM • *See* Ethacrynic Acid.

ETHACRYNIC ACID (Rx) • **Edecrin. Ethacrynate Sodium.** A potent loop diuretic (*see*), it is used to treat congestive heart failure, cirrhosis of the liver, kidney dysfunction, high blood pressure, and other conditions in which excessive fluid must be relieved. Potential adverse reactions include nausea, vomiting, diarrhea, inflammation of the pancreas, dizziness, headache, blurred vision, ringing in the ears, anemia, kidney dysfunction, stomach pains, dry mouth, impotence, muscle weakness or cramps, joint pains, low blood pressure, irregular heartbeat, chest pains, and hearing loss. Severe diarrhea may necessitate discontinuation of the drug. An interaction with aminoglycoside antibiotics may increase the possibility of adverse effects on the ear. Warfarin may increase ethacrynate's blood-thinning effects. Contraindicated in the absence of urine formation and in infants. Should be used cautiously in electrolyte abnormalities. Excessive use can cause a serious drop in chloride, sodium, and potassium; sodium and potassium chloride supplements may be needed during therapy. May be taken with meals to avoid gastrointestinal upset.

ETHAMBUTOL (Rx) • **Myambutol.** An adjunctive (*see* Adjunct) treatment for tuberculosis. May cause headache, dizziness, mental confusion, numbness in arms and legs, vision loss, loss of appetite, nausea, vomiting, abdominal pain, elevated uric acid, and severe allergic reactions; also fever, malaise, and bloody sputum. The medication must be taken for the full course if TB is to be eliminated.

ETHAMOLIN • *See* Ethanolamine Oleate.

ETHANOIC ACID • *See* Acetic Acid.

ETHANOLAMINE OLEATE (Rx) • **Ethamolin.** A mild sclerosing (scar-forming) agent used for bleeding esophageal veins. Introduced in 1989, it is also used for the treatment of re-bleeding in patients suffering from swollen veins in the esophagus.

ETHAQUIN • *See* Ethaverine Hydrochloride.

ETHATAB • *See* Ethaverine Hydrochloride.

ETHAVERINE HYDROCHLORIDE (Rx) • **Ethaquin. Ethatab. Ethavex-100. Isovex.** A vasodilator that directly relaxes smooth muscles, it is used in the long-term treatment of peripheral and cerebrovascular insufficiency associated with spasms of the artery and spastic conditions of the gastrointestinal and genitourinary tracts. Potential adverse effects include headache, drowsiness, low blood pressure, flushing, sweating, dizziness, slowed heartbeat, irregular heartbeat, nausea, loss of appetite, abdominal distress, dry throat, constipation, diarrhea, jaundice, rash, respiratory difficulties, and malaise. Should be used with caution in glaucoma, pulmonary embolus, and pregnant women or women of childbearing age. Contraindicated in certain heart conditions and in severe liver disease. *See* Pulmonary Embolism.

ETHAVEX-100 • *See* Ethaverine Hydrochloride.

ETHCHLORVYNOL (Rx) • **Placidyl.** A sleeping medication; the mechanism of its effect is unknown. Potential adverse reactions include reduction of blood platelets, facial numbness, fatigue, nightmares, dizziness, daytime drowsiness, muscular weakness, faintness, loss of balance, low blood pressure, bad taste in the mouth, blurred vision, abdominal distress, nausea, vomiting, rash, and hives. Increased central nervous system depression may occur if ethchlorvynol is taken with alcohol, narcotic analgesics, tricyclic antidepressants, and MAO inhibitors (*see*). Ethchlorvynol may make blood thinners less effective. Contraindicated in uncontrolled pain and porphyria (*see*). Should be taken with food or milk. Effective for short-term use and should not be taken for more than one week.

ETHER (RX) (OTC) • An anesthetic. Has been used in digestive-aid products. In 1992, the FDA issued a notice that ether had not been shown to be safe and effective as claimed in OTC digestive-aid products.

ETHINYL ESTRADIOL; ETHYNODIOL DIACETATE; LEVONORGESTREL; NORETHINDRONE (Rx) • **Brevicon. Demulen. Estinyl. Feminone. Genora. Levlen. Modicon. Nelova. Norcept-E. Norgestrel. Norinyl. Norlestrin. Ortho-Novum. Ovcon. Tri-Levlen. Triphasil.** Oral contraceptive combinations of estrogen and progestin that inhibit ovulation through a negative feedback directed at the hypothalamus in the brain. They may also prevent transport of the ovum through the fallopian tubes. Estrogen in the contraceptives suppresses secretion of follicle-stimulating hormone, blocking the development and release of the eggs. Progestin suppresses luteinizing-hormone secretion so that ovulation can not occur even if the follicle develops. Progestin thickens the mucus that lines the cervix and interferes with the sperms' journey; and progestin also causes changes in the lining of the uterus, making it unfriendly to implantation of the fertilized ovum. Potential adverse reactions include nausea, vomiting, depression, high blood pressure, dizziness, migraine, libido changes, water retention, increased risk of stroke, blood clots to the lungs, and heart attack. May worsen nearsightedness, cause intolerance to contact lenses, and lead to loss of appetite, increased appetite, excessive thirst, pancreatitis, bloating, and abdominal cramps. May also cause breakthrough bleeding, altered menstrual flow, painful or absent menstruation, enlargement of benign tumors of the uterus, cervical erosion, abnormal secretions, and vaginal candidiasis. There may be jaundice, high blood sugar, high calcium in the blood, folic-acid deficiency, dark spots appearing on the skin, hives, acne, oily skin, and breast tenderness, enlargement, and secretion. Contraindicated in persons with blood-clot disorders, cancer of the breast, reproductive organs, or genitals, in those with undiagnosed abnormal genital bleeding, and in pregnancy. Should be used with caution in high blood pressure, asthma, mental depression, bone disease, blood problems, gallbladder disease, migraine, seizures, diabetes, absence of menstruation, heart failure, liver or kidney dysfunction, and a family history of breast or genital-tract cancer. Also contraindicated in women thirty-five years or older who smoke more than fifteen cigarettes a day, and in all women over forty years of age. Prolonged use of these contraceptives is not recommended for those who plan to become pregnant. Estrogens and progestins may alter glucose-tolerance tests.

ETHIONAMIDE (Rx) • **Trecator-SC.** An adjunctive (*see* Adjunct) treatment for tuberculosis after primary therapy with streptomycin or isoniazid (*see both*) has failed or cannot be used. Potential adverse reactions include nerve irritation, psychological disturbances (especially depression), a drop in blood pressure, loss of appetite, metallic taste in the mouth, nausea, vomiting, excessive secretion of saliva, abdominal pain, diarrhea, and weight loss.

ETHMOZINE • *See* Moricizine Hydrochloride.

ETHOPROPAZINE (Rx) • **Parsidol. Profenamine.** Although chemically a phenothiazine derivative, it is distinct from other drugs of its class. It is an anticholinergic agent with some anthistamine action and is used to treat the symptoms of Parkinson's disease.

ETHOSUXIMIDE (Rx) • **Zarontin.** An anticonvulsant introduced in 1960 that increases seizure threshold and reduces abnormal patterns of nerve transmission in the motor-control area of the brain. Derived from succinimide (*see*). Potential adverse reactions include anemia, drowsiness, headache, fatigue, dizziness, loss of balance, irritability, hiccups, euphoria, lethargy, nearsightedness, nausea, vomiting, diarrhea, swollen gums, swollen tongue, weight loss, cramps, loss of appetite, epigastric and abdominal pain, vaginal bleeding, hives, itching, rash, and hairiness. Contraindicated in hypersensitivity to succinimide derivatives, and should be used cautiously in kidney

and liver disease. Should not be withdrawn suddenly. Should be taken with food to minimize GI distress.

ETHOTOIN (Rx) • **Peganone.** An anticonvulsant drug derived from hydantoin (*see*). It limits seizures by controlling the passage of salt across cell membranes in the motor cortex of the brain during generation of nerve impulses. Ethotoin's reported benefit is that it causes less central nervous system depression than other anticonvulsant drugs. Potential adverse reactions include anemia, fatigue, insomnia, dizziness, headache, numbness, chest pain, double vision, nausea, vomiting, diarrhea, swollen glands, swollen gums, rash, and fever. Alcohol and folic acid make it less effective. Oral blood thinners, antihistamines, chloramphenicol, cimetidine, diazepam, diazoxide, disulfiram, isoniazid, salicylates, sulfamethizole, and valproate may make ethotoin more toxic. Contraindicated in hydantoin hypersensitivity, and in liver and blood disorders. Should not be withdrawn suddenly. Should be taken after meals. Ethotoin generally produces milder adverse reactions than phenytoin (*see*); however, the large doses required may cause GI distress.

ETHOXYZOLAMIDE (Rx) • Related to acetazolamide (*see*), it is a thiazide diuretic (*see*) used as an added treatment along with other medications for glaucoma and epilepsy.

ETHRANE • *See* Enflurane.

ETHYL ACETATE • A colorless liquid with a pleasant fruity odor that occurs naturally in apples, bananas, grape juice, pineapple, raspberries, and strawberries. It is used as a solvent and as an artifical scent. It is a mild local irritant and central nervous system depressant. Irritating to the skin.

ETHYL ALCOHOL (OTC) • **Anbesol. P & S Tar Gel. X-Seb T Shampoo.** Contains ethanol, grain alcohol, and neutral spirits. Rapidly absorbed through the gastric and intestinal mucosa. Anbesol is used for the temporary relief of pain due to braces, dentures, and other orthodontic irritation, toothache, sore gums, cold and canker sores, and fever blisters. Temporarily deadens sensations of nerve endings to provide relief. Also reduces oral bacteria. It is for temporary relief only and should be discontinued if irritation develops. The tar gel and shampoo are used to relieve the itching, irritation, and skin-flaking associated with dandruff and psoriasis; for external use only and should not be used for a prolonged period of time.

ETHYL AMINOBENZOATE • *See* Benzocaine.

ETHYL CHLORIDE (Rx) • **Chloroethane.** Prepared by the action of chlorine on ethylene in the presence of hydrochloric acid and light. Used as a topical anesthetic in minor operative procedures, and to relieve pain caused by insect stings, burns, and skin irritation. Mildly irritating to mucous membranes. High concentrations of vapors cause unconsciousness.

ETHYL NITRITE (OTC) • **Sweet Spirit of Niter.** Used as a synthetic flavoring in foods. In 1992, the FDA proposed a ban on ethyl nitrite in oral menstrual drug products because it had not been shown to be safe and effective as claimed.

ETHYLNOREPINEPHRINE HYDROCHLORIDE (Rx) • **Bronkephrine.** Used in bronchial asthma and reversible bronchospasm.

ETHYNODIOL • *See* Progesterone and Oral Contraceptives.

ETHYOL • *See* Amifostine.

ETIBI • *See* Ethambutol.

ETIDOCAINE (Rx) • **Duranest.** A local anesthetic that blocks nerve signals. Onset is in two to eight minutes, and duration from three to six hours. Potential adverse reactions include skin reactions, swelling, continuous asthma attacks, severe allergic reactions, anxiety, nervousness, seizures followed by drowsiness, unconsciousness, tremors, twitches, shivering, and respiratory arrest. Other potential reactions include blurred vision, ringing in the ears, nausea, and vomiting.

Should be used with extreme caution if MAO inhibitors or cyclic antidepressants are being taken by the patient.

ETIDRONATE (Rx) • **Didronel. EHDP. Sodium Etidronate.** A phosphoric acid preparation used to treat Paget's disease, high blood calcium due to malignancy, and to help build up bone after total hip replacement or in spinal cord injuries. Potential adverse reactions include diarrhea, nausea, increased or recurrent bone pain, elevated phosphate in the blood, and increased risk of fracture. Prolonged use may increase the risk of liver damage. Used cautiously in persons with colitis or impaired kidney function. Calcium in the diet may prevent the absorption of oral etidronate.

ETIOLOGY • The origin of a disease.

ETODOLAC (Rx) • **Lodine.** Introduced in 1991, it is indicated for acute and long-term use in the management of osteoarthritis, and for the management of pain. Contraindicated for those with hypersensitivity to etodolac. Should not be taken by those sensitive to aspirin or other NSAIDs (*see*), or those having induced asthma, stuffy nose, hives, or other allergic reactions, since fatal asthmatic reactions have been reported in such patients. Potential adverse reactions include risk of GI ulceration, bleeding, and perforation, which can occur at any time without warning. Those who have had a problem with alcohol, previous peptic ulcers, who smoke or are elderly or debilitated, are at high risk for such problems. Other potential adverse reactions include kidney and liver dysfunction, chills, fever, heartburn, abdominal pain, diarrhea, gas, nausea, constipation, vomiting, weakness, dizziness, depression, nervousness, skin rash and itching, blurred vision, ringing in the ears, painful and/or frequent urination, high blood pressure, palpitations, faintness, congestive heart failure, anemia, asthma, sweating, light bothering the eyes, blood loss, fluid retention, and bleeding. Should not be used with aspirin. Etodolac may increase the toxicity of cyclosporine, digoxin, lithium carbonate, and methotrexate (*see all*). May cause false readings on certain laboratory tests.

ETOMIDATE (Rx) • Amidate. Hypnomidate. A general anesthetic with a rapid onset of about one minute and a duration of effect as short as three minutes. It has a much lower incidence of heart and respiratory effects than other general anesthetics and is therefore often used in high-risk surgical patients. Potential side effects include movement disorders, transient respiratory problems, high blood pressure, low blood pressure, rapid heartbeat, slow heartbeat, throat spasms, nausea or vomiting, inhibition of adrenal steroid hormone, hiccups, and snoring.

ETOPOSIDE (Rx) • VePesid. VP-16. An anticancer drug, a semisynthetic derivative of podophyllotoxin, that arrests cell division. Used to treat small-cell carcinoma of the lung, acute nonlymphocytic leukemia, lymphosarcoma, Hodgkin's disease, and testicular cancer. Potential adverse reactions include nausea, vomiting, suppression of bone marrow, a drop in white blood cells, low blood pressure, headache, reversible hair loss, and rarely, severe allergic reactions. Warfarin (*see*) may increase bleeding time.

ETRAFON • *See* Amitriptyline and Perphenazine.

ETRETINATE (Rx) • Tegison. A drug introduced in 1976 used to treat severe, unresponsive psoriasis. Potential adverse reactions include nausea, dry mouth, appetite change, blood disorders, pressure on the brain, fatigue, headache, dizziness, lethargy, blood clots, eye pain, sore tongue, chapped lips, hepatitis, blood in urine, irregular menstrual periods, high blood fats, skin peeling, itching, bone pain, shortness of breath, and sensitivity to light. May lower high blood potassium. Alcohol increases the risk of high blood fats. Drugs that affect the liver increase the risk of liver toxicity. Milk and a high-fat diet increase the absorption of etretinate. Tetracycline increases the risk of brain pressure. Vitamin A adds to its toxic effects. Contraindicated in patients who are pregnant or who intend to become pregnant. Significant residual blood levels of etretinate have been reported nearly three years after cessation of treatment. Etretinate should be taken with milk immediately after meals. The tablets should be swallowed whole.

ETS-2% • *See* Erythromycin.

EU- • Prefix meaning well and good, as in *euphoria.*

EUCALYPTUS (OTC) (H) • *Eucalyptus globulus.* Blue Gum Tree. Dinkum Oil. Halls Mentho-Lyptus Cough Suppressant Tablets. Listerine Antiseptic. Vicks VapoRub. The colorless to pale yellow volatile liquid from the fresh leaves of the tree has a camphorlike odor and is used as a local antiseptic. The chief constituent of eucalyptus, eucalyptol, is used as an antiseptic, antispasmodic, and expectorant. Herbalists maintain that as a disinfectant, it destroys bacteria, fungi, and viruses. Most commonly, the oil is rubbed directly on the chest or back for respiratory problems. It is also used in liniments to treat arthritic pains. In 1992, the FDA proposed a ban for the use of eucalyptus oil to treat fever blisters and cold sores, poison ivy, poison sumac, and poison oak, and in astringent (*see*) drugs because it had not been shown to be safe and effective as claimed in OTC products.

EUCATROPINE (Rx) • A drug used to dilate the pupil of the eye. It produces no anesthesia, pain, or increased inside eye pressure.

EUGENIA CARYOPHYLLATA • *See* Clove.

EUGENOL (OTC) (H) • Clove Oil. Occurs naturally in cloves, allspice, basil, bay, laurel, and calamus. Acts as a local antiseptic. When ingested, may cause vomiting and gastric irritation. Many people are allergic to eugenol. In 1992, the FDA proposed a ban for the use of eugenol to treat fever blisters and cold sores, poison sumac, poison ivy, and poison oak, and in astringent (*see*) drugs because it had not been shown to be safe and effective as claimed in OTC products.

EULEXIN • *See* Flutamide.

EUPATORIUM PERFOLIATUM • *See* Boneset.

EUPATORIUM PURPUREUM (H) • Used as a homeopathic medicine for aching bones. *See* Joe-Pye Weed.

EUPHORIA • An exaggerated feeling of emotional and physical well-being, usually of psychological origin. This condition is seen in organic mental disorders, toxic and drug-induced states, and mania.

EUPHR • The abbreviation used in homeopathy to designate euphrasia (*see*).

EUPHRASIA (H) • A homeopathic medicine to treat sore eyes. *See* Eyebright.

EUP-P. • Homeopathic abbreviation for eupatorium perfoliatum. *See* Boneset.

EURAX • *See* Crotamiton.

EUTHROID (Rx) • *See* Levothyroxine, Liothyronine, and Liotrix.

EVAC-Q-KIT (OTC) • A combination of magnesium citrate, phenolphthalein, and laxatives (*see all*).

EVAC-U-LAX (OTC) • *See* Phenolphthalein and Laxative.

EVENING PRIMROSE (H) • *Oenothera biennis.* **Sundrops.** The leaves and oil from the seed are used by herbalists to treat liver and kidney dysfunctions. The oil has a high content of linoleic acid, an essential polyunsaturated fatty acid that is converted into prostaglandins (*see*) and hormones. Used as a tonic for inflammatory conditions. It reputedly lowers cholesterol and is said to relieve premenstrual tension, high blood pressure, and anxiety associated with inflammatory conditions. Has been recommended for infantile eczema, painful breasts, arthritis, and neurosis. An article in the January 28, 1995, issue of *Lancet* pointed out that evening primrose oil is a rational treatment for atopic eczema because in this skin condition, the body's processing of dietary linoleic acid is apparently impaired. A subject of great controversy, some scientists say it is used in many conditions with little justification. Others say that it may be helpful in the treatment of diabetic nerve damage, atopic dermatitis (*see*), rheumatoid arthritis, and premenstrual syndrome. Pharmaceutical companies say they will not pursue the confirming research unless they can patent the formulation.

EVERONE • *See* Testosterone.

E-VISTA • *See* Hydroxyzine.

EWING'S SARCOMA • A malignant tumor that usually occurs before the age of twenty, about twice as frequently in males. In about 75 percent of patients it involves bones of the extremities, including the shoulder.

EXCEDRIN (OTC) • Excedrin contains 65 mg of caffeine. *See* Acetaminophen, Aspirin, and Caffeine.

EXELDERM • *See* Sulconazole Nitrate.

EXFOLIATION • Falling off in scales or layers.

EX-LAX (OTC) • *See* Phenolphthalein and Laxative.

EXNA • *See* Benzthiazide.

EXOGENOUS • Introduced from or produced outside the body.

EXPECTORANT • Medication that helps thin and loosen the thick mucus of the respiratory tract, making it easier to expel. Among the herbs used for this purpose are pleurisy root, horehound, and wild cherry (*see all*). Among the Rx and OTC products, guaifenesin (*see*) is widely used.

EXPIRATION DATE • The date prior to which a product can be expected to retain its full strength as stated on the label, according to the manufacturer.

EXSEL • *See* Selenium.

EXTEND • *See* Dextromethorphan.

EXTENDRYL SR. • *See* Chlorpheniramine, Phenylephrine, and Methscopolamine.

EXTRACT • A highly concentrated alcohol base in liquid form, derived from herbs.

EXTRA-STRENGTH DOAN'S (OTC) • *See* Magnesium Salicylate.

EXTRA STRENGTH GAS-X • *See* Simethicone.

EXUDATE • A substance that is exuded, oozed, trickled, or pushed out of the body or tissue.

EYEBRIGHT (H) • *Euphrasia officinalis.* **Euphrasia.** An annual herb native to Europe and western Asia and grown in the United States, it belongs to the figwort family. Contains tannins, iridoid glycosides, phenolic acids, and volatile oil. It has been mentioned in medical literature since the early 1300s. It had the reputation of being able to restore eyesight in very old people and is still used today as an eyewash for inflamed and tired eyes, and to treat sinus congestion. Astringent infusions are made by herbalists for coughs, colds, and sore throats. Also occasionally used to treat jaundice, loss of memory, and dizziness.

EYE-SED • *See* Zinc Sulfate.

EYEWASH • A sterile solution used to bathe the eye or dilute and flush out irritating foreign matter.

EZ-DETECT (OTC) • A diagnostic test for blood in feces.

F

FACT (OTC) • A pregnancy test.

FACTOR IX COMPLEX (Rx) • **Konyne-HT. Profilnine. Proplex T.** Directly replaces deficient clotting factor. Used to prevent hemorrhage in patients with hemophilia. Potential adverse reactions include headache, transient fever, chills, flushing, tingling, and allergic reactions. Contraindicated in liver disease.

FALSE HELLEBORE • *See* Hellebore.

FALSE UNICORN ROOT (H) • *Chamaelirium luteum. Aletris farinosa.* **Blazing Star. Helonias.** The North American Indians used this herb as a tonic and to strengthen the reproductive system. Used by herbalists today to treat painful and irregular menstruation, threatened miscarriage, and nausea during pregnancy. Also used to treat worms and parasites, and as a general tonic for the genitourinary tract, heartburn, and loss of appetite. Large doses will cause nausea and vomiting.

FAMCICLOVIR • **Famvir.** An oral medication introduced in 1994 for the treatment of uncomplicated shingles (*see* Herpes Varicella-Zoster Virus). Famciclovir is given three times a day, which is less than existing therapies. The manufacturer says famciclovir, when given during acute shingles, effectively reduces the duration of postherpetic neuralgia, the chronic, often debilitating pain that persists after shingles lesions have healed. It has been used in the United Kingdom since 1993 and was approved by the FDA after a review of twelve months. It has not been studied in eye zoster infections, disseminated zoster, or in immune-deficient patients. The most common potential adverse effects reported were headache, nausea, and fatigue.

FAMOTIDINE (Rx) (OTC) • **Pepcid. Pepcid AC.** An antiulcer medication introduced in 1986 that blocks the action of histamine, decreasing gastric-acid secretions. Gastric cancer must be ruled out before famotidine therapy. Potential adverse reactions include nausea, headache, dizziness, hallucinations, diarrhea, constipation, gas, kidney dysfunction, acne, itching, swelling of the eyelids, and rash. The drug should not be taken for longer than eight weeks unless specifically ordered by a physician. Famotidine was relabeled after its introduction because it was associated with liver damage and anaphylaxis, an allergic reaction that could produce life-threatening shock. Famotidine may inhibit the absorption of ketoconazole (*see*) and vitamin B_{12}. Should be taken with or immediately following meals. If needed, antacids can be taken with this medication to reduce ulcer pain. It was approved in 1995 for OTC status to relieve heartburn, indigestion, and upset stomach.

FAMVIR • *See* Famciclovir.

FANG-FENG • *See* Sileris.

FAN JIA • *See* Pepper, Black.

FAN MUC GUA • *See* Papaya.

FANSIDAR (Rx) • A combination of pyrimethamine and sulfadoxine. *See* Pyrimethamine with Sulfadoxine, a drug to prevent malaria.

FASTIN • *See* Phentermine.

FATTY ACID • A compound of carbon, hydrogen, and oxygen that combines with glycerol to make a fat.

FDA • The Food and Drug Administration, a branch of the U.S. government's Department of Health and Human Services. The FDA is responsible for reviewing data required to establish safety, effectiveness, and proper labeling and manufacturing practices for all nonprescription and prescription medications prior to marketing. It also regulates foods, cosmetics, and medical devices.

FD&C ACT • The Food, Drug, and Cosmetic Act, passed in 1938, is the primary law governing drugs sold in the United States. Included in the act is the sales prohibition on drugs that are contaminated, misbranded, or otherwise a hazard to health. It also establishes minimum standards of strength, quality, and purity for many drugs and sets up specifications for drug labeling.

FD&C BLUE NO. 1 • Brilliant Blue FCF.
A coal tar derivative, triphenylmethane, used for hair colorings, face powders, and other cosmetics. Also used as a coloring in bottled soft drinks, gelatin, desserts, cereals, and other foods. May cause allergic reactions. On the FDA permanent list of color additives. Rated 1A, that is, completely acceptable for nonfood use, by the World Health Organization. However, it produced malignant tumors at the site of injection and by ingestion in rats.

FD&C BLUE NO. 2 • Moderate bright green.
A coal tar derivative, triphenylmethane, used in hair rinses, mint-flavored jelly, frozen desserts, candy, confections, and cereals. It is a sensitizer in the allergic. Permanently listed for surgical sutures in 1971, and for food and ingested-drug use in 1987. Produced malignant tumors at the site of injection when introduced under the skins of rats.

FD&C BRILLIANT BLUE NO. 1 ALUMINUM LAKE • Aluminum salt of certified Brilliant Blue No. 1 (see).

FD&C COLORS • (Food, Drug, and Cosmetic Colors.)
A *color additive* is a term to describe any dye, pigment, or other substance capable of coloring a food, drug, or cosmetic, on any part of the human body. In 1900, more than eighty dyes were used to color foods. There were no regulations, and the same dye used to color clothes could also be used to color candy. In 1906, the first comprehensive legislation for food colors was passed. Only seven colors, when tested, were shown to be composed of known ingredients that demonstrated no harmful effects. Those colors were orange, erythrosin, Ponceau 3R, amaranth, indigotin, naphthol yellow, and light green. A voluntary system of certification for batches of color dyes was set up. In 1938, new legislation was passed, superseding the 1906 act. The colors were given numbers instead of chemical names, and every batch had to be certified. Fifteen food colors were in use at the time. In 1950, children were made ill by certain colorings used in candy and popcorn. These incidents led to the delisting of FD&C Orange No. 1 and Orange No. 2, and FD&C Red No. 32. Since that time, due to experimental evidence of possible harm, FD&C Red No. 1, and Yellow Nos. 1, 2, 3, and 4 have also been delisted. FD&C Violet No. 1 was removed in 1973. In 1976, one of the most widely used of all colors, FD&C Red No. 2, was removed because it was found to cause tumors in rats. In 1976, FD&C Red No. 4, last used for coloring maraschino cherries, and carbon black were banned at the same time because they contain cancer-causing agents. Earlier, in 1960, scientific investigations were required by law to determine the suitability of all colors in use for permanent listing. Since then, FD&C Citrus Red No. 2 (limited to 2 ppm), for coloring the skins of oranges, has been permanently listed; FD&C Blue No. 1, Red No. 3, Yellow No. 5, and Red No. 40 have been permanently listed without any restrictions. The other food coloring additives are still on the "temporary list." In 1959, the FDA approved the use of "lakes" (*see*), organic solutions in which the dyes have been mixed with alumina hydrate in order to make them insoluble. The safety of colors in food is now being questioned by the FDA and regulatory agencies in other countries, as well as the World Health Organization. There are inconsistencies in safety data and in the banning of some colors, which, in turn, affect international commerce. *See also* other D&C colors and Lakes, Color.

FD&C GREEN NO. 3 • Permanently listed in 1982 by the FDA for use in foods, drugs, and cosmetics, except in the area of the eye.

FD&C RED NO. 2 • Amaranth.
Formerly one of the most widely used cosmetic and food colorings, the dye was banned by the FDA in January 1976.

FD&C RED NO. 3 • Erythrosin.
Bluish pink. A coal tar derivative, a xanthene color, it has been determined a carcinogen. The FDA postponed the closing date for FD&C to allow the agency additional time to study complex scientific and legal questions about the color before deciding to approve or terminate its use. FD&C Red No. 3 is

permanently listed for use in food and ingested drugs, but only provisionally listed for cosmetics and externally applied drugs.

FD&C RED NO. 3 ALUMINUM LAKE • The aluminum salt of certified FD&C Red No. 3 (*see*). *See also* Colorings.

FD&C RED NO. 4 • A monoazo color and coal tar dye. Used in mouthwashes, bath salts, and hair rinses. It was banned for use in foods by the FDA in 1964 when it was shown to damage the adrenal glands and bladders of dogs. The agency relented and gave it provisional license for use in maraschino cherries. In 1976, it was banned for use in all foods because it was shown to cause urinary bladder polyps and atrophy of the adrenal glands in animals. It was also banned in orally taken drugs, but is still permitted in cosmetics for external use only.

FD&C RED NO. 20 • Permanently listed by the FDA in 1983 for general use in drugs and cosmetics, except in areas around the eyes.

FD&C RED NO. 22 • Permanently listed by the FDA in 1983 for general use in drugs and cosmetics, except in areas around the eyes.

FD&C RED NO. 40 • Allura Red AC. Newest color. Used widely in the cosmetics industry. Approved in 1971, Allied Chemical has an exclusive patent on this dye. It is substituted for FD&C Red No. 4 in many cosmetics, foods, and drug products. Permanently listed in 1971 because, unlike the producers of "temporary" colors, this producer supplied reproductive data. However, many American scientists feel that the safety of Red No. 40 is far from established, particularly because all the tests were conducted by the manufacturer. Therefore, the dye should not have received a permanent safety rating. The National Cancer Institute reported that P-credine, a chemical used in the preparation of Red No. 40, was carcinogenic in animals. *See also* Azo Dyes.

FD&C YELLOW NO. 5 • Tartrazine. A coal tar derivative that causes allergic reactions in persons sensitive to aspirin. The certified color industry petitioned for permanent listing of this color in February 1966, with no limitations other than sound manufacturing practice. However, in February 1966, the FDA proposed the listing of this color with a maximum rate of use of 300 ppm in food. The color industry objected to the limitations. Yellow No. 5 was thereafter permanently listed as a color additive without restrictions. Rated 1A by the World Health Organization—acceptable in food. It is estimated that half the aspirin-sensitive people, plus 47,000 to 94,000 others in the nation, are sensitive to this dye. It is used in about 60 percent of both over-the-counter and prescription drugs. Efforts were made to ban this color in over-the-counter pain relievers, antihistamines, oral decongestants, and prescription anti-inflammatory drugs. Aspirin-sensitive patients have been reported to develop life-threatening asthmatic symptoms with ingestion of this yellow. Since 1981, it is supposed to be listed on the label if it is used.

FD&C YELLOW NO. 5 ALUMINUM LAKE • *See* FD&C Yellow No. 5 and Lakes, Color.

FD&C YELLOW NO. 6 • Sunset Yellow FCF. A coal-tar, monoazo color. It is not used in products that contain fats and oils. May cause allergic reactions. Permanently listed in 1986 for use in foods, drugs, and cosmetics. Labeling requirements began in 1989 because of its potential for causing allergic reactions. *See* Colorings.

FD&C YELLOW NO. 6 ALUMINUM LAKE • *See* FD&C Yellow No. 6.

FEBRIFUGE • Any medicine that mitigates or dispels fever. Aspirin is used for this purpose. Herbs that are said to lower fever include cayenne, elderflower, and eucalyptus (*see all*).

FEDAHIST TIMECAPS and GYROCAPS (Rx) • A combination of chlorpheniramine and pseudoephedrine (*see both*) used to treat symptoms of allergies. The Timecaps contain 120 mg of pseudoephedrine while the Gyrocaps contain 65 mg. The Timecaps also contain 8 mg of chlorpheniramine while the Gycrocaps contain 10 mg.

FEEN-A-MINT (OTC) • *See* Phenolphthalein.

FELBAMATE (Rx) • **Felbatol.** An antiepileptic drug approved in the early 1990s for adults and as an adjunct therapy in children with Lennox-Gastaut syndrome, in which there is brain damage and repeated epileptic seizures. The producers of felbamate warn that the drug should be used in patients whose epilepsy is so severe that the risk of aplastic anemia is deemed acceptable in light of the benefits conferred by its use.

FELDENE • *See* Piroxicam.

FELODIPINE (Rx) • **Plendil.** A calcium channel blocker (*see*) introduced in 1991 that provides once-a-day dosing for the treatment of mild to moderate high blood pressure. Promoted as acting more on vascular smooth muscle than on heart muscle. Expected to be approved to treat heart failure. Potential adverse effects include a drop in blood pressure, swelling, palpitations, headache, swollen gums, flushing, dizziness, upper-respiratory infection, weakness, cough, numbness, heartburn, chest pain, nausea, muscle cramps, abdominal pain, constipation, diarrhea, sore throat, stuffy nose, back pain, and rash. Contraindicated in patients who are hypersensitive to the product. Used cautiously in persons with heart failure, the elderly, and those with impaired liver function. The drug should be swallowed whole and not chewed or crushed. Grapefruit juice may cause potentially dangerous, increased levels of this medication in the blood.

FEMININE GOLD ANALGESIC RELIEVING RUB (OTC) • *See* Camphor.

FEMINONE • *See* Ethinyl Estradiol.

FEMIRON (OTC) • *See* Ferrous Fumarate.

FEMSTAT • *See* Butoconazole.

FEMTROL NO. 818 P.S.E. (H) • A dong quai (*see*) formulation containing vitamin C, hesperidin, licorice root extract, chaste berry, black cohosh, false unicorn, and fennel (*see all*). Contains phytoestrogen (*see*), which is said to help menopausal symptoms.

FENESIN • *See* Guaifenesin.

FENFLURAMINE (Rx) • **Ponderal. Ponderaz. Pondimin.** An appetite suppressant related to the amphetamines. Also used to treat autistic children. It stimulates the hypothalamus. Potential adverse reactions include drowsiness, dizziness, incoordination, headache, euphoria or depression, anxiety, insomnia, weakness, fatigue, agitation, palpitations, low or high blood pressure, chest pain, eye irritation, blurred vision, diarrhea, dry mouth, nausea, vomiting, abdominal pain, constipation, painful urination, increased urination, impotence, hives, rash, sweating, chills, fever, and increased libido. Alcohol and central nervous system depressants may add to central nervous system depression. High blood pressure medications that act on the brain may be less effective. MAO inhibitors (*see*) may cause severe high blood pressure. Contraindicated in glaucoma, some heart conditions, alcoholism, and history of drug abuse. Should be used with caution in patients with high blood pressure, mental depression, or diabetes. Differs from amphetamines in that it causes central nervous system depression rather than stimulation.

FENNEL (OTC) (H) • *Foeniculum vulgare.* A perennial herb of the carrot family, fennel is native to southern Europe and Asia Minor. Fennel, used by the Anglo-Saxons, is said to be good for jaundice, flatulence, hiccups, and as a laxative. Hippocrates used it to increase the secretion of milk in nursing mothers. Pliny recommended its use in eye problems because of the observation that serpents, when they shed their skins, eat the plant to restore their eyesight. It contains oils similar to catnip and peppermint (*see both*). American Indians used fennel tea for childhood colic. Used today as an herbal tea for digestive problems, and as an eyewash. It has been reported to have antibiotic properties and is used topically by some herbalists to treat toothaches, earaches, tumors, and chronic swellings. Fennel was in the USP (*see*) for many years and is still listed in many pharmacopeias worldwide. In 1992, the FDA issued a notice that fennel had not been shown to be safe and effective as claimed in OTC digestive-aid products.

FENOLDOPAM (Rx) • An orally active, potent dopamine (*see*) increaser, it lowers blood pressure and systemic vascular resistance. Used in congestive heart failure to decrease arterial pressure.

FENOPROFEN (Rx) • **Nalfon.** Produces anti-inflammatory, analgesic, and fever-reducing effects, possibly through inhibition of prostaglandins (*see*). Introduced in 1976, it is used to treat arthritis and mild to moderate pain. Potential adverse reactions include headache, drowsiness, dizziness, swelling, stomach distress, nausea, vomiting, occult blood loss, peptic ulceration, constipation, reversible renal failure, liver dysfunction, rash, and hives. Effects of oral blood thinners and sulfonylureas (*see*) are enhanced by fenoprofen. Serious GI toxicity can occur at any time in patients taking NSAIDs (*see*) or ingesting alcohol. Fenoprofen increases the effects of phenytoin, sulfa drugs, antidiabetes drugs, and blood thinners. Contraindicated in asthmatics with nasal polyps and in patients allergic to aspirin. Should be used cautiously by elderly patients, and those with GI disorders, cardiovascular diseases, or allergy to other NSAIDs. Most effective when taken thirty minutes before or two hours after meals. If stomach upset is a problem, it can be taken with milk or meals.

FENOTEROL (Rx) • **Berotec.** A beta-blocker (*see*) that is, as of this writing, being investigated in the United States as a bronchodilator. It has been available outside the United States since the early 1970s in a metered-dose inhaler and in oral dosage form. Clinical studies have shown it is effective for maintenance therapy in patients with moderate to severe asthma. Potential side effects are rare in inhalation doses. In oral medication, there may be muscle tremor, rapid heartbeat, palpitations, and nervousness. It is contraindicated in patients with overactive thyroid glands and is used with caution in those with heart disease, diabetes, and liver or kidney dysfunction.

FENTANYL (Rx) • **Duragesic. Innovar. Sublimaze.** A narcotic analgesic often used as an adjunct to general anesthesia, it alters through an unknown mechanism the perception of an emotional response to pain. May also be used by applying a transdermal (*see*) patch to relieve chronic pain. Potential adverse reactions include sedation, sleepiness, euphoria, dizziness, seizures, low blood pressure, irregular heartbeat, nausea, vomiting, constipation, urine retention, itching, redness, respiratory depression, and muscle rigidity. Alcohol and central nervous system depressants are additive and may depress the central nervous system too much. Contraindicated in patients who have been receiving MAO inhibitors (*see*) within fourteen days, or who have myasthenia gravis (*see*). Must be used cautiously in patients with head injury, increased pressure on the brain, asthma, chronic obstructive pulmonary disease, respiratory depression, seizures, liver or kidney dysfunction, low thyroid hormone, Addison's disease, a history of alcoholism, shock, and in elderly or debilitated patients. May be addictive.

FENUGREEK (H) • *Trigonella foenumgraecum.* One of the oldest-known medicinal plants. The use of fenugreek dates back to the ancient Egyptians, and Hippocrates. A folk remedy for sore throats and colds, this herb is also reputed to be an aphrodisiac. Fenugreek may also be used against diabetes. In a study done in India involving insulin-dependent diabetics on low doses of insulin, pulverized seeds of fenugreek were shown to reduce blood sugar and harmful fats. Used externally, fenugreek seeds may help soothe skin irritation and reduce the pain of neuralgia, swollen glands, and tumors. The saponin-containing plant fibers of fenugreek may inhibit the intestinal absorption of cholesterol.

FEOSOL (OTC) • *See* Ferrous Sulfate.

FEOSTAT • *See* Ferrous Fumarate.

FEP CREME • *See* Hydrocortisone and Pramoxine Hydrochloride.

FERANCEE (OTC) • A combination of vitamin C and ferrous fumarate (*see both*), used for the prevention and treatment of iron-deficiency anemias.

FERGON (OTC) • *See* Ferrous Gluconate.

FER-IN-SOL (OTC) • *See* Ferrous Sulfate.

FERMALOX (OTC) • A combination of aluminum hydroxide, magnesium hydroxide, and ferrous sulfate (*see all*), used to prevent and treat iron-deficiency anemias. Has antacids included to help prevent stomach upset.

FERMYCIN SOLUBLE • *See* Chlortetracycline.

FERNDEX • *See* Dextroamphetamine.

FERO-FOLIC-500 (OTC) • A combination of folic acid and ferrous sulfate (*see both*), used to treat and prevent iron-deficiency anemias.

FERO-GRAD-500 (OTC) • A combination of ferrous sulfate and vitamin C (*see both*), used to treat and prevent iron-deficiency anemia.

FERO-GRADUMET (OTC) • *See* Ferrous Sulfate and Sodium Ascorbate.

FERONIM (OTC) • *See* Iron and Dextran.

FEROSPACE (OTC) • *See* Ferrous Sulfate.

FERRALET PLUS (OTC) • *See* Ferrous Gluconate.

FERRA-TD (OTC) • *See* Ferrous Sulfate.

FERRIC CHLORIDE (OTC) • In 1992, the FDA proposed a ban on the use of ferric chloride to treat insect bites and stings, in poison ivy, poison oak, and poison sumac drugs, and in oral menstrual drugs because it had not been shown to be safe and effective as claimed in OTC products.

FERRIC PYROPHOSPHATE (OTC) • **Troph-Iron.** A nutrient supplement.

FERR-M • Homeopathic abbreviation for ferrum metallicum. *See* Iron.

FERRO-SEQUELS (OTC) • *See* Docusate and Ferrous Fumarate.

FERROUS FUMARATE (OTC) • **Bugs Bunny Plus Iron. Caltrate. Centrum, Jr. Cpiron. Erco-Fer. Femiron. Feostat. Ferancee. Ferancee Chewable Tablets. Fero-Grad-500. Ferrofume. Ferronat. Ferrone. Ferro-Sequels. Ferrotemp. Ferroton. Flintstones. Fumerin. Fumiron. Hemaspan FA. Hemocyte. Poly-Vi-Sol with Iron.** An iron preparation containing a minimum of 31.2 percent iron and not less than 2 percent ferric iron. Used to build up the red blood cells. *See* Iron.

FERROUS GLUCONATE (Rx) (OTC) • **Fergon. Ferralet. Ferralet Plus. Ferronicum. Gluco-Ferrum. Simron.** An iron preparation used in severe iron-deficiency anemia. Stable in solution. *See* Iron.

FERROUS SULFATE (OTC) • **Dayalets Plus Iron. Feosol Elixir. Feostat. Fer-In-Soc. Fermalox. Fero-Folic-500. Fero-Gradumet. Ferospace. Ferralyn Lanacaps. Ferra-TD. Mol Iron. Poly-Vi-Sol. Slow Fe Tablets.** An iron preparation that occurs in nature, it is used to build up red blood cells. May cause GI disturbances. In children, ingestion of large amounts may cause vomiting, liver damage, rapid heartbeat, and blood-vessel collapse. Contraindicated in persons with stomach upset, peptic ulcer, or ulcerative colitis. Should be taken with food. In 1992, the FDA proposed a ban on ferrous sulfate in oral menstrual drug products because it had not been shown to be safe and effective as claimed. *See* Iron.

FERR. PHOS. • **Ferrum Phosphoricum.** A homeopathic medicine (*see*) composed of iron phosphate. Iron is an essential mineral and carries oxygen in the blood. Phosphate helps maintain the acid/alkali balance. Homeopaths use it to overcome complaints from overexertion and for general weakness and nosebleeds. *See* Tissue Salts.

FERRUM METALLICUM • *See* Iron.

FERRUM PHOSPHORICUM • *See* Ferr. Phos.

FERULA ASAFETIDA • *See* Asafetida.

FESTAL (Rx) • *See* Pancrelipase.

FEVERALL (OTC) • *See* Acetaminophen.

FEVER BLISTER • A common term for herpes of the lip. *See* Herpes Simplex Virus I.

FEVERFEW (H) • *Chrysanthemum parthenium. Pyrethrum parthenium. Tanacetum parthenium.* **Bachelor's Buttons. Flirtwort. Maydes' Weed. Wild Quinine.** A small, hardy perennial herb, a member of the chamomile (*see*) family, it was introduced into Britain from Southeast Asia. Since ancient times it has been used by physicians for its action on the uterus. It was thought to promote menstrual evacuation and to aid in the expulsion of the placenta after childbirth. It was prescribed as an antidote against narcotic poisoning and was also considered to be a poultice herb with cooling and analgesic properties. Herbalists today use feverfew as a laxative, and to treat stings and bites. The name *feverfew* is derived from *febrifuge,* meaning "to lower fever," the most common use for the herb by ancient Greek physicians. It is now being investigated as a preventative for migraine. It has low toxicity but can stimulate the uterus and should therefore be avoided during pregnancy. It may also cause mouth ulcer with chronic use.

FEVERWORT • *See* Boneset.

FIBER • Nondigestible food content that adds roughage to the diet and bulk to the stool. Used to promote regular bowel movement. The various types of fiber can be divided into two broad categories: soluble and insoluble. Most soluble fiber is derived from fruits and vegetables. Specific types of soluble fiber include lignin, pectin, and gums. Insoluble fiber is derived primarily from grains. The main forms are cellulose, and hemicellulose, as well as some forms of lignin.

FIBERALL (OTC) • *See* Psyllium.

FIBERALL TABLETS (OTC) • *See* Calcium Polycarbophil.

FIBERCON (OTC) • *See* Calcium Polycarbophil.

FIBER-LAX (OTC) • *See* Calcium Polycarbophil.

FIBRILLATION • Rapid, uncoordinated contractions and chaotic beating of the heart.

FIBRIN • An insoluble protein formed in blood as it clots. Derived from fibrinogen (*see*).

FIBRINOGEN • A clotting factor; an inactive plasma protein that is activated by thrombin to form fibrin (*see*).

FIBRINOLYSIN (Rx) • **Elase.** A preparation containing plasmin, an agent that breaks down blood clots. Used topically to treat skin ulcers, surgical wounds, second- and third-degree burns, circumcision, episiotomy, inflammation of the cervix or vagina, abscesses, and fistulas. Potential adverse reactions include allergy and increased blood in an organ or body part.

FIBRINOLYSIS • The dissolution of fibrin (*see*) by enzymes.

FIBROCYSTIC • Pertaining to fibrocysts, lesions surrounded by or situated within fibrous connective tissue.

FIBROCYSTIC BREAST DISEASE • A benign condition that is the most common disorder of the female breast. The fact that new cysts usually do not appear after menopause suggests that ovarian hormones are involved in this disease.

FIBROSIS • The replacement of normal tissue with fibrous connective tissue in scar-tissue formation.

FIBROSITIS • Inflammation of connective tissue, often combined with inflammation of muscle tissue, producing pain, tenderness, and stiffness.

FIGWORT (H) • *Scrophularia nodosa.* A perennial plant native to Britain and the United States, it used to be hung in houses and barns to ward off witches. Homeopathic physicians use it as an ointment to remove freckles, and to treat eczema, rashes, bruises, scratches, and small wounds. It has also been used as a diuretic and to get rid of worms. It is contraindicated in heart disease, especially if irregular heartbeat is present. It is highly toxic in large doses.

FILGRASTIM (Rx) • **Neupogen.** A recombinant granulocyte colony stimulating factor (*see* G-CSF), it was introduced in 1991. It is used for the prevention of chemotherapy-induced neutropenia (*see*). It reduces the risk of infections. Contraindicated in patients with known hypersensitivity to *Escherichia coli*–derived proteins. Potential adverse reactions include nausea, vomiting, skeletal pain, loss of hair, diarrhea, fever, fatigue, loss of appetite, shortness of breath, rash, weakness, sore throat, sore tongue, constipation, and nonspecific pain. It is administered by injection. The safety and efficacy of filgrastim given simultaneously with other chemotherapy has not been established. A growth factor, filgrastim primarily stimulates infection-fighting white blood cells. However, it can possibly act as a growth factor for any tumor type, particularly bone-marrow malignancies; therefore, it is not recommended for use with any malignancy involving bone marrow.

FINASTERIDE (Rx) • **Proscar.** A drug introduced in 1992 to treat enlarged prostate glands. A daily dose of the pill can shrink an enlarged prostate gland in some men, but six months of treatment is needed before it is known whether they will respond. Regression has been maintained for as long as three years. The drug is also being tested in treating male baldness. It is believed to have the potential to grow hair by blocking the formation of the male hormone dihydrotestosterone. Men born with reduced levels of this hormone rarely become bald. Proscar apparently shrinks enlarged prostates by blocking the formation of the same hormone. Among the adverse reactions of finasteride are impotence and decreased libido. The crushed tablets should not be handled by women who are or who may become pregnant. The drug can be absorbed through the skin and pose a subsequent risk to the male fetus. For the same reason, the sperm of a man taking this drug should not be used to impregnate.

FIOGESIC (OTC) • A combination of aspirin, phenylpropanolamine, pheniramine, and pyrilamine (*see all*) used to treat symptoms of allergy, especially headache.

FIORICET • *See* Butalbital Compounds.

FIORINAL (Rx) • **Butalbital Compound. Fiorgen PF. Lanorinal. Marnal.** A combination of aspirin, butalbital, and caffeine (*see all*), it is used to treat headache and other types of pain. Potential adverse reactions include nausea, vomiting, light-headedness, dizziness, sedation, sweating, stomach upset, loss of appetite, weakness, headache, insomnia, agitation, tremor, incoordination, mild hallucinations, disorientation, visual disturbances, euphoria, dry mouth, loss of appetite, constipation, flushing, irregular heartbeat, difficulty in urination, rash, itching, rapid breathing, and diarrhea. Interaction with alcohol, tranquilizers, barbiturates, sleeping pills, or other drugs that produce central nervous system depression can cause increased depressive effects. Should be taken with a full glass of water or food to reduce possible GI distress.

FIORINAL WITH CODEINE (Rx) • A combination of aspirin, codeine phosphate, and butalbital (*see all*) used to treat headache pain.

FIRST AID PLANT • *See* Aloe Vera.

FIRST RESPONSE (OTC) • A pregnancy test.

FIRST RESPONSE OVULATION PREDICTOR (OTC) • A kit to determine ovulation.

FISALAMINE • *See* Mesalamine.

FISH OIL (OTC) • Large amounts of long-chain, highly unsaturated, omega-3 fatty acids that are present in cold-water fish have been found to decrease fats in the blood, including cholesterol. A two-year study in male survivors of heart attacks showed that a moderate intake of fatty fish or fish oil decreased total mortality by 29 percent. This effect occurred without any reduction in serum cholesterol levels. Omega-3 fatty acids from fish can interfere with blood clotting.

FISTULA • An abnormal passage from an internal organ, such as the bladder or intestine, to the body's surface.

5-FC • *See* Flucytosine.

5-FORMYL TETRAHYDROFOLATE • *See* Leucovorin.

5-FU • *See* Fluorouracil.

FLAG • Symbol, phrase, or notation on a package alerting consumers to significant product changes, including new ingredients, dosage instructions, or warnings.

FLAG LILY • *See* Blue Flag.

FLAGYL • *See* Metronidazole.

FLAMAZINE • *See* Silver Sulfadiazine.

FLATULEX (OTC) • A combination of simethicone and activated charcoal (*see both*). Indicated for the relief of acute severe pain due to gas resulting from swallowing air, postoperative distension, heartburn, or food intolerance. Also used as an adjunctive treatment in which increased gas retention and/or production is a consequence of peptic ulcers, malabsorption syndromes, spastic colon, irritable colon, diverticulosis, and certain types of medications. Promoted as formulated to release simethicone at the stomach level, alleviating upper-GI gas retention, and to release the charcoal at the intestinal level, alleviating lower-GI gas retention.

FLAVONES • One of a group of plant pigments that produces ivory and yellow colors. They are reputed to have a wide range of activities, including reducing excess fluid and stimulating the heart. Some, such as rutin and hesperidin, are said to increase the strength of the capillaries and to lower blood pressure. The bioflavonoids (*see*) reputedly aid immunity.

FLAVONOIDS (H) • A compound in a plant such as a pigment. They constitute most of the yellow, red, and blue colors in flowers and fruits. Bioflavonoids have biological effects. Rutin, for example, has chelating properties (*see* Chelation) and influences the functioning of minute blood vessels. Most plants and vegetables contain flavonoids. It is believed flavonoids block receptor sites for certain hormones that promote cancers. *See also* Bioflavonoids.

FLAVORCEE • *See* Vitamin C.

FLAVOXATE (Rx) • **Urispas.** A drug that has a direct antispasmodic effect on the smooth muscles of the urinary tract. It also provides some local pain relief. Used to treat painful urination, frequency, urgency, need to urinate during the night, incontinence, and pain associated with urologic disorders. Potential adverse reactions include confusion, nervousness, dizziness, headache, drowsiness, rapid heartbeat, palpitations, dry mouth and throat, blurred vision, abdominal pain, constipation, nausea, vomiting, hives, rash, and fever. Contraindicated in stomach, intestinal, or urinary obstructions. Must be used cautiously in patients suspected of having glaucoma.

FLAX (H) • *Linum usitatissimum.* **Linseed. Lint Bells.** A native of the Mediterranean countries, it was cultivated in Mesopotamia in prehistoric times. It was widely grown in ancient Egypt. Flaxseed or linseed has been used in medicine since ancient times, being valued for poultices for pleurisy, ripening boils, softening tumors, and drawing out thorns and splinters, in cough medicines, and as a liniment for burns. Flaxseed contains important demulcent and emollient qualities.

Flax is combined with other herbs today by herbalists as a laxative, and to treat kidney stones and edema. Listed in the USP (*see*). Widely used in household medicine.

FLEABANE OIL • *See* Erigeron.

FLECAINIDE ACETATE (Rx) • **Tambocor.** An antiarrhythmic drug introduced in 1985 used for premature ventricular contractions (*see* PVC) and nonsustained ventricular irregular heart palpitations. Flecainide produces its helpful effects by slowing nerve impulses in the heart and making the heart tissue less sensitive. There is a chance that flecainide may worsen heart-rhythm problems. Potential adverse reactions include dizziness, headache, fatigue, tremor, new or worsened heart irregularities, chest pain, cardiac heart failure, visual disturbances, nausea, constipation, abdominal pain, shortness of breath, water retention, and rash. May interact with amiodarone, cimetidine, digoxin, and propranolol and increase toxicity. Contraindicated in people with heart blocks or allergy to the drug. Urine acidifying and alkalinizing agents may alter excretion of flecainide. May be taken with food.

FLEET BABYLAX (OTC) • *See* Glycerin.

FLEET BISACODYL (OTC) • *See* Bisacodyl.

FLEET MINERAL OIL (OTC) • *See* Mineral Oil.

FLEET PHOSPHO-SODA (OTC) • *See* Sodium Phosphate.

FLEET RELIEF (OTC) • *See* Pramoxine Hydrochloride.

FLETCHER'S CASTORIA • *See* Senna.

FLEUR-DE-LIS • *See* Blue Flag.

FLEXERIL • *See* Cyclobenzaprine.

FLEXOJECT • *See* Orphenadrine.

FLEXON • *See* Orphenadrine.

FLEXURAL • Pertaining to the point or area of bending.

FLINT SSD • *See* Silver Sulfadiazine.

FLINTSTONES (OTC) • A multivitamin preparation.

FLOLAN (Rx) • *See* Epoprostenol.

FLONASE NASAL SPRAY (Rx) • A synthetic steroid available overseas since 1991, this product is used to treat seasonal and perennial allergic rhinitis that results in inflammation of the nasal passages. The FDA gave permission for its marketing in the United States in 1994. *See* Steroids.

FLORINEF • *See* Fludrocortisone.

FLORONE • *See* Diflorasone.

FLOROPRYL • *See* Isoflurophate.

FLORVITE (OTC) • A vitamin supplement.

FLOXIN • *See* Ofloxacin.

FLOXURIDINE (Rx) • **Fluorodeoxyuridine. FUDR.** An anticancer drug used to treat brain, breast, head, neck, liver, gallbladder, and bile-duct malignancies. Potential adverse reactions include nausea, vomiting, diarrhea, sore mouth, cramps, bleeding, anemia, loss of balance, dizziness, seizures, depression, paralysis, hiccups, lethargy, blurred vision, rash, itching, jaundice, and inflammation of the bile duct.

FLUBENISOLONE • *See* Betamethasone.

FLUCONAZOLE (Rx) • **Diflucan.** An antifungal medication used to treat oral and throat candidiasis, systemic candidiasis, and cryptococcal meningitis. In 1995, it was also approved for treatment of vaginal candidiasis (yeast) infection. The product is the first one-dose oral treatment in the United States. Potential adverse reactions include headache, nausea, vomiting, abdominal pain, diarrhea, rash, and rarely, liver problems. Fluconazole interacts with cyclosporine, phenytoin, and oral antidiabetic agents causing possible increased blood concentrations of these drugs. May cause increased liver enzymes when taken with isoniazid, phenytoin, rifampin, valproic acid, or sulfonylureas. May counteract the action of the anticoagulant warfarin and may be less effective when taken with rifampin. It is a candidate for OTC status.

FLUCYTOSINE (Rx) • Ancobon. 5-FC. Used for severe fungal infections caused by *Candida* and *Cryptococcus.* Potential adverse reactions include anemia, dizziness, drowsiness, confusion, headache, nausea, vomiting, diarrhea, abdominal bloating, elevation of liver enzymes, and rash. Because this drug may make you sensitive to sunlight, apply a sunblock that has a skin protection factor of at least 15; include protecting your lips.

FLUDARA • *See* Fludarabine.

FLUDARABINE (Rx) • Fludara. An anticancer drug introduced in 1991, it is used in the treatment of chronic lymphocytic leukemia (B cell) in patients who have not responded to standard therapies. Fludarabine attacks and destroys the abnormal cells, allowing normal cells to reproduce.

FLUDEOXYGLUCOSE F18 (Rx) • A PET scan imaging agent for defining the location and origin of epileptic seizures in the brain. Introduced in 1994 after a nineteen-month review by the FDA. A PET (position emission tomography) is a machine that shows the brain's metabolism of blood sugar.

FLUDROCORTISONE (Rx) • Florinef. A powerful synthetic adrenocorticosteroid, it is used to treat adrenal insufficiency, and severe orthostatic low blood pressure; otherwise, used only topically. Potential adverse reactions include sodium and water retention, high blood pressure, enlarged heart, swelling, and low potassium. Contraindicated in high blood pressure, congestive heart failure, or other heart diseases. Should be used with caution in Addison's disease (*see*).

FLUID EXTRACT • Alcohol is used as a solvent to extract the active agent or agents in an herb.

FLUMAZENIL (Rx) • Mazicon. An injectable drug introduced in 1991 for the complete or partial reversal of benzodiazepine-induced anesthesia or sedation, and as an adjunct in the management of benzodiazepine (*see*) overdose.

FLUNISOLIDE (Rx) • AeroBid Inhaler. Nasalide. Rhinalar Nasal Mist. A corticosteroid (*see*) used to treat lung disorders, particularly asthma. In a nasal spray, it decreases inflammation for relief of stuffy nose from allergies. Potential adverse reactions include headache, mild temporary nasal burning, stuffy nose, sneezing, watery eyes, bloody nose, nausea, vomiting, and development of fungal infections of the nose and throat. Should not be used if any infections are present unless anti-infectives are also used under medical supervision.

FLUOCET • *See* Fluocinolone.

FLUOCINOLONE (Rx) • Fluocet. Fluonid. Flurosyn. Synalar. Synemol. A corticosteroid (*see*) cream, ointment, or topical solution used to treat skin inflammation. Potential adverse reactions include burning, itching, irritation, dryness, inflammation of the hair follicles, acne, rash around the mouth, spots of pigment loss, hairiness, allergic contact dermatitis, and if covered with a dressing, secondary infection, atrophy, streaks, and blisters. Should be used cautiously in skin problems caused by viruses such as herpes, and in fungal or bacterial skin infections. Should not be used for more than two weeks due to potential absorption into the system, consequently causing an effect on the hypothalamus, and pituitary and adrenal glands, as well as a permanent thinning of the skin. Fluocinolone should not be applied near the eyes or mucous membranes, under the arms, on the face, groin, or under the breast unless medically specified.

FLUOCINONIDE (Rx) • **Fluocin. Licon. Lidex. Vasoderm.** A potent corticosteroid (*see*) cream, gel, ointment, or topical solution used to treat skin inflammation. Potential adverse reactions include burning, itching, irritation, dryness, inflammation of the hair follicles, acne, rash around the mouth, spots of pigment loss, hairiness, allergic contact dermatitis, and if covered with a dressing, secondary infection, atrophy, streaks, and blisters. Should be used cautiously in skin problems caused by viruses such as herpes, and in fungal or bacterial skin infections. Should not be used for more than two weeks due to potential absorption into the system, consequently causing an effect on the hypothalamus, and pituitary and adrenal glands. Should not be applied near the eyes or mucous membranes, under the arms, on the face, groin, or under the breast unless medically specified.

FLUONID • *See* Fluocinolone.

FLUOR-A-DAY • *See* Sodium Fluoride.

FLUORAN • A luminescent coal-tar-derived color.

FLUORESCEIN (Rx) • **AK-Fluor. Fluorescite. Fluor-l-Strip. Fluor-l-Strip A.T. Ful-Glo. Funduscein-25.** A yellow granular or red crystalline dye giving a brilliant yellow-green fluorescence in an alkaline solution. Fluorescein eyedrops are used to diagnose corneal abrasions and foreign bodies, to check tear ducts, and for other diagnostic procedures. Instillation may cause stinging, burning, and yellowish streaks from tears. If given intravenously, potential adverse reactions may include headache persisting for more than two days, dizziness, faintness, seizures, low blood pressure, shock, cardiac arrest, nausea, vomiting, temporary bright yellow urine, and skin and hypersensitivity reactions, including hives and anaphylaxis. Should be used with caution in patients with a history of allergy or bronchial asthma. Should not be instilled while patient is wearing soft contact lenses because the drug will destroy them.

FLUORESCITE • *See* Fluorescein.

FLUORIDE (OTC) • **Act. Fluorigard. Fluorineed. Fluoritab. Flura. Gel-Kam. Gel-Tin. Karidium. Karigel. Luride. Pediaflor. Phos-Flur. PreviDent. Thera-Fluor.** An acid salt used in toothpaste and drinking water to prevent tooth decay. It is believed to work on the teeth by strengthening the mineral content of tooth enamel, making it more resistant to decay. It may also strengthen developing bones. Fluoride can cross the placental barrier; the effects on the fetus are unknown. Kidney disturbance is reportedly due to the amount of fluoride in the blood. Not to be used as a dietary supplement. Prolonged intake of large quantities of fluoride or water containing more than 2 ppm may cause fluorosis, causing mottled or discolored enamel in teeth. Very high levels—more than 8 ppm—may also lead to bone disorders, kidney dysfunction, and degenerative changes in the liver, adrenal glands, heart, central nervous system, and reproductive organs. The use of supplements is being studied as a means to preventing and treating osteoporosis, fragile bones. *See* Sodium Fluoride.

FLUORIGARD • *See* Sodium Fluoride.

FLUORINSE • *See* Sodium Fluoride.

FLUORITAB • *See* Fluoride.

FLUORODEOXYURIDINE • *See* Floxuridine.

FLUOROMETHOLONE (Rx) • **AK-Metholone. Fluor-Op. FML. Liquifilm Ophthalmic.** An ointment or solution of a steroid preparation used to treat inflammatory and allergic conditions of the eye. Potential adverse reactions include increased pressure within the eye, thinning of the cornea, interference with corneal wound healing, corneal ulcerations, increased susceptibility to viral or fungal eye infections, and with excessive or long-term use, worsening of glaucoma, cataracts, decreased visual acuity, optic nerve damage, and systemic effects such as adrenal-gland suppression. Contraindicated when fungal or viral infections are present.

FLUOR-OP • *See* Fluorometholone.

FLUOROPLEX • *See* Fluorouracil.

FLUOROURACIL (Rx) • **Adrucil. Efudex. 5-Fluorouracil. 5-FU. Fluoroplex.** An anticancer drug used to treat colon, rectal, breast, ovarian, cervical, bladder, liver, and pancreatic cancer. Introduced in 1962, it interferes with the growth of cancer cells, which are eventually destroyed. Since the growth of normal body cells also may be affected by fluorouracil, other undesirable effects will also occur, including nausea, vomiting, diarrhea, sore mouth, GI ulcers, anemia, a drop in platelets, loss of balance, rash, dark spots on the skin, redness, pain, burning, scaling, loss of hair, weakness, and malaise. Cimetidine and amphotericin B (*see both*) may increase the adverse effects of fluorouracil, as may a number of other drugs. A topical cream is used to treat skin cancer; potential adverse reactions include a burning sensation when the cream is applied, increased sensitivity of skin to sunlight, itching, oozing, rash, soreness or tenderness of skin, darkening of skin, and tearing eyes.

FLUOSTIGMINE • *See* Isoflurophate.

FLUOTHANE • *See* Halothane.

FLUOXETINE HYDROCHLORIDE (Rx) • **Prozac. Pulvules.** This is one of the most popular drugs in the world for the short-term management of depression. In 1994, sales jumped 39 percent to $1.67 billion worldwide. A nontricyclic antidepressant introduced in 1978, it increases serotonin (*see*). In 1994, the FDA also approved it for the treatment of the eating disorder bulimia (*see*). May also relieve the symptoms of obsessive-compulsive disorders. It also reportedly helps alleviate premenstrual syndrome (PMS). Potential adverse reactions include chills, a hangover effect, jaw pain, nervousness, anxiety, insomnia, headache, drowsiness, tremor, dizziness, abnormal dreams, palpitations, flushing, slow heartbeat, irregular heartbeat, flulike syndrome, stuffy nose, upper-respiratory infection, sore throat, cough, sinusitis, visual disturbances, ringing in the ears, respiratory distress, nausea, diarrhea, dry mouth, loss of appetite, heartburn, constipation, abdomi-nal pain, vomiting, taste change, gas, increased appetite, muscle pain, weight loss, rash, itching, hives, weakness, water retention, and swollen glands. Tryptophan may cause agitation and GI distress when taken with fluoxetine. Diazepam blood levels may be increased. Warfarin and digitoxin may cause toxic effects. In 1991, after careful review of pertinent scientific data, the FDA rejected the Scientologists' petition seeking removal of fluoxetine from the market. According to FDA findings, a Scientology-founded group, the Citizens Commission for Human Rights, had not demonstrated links between the drug and suicidal thinking or violent behavior. The FDA also found no demonstrable connection between the drug and tardive dyskinesia (*see*). In *Biomedical Inquiry,* summer 1992 issue, researchers at the University of Texas Medical Branch at Galveston reported fluoxetine to be one of the safest antidepressants on the market. They said even when taken in overdosage, it is less toxic than most other antidepressant medications. They also reported that side effects associated with the use of tricyclic antidepressants—such as weight gain, dry mouth, dizziness, and cardiac toxicity—are rarely experienced by patients using fluoxetine. Manifestation of the full beneficial antidepressant effects may take as long as four weeks after treatment begins. Fluoxetine should be taken in the morning to avoid its effects on sleep. May be taken with or without food.

FLUOXYMESTERONE (Rx) • **Android-F. Halodrin. Halotestin. Ora-Testryl.** A potent androgen (*see*) used to treat hypogonadism and impotence caused by testicular deficiency, postpartum breast engorgement, and cancer. Potential adverse reactions in women include acne, edema, oily skin, weight gain, hairiness, hoarseness, clitoral enlargement, changes in libido, flushing, sweating, and vaginitis with itching. In males, prepubescent, premature epiphyseal closure, priapism, growth of body and facial hair, phallic enlargement; postpubescent, testicular atrophy, scanty sperm, decreased ejaculatory volume, impotence, enlargement of breasts, and epididymitis. In both sexes, edema, gastroenteritis, nausea, vomiting, constipation, change in appetite, diarrhea, bladder irritability, and jaundice. Contraindicated in men with enlarged or cancerous prostates; carcinoma of the male breast; high levels of calcium in the blood; heart, liver, or kidney dysfunction; and in premature infants. Should be used cautiously in prepubescent males, patients with diabetes or heart disease, and those taking ACTH, corticosteroids, or anticoagulants. Should be taken with food or meals.

FLUPHENAZINE HYDROCHLORIDE, DECANOATE, or ENANTHATE (Rx) • **Decanoate. Enanthate. Modecate. Moditen. Permitil. Prolixin.** A drug introduced in 1959 used to treat psychotic disorders. (The enanthate and decanoate compounds prolong the duration of effects.) Potential adverse reactions include a drop in white blood cells, extrapyramidal reactions, sedation, pseudoparkinsonism, dizziness, a drop in blood pressure when rising from a seated or prone position, irregular heartbeat, dry mouth, vision changes, constipation, urine retention, menstrual irregularities, enlargement of male breast, inhibited ejaculation and male orgasm, depressed male libido, increased female libido, impotence, liver dysfunction, mild photosensitivity, allergic skin reactions, weight gain, increased appetite, fever, and sweating. Tardive dyskinesia (*see*) may occur with long-term use. Abrupt withdrawal may cause gastritis, nausea, vomiting, dizziness, tremors, sweating, headache, and insomnia. Use with alcohol and other central nervous system depressants may increase central nervous system depression. Antacids inhibit its absorption. Barbiturates and lithium may make it less effective. High blood pressure medications that act on the brain may be less effective. Contraindicated in coma, enlarged prostate, central nervous system depression, bone-marrow depression, liver, lung, or kidney damage, and with the use of spinal or epidural anesthetics or adrenergic-blocking agents (*see*). Should be used cautiously in combination with barbiturates, alcohol, sleeping pills, narcotics, antihistamines, or any central nervous system depressant. Patients taking fluphenazine should use sunscreens to avoid photosensitivity skin reactions and be cautious about exposure to hot weather because this drug can increase the possibility of heatstroke. May be taken with meals to reduce stomach upset.

FLURA • *See* Fluoride.

FLURA-DROPS • *See* Sodium Fluoride.

FLURANDRENOLIDE (Rx) • **Flurandrenolone. Cordran. Cordran Tape. Drenison. Drenison Tape.** A corticosteroid ointment, cream, lotion, or tape used to treat skin inflammation. Potential adverse reactions include burning, itching, irritation, dryness, inflammation of the hair follicles, acne, rash around the mouth, spots of pigment loss, hairiness, allergic contact dermatitis, and if covered with a dressing, secondary infection, atrophy, streaks, and blisters. Reactions with tape include striping of the skin, infection of the hair follicles, and tiny skin hemorrhages. Should be used cautiously in skin problems caused by viruses such as herpes, and in fungal or bacterial skin infections. Should not be used for more than two weeks due to potential absorption into the system, consequently causing an effect on the hypothalamus, and pituitary and adrenal glands. Should not be applied near the eyes or mucous membranes, under the arms, on the face, groin, or under the breast unless medically specified.

FLURANDRENOLONE • *See* Flurandrenolide.

FLURAZEPAM (Rx) • **Dalmane. Durapam.** A benzodiazepine (*see*) sleeping medication introduced in 1970, it works on the limbic system, thalamus, and hypothalamus of the brain. May cause a decline in white blood cells, daytime sedation, dizziness, drowsiness, incoordination, lethargy, confusion, headache, nausea, vomiting, heartburn, and liver dysfunction. Use with alcohol, narcotic analgesics, and other central nervous system depressants may cause excessive central nervous system depression. Use with cimetidine (*see*) increases sedation. Flurazepam should be used cautiously in patients with impaired kidney or liver function, mental depression, suicidal tendencies, or a history of drug abuse. Elderly patients are more sensitive to the drug's adverse central nervous system effects. More effective by the second, third, or fourth nights of use because active metabolite accumulates. Dependence is possible with long-term use.

FLURBIPROFEN (Rx) • **Ansaid. Ocufen.** A nonsteroidal anti-inflammatory drug introduced in 1977 that interferes with prostaglandins (*see*), it is used to treat arthritis. Also used in an eye solution to keep the pupil from constricting. Recommended for relief of menstrual cramps. The most frequent side effect is gastrointestinal disturbance. Potential adverse reactions include headache, anxiety, insomnia, increased reflexes, tremors, amnesia, weakness, drowsiness, malaise, depression, dizziness, stuffy nose, ringing in the ears, visual changes, heartburn, diarrhea, abdominal pain, nausea, constipation, GI bleeding, gas, vomiting, symptoms suggesting urinary-tract infection, rash, weight changes, and elevated liver enzymes. The liver side effects may mimic hepatitis symptoms. Flurbiprofen reduces effectiveness of diuretics and may cause increased bleeding tendencies when used with oral anticoagulants. Aspirin decreases flurbiprofen levels; concomitant use is not recommended. Contraindicated in patients allergic to aspirin. Serious GI toxicity can occur with patients taking NSAIDs (*see*), including aspirin. Alcoholic beverages also may cause serious problems while taking this drug. The elderly, debilitated, or those with liver or kidney dysfunction must be carefully monitored if taking the drug. In the eye solution, it causes transient burning and stinging upon instillation and may cause eye irritation. If used with acetylcholine or carbachol (*see both*), it may be ineffective. The drug may render epinephrine (*see*) or other antiglaucoma agents less effective in lowering eye pressure. Contraindicated if the virus herpes simplex is affecting the eyes. Should be taken with food, milk, or antacid.

FLUROSYN • *See* Fluocinolone.

FLUTAMIDE (Rx) • **Eulexin.** An anticancer drug that inhibits androgen (*see*) uptake and is used to treat metastatic prostate cancer in combination with luteinizing hormone-releasing hormone (*see* LHRH). Potential adverse reactions include nausea, vomiting, diarrhea, high blood pressure, impotence, rash, sensitivity to light, hot flashes, enlargement of male breasts, fluid retention, liver dysfunction, and loss of interest in sex.

FLUTEX • *See* Triamcinolone.

FLUTICASONE (Rx) • **Cutivate. Flonase.** Used in the relief of inflammation and itching associated with corticosteroid-responsive skin rashes. A nasal-spray formulation has been approved by the FDA for the treatment of seasonal and perennial allergic rhinitis in adults and children over twelve years. The topical application of corticosteroids decreases inflammation in the nasal mucosa. Potential adverse effects in the nasal spray may include irritation of the nasal mucosa. As with other corticosteroid nasal sprays, subclinical suppression of bone mineralization and the hypothalamus-pituitary-adrenal axis (*see*) occurs. The manufacturer recommends beginning with two sprays in each nostril once a day or one spray in each nostril twice a day, but suggests that after a few days some patients may be able to reduce the dosage to one spray in each nostril once daily. *See* Corticosteroids.

FLUVASTATIN • **Lescol.** A water-soluble cholesterol-lowering agent that acts through the inhibition of certain liver enzymes that affect the production of cholesterol. Administration of fluvastatin lowered low-density lipids in the blood by as much as 22 percent after nine weeks. Increases in the good cholesterol, HDL, and reduction in triglycerides were also noted in clinical studies. Contraindicated in persons with active liver disease. Biochemical liver abnormalities have been associated with cholesterol-lowering drugs of this type. Liver-function tests should be done before the initiation of treatment, at six and twelve weeks after initiation of therapy or elevation in dose, and periodically thereafter. Such drugs may also cause muscle pain and a serious condition, rhabdomyolysis with kidney dysfunction. The risk of muscle problems is increased if therapy with cyclosporine, gemfibrozil, erythromycin, or niacin is also taken. Other potential adverse effects include dysfunction of certain cranial nerves, impairment of eye movement, facial paresis, tremor, dizziness, memory loss, numbness, anxiety, insomnia, and depression. There may also be hypersensitivity reactions, skin rash, dryness of skin and mucous membranes, changes to hair and nails, swelling of the breast, loss of libido, erectile dysfunction, progression cataracts, and insomnia. The medication should be taken at bedtime.

FLUVOXAMINE (Rx) • **Luvox.** An oral medication used to treat obsessive-compulsive disorder (*see*), introduced in 1994 after a thirty-five-month review by the FDA. It has been used in Switzerland since 1983 and is approved in thirty-five other countries. It is an oral selective serotonin (*see*) reuptake inhibitor. Serotonin sends nerve impulses from one nerve cell to another. Potential adverse effects of fluvoxamine include insomnia, sleepiness, nausea, weakness, abnormal ejaculation, nervousness, dry mouth, and constipation. It may also impair judgment, thinking, or motor skills. Adverse interactions with psychiatric and other drugs have been reported, especially with MAO inhibitors (*see*). Fluvoxamine also reportedly reduces the clearance of Xanax (*see* Alprazolam), initial doses of which should be reduced by half. It should also not be taken in combination with the prescription antihistamines terfenadine and astemizole (*see both*).

FLY AGARIC • *See* Agaricus.

FML • *See* Fluorometholone.

FOILLE (OTC) • A combination of bacitracin, benzocaine, neomycin, and polymyxin B (*see all*), used to treat skin inflammations and infections.

FOILLE PLUS (OTC) • *See* Benzocaine.

FOLACIN • *See* Folic Acid.

FOLATE • *See* Folic Acid.

FOLDAN • *See* Thiabendazole.

FOLEX • *See* Methotrexate.

FOLIC ACID (OTC) • **Vitamin B$_9$. Fero-Folic-500. Folacin. Folate. Folvite. Hemaspan FA. Novofolacid.** Aids cell growth and regeneration, red blood cell formation, and protein metabolism. It is used to treat folic-acid deficiency caused by alcoholism, anemia, diarrhea, fever, hemodialysis, prolonged illness, intestinal diseases, liver disease, prolonged stress, and surgical removal of the stomach. The recommended daily allowance (RDA) for adults is 0.4 mg. Deficiency symptoms include gastrointestinal problems and anemia. Current research indicates that folic acid may prevent cervical cancer and reduce the risk of birth defects such as spina bifida. In a study reported in the *Journal of the American Medical Association,* January 22, 1992, a new link was identified between low blood levels of this vitamin and cervical cancer. In 1996, it was reported in the same journal that it reduced the risk of fatal heart disease. Recommended daily allowance: newborns and infants to six months, 25 mcg; infants six months to one year, 35 mcg; children one to three years, 50 mcg; four to six years, 75 mcg; seven to eleven years, 100 mcg; eleven to fourteen years, 150 mcg; males fifteen years and over, 200 mcg; females fifteen years and over, 180 mcg; pregnant women, 400 mcg; lactating women, 260 to 280 mcg. The FDA is proposing, at this writing, to require folic acid fortification of such products as enriched breads, rolls, and buns, enriched flour and enriched self-rising flour, enriched cornmeal, rice, and macaroni. The fortification level would be 140 mg/100 g of the product. The FDA is proposing this action as one measure to reduce the risk of neural-tube defects. Potential adverse reactions include rash, itching, redness, allergic bronchospasms, and general malaise.

FOLINIC ACID • *See* Leucovorin.

FOLLICULITIS • A bacterial infection of the hair follicles, characterized by small red bumps appearing on the scalp, arms, legs, eyelids, and under beards.

FOLLUTEIN • *See* Gonadotropin, Human Chorionic.

FOLVITE • *See* Folic Acid.

FOMENTATION • An external application of herbs, generally used to treat swelling, pain, colds, and flu. A towel or cloth is soaked in the desired tea and applied to the affected area.

FOOTWORK • *See* Tolnaftate.

FORMALDEHYDE • An inexpensive and effective disinfectant. However, there are questions about its safety. It is a highly reactive chemical that is damaging to the hereditary substances in the cells of several animal species.

FORMIC ACID • Colorless, pungent, highly corrosive, it occurs naturally in apples and other fruits. Used as a flavoring. Chronic absorption is known to cause protein in urine. When administered orally, it caused cancer in rats, mice, and hamsters. In 1992, the FDA proposed a ban on formic acid in lice-killing products because it had not been shown to be safe and effective as claimed.

FORTAZ • *See* Ceftazidine.

FORTEL OVULATION TEST (OTC) • A diagnostic test for ovulation.

FOSAMAX (Rx) • *See* Alendronate.

FOSCARNET (Rx) • **Foscavir.** An AIDS drug introduced in 1991. An injectable medication to treat cytomegalovirus, an opportunistic infection that can cause blindness and be fatal to AIDS patients.

FOSCAVIR • *See* Foscarnet.

FOSINOPRIL (Rx) • **Monopril.** An ACE inhibitor (*see*) introduced in 1991, it is used in the treatment of high blood pressure, either alone or in combination with other antihypertensive medications. In 1995 it was approved by the FDA for treatment of heart failure. It is claimed that it has a lower incidence of orthostatic hypotension (drop in blood pressure upon standing) than other high blood pressure drugs. Some hypertensive patients with no apparent preexisting kidney disease have developed increases in blood urea nitrogen and serum creatinine, usually minor and transient, especially when fosinopril has been given with a diuretic. Fosinopril is contraindicated in patients who are hypersensitive to this product. Swelling of the face, lips, tongue, glottis, or larynx has been reported in patients receiving ACE inhibitors. When used in pregnancy during the second and third trimesters, ACE inhibitors can cause injury and even death to the developing fetus, and thus fosinopril should be discontinued as soon as possible. Among other potential adverse effects are headache, cough, dizziness, diarrhea, fatigue, nausea, vomiting, and sexual dysfunction.

FOSTEX (OTC) • A combination of benzoyl peroxide, salicylic acid, and sulfur (*see all*), used as a therapeutic shampoo and acne wash.

FO-TI (H) • *Polygonum multiforum.* **Ho Shou Wu.** One of the most popular herbs in China. Employed to treat skin ulcers and stomach ulcers, as well as abscesses. The Chinese claim this herb has rejuvenating properties and can prevent gray hair and other premature signs of aging. It is also believed to increase fertility and maintain strength and vigor. Modern animal tests using fo-ti extract have demonstrated antitumor activity. This herb also shows heart-protecting possibilities. Studies in humans have shown fo-ti to reduce high blood pressure, high blood cholesterol, and the incidence of heart disease among people prone to these conditions. It is used by herbalists as a purgative and emetic. In India it is used against colic and stomach upsets; in Brazil, to treat hemorrhoids and gout.

FOTOTAR • *See* Coal Tar.

4-WAY FAST ACTING NASAL SPRAY (OTC) • A combination of phenylephrine hydrochloride, naphazoline hydrochloride, and pyrilamine maleate. Also in a mentholated formula. For prompt, temporary relief of nasal congestion due to the common cold, sinusitis, hay fever, or other upper-respiratory allergies. May cause burning, stinging, sneezing, or increased nasal discharge if recommended dosages are exceeded. Should not be used by children under twelve. Also contraindicated for people with heart disease, high blood pressure, thyroid disease, diabetes, or difficulty in urination due to the enlargement of the prostate gland, unless directed by a doctor. The spray container should not be used by more than one person to avoid cross-contamination.

4-WAY LONG ACTING NASAL SOLUTION • *See* Oxymetazoline. (Contains phenylmercuric acetate as a preservative.)

FOXGLOVE (Rx) (H) • *Digitalis purpurea.* Found growing wild in the English countryside and along the western coast of the United States, it is the plant from which the heart drug digitalis (*see*) is derived. Foxglove is often cited as an example of an herbal medicine that became a widely used prescription medication. A Welsh woman used it to treat dropsy, fluid retention caused by congestive heart failure. An English botanist, Dr. William Withering, observed this use in 1775 and isolated digitalis from the leaves. Digitalis, the active principle of foxglove, is widely used today as a diuretic, a stimulant for heart failure, and a tonic for chronic heart disorders. Prior to the discovery of its effect on the heart, foxglove was used in folk medicine as an expectorant, in epilepsy, and to reduce swollen glands. In Italy, it was used externally to heal wounds and reduce swelling. The herb, however, contains a deadly poison and should be used only under proper medical supervision.

FRAGARIA VESCA • *See* Strawberry.

FRAGMIN • *See* Dalteparin Sodium.

FRANGULA • Banned as an ingredient in laxatives by the FDA, May 1992.

FREE RADICAL • Any molecule that is "single" and looking for a partner. The most commonly and potentially hazardous free radicals are oxygen singles that look for a mate by stealing someone else's partner or by attaching themselves to a couple. They damage cells lining blood vessels and arteries. They are also believed to play a role in the development of cancer and in aging.

FRINGE TREE (H) • *Chionanthus virginica.* The root bark is used to treat liver problems, including jaundice. It is used by herbalists to treat gallbladder inflammation. Acts as a gentle laxative.

FRUCTOSE (OTC) • **Emetrol. Levulose.** A sugar occurring naturally in honey and many varieties of fruits. Researchers at the General Clinical Research Center at the University of Colorado School of Medicine, Denver, report that fructose is absorbed in the gastrointestinal tract more slowly than sugars such as sucrose. Fructose is used in combination with dextrose and phosphoric acid to treat nausea and vomiting.

FRUSEMIDE • *See* Furosemide.

FTC • Federal Trade Commission, the federal agency responsible for preventing unfair and deceptive advertising. Along with the FTC, the FDA also has a say in how drugs are presented to physicians and to the public.

FUCUS VESICULOSUS (H) • *See* Bladder Wrack.

FUDR • *See* Floxuridine.

FUL-GLO • *See* Fluorescein.

FU LING (H) • *Poria cocos.* **Muk Sheng.** A fungus reputed to be an effective diuretic, it is used to rid the body of excess fluid. Also used to treat kidney dysfunction, lung congestion, and insomnia, to expel mucus, and to treat hyperactivity in children. Reported to be a nerve tonic, it is prescribed in wasting diseases.

FULVICIN-U/F • *See* Griseofulvin.

FUMITORY (H) • *Fumaria officinalis.* **Earth Smoke. Horned Poppy. Wax Dolls.** An abundant weed in fields, herbalists use it in drinks for clearing obstructions from the liver or kidneys, and to cure many diseases of the skin. May also be used as an eyewash to ease conjunctivitis (*see*). It is considered harmless in low doses, but in excessive or long-term use it can cause stomach irritation. An excessive dose can cause uterine contractions, therefore fumitory should not be used during pregnancy.

FUNGATIN • *See* Tolnaftate.

FUNGI • A group of simple plantlike organisms that can cause disease. Fungal diseases in humans often affect the outer surfaces of the body (ringworm, athlete's foot) and the epithelial surfaces of interior structures (vaginitis, thrush). Fungi include mushrooms, yeasts, rusts, molds, and smuts.

FUNGIZONE • *See* Amphotericin B.

FUNGOID • *See* Triacetin.

FURACIN • *See* Nitrofurazone.

FURADANTIN • *See* Nitrofurantoin.

FURALAN • *See* Nitrofurantoin.

FURAN • *See* Nitrofurantoin.

FURANITE • *See* Nitrofurantoin.

FURAZOLIDONE (Rx) • **Furoxone.** An antiprotozoal drug used in diarrhea and enteritis caused by *Giardia lamblia* and *Vibrio cholerae*. Taken by mouth, it works inside the intestines to counteract cholera, colitis, and/or diarrhea caused by these bacteria. Potential adverse reactions include joint pain, fever, itching, skin rash or redness, nausea, vomiting, diarrhea, stomach pain, headache, and sore throat. Severe high blood pressure and other side effects may occur if MAO inhibitors (*see*), ephedrine, and tricyclic antidepressants are combined with this drug. Severe high blood pressure and other undesirable side effects may occur if the following are eaten or drunk while taking this drug: aged cheese, caviar, yeast or protein extracts, fava or broad beans, smoked or pickled meat, poultry or fish, fermented sausages (bologna, pepperoni, salami, summer sausage) or other fermented meat, any overripe fruit, dark beer, red wine, sherry, or liqueurs. The above foods and drinks should be avoided for at least two weeks after discontinuing furazolidone.

FURAZOSIN • *See* Prazosin Hydrochloride.

FUROMIDE • *See* Furosemide.

FUROSEMIDE (Rx) • **Furomide. Lasix. Lo-Aqua. Myrosemide.** A potent diuretic introduced in 1964, used to treat fluid in the lungs and edema. Potential adverse reactions include a drop in red blood cells and platelets, dehydration, abdominal discomfort, rash, impotence, potassium, low-chloride, and other fluid and electrolyte imbalances, and high blood sugar. An interaction with aminoglycoside antibiotics may increase the possibility of adverse effects on the ear. Chloral hydrate may cause sweating or flushing when used with furosemide. Clofibrate enhances furosemide's effects. Furosemide may increase levels of lithium in the blood, leading to an increased risk of lithium poisoning. NSAIDs (*see*) may reduce the diuretic effects of furosemide. Indomethacin makes it less effective. Furosemide will potentiate the effects of other blood-pressure-lowering drugs. It must be used cautiously in heart shock complicated by fluid in the lungs, in the absence of urine formation, in coma due to liver dysfunction, and in electrolyte imbalances. Not usually given to women of childbearing age because its safety in pregnancy has not been established. Sulfonamide-sensitive patients may have allergic reactions to furosemide. A high-potassium diet should be followed, including such foods as citrus fruits, tomatoes, bananas, dates, and apricots. Usually taken after breakfast.

FUROXONE • *See* Furazolidone.

FURUNCLES • Hard, painful red nodules that develop most commonly on the face, neck, armpits, and buttocks; may eventually enlarge and exude pus.

GABA • Abbreviation for gamma-aminobutyric acid (*see*).

GABAPENTIN (Rx) • **Neurontin.** A medication used in addition to other drugs to treat epileptic seizures; approved by the FDA in 1994. Structurally related to the brain chemical GABA, its exact mode of controlling seizures is unknown. During the course of premarket development, 8 sudden, unexplained deaths occurred among 2,203 patients. Although this rate exceeds that expected in a healthy population matched for age and sex, it is within the range of estimates for the incidence of sudden, unexplained deaths in patients with epilepsy not receiving gabapentin, according to the manufacturer. The most common adverse effects associated with the use of gabapentin in combination with other antiepileptic drugs were sleepiness, dizziness, ataxia, fatigue, and nystagmus (*see*). Antacids reduce the effectiveness of gabapentin by about 20 percent and should be taken at least two hours later. Gabapentin should be taken exactly as prescribed and should not be stopped suddenly. May be taken with or without food.

GALACTAGOGUE • A compound that aids the flow of milk in breast-feeding mothers. Among the herbs used for this purpose are blessed thistle and vervain (*see both*).

GALANGAL (H) • *Alpinia officinarum.* **Lesser Galangal.** An herb native to China, the rhizomes are unearthed in late summer and early autumn, cut into segments, and dried. Used by some Chinese herbalists to break up intestinal gas, and to treat heartburn and nausea.

GALEGA (OTC) • *Galega officinalis.* In 1992, the FDA issued a notice that galega, a Eurasian herb, had not been shown to be safe and effective as claimed in OTC digestive-aid products. The herb's seeds have long been used by herbalists to treat stomach disorders. *See* Goat's Rue.

GALLIUM APARINE • *See* Cleavers.

GALLAMINE (Rx) • **Flaxedil.** A muscle relaxant used as an adjunct to anesthesia. Potential adverse reactions include rapid heartbeat, respiratory paralysis, muscle weakness, and allergic or unusual hypersensitivity.

GALLSTONES • Solid material that forms in the gallbladder or bile ducts. The gallbladder is a saclike organ underlying the liver, in which bile, which helps to process fats, is stored and concentrated, then delivered to the digestive tract as needed.

GAMASTAN • *See* Immune Serum Globulin.

GAMBOGE • Banned as an ingredient in laxatives by the FDA, May 1992.

GAMIMUNE N • *See* Immune Serum Globulin.

GAMMA-AMINOBUTYRIC ACID • **GABA.** An amino acid that serves as the principal inhibitor of nerve message transmission in the brain.

GAMMA BENZENE HEXACHLORIDE • *See* Lindane.

GAMMACORTEN • *See* Dexamethasone.

GAMMAGARD • *See* Immune Serum Globulin.

GAMMA GLOBULIN (Rx) • **Immune Globulin.** A type of blood protein that includes antibodies (*see*). Gamma globulins can be extracted from donated blood to treat infections such as hepatitis. *See also* Immune Serum Globulin.

GAMMAR • *See* Immune Serum Globulin.

GAN CAO • *See* Licorice.

GANCICLOVIR (Rx) • **Cymevene. Cytovene. GCV Sodium.** An antiviral introduced in 1989 used to treat cytomegalovirus (CMV) (*see*) infection of the eyes, including in those with AIDS. Ganciclovir does not cure the eye infection, but helps to keep it under control. It should be administered under supervision of experienced medical personnel. It has only been administered intravenously. An oral formulation was approved for marketing in 1994. The oral medication is indicated for maintenance therapy of CMV retinitis. In clinical studies, oral ganciclovir was associated with a moderately faster progression of CMV than with the IV formulation, and a decision has to be made whether more rapid disease progression is balanced by the benefit associated with avoiding daily IV infusions. Potential side effects of ganciclovir include blood problems including anemia, confusion, dizziness, headache, nausea, vomiting, diarrhea, loss of appetite, blood in the urine, injection-site inflammation, and retinal detachment. Probenecid increases ganciclovir blood levels. Zidovudine increases its blood side effects. Ganciclovir may increase seizure activity if used with imipenem or cilastatin.

GANGLION • A cluster of nerve cells.

GANGRENE • Death of tissue due to loss of nutritive supply followed by bacterial invasion.

GAN JIANG • *See* Ginger.

GANTANOL • *See* Sulfamethoxazole.

GANTRISIN • *See* Sulfisoxazole.

GARAMYCIN • *See* Gentamicin.

GARDEN HELIOTROPE • *See* Valerian.

GARLIC (H) • *Allium sativum.* **Hu Suan. Kyolic.** A member of the onion family, garlic has been cultivated in Egypt from earliest times and was known in China more than two thousand years ago. Herbalists have long used garlic to treat respiratory infections and flu. Ancient herbalists made a syrup of garlic and honey to treat colds, coughs, asthma, and bronchitis. Hippocrates used garlic to treat pneumonia and infected wounds. Garlic was used during the Great Plague in Europe, and during World War I in the treatment of typhus and dysentery. Albert Schweitzer used garlic effectively against typhus, cholera, and typhoid. Garlic contains lots of potassium, fluorine, sulfur, phosphorus, and vitamins A and C. It has recently been found to contain antibiotic, antiviral, and antifungal ingredients. Many modern studies have reported that garlic can lower blood serum cholesterol and triglyceride levels, decrease the ability of platelets to clot, and possibly lower high blood pressure. It is theorized that garlic expands blood vessels. It has also been reported in scientific literature that garlic may decrease nitrosamine formation (a powerful cancer-causing agent created when nitrates combine with natural amines in the stomach), modulate cancer-cell multiplication, increase immunity, and protect the body against ionizing radiation. In 1992, at the American Chemical Society meeting in Washington, D.C., three Rutgers University researchers reported that chemicals in garlic may protect the liver from damage caused by large doses of the painkiller acetaminophen and may prevent growth of lung tumors associated with tobacco smoke. Such research reports have been criticized by other scientists, who say that it is difficult to do double-blind studies in which neither the subjects nor the scientists know which compound contains the placebo and which the garlic.

GASTR-, GASTRO- • Prefixes meaning pertaining to the stomach.

GASTRIC (STOMACH) ULCER • An open sore on the lining of the stomach.

GASTRITIS • Inflammation of the stomach lining.

GASTROCROM • *See* Cromolyn Sodium.

GASTROENTERITIS • An inflammation of the stomach and intestines, producing symptoms such as diarrhea, abdominal cramps, nausea, vomiting, and fever. Among the causes are infections, food poisoning, parasites, allergies, bacteria, viruses, and toxins.

GASTROESOPHAGEAL REFLUX DISEASE (GERD) • A chronic condition that occurs when stomach acid abnormally backs up into the esophagus. Symptoms include chronic heartburn, regurgitation of acid in the mouth, pain or difficulty in swallowing, or cough.

GASTROINTESTINAL • Pertaining to the stomach and intestines.

GASTROSED • *See* Hyoscyamine.

GAS-X • *See* Simethicone.

GAVISCON (OTC) • **Algenic Alka Liquid. Parviscon.** An antacid compound that contains aluminum hydroxide, alginic acid, and sodium bicarbonate (*see all*), it is promoted as covering the esophagus (*see*) 50 percent better than other antacids and allowing fewer acid refluxes (backup of acid in the throat). Because Gaviscon floats, it is said to remain in the stomach longer, thus neutralizing acid longer. The FDA approves it for relief of heartburn, sour stomach, and/or acid indigestion, and upset stomach associated with heartburn. It contains salt and should not be used by those on sodium-restricted diets. Prolonged use of aluminum-containing antacids in patients with kidney failure may result in worsening of bone-softening and pain and may cause brain dysfunction in patients on dialysis. It may also reduce the amount of phosphate in normal people, potentially leading to muscle weakness, loss of appetite, malaise, and softening of the bones. Gaviscon should not be taken with tetracycline, digoxin, phenytoin, quinidine, warfarin, or oral iron supplements because it affects absorption of these and other drugs. If necessary, Gaviscon should be taken one to two hours before taking another medication so that it does not affect absorption of the latter. For best effects, tablets should be chewed or the liquid form taken, followed by half a glass of water.

GBH • *See* Lindane.

G-CSF (Rx) • **Granulocyte-Colony Stimulating Factor. Amgen. Filgrastim.** A protein that stimulates proliferation of white blood cells from bone marrow. It is used to fight infections in patients with malignant and infective diseases. Potential adverse reactions include bleeding, loss of hair, worsening of preexisting conditions, skeletal pain, fever, enlargement of the spleen, and osteoporosis.

GCV SODIUM • *See* Ganciclovir.

GDNF • *See* Glial Cell–Derived Neurotrophic Factor.

GEE-GEE • *See* Guaifenesin.

GELIDIUM POLYPORUS • *See* Agar.

GEL II • *See* Sodium Fluoride.

GEL-KAM • *See* Sodium Fluoride.

GELS • Homeopathic abbreviation for gelsemium (*see*).

GELSEMIUM (H) • **False Jasmine. Wild Jamine. Yellow Jessamine.** A woody evergreen, *Gelsemium sempervirens,* native to North America. Its root contains indole alkaloids. A homeopathic medicine to treat fear, anxiety, congestive headaches, arthritis, and weariness. Herbalists used it as a sedative and antispasmodic, but it is rarely used now because it is highly toxic in overdose. Symptoms of poisoning include dilated pupils, double vision, difficulty swallowing and talking, shortness of breath, respiratory failure, and death. Children have been poisoned sucking nectar from this plant.

GEL-TIN • *See* Sodium Fluoride.

GELUCAST • *See* Zinc Gelatin.

GELUSIL (OTC) • *See* Aluminum Hydroxide and Simethicone.

GEMFIBROZIL (Rx) • **Lopid.** A fat-regulating agent introduced in 1976 that decreases serum triglycerides and low-density lipoprotein (LDL) cholesterol and increases high-density lipoprotein (HDL) cholesterol. In some patients with elevated triglycerides due to Type IV hyperlipoproteinemia, the drug often results in a rise in low-density cholesterol. It should not be used in patients with liver or severe kidney dysfunction, gallbladder disease, or hypersensitivity to gemfibrozil. The potential benefit of gemfibrozil in treating elevations of cholesterol has to be carefully evaluated to outweigh the risks due to potential adverse effects such as malignancy, gallbladder disease, abdominal pain leading to appendectomy and other abdominal surgeries, an increased incidence in noncoronary mortality, and a 39 percent increase in all-cause mortality seen with the chemically and pharmacologically related drug clofibrate. Other potential adverse reactions include heartburn, abdominal pain, diarrhea, fatigue, nausea and vomiting, eczema, dizziness, constipation, headache, jaundice, depression, blurred vision, impotence, muscle pain, anemia, depressed libido, allergic reactions, and rash. Concomitant therapy with gemfibrozil and lovastatin (Mevacor) has been associated with kidney failure, and with rhabdomyolysis, an acute, fulminating, potentially fatal disease of skeletal muscle. The effects of oral blood thinners may be increased with gemfibrozil. Gemfibrozil may raise blood sugar levels, reducing the effectiveness of diabetes medications. Most effective when taken on an empty stomach. Gemfibrozil is produced generically.

GEMONIL • *See* Metharbital.

-GEN- • Producing, begetting, as in *generating*.

GENABID • *See* Papaverine Hydrochloride.

GENAC • *See* Triprolidine and Pseudoephedrine.

GENAGESIC • *See* Propoxyphene and Acetaminophen.

GENALAC • *See* Calcium Carbonate.

GENALLERATE • *See* Chlorpheniramine.

GENAPAP (OTC) • *See* Acetaminophen.

GENAPAX (Rx) • Vaginal tampons containing gentian violet (*see*).

GENASAL NASAL SOLUTION (OTC) • *See* Oxymetazoline.

GENE • The smallest genetic unit of a chromosome. It is a piece of DNA that contains the hereditary information for the production of a protein.

GENEBS • *See* Acetaminophen.

GENE MAPPING • Locating genes on a chromosome so scientists know which genes control which traits.

GENERIC DRUG • Drug not protected by a trademark. The generic name is distinct from a brand name chosen by a manufacturer for a particular product. Generic names are coined by committees of officially appointed drug experts and are approved by government agencies for national and international use.

GENETIC ENGINEERING • A type of biotechnology (*see*) that involves the alteration of genetic material carried by a living organism to produce some desired change in that organism or to influence the products it makes. Production of a particular protein in a living cell is under the control of specific genes. Most genetic engineering, as of this writing, has been used to mass produce large therapeutic pharmaceutical molecules. Some of the medical treatments developed through genetic engineering include human hormones, such as insulin and growth hormone; a protein—factor VIII—used to treat hemophilia; and tissue plasminogen activator (T-PA), which dissolves blood clots.

GENISTEIN (Rx) (H) • A plant estrogen found in the urine of people with diets rich in soybeans and to a lesser extent in the cabbage-family vegetables, this compound seems to block the growth of new blood vessels, essential for some tumors to grow and spread. Sheep grazing on some clovers are prone to reproductive failure because of genistein in the plants. It is now being tested against breast cancer in the United States.

GEN-K • *See* Potassium Chloride.

GENOME • The genetic information contained in one complete set of chromosomes.

GENOPTIC • *See* Gentamicin.

GENORA • *See* Estradiol and Norethindrone.

GENOTROPIN • *See* Somatotropin.

GENOTYPE • The hereditary makeup or genetic constitution of an individual organism, distinguished from its physical appearance or visible traits (phenotype).

GENPRIL • *See* Ibuprofen.

GENTACIDIN • *See* Gentamicin.

GENTAFAIR • *See* Gentamicin.

GENTAK • *See* Gentamicin.

GENTAMICIN (Rx) • **Garamycin. Genoptic. Gentacidin. Gentafair. Gentamicin Sulfate. Gentrasul. I-Gent. Jenamicin. Ocu-Mycin. Spectro-Genta.** An antibiotic used against serious infections caused by *Pseudomonas aeruginosa, Escherichia coli, Porteus, Klebsiella, Serratia, Enterobacter, Citrobacter,* and *Staphylococcus* (*see all*). In eyedrops and ointments, it is used to treat eye and eyelid infections. In skin creams or ointments, it is used to treat superficial burns, infected insect bites and stings, infected lacerations, and abrasions and wounds from minor surgery. Potential adverse reactions include headache, lethargy, muscle dysfunction, kidney dysfunction, urinary-tract problems, liver damage, and allergic reactions. In eye preparations, it may cause burning, stinging, blurred vision, transient irritation, overgrowth of resistant organisms with long-term use, and allergic reactions. In skin preparations, it may cause minor skin irritation, possible sensitivity to light, and allergic rash. A wide range of drugs increase the risk of hearing loss and/or kidney failure with gentamicin. Such drugs include aminoglycosides (*see*), cephalothin, dimenhydrinate, general anesthetics, local anesthetics, loop diuretics such as furosemide (*see*), and penicillins given intravenously.

GENTIAN, YELLOW (H) • *Gentiana lutea.* **Baldmoney. Felwort. Field Gentian.** An annual plant that grows in dry, chalky soil in Great Britain, it is used in modern medicine. Herbalists make an infusion of the root and rhizome as a digestive tonic for heartburn or gas after eating. They also use it to stimulate the appetite. In 1992, the FDA proposed a ban on *Gentiana lutea* in oral menstrual drug products because it had not been shown to be safe and effective as claimed.

GENTIANA LUTEA • *See* Gentian, Yellow.

GENTIAN VIOLET (OTC) • **Genapax. Methylrosaniline Chloride Crystal Violet.** A tampon and topical dye solution obtained from coal tar. Used to treat fungus and bacterial infections of the skin, face, and vagina. Potential adverse reactions include permanent discoloration if applied to roughened tissue, and irritation or ulceration of mucous membranes.

GENTLE NATURE • *See* Senna.

GENTRAN 40 • *See* Dextran.

GENTRASUL • *See* Gentamicin.

GEN-XENE • *See* Clorazepate.

GEOCILLIN • *See* Carbenicillin Disodium.

GEOPEN • *See* Carbenicillin Disodium.

GERAVITE (OTC) • A multivitamin preparation.

GERD • Abbreviation for gastroesophageal reflux disease (*see*).

GERIATRICS • From the Greek *geras,* meaning old age, and *iatrikos,* meaning healing; a branch of medicine concerned with the problems and care of older people.

GERIDIUM • *See* Phenazopyridine Hydrochloride.

GERIMAL • *See* Ergoloid Mesylates.

GERIMED (OTC) • A multivitamin and multimineral supplement targeted at older people.

GERIPLEX (OTC) • A multivitamin preparation with iron targeted at older people.

GERITOL (OTC) • A multivitamin preparation with iron targeted at older people.

GERMANDER (H) • *Teucrium chamaedrys.* **Wall Germander.** A member of the mint family, it has long been used by herbalists, as far back as Hippocrates and Pliny. The Greeks used it as a tonic. In the mid-eighteenth century, herbalists used it to treat gout. It is an astringent, antiseptic, diuretic, and stimulant and has been used in the treatment of jaundice, excess fluid due to heart failure, and ailments of the spleen. It continues to be used in folk medicine to heal ulcers and sores. Cases of its use in tea or capsules have been reported to the Centers for Disease Control as causing liver toxicity.

GERMANIUM (Rx) (H) • **Suma.** A naturally occurring isotope in the earth's crust, it is recovered from residues from the refining of zinc and from other sources. It is also present in some coals. It is used in infrared transmitting glass and electronic devices.

GERMPLASM • The total genetic variability available in particular populations of an organism, usually represented by the seeds or reproductive cells, such as eggs and sperm—also called germ cells.

GER-O-FOAM • *See* Benzocaine and Methyl Salicylate.

GESTEROL 50 • *See* Progesterone.

GESTEROL LA • *See* Hydroxyprogesterone.

GG • *See* Guaifenesin.

GG-CEN • *See* Guaifenesin.

GHRH • Abbreviation for growth hormone–releasing hormone. *See* Growth Hormone.

GI • Abbreviation for gastrointestinal, relating to the stomach and the intestines.

GINGER (OTC) (H) • *Zingiber officinale.* **Gan Jiang.** Native to Asia but cultivated in many parts of the tropics. Hippocrates used ginger as a medicine. Ginger tea is soothing for colds and sore throats. The herb is used to treat low blood sugar. It increases the availability of dietary nutrients for digestion and metabolism. Gingerroot is used by herbalists to treat headaches, diarrhea, and nausea, including motion sickness. Some studies have shown that gingerroot is a mild stimulant for the heart and brain and may even help ease learning. Ginger tea is widely used as a remedy for colds, producing perspiration, and for inducing menstruation if suppressed by a cold. Externally, ginger is a rubefacient (*see*) and has been credited with relieving toothache. Modern studies have shown that ginger inhibits prostaglandins, as do NSAIDs (*see both*), and thus reduces inflammation. Japanese scientists have found that extract of ginger inhibits stomach lesions. They concluded that the use of ginger in folk medicine was effective because of a constituent, zingiberone. Scientists have also found that ginger slows the formation of platelet clumping and thus may help to prevent blood clots. In 1992, the FDA issued a notice that ginger had not been shown to be safe and effective as claimed in OTC digestive-aid products. Contraindicated in persons with acute bowel disorder. It should also be avoided in individuals suffering from skin disease. An excessive dose can cause irritation of the mucous membrane lining of the stomach. It can also promote menstruation.

GINGIVITIS • Condition in which the gums are red, swollen, and bleeding. It most often results from poor oral hygiene and development of plaque on the teeth. If untreated, gingivitis can cause infection and tooth loss.

GINKGO (H) • *Ginkgo biloba.* **Ginkgold. Maidenhair.** The leaves and nuts are used in an ancient Chinese remedy for upper-respiratory problems, including asthma and allergies. The ginkgo is supposedly the oldest living species of tree, having survived some 200 million years. It is reportedly the only tree that survived the effects of atomic radiation in Hiroshima. Ginkgo has been found to improve circulation, mental functioning, relieve ringing in the ears, and to relieve symptoms of Alzheimer's disease, coldness, emotional depression, Raynaud's disease, arthritic problems, hardening of the arteries, dizziness, and anxiety. It was synthesized at Harvard into a compound, ginkgolide B, that is being studied as a potential drug to prevent rejection of transplanted organs and combat toxic-shock syndrome. A report in the *Journal of Urology,* 1989, described a study of sixty patients suffering from impotence due to insufficient blood supply to the penis. After six months of daily treatment with an extract of ginkgo, 50 percent of the subjects were again able to achieve erections. Nearly 45 percent of the remaining subjects showed some improvement. Ginkgo has also been reported in recent years in such publications as the British medical journal *Lancet* to have antihistamine properties. Excessive use can cause itching and gastrointestinal upset. In rare instances, excessive doses can induce shortness of breath and convulsions.

GINSENG (H) • *Panax ginseng* **(Asia).** *Panax quinquefolium* **(North America).** *Eleutherococcus senticosus* **(Siberian Ginseng). Jen Shang.** Chinese esteem ginseng as an herb of many uses. *Panax* comes from the Greek word *panakos,* meaning panacea. Among ginseng's active ingredients are amino acids, essential oils, carbohydrates, peptides, vitamins, minerals, enzymes, and sterols. It has been found to normalize high or low blood sugar. In Asia, ginseng is esteemed for its abilities to preserve health, invigorate the system, and prolong life. It is taken in an herbal tea as a daily tonic. North American Indians used ginseng as a love potion. Russian scientists are studying ginseng for the treatment of insomnia and general debility. Japanese scientists recently reported isolating a number of compounds—rare in nature—from ginseng, some of which have anticancer properties, tranquilizing effects, or aphrodisiac properties.

GLAUCIUM (Rx) (H) • *Glaucium flavum.* **Yellow Horned Poppy.** An erect, branched biennial or perennial native to Europe and cultivated in moderate zones. The plant is a source of the alkaloid glaucine, which has been used in the form of tablets in conventional medicine to treat dry cough and asthma. A mixture of alkaloids isolated from this plant has been used to treat gallbladder problems. It has also been used as an antispasmodic and anti-inflammatory. Contraindicated in persons with low blood pressure.

GLAUCOMA • The most common cause of blindness in adults, produced by destructive fluid pressure within the eye. *See* Narrow Angle Glaucoma.

GLAUCON • *See* Epinephrine.

GLIAL CELL–DERIVED NEUROTROPHIC FACTOR • **GDNF.** A substance discovered in 1994 that reportedly preserves and restores two kinds of nerve cells, one in the brain and one in the spinal cord, that activate muscle movement. The substance is now being tested for its potential in the treatment of Parkinson's disease, amyotrophic lateral sclerosis, and Alzheimer's disease (*see all*).

GLIBENCLAMIDE • *See* Glyburide.

GLIMEPIRIDE (Rx) • **Amaryl.** An insulin-sparing sulfonyurea (*see*) agent introduced in 1995. It is a first-line therapy to lower blood glucose in Type II diabetes (*see*) when diet and exercise alone cannot control high blood sugar levels. Amaryl (*see*) is used alone or in combination with insulin.

GLIPIZIDE (Rx) • Glucotrol. Glucotrol XL. A member of the sulfonylurea (*see*) family, introduced in 1972, it is prescribed to reduce blood glucose levels by stimulating the pancreas to produce insulin. Adjunct to diet to lower blood sugar in patients with non-insulin-dependent diabetes. Has a mild diuretic effect. Potential adverse reactions include nausea, vomiting, dizziness, jaundice, low blood sugar, rash, itching, facial flushing, and hypersensitivity reactions. It is a second-generation sulfonylurea and is promoted as having fewer side effects than earlier sulfonylureas. Anabolic steroids (*see*), chloramphenicol, clofibrate, guanethidine, MAO inhibitors (*see*), oral blood thinners, phenylbutazone, salicylates, and sulfonamides increase blood-sugar-lowering activity. Beta-blockers (*see*) and clonidine prolong the low blood sugar effect and may mask symptoms of low blood sugar. Corticosteroids, glucagon, rifampin, and thiazide diuretics decrease the blood-sugar-lowering effect. Contraindicated in treating insulin-dependent diabetes, in diabetes adequately controlled by diet, and in Type II diabetes complicated by ketosis, acidosis, diabetic coma, Raynaud's disease, gangrene, liver or kidney dysfunction, or thyroid or other endocrine dysfunction. The possibility of increased heart deaths is associated with the use of sulfonylureas. If two doses of glipizide are to be taken, one should be with breakfast and the other with dinner. As of this writing, glipizide is scheduled to be produced as a less expensive generic drug. Glucotrol XL is a once-a-day oral treatment for Type II diabetes.

GLON • Homeopathic abbreviation for glonoine (*see*).

GLONOINE (H) • Glon. Nitroglycerine. Homeopaths use it to treat confusion, forgetfulness, and headache. The homeopathic remedy is made from nitroglycerin diluted with alcohol. *See* Nitroglycerin.

GLOSSA-, GLOSSO- • Prefixes from the Greek word *glossa,* meaning tongue.

GLUCAGON (Rx) • Used to treat hypoglycemia, it is a pancreatic enzyme with action opposite to that of insulin. It is involved in glucose metabolism and hunger. Used in insulin-shock therapy for depression, for severe insulin-induced low blood sugar during diabetic therapy; also as a diagnostic aid for X-ray examination. Potential adverse reactions include nausea, vomiting, drowsiness, and hypersensitivity. Phenytoin inhibits glucagon's ability to cause insulin release.

GLUCAMIDE • *See* Chlorpropamide.

GLUCOALKALOID • An organic compound of vegetable origin that has a sugar component.

GLUCOBAY • *See* Acarbose.

GLUCOCORTICOIDS • Introduced in the 1940s, they are synthetic versions of the steroids produced by the adrenal glands. These cortisone-like hormones influence carbohydrate, protein, and fat metabolism. Among the conditions for which glucocorticoids are prescribed are arthritis, asthma, allergies, ulcerative colitis, liver disease, lupus, cancer, and organ transplants. Although one of the most useful and widely prescribed class of drugs, they leach calcium from bone, leading to fragility and fractures. *See* Steroids.

GLUCOPHAGE • *See* Metformin HCL.

GLUCOSAMINE (OTC) (H) • Chitosamine. An amino acid found in chitin (*see*), cell membranes, and protein-b-sugar complexes as found in blood. Research is under way at Dartmouth-Hitchcock Medical Center in the United States and in institutions in Paris, France, to determine if faulty glucosamine metabolism may play a part in the development of osteoarthritis and whether supplementation with glucosamine may be therapeutic.

GLUCOSE • Glutose. Sugar that occurs naturally in blood, grapes, and corn. A source of energy for animals and plants. Sweeter than sucrose. Used medicinally for nutritional purposes and in the treatment of diabetic coma. Also used to soothe the skin.

GLUCOSE TOLERANCE FACTOR • *See* Chromium.

GLUCOSIDES • Compounds with sugar and alcohol.

GLUCOSTIX (OTC) • A diagnostic test for glucose in blood.

GLUCOTROL • *See* Glipizide.

GLUCOTROL XL (Rx) • A newer once-a-day medication for Type II (adult onset) diabetes. *See* Glipizide.

GLU-K • *See* Potassium Gluconate.

GLUKOR • *See* Chorionic Gonadotropin.

GLUTAMIC ACID • **Acidulin.** A nonessential amino acid.

GLUTARAL • An amino acid (*see*) that occurs in green beets. Used in creams and emollients as a skin antiseptic.

GLUTATHIONE S-TRANSFERASE • **GST.** Cloves, caraway, dill weed, parsley, lemongrass oil, and celery have been found to have significant amounts of substances that stimulate the production of glutathione S-transferase in the body, a detoxifying enzyme that can combat cancer-causing agents.

GLUTEN INTOLERANCE • *See* Celiac Sprue.

GLUTETHIMIDE (Rx) • **Doriden. Doriglute.** A sleep medication whose mechanism of action is unknown. Potential adverse reactions include hangover, dizziness, loss of balance, paradoxical excitation, headache, dizziness, dry mouth, blurred vision, stomach irritation, nausea, bladder problems, rash, and hives. Contraindicated in uncontrolled pain, severe kidney impairment, or porphyria (*see*). Must be used cautiously in mental depression, suicidal tendencies, history of drug abuse, enlarged prostate, peptic ulcer, bladder-neck obstruction, glaucoma, and irregular heart-beat. Abrupt withdrawal may produce nausea, vomiting, nervousness, tremors, chills, fever, nightmares, insomnia, numbness of the limbs, and seizures. Use with alcohol or other central nervous system depressants, including narcotic analgesics, may cause increased central nervous system depression. May decrease the effectiveness of oral blood thinners. Glutethimide is effective for short-term use only.

GLUTOSE • Used to treat low blood sugar. *See* Glucose.

GLYATE • *See* Guaifenesin.

GLYBURIDE (Rx) • **DiaBeta. Glibenclamide. Glynase-PresTab. Micronase.** An oral antidiabetes sulfonylurea (*see*) medicine introduced in 1970 for long-term blood sugar control. It stimulates insulin release from the pancreatic beta cells and reduces glucose output by the liver. Also reportedly reduces liver sugar production and enhances tissue uptake of blood glucose. The administration of oral diabetes medications has been reported to be associated with increased heart and blood-vessel deaths as compared to treatment with diet alone or diet plus insulin. The blood-sugar-lowering effects of glyburide may be potentiated by certain drugs, including NSAIDs, salicylates, sulfonamides, chloramphenicol, probenecid, coumarin, monoamine oxidase inhibitors, and beta-blockers (*see all*). Among other potential adverse reactions are jaundice, nausea, bloating, heartburn, liver dysfunction, allergic skin reactions, low sodium, and disulfiram-like reactions. Contraindicated in patients with known hypersensitivity to glyburide or in diabetic ketoacidosis with or without coma. Most effective when taken on an empty stomach. As of this writing, glyburide is scheduled to be produced as a less expensive generic drug.

GLYCATE (OTC) • *See* Calcium Carbonate.

GLYCERIDES • Any of a large class of compounds that are esters (*see*) of the sweet alcohol glycerin. They also are made synthetically. Used in cosmetic creams as texturizers and emollients.

GLYCERIN (Rx) (OTC) • Glycerol. Glyrol. Osmoglyn. Aqua Care Cream. Clear Eyes Lubricating. Collyrium Fresh. Dry Eye Therapy. Fleet Babylax. Moisture Drops. Neutrogena Cleansing Wash. Ophthalgan. Sani-Supp. Any by-product of soap manufacture, it is a sweet, warm-tasting, oily fluid obtained by adding alkalies (*see*) to fats and fixed oils. An ingredient in cough mixtures, bases for skin preparations, artificial tears (*see*), suppositories, earwax-softening drips, enemas, and laxative suppositories. (Glycerin draws water from the tissues into the feces, thus stimulating evacuation. Potential adverse reactions include cramping, rectal discomfort, and irritation of the rectal mucosa. Suppositories or enemas should be retained for at least fifteen minutes. Acts usually within one hour.) In eyedrops, it is used to remove excess fluid from the cornea. In concentrated solutions, glycerin is irritating to the mucous membranes, but in gentle solutions it is nontoxic, nonirritating, and nonallergenic. In eye solutions, however, it can cause pain if instilled without a topical anesthetic. In 1992, the FDA issued a notice that glycerin had not been shown to be safe and effective as claimed in OTC poison ivy, poison oak, and poison sumac products, as well as in diaper rash drug products.

GLYCEROL • *See* Glycerin.

GLYCERYL GUAIACOLATE • *See* Guaifenesin.

GLYCERYL TRIACETATE • *See* Triacetin.

GLYCERYL TRINITRATE • *See* Nitroglycerin.

GLYCINE • A nonessential amino acid, usually derived from gelatin. In 1992, the FDA issued a notice that glycine had not been shown to be safe and effective as claimed in OTC digestive-aid products.

GLYCO- • Prefix from the Greek word *glyks,* for sweet, referring to sugar.

GLYCOGEN • The liver manufactures glycogen from sugar, stores it, then releases it to meet the body's energy requirements.

GLYCOL SALICYLATE (OTC) • A compound made up of glycerin, alcohol, and salicylate (*see all*). In 1992, the FDA proposed a ban for the use of glycol salicylate to treat fever blisters and cold sores, and poison ivy, poison oak, and poison sumac, because it had not been shown to be safe and effective as claimed in OTC products.

GLYCOPYRROLATE (Rx) • **Robinul.** An anticholinergic, antispasmodic drug used to treat irritable bowel syndrome, and as an adjunctive therapy in peptic ulcers and other GI disorders. Potential adverse reactions include disorientation, irritability, incoherence, weakness, nervousness, drowsiness, dizziness, headache, palpitations, rapid heartbeat, slow heartbeat, blurred vision, sensitivity to light, increased eye pressure, difficulty in swallowing, constipation, dry mouth, nausea, vomiting, epigastric distress, urinary retention, impotence, hives, decreased sweating, and fever. Contraindicated in glaucoma, obstructions in the urinary or GI tract, myasthenia gravis (*see*), paralytic ileus (*see*), intestinal flaccidity, unstable cardiovascular status in acute hemorrhage, and toxic megacolon. Should be used with caution in patients with nerve damage, overactive thyroid, coronary artery disease, irregular heartbeat, congestive heart failure, high blood pressure, hiatal hernia, liver or kidney disease, and ulcerative colitis. Should also be used with caution in people over forty years of age due to the possibility of glaucoma. Should be taken thirty minutes to one hour before meals.

GLYCOSIDES (Rx) (H) • A class of drugs used in heart failure. Many flowering plants contain cardiac glycosides. The best known are foxglove, lily of the valley, and squill. Cardiac glycosides increase the force and power of the heartbeat without increasing the amount of oxygen needed by the heart muscle. Among the glycosides in plants are cyanogens, goitrogens, estrogens, and saponins. They are found in lima beans, cassava, flax, legumes, broccoli and other brassicas, and grasses.

GLYCOSURIA • The presence of an abnormal amount of glucose (sugar) in the urine.

GLYCOTUSS (OTC) • An expectorant cough medication containing guaifenesin (*see*).

GLYCYRRHIZA GLABRA • *See* Licorice.

GLYNASE-PRES TAB (Rx) • A formulation with glyburide, introduced in 1992, that is easy to divide and reportedly allows a more consistent dose of the drug. *See* Glyburide.

GLY-OXIDE • *See* Carbamide Peroxide.

GLYROL • *See* Glycerin.

GM-CSF (Rx) • Granulocyte-macrophage colony stimulating factor; a cytokine (*see*) that promotes the growth and differentiation of infection-fighting white blood cells.

GnRH • Abbreviation for gonadotropin-releasing hormone. *See* Gonadotropin, Human Chorionic.

GOAT'S RUE (H) • *Galega officinalis.* This plant contains alkaloids, saponins, flavones, glycosides, bitters, and tannin (*see all*). It is used to reduce blood sugar levels. Also a powerful milk inducer in breast-feeding women. It has long been used to treat early stages of diabetes. The plant extract reduces blood sugar level, but its action is weak and the effect gradual. Goat's rue preparations show synergistic effects with some synthetic antidiabetic agents.

-GOGUE • Suffix that means eliciting a flow, such as in *cholagogue,* stimulating the emission of bile.

GOITER • An enlargement of the thyroid gland.

GOLD-50 • *See* Aurothioglucose.

GOLDENROD (H) • *Solidago virgauria.* A perennial that includes 125 species, it was valued for its medicinal properties by herb women in Elizabethan London. The name *Solidago* means "makes whole" and herbalists claim it helps to heal wounds, and in fact, at one time it was called woundwort. It is used by herbalists as an antiseptic. Used in an herbal tea as a tonic to improve general health and to allay morning sickness. The pulped leaves, stalks, and flowers are good for staunching blood. The American Indians used goldenrod to treat bee stings.

GOLDENSEAL (H) • *Hydrastis canadensis.* **Yellow Puccoon. Yellow Root.** The American Indians were the first to use it for sore eyes. Early pioneers, along with many Indian tribes, used it as a general tonic. The rhizome and root are used by herbalists to treat heartburn and acid indigestion, colitis, duodenal ulcers, heavy menstrual periods, and as a general tonic for the female reproductive tract. Goldenseal is also used for penile discharge, eczema, and skin disorders. Herbalists claim it dries and cleanses the mucous membranes and is good for liver dysfunction, and for all inflammations. It contains berberine (*see*) and reputedly has potent antibiotic and antiseptic properties. Contraindicated during pregnancy and for persons suffering from high blood pressure and ischemia (insufficient blood flow). In 1992, the FDA issued a notice that *Hydrastis canadensis* and hydrastis fluid extract have not been shown to be safe and effective as claimed in OTC digestive-aid products and oral menstrual products. It should be used on the skin with caution because strong extracts may cause ulceration.

GOLD SALTS (Rx) • **Myochrysine. Ridaura. Solganal.** Gold can be effective for active rheumatoid arthritis and may delay or prevent progression of joint erosion in some patients. Gold sodium thiomalate (Myochrysine) and aurothioglucose (Solganal) are two injectable preparations available in the United States. An oral preparation, auranofin (Ridaura), is also available, but is reportedly less effective than injectable gold and frequently causes diarrhea. Injectable gold causes many adverse effects. The most common are inflammation of the mucous membranes of the mouth, rash, kidney dysfunction, potentially fatal colitis, inflammation of the lungs, aplastic anemia, flushing, weakness, nausea, and dizziness.

GOLD SODIUM THIOMALATE • *See* Aurothioglucose.

GoLYTELY (Rx) • A preparation for cleansing the bowel before investigative procedures; contains polyethylene glycol (*see*) and salts of sodium and potassium. *See also* Laxative.

GONADORELIN (Rx) • **LRA. Lutrepulse.** An injectable gonadotropin, it mimics the action of gonadotropin-releasing hormone (*see*), which releases luteinizing hormone from the pituitary gland, thus enabling the reproductive organs to regulate hormone production. Used to induce ovulation in women with primary hypothalamic absence of menstruation. Potential adverse reactions include overstimulation of the ovary and multiple pregnancy. Contraindicated in patients hypersensitive to the drug, any women with conditions that could be complicated by pregnancy, patients who are without functioning ovary from any cause other than hypothalamic disorder, and in patients with ovarian cysts.

GONADORELIN (Rx) • **Factrel. Gonadotropin-Releasing Hormone, GnRH. Luteinizing Hormone-Releasing Hormone.** A synthetic injectable gonadotropin used to evaluate the functional capacity of the gonadotropins in the pituitary gland. It mimics the action of gonadotropin-releasing hormone, which releases luteinizing hormone from the pituitary gland, thus enabling the reproductive organs to regulate hormone production. Potential adverse reactions include headache, flushing, light-headedness, nausea, abdominal discomfort, and local swelling and itching. Digoxin and oral contraceptives may depress gonadotropin levels.

GONADOTROPIN, HUMAN CHORIONIC (Rx) • **HCG. Antuitrin. A.P.L. Chorex. Follutein. Gonic. Pregnyl. Profasi HP.** An injectable substitute for luteinizing hormone, to stimulate ovulation of a human menopausal gonadotropin-prepared follicle. Also promotes secretion of gonadal steroid hormones by stimulating production of androgen by the interstitial cells of the testes. Used to treat infertility, lack of ovulation, and hypogonadism (*see*) in males. Potential adverse reactions include headache, fatigue, irritability, restlessness, depression, early puberty, enlargement of male breast, and edema. Contraindicated in pituitary problems, prostatic cancer, and early puberty (usually between ten and thirteen years of age). Should be used cautiously in epilepsy, migraine, asthma, and heart or kidney disease. Chorionic gonadotropin is banned and tested for by the United States Olympic Committee and the National Collegiate Athletic Association.

GONADS • The primary sex glands, ovaries and testes.

GONAK • *See* Hydroxypropyl Methylcellulose.

G-1 (Rx) • A combination of acetaminophen, butalbital, and caffeine (*see all*), used as a painkiller.

GONIC • *See* Gonadotropin.

GONIOSOL • *See* Hydroxypropyl Methylcellulose.

GONORRHEA • The most common venereal disease, an infection produced by sphere-shaped bacteria.

GORDOLOBO YERBA TEA (H) • Has been reported to be toxic to the liver. *See* Yerba Santa Fluid Extract.

GOSERELIN (Rx) • **Zoladex.** A luteinizing hormone-releasing hormone (*see* LHRH) analog that acts on the pituitary gland to decrease the release of hormones affecting the ovary. A new version has an implant that lasts for three months. In males, the result is to dramatically lower blood levels of the male hormone testosterone. Used in the palliative treatment of advanced cancer of the prostate and breast cancer. Potential adverse reactions include anemia, lethargy, pain, dizziness, insomnia, anxiety, depression, headache, chills, fever, fluid retention, congestive heart failure, irregular heartbeat, stroke, high blood pressure, heart attack, blood-vessel disorders, chest pain, upper-respiratory infection, nausea, vomiting, diarrhea, constipation, ulcer, decreased erections, lower-urinary-tract symptoms, kidney dysfunction, rash, sweating, hot flashes, sexual dysfunction, gout, high blood sugar, weight increase, and breast swelling and tenderness.

GOTU COLA • *See* Gotu Kola.

GOTU KOLA (H) • *Centella asiatica.* **Asiatic Pennywort. Gotu Cola. Thickleaved.** An herb grown in Pakistan, India, Malaysia, and parts of Eastern Europe, it is commonly used for diseases of the skin, blood, and nervous system. In homeopathy, it is used for psoriasis, cervicitis, pruritus vaginitis, blisters, and other skin conditions. Gotu kola is used in the Far East to treat leprosy and tuberculosis. Also used as a sedative. It is toxic in large overdose or as a result of long-term use. It can produce narcotic effects, headache, vertigo, and in some sensitive individuals may even lead to coma. It can also cause photosensitivity (*see*).

GOUT • **Arthritis Nodosa.** An inherited disorder of purine metabolism, occurring mostly in men. Involves a high level of uric acid and sudden, severe onset of arthritis resulting from deposits of crystals of sodium urate in connective tissue and cartilage. The feet, ankles, and knees are commonly affected.

GRAMICIDIN (Rx) • **Cortisporin Cream. Mycolog II Cream. Neosporin. Neosporin Ophthalmic Solution. Spectrocin Ointment.** Introduced in 1949, it is a naturally occurring antibiotic produced by bacteria. Available only in combined preparations, it is used with other antibiotics to treat skin and eye infections. Some gramicidin medications contain corticosteroids (*see*) to relieve itching and inflammation. Gramicidin is also combined with antifungal drugs such as nystatin (*see*) to treat mixed fungal and bacterial infections. Potential adverse reactions include rash and irritation.

GRAM-POSITIVE, -NEGATIVE • A classification of bacteria according to whether or not they accept a stain named after Hans Gram, a Danish bacteriologist. Different life processes and vulnerabilities of germs are reflected by their gram-positive or gram-negative characteristics. An antibiotic may be effective against certain gram-positive germs and have no effect on gram-negative ones and vice versa.

GRANISETRON (Rx) • An adjunct to chemotherapy for cancers of the breast, colon, lung, pancreas, and prostate. Expected to be approved.

GRANULOCYTE • A type of white blood cell produced in bone marrow that destroys bacteria.

GRANULOMATOUS DISEASE • Small nodular inflammatory lesions caused by bacteria, fungi, and parasites.

GRANULOCYTE COLONY STIMULATING FACTOR • *See* G-CSF.

GRATIOLA (H) • *Gratiola officinalis.* **Hedge Hyssop.** A hairless perennial native to Europe and introduced to western Asia and North America, it is used by homeopathic physicians for the treatment of arthritis and urinary-tract ailments. It is also used by herbalists to treat constipation and eczema. Contraindicated during pregnancy. It can cause miscarriage. The plant is a hazardous heart poison and should be used only under medical supervision.

GRAVELROOT (H) • *Eupatorium purpureum.* **Joe-Pye Weed. Queen-of-the-Meadow.** The root is used by herbalists to treat kidney, bladder, stomach, and liver complaints. It is used particularly to treat gravel stones in the urinary tract and to reduce the frequency of nighttime urination.

GRAVOL • *See* Dimenhydrinate.

GREAT BURNET (H) • *Sanguisorba officinalis.* Used in medieval medicine as an astringent herb to stop hemorrhage. Also used in salves for ulcers and wounds.

GREATER CELANDINE • *See* Celandine.

GRECORT • *See* Hydrocortisone.

GREEN TEA • *See* Tea.

GRIFULVIN V • *See* Griseofulvin.

GRINDELIA (H) • *Grindelia camporum.* California Gum. Curly Cup. The genus *Grindelia* contains some twenty-five species. They are coarse perennial or biennial herbs. The principal use of grindelia is for the treatment of inflammation of the bronchial tubes, particularly in asthma. It is reputed to act as an expectorant and antispasmodic. In topical poultices and solution, grindelia is used by herbalists to treat burns, vaginitis, and genitourinary membrane infections and inflammations. Also used to treat poison ivy and other rashes. Excessive doses can cause irritation of the urinary tract and kidney and disrupt the heart rhythm. Contraindicated in persons with kidney disorders, heart failure, or gastrointestinal inflammation.

GRISACTIN • *See* Griseofulvin.

GRISEOFULVIN (Rx) • Fulvicin P/G. Fulvicin-U/F. Grifulvin V. Grisactin. Grisactin Ultra. Griseostatin. Grisovin 500. Grisovin-FP. Gris-PEG. Arrests fungal-cell activity. Introduced in the late 1950s, it is used to combat ringworm infections of skin, scalp, and nails (tinea corporis, tinea capitis, and tinea unguium) when caused by *Trichophyton, Microsporum,* or *Epidermophyton.* Adverse reactions include a drop in white blood cells, headache, temporary hearing problems, fatigue, occasional mental confusion, impaired performance of routine activities, psychotic symptoms, dizziness, and insomnia. May also cause nausea, vomiting, thirst, bloating, and diarrhea. In addition to rashes and hives, it may cause estrogenlike effects in children and oral thrush (*see*) and may also aggravate lupus erythematosus (*see*). May interact with alcohol, barbiturates, blood thinners, and oral contraceptives. Because it may cause liver dysfunction and affect bone marrow, it is prescribed only when other less toxic drugs have failed.

GRIS-PEG • *See* Griseofulvin.

GROUND IVY (H) • *Glechoma hederacea.* Alehoof. Benth. Cat's Foot. Devil's Candlesticks. Hale House. Hay House. Hay Maids. Hedge Maids. May House. Thunder Vine. Tun-Hoof. A common plant on wastelands, it contains tannin, volatile oil, bitter principle, and saponin (*see all*). It is used by herbalists for cough, headache, and backache caused by sluggishness of the liver or obstruction of the kidneys. Also used to treat bronchitis. Mixed with yarrow, the herb makes a poultice that has been used by folk doctors for "gathering tumors," clearing the head, and relieving backache. The astringency of the herb helps in the treatment of diarrhea and hemorrhoids.

GROUNDSEL (H) • *Senecio vulgaris.* An enormous worldwide genus of between two thousand and three thousand species, groundsel was used in European and American folk medicine to ease painful menstruation. American Indians used it to speed childbirth. In general, the plant has been used to induce sweating, to rid the body of excess fluid, and as a tonic. In dentistry, it is employed to treat bleeding gums. It is also used to induce delayed menstruation, ease urinary tract inflammation, and to treat the common cold. Cases of liver toxicity from its use have been reported by the Centers for Disease Control. It is also a potential cancer-causing agent.

GROWTH FACTORS (Rx) • The body's own growth factors are produced by almost all tissues. Like hormones, growth factors trigger a variety of bodily functions. Some regulate normal processes, such as maintaining blood supply, while others come into play when things go awry during illness. Although the distinction between growth factors and hormones is unclear, hormones typically travel from the organ that produces them to distant areas of the body; most growth factors have only a short jaunt through the bloodstream to their target, where they bind to proteins on cell surfaces. Scientists have now been able to produce bioengineered growth factors in the laboratory. The first bioengineered growth factor to hit the market was erythropoietin (*see*). Several other growth factors are in wide experimental use.

GROWTH HORMONE (Rx) • GHRH. HGH. Protropin. Somatonorm. Somatrem. Somatropin.
A hormone produced in the front of the pituitary gland that stimulates the production of bone-forming cells and growth. A child whose body produces insufficient HGH will not reach normal height as an adult. Beginning in the late 1950s, such children were treated with HGH extracted from cadaver pituitaries. This was not only extremely expensive, but exposed youngsters to the risk of infection from viral contamination of the hormone. Today, genetic engineering technology makes available pure supplies of HGH. Somatrem and somatropin are laboratory-created versions of growth hormone. Research is continuing to find other beneficial applications of this product. In rare instances, growth hormone may induce the onset of diabetes mellitus or thyroid dysfunction. Corticosteroids (*see*) may make growth hormone less effective. *See also* Human Growth Gonadotropin HGH.

GUAIAC (Rx) (H) • *Guaiacum officinale. Lignum vitae.* Guaiacum.
An evergreen tree native to the West Indies and South America formerly used to treat arthritis and constipation. It is now used in conventional medicine as a reagent used to test for hidden blood. *See* Guaiacum.

GUAIACOL (OTC) (H) •
Isolated from the resin of the wood of *Guaiacum officinale* or *Guaiacum sanctum.* It is used as an expectorant in many cough medicines.

GUAIACOLSULFONATE • *See* Guaiacol.

GUAIACUM (H) • *Guaiacum officinale.*
The resin of the wood from this Mexican tree exudes naturally from the trunk and is collected to treat arthritis and gout. It contains guaiac acid, saponins (*see both*), and vanillin. Now used in conventional medicine for a variety of tests. *See* Guaiac.

GUAIAHIST (OTC) •
See Phenylephrine, Pyrilamine, and Guaifenesin.

GUAIFED (OTC) •
See Pseudoephedrine and Guaifenesin.

GUAIFENESIN (OTC) • Glyceryl Guaiacolate. Amonidrin. Anti-Tuss. Baytussin. Benylin Expectorant. Breonesin. Bronkaid. Bronkotabs. Cheracol D. Colrex Expectorant. Comtrex Cough Formula. Congestac Caplets. Contac Cough and Chest Cold. Cremacoat 2. Dimacol Caplets. Dorcol Children's Cough Syrup. Fenesin. Gee-Gee. G.G. GG-CEN. Glyate. Glycotuss. Glytuss. Guaiahist. Guaifed Syrup. Guaitab. Guaituss. Guaituss AC. Guaituss DM. Halotussin. Humibid L.A. Hycotuss. Hytuss. Malotuss. Medi-Tuss. Mytussin. Naldecon Senior EX. Nortussin. Novahistine DX. Organidin NR. Robafen. Robitussin. Scot-Tussin. S-T Expectorant. Theolair. Triaminic Expectorant. Vicks Children's Cough Syrup.
An expectorant drug used in many over-the-counter and prescription cough medicines. It reduces the viscosity of thick, tenacious secretions. Potential adverse reactions include nausea, vomiting, diarrhea, stomach pain, and drowsiness. Its use with heparin may increase the risk of bleeding. Guaifenesin is most effective if taken on an empty stomach, but to gain maximum effect to help loosen mucus, drink a glass of water after each dose.

GUAITUSS (OTC) • *See* Guaifenesin.

GUIATUSS AC • *See* Guaifenesin and Codeine Phosphate and Sulfate.

GUAITUSS DM (OTC) • *See* Guaifenesin and Dextromethorphan.

GUANABENZ (Rx) • **Wytensin.** An antihypertensive drug that blocks the nerve signals that trigger constriction of blood vessels. Potential adverse reactions include drowsiness, dizziness, weakness, headache, loss of balance, depression, severe rebound hypertension, dry mouth, and sexual dysfunction. Interaction with central nervous system depressants may cause increased sedation. Tricyclic antidepressants and MAO inhibitors (*see both*) may decrease its antihypertensive effects.

GUANADREL (Rx) • **Hylorel.** An antihypertensive drug that blocks the nerve signals that trigger constriction of blood vessels. Potential adverse reactions include fatigue, dizziness, drowsiness, faintness, a drop in blood pressure upon standing up, edema, diarrhea, impotence, and ejaculation disturbances. MAO inhibitors (*see*), ephedrine, norepinephrine, methylphenidate, tricyclic antidepressants, amphetamines, and phenothiazines may inhibit the blood-pressure-lowering effects of guanadrel. Care must be taken when getting up from a sitting or prone position, and when exercising. Most effective when taken on an empty stomach, but may be taken with a small amount of food if stomach upset is a problem.

GUANETHIDINE (Rx) • **Esimil. Ismelin.** An antihypertensive drug introduced in the early 1960s that blocks the nerve signals that trigger constriction of blood vessels. Potential adverse reactions include dizziness, weakness, faintness, a drop in blood pressure when rising from a sitting or prone position, congestive heart failure, and irregular heartbeat. May cause nasal stuffiness, diarrhea, water retention, and inhibition of ejaculation. Levodopa and alcohol may increase the low-blood-pressure effect of guanethidine. MAO inhibitors (*see*), ephedrine, norepinephrine, methylphenidate, tricyclic antidepressants, amphetamines, and phenothiazines may inhibit the antihypertensive effect of guanethidine. Strenuous exercise and hot showers may cause the blood pressure to fall too low. A low-sodium diet is also indicated. Most effective when taken on an empty stomach, but may be taken with a small amount of food if stomach upset is a problem.

GUANETHIDINE AND HYDROCHLOROTHIAZIDE (Rx) • **Esimil.** A combination drug to treat high blood pressure. *See both* Guanethidine and Hydrochlorothiazide.

GUANFACINE (Rx) • **Tenex.** An antihypertensive drug introduced in 1980 that works on the brain centers that control blood-vessel size. Used to treat mild to moderate high blood pressure, it need be taken only once a day. It reportedly has no effect on blood lipids. Recommended for people who are already receiving a thiazide diuretic (*see*). Potential adverse effects include drowsiness, dizziness, fatigue, headache, insomnia, a drop in blood pressure upon rising from a sitting or prone position, rebound hypertension, dry mouth, constipation, diarrhea, nausea, and rash. When used with other central nervous system depressants such as tranquilizers or alcohol, sedation is increased. The drug should not be discontinued abruptly. May be taken with or without food, but is recommended that it be taken at night to reduce the side effect of daytime drowsiness.

GUANIDINE HYDROCHLORIDE (Rx) • Used to reduce the symptoms of muscle weakness associated with myasthenic syndrome of Eaton-Lambert; not for myasthenia gravis.

GUARANÁ (H) • **Paullinia cupana.** A native of tropical America, the seeds of this wood vine are used by Brazilian Indians in a traditional beverage. The caffeine content of the plant is two and a half times that of coffee. It also contains tannins (*see*). Guaraná was introduced into France by a physician who had been working in Brazil. It came to be used to treat migraine and nervous headaches, neuralgia, paralysis, urinary tract irritation, and other ailments, as well as for chronic diarrhea. The caffeine (*see*) is assumed to be effective for migraine relief, and the tannins for the beneficial effects on diarrhea.

GUAR GUM (H) • A gum derived from the nutritive seed tissue of guar plants cultivated in India, it has five to eight times the thickening power of starch. It is employed by herbalists as an appetite suppressant, and to treat peptic ulcers. Banned by the FDA as an ingredient in laxatives, May 1992. Also banned in diet products because it can cause swelling and obstruction of the esophagus.

GUDUCHI (H) • *Tinosphora cordifolia.* An herb used in India to treat diabetes and ulcers.

GUGULPLUS (H) • Combines niacin, vitamin C, and chromium with guglipid extract, from an ornamental plant long used in India's Ayuredic health care system. Used to strengthen the heart.

GUM • True plant gums are the dried exudates from various plants obtained when the bark is cut or other injury is suffered. Gums are soluble in hot or cold water, and sticky. Today, the term *gum,* both for natural and synthetic sources, usually refers to resins (*see*). Gums are also used as emulsifiers, stabilizers, and suspending agents.

GUM ARABIC • *See* Acacia Gum.

GUM BENJAMIN • *See* Benzoin.

GUM BENZOIN • *See* Benzoin.

GUSPERIMUS • *See* Deoxyspergualin.

GUSTALAC • *See* Calcium Carbonate.

GUTOKOLA (H) • *See* Kola Nut.

GYN- • Prefix from the Greek word *gyne,* meaning woman.

GYNECOMASTIA • An abnormal enlargement of the male breast.

GYNECORT • *See* Hydrocortisone.

GYNE-LOTRIMIN (OTC) • *See* Clotrimazole.

GYNE-SULF (Rx) • *See* Sulfabenzamide, Sulfacetamide, and Sulfathiazole.

GYNOGEN LA • *See* Estradiol.

GYNOL II (OTC) • A spermicide gel containing nonoxynol-9 (*see*).

H

H₂O₂ • *See* Hydrogen Peroxide.

HABITROL (Rx) • **Nicoderm.** A transdermal (*see*) patch with nicotine, used as an aid to help people stop smoking cigarettes. From 7- to 21-mg doses per twenty-four hours. One double-blind, placebo-controlled trial in 220 smokers treated for eighteen weeks with a sixteen-hour nicotine patch without intensive group counseling found that 25 percent of those who received nicotine were not smoking one year later, compared to 9 percent of those who received placebo. Manufacturers recommend wearing the patches for four to twelve weeks, but the optimal duration of patch use is unknown. Nicoderm should be used during pregnancy only if the likelihood of smoking cessation justifies the potential risk of use of nicotine replacement by the patient, who may continue to smoke. Smoking while using Nicoderm can be extremely dangerous. Habitrol should be used with caution in patients with overactive thyroid, pheochromocytoma, or insulin-dependent diabetes. Nicotine delays the healing of peptic ulcer and should be used by those with active ulcers only if nicotine-replacement therapy outweighs the risks of smoking. Spontaneous abortion during nicotine-replacement therapy has been reported; as with smoking, nicotine as a contributing factor cannot be excluded. Although it has been difficult to separate out the effects of nicotine replacement therapy from the withdrawal symptoms of smoking cessation, reported probable adverse reactions include diarrhea, heartburn, dry mouth, joint and muscle aches, abnormal dreams, insomnia, nervousness, and sweating. Possible but unproven effects may be weakness, back, chest, or abdominal pain, constipation, nausea, vomiting, dizziness, headache, numbness, increased cough, sore throat, sinusitis, rash, taste perversion, and painful menstruation. A candidate for OTC status.

HAEMOPHILUS INFLUENZAE—TYPE B (Rx) • **HibTITER. PedvaxHIB. ProHIBIT.** Haemophilus influenza type B is the cause of more than half the cases of bacterial meningitis in children. It attacks the area around the brain and spinal cord and is fatal to about 5 to 10 percent infected. It may cause another life-threatening disease, epiglottitis, an infection that swells the flap at the back of the throat. Approximately 30 percent of children who survive the infection are left with some type of serious permanent damage, such as mental retardation, deafness, epilepsy, or partial blindness. It can be prevented by a vaccine given to infants in a series at two, four, and six months, followed by a booster dose at fifteen months. Potential adverse reactions include vomiting, drowsiness, fever, lack of appetite, redness at place of injection, reduced physical activity, fatigue, diarrhea, itching, and irritability.

HAIRY TONGUE • A rare condition that may occur after use of antibiotics, or from unknown causes. Black hairy filaments form on the surface of the tongue.

HALAZEPAM (Rx) • **Paxipam.** A benzodiazepine (*see*) minor tranquilizer that depresses the central nervous system at the area of the brain controlling emotions. Used to treat anxiety, tension, and agitation. Potential side effects include drowsiness, lethargy, hangover, fainting, transient low blood pressure, dry mouth, nausea, vomiting, and abdominal discomfort. Should not be used with central nervous system depressants, including antihistamines, sleeping pills, and alcohol. Cimetidine may increase sedation. Contraindicated in glaucoma and psychoses. Should be used cautiously in persons with kidney or liver dysfunction. Use of halazepam is not recommended for more than four months, but it should not be discontinued abruptly. Most effective when taken on an empty stomach.

HALCINONIDE (Rx) • **Halog.** A corticosteroid (*see*) cream, ointment, or solution used to treat skin inflammation. Potential adverse reactions including burning, itching, irritation, dryness, inflammation of the hair follicles, acne, rash around the mouth, spots of pigment loss, hairiness, allergic contact dermatitis, and if covered with a dressing, secondary infection, atrophy, streaks, and blisters. Should be used cautiously in skin problems caused by viruses such as herpes, and in fungal or bacterial skin infections. Should not be used for more than two weeks due to potential absorption into the system, consequently causing an effect on the hypothalamus, and pituitary and adrenal glands. Should not be applied near the eyes or mucous membranes, under the arms, on the face, groin, or under the breast unless medically specified.

HALCION • *See* Triazolam.

HALDOL DECANOATE • *See* Haloperidol Decanoate.

HALDRONE • *See* Paramethasone.

HALENOL • *See* Acetaminophen.

HALEY'S M-O (OTC) • A combination of magnesium hydroxide and mineral oil (*see both*) used to treat constipation.

HALFAN • *See* Halofantrine.

HALF-LIFE • The time it takes for half a dose of a drug to be eliminated from the bloodstream, a factor used to determine how frequently a medicine should be taken.

HALFPRIN (OTC) • An enteric-coated, low-dose aspirin taken as a preventative against heart attacks. *See* Aspirin.

HALLS MENTHO-LYPTUS • *See* Eucalyptus.

HALLUCINATION • The false perception of a sight, sound, taste, smell, or touch when no actual stimulus is present. Hallucination also refers to the imaginary object apparently seen or heard.

HALLUX • Big toe.

HALLUX VALGUS • Bunion.

HALOBETASOL PROPIONATE (Rx) • Ultravate. Used for the relief of inflammation and itching in skin problems responsive to corticosteroids (*see*).

HALODRIN • *See* Estradiol and Fluoxymesterone.

HALOFANTRINE (Rx) • **Halfan.** A drug introduced in the United States in 1992 for the treatment of multidrug-resistant strains of malaria. Introduced in France in 1988, it is currently being used in fifty-one countries.

HALOFED • *See* Pseudoephedrine.

HALOG • *See* Halcinonide.

HALOPERIDOL DECANOATE or LACTATE (Rx) • **Haldol Decanoate. Haloperon.** An antipsychotic drug introduced in 1958, it is used to treat patients who require prolonged therapy. Also used to treat Tourette's syndrome (*see*) and for short-term treatment of hyperactive children, and nervous, mental, and emotional conditions. Haloperidol is effective in reducing the violent, aggressive manifestations of schizophrenia and mania. Potential adverse reactions include a drop in white blood cells, high incidence of severe toxic effects on the brain including movement disorders and low incidence of sedation, blurred vision, dry mouth, urine retention, menstrual irregularities, decreased libido, impotence, enlargement of male breast, rash, fever, irregular heartbeat, and sweating. Use with alcohol and other central nervous system depressants increases central nervous system depression. Lithium may cause confusion and lethargy. Methyldopa may cause symptoms of dementia. Contraindicated in parkinsonism, coma, or central nervous system depression. Should be used with caution in elderly and debilitated patients, in severe cardiovascular disorders, allergies, glaucoma, urine retention, and in conjunction with anticonvulsant, anticoagulant, antiparkinsonian, or lithium medications. Haloperidol should not be withdrawn suddenly. Most effective when taken on an empty stomach, but may be taken with a small amount of food to avoid stomach upset.

HALOPROGIN (OTC) • **Halotex.** A drug used to treat fungal skin conditions. Changed from Rx to OTC. Potential adverse reactions include burning sensation, irritation, blisters, itching, and worsening of existing lesions. If the skin problem does not clear up in four weeks or if it becomes worse, consult your physician.

HALOTESTIN • *See* Fluoxymesterone.

HALOTEX • *See* Haloprogin.

HALOTHANE (Rx) • **Fluothane.** A gas used to induce general anesthesia.

HALOTUSSIN (OTC) • *See* Guaifenesin.

HALTRAN (OTC) • *See* Ibuprofen.

HAM • The homeopathic abbreviation for hamamelis water (*see*).

HAMAMELIS WATER • *See* Witch Hazel.

HAPONAL (Rx) • A combination of phenobarbital, atropine, and hyoscyamine (*see all*) used to treat spasms of the bowel and bladder and to help in the treatment of peptic ulcer.

HARMONYL • *See* Deserpidine.

HARVIX • *See* Hepatitis A Vaccine.

HAW BARK • *See* Viburnum Extract.

HAWKWEED • *See* Mouse-Ear.

HAWTHORN BERRY (H) • *Crataegus oxyacantha.* A spring-flowering shrub or tree. A number of scientific studies in Central Europe and in the United States have found that hawthorn berries can dilate the blood vessels and lower blood pressure. The berries reportedly can also increase the enzyme metabolism of the heart and make the heart's use of oxygen during exercise more efficient. Hawthorn extracts are also believed to have some diuretic properties. In the 1800s, the berries were used to treat digestive problems and insomnia. They contain bioflavonoids, compounds that are necessary for vitamin C function and also help strengthen blood vessels. *See* Bioflavonoids.

HCG • Abbreviation for human chorionic gonadotropin (*see*).

HCG PREGNANCY TESTS (OTC) • **Advance Pregnancy Test. e.p.t. Early Pregnancy Test. Fact Plus Pregnancy Test.** When a woman becomes pregnant, her body produces a special hormone, human chorionic gonadotropin (HCG), which appears in the urine. Pregnancy tests can detect HCG as early as the day the period should have started.

HCL • Abbreviation for hydrochloride (*see*).

H-CONT • *See* Hydrocortisone.

HCRF • *See* human corticotropin-releasing factor.

HCTZ • *See* Hydrochlorothiazide.

HCV CREAM (Rx) • *See* Hydrocortisone and Clioquinol.

HDL • The abbreviation for high-density lipoprotein. HDL is believed to pick up excess cholesterol in the blood and help the body eliminate it.

HEAD & SHOULDERS ANTIDANDRUFF SHAMPOO (OTC) • *See* Pyrithione Zinc.

HEALON • *See* Hyaluronate.

HEALTHY HEART • A dietary supplement with nutrients intended to improve heart health by lowering homocystein, an amino acid, in the blood that is linked to risk for heart attack. It contains large doses of Vitamin E as well as B vitamins. It has not been evaluated or approved by the FDA.

HEART BLOCK • A condition in which electrical signals from the heart's natural pacemaker in the right atrium are blocked from traveling to the heart's ventricles, the lower chambers of the heart.

HEARTBURN • **Pyrosis. Reflux Esophagitis.** An unpleasant burning sensation in the chest due to inflammation of the esophagus, which is due to the backwash of stomach contents into the esophagus.

HEART FAILURE • A condition in which the heart is unable to pump enough blood to meet the metabolic needs of the body.

HEART RATE • The rate at which the heart pumps.

HEB-CORT • *See* Hydrocortisone.

HECTORITE (OTC) • A clay consisting of silicate magnesium and lithium. In 1992, the FDA issued a notice that hectorite had not been shown to be safe and effective as claimed in OTC digestive-aid products, and poison ivy, poison sumac, and poison oak products.

HELICOBACTER PYLORI • The bacteria now targeted as mainly responsible for the development of peptic ulcer disease. The organism is known to reside underneath the mucous layer in the stomach and promote ulcer formation.

HELIOTROPE (H) • *Heliotropium europaeum.* **Desert Heliotrope.** Bluish purple flowers on a stem that coils in the shape of a fiddle neck. It grows throughout the southwestern United States and is a frequent cause of allergic contact dermatitis on the legs and ankles of persons walking through the desert. It also grows in Europe as a weed. Used in folk medicine as a diuretic, to treat gallbladder problems, and to induce delayed menstruation. All parts of the plant are highly toxic. Prolonged use can cause severe liver damage and may be lethal.

HELLEBORE (H) • *Veratrum viride. Helleborus niger.* **American Hellebore. Black Hellebore. Christmas Rose. False Hellebore. Green Hellebore. Indian Poke. Itch Weed. Veratrum.** Black hellebore was employed by ancient physicians to treat insanity. The doctors believed that patients brought near death by the medication would be shocked into sanity. American hellebore is used by homeopathic physicians as a means to slow heartbeat. Herbalists use it for its irritant and sedative action to treat pneumonia, gout, rheumatism, typhoid, rheumatic fever, and local inflammation. Black hellebore is used to treat fluid retention associated with heart failure. Hellebore is toxic and can cause severe nausea and extreme depression of the nervous system.

HELMEX • *See* Pyrantel, Embolate, and Pomoate.

HELMIZIN • *See* Piperazine.

HELONIAS • *See* False Unicorn Root.

HELPER T CELLS • A subset of T cells (*see*) that are essential for turning on antibody production, activating killer T cells, and initiating many other immune responses.

HEM-, HEMA-, HEMATO- • Prefixes from the Greek word *haima*, meaning blood.

HEMABATE • *See* Carboprost.

HEMACHEK (OTC) • A diagnostic test for blood in feces.

HEMANGIOMA • An aggregation of multiple, dilated blood vessels.

HEMASPAN FA (Rx) • A combination of folic acid, vitamin C, ferrous fumarate, and docusate (*see all*), used to treat iron and vitamin deficiency.

HEMASTIX (OTC) • A diagnostic test for blood in urine.

HEMATEST (OTC) • A diagnostic test for blood in feces.

HEMATOCRIT • Measurement of the percentage of red blood cells in a volume of blood.

HEMATOLOGICAL • Relating to the blood.

HEMATOMA • A swelling that contains blood, usually clotted.

HEMATURIA • Presence of blood in urine, sometimes due to infarction of a segment of the kidney.

HEMI- • Prefix meaning half.

HEMIANOPIA • Loss of vision in one-half of the visual field.

HEMIN (Rx) • **Panhematin.** A drug used for recurrent attacks of porphyria (*see*).

HEMIPLEGIA • Paralysis of one side of the body.

HEMLOCK (H) • *Conium maculatum.* **Poison Hemlock. Poison Parsley.** Found in many parts of Europe and the Americas, the hemlock is related to parsnip, carrot, celery, fennel, and parsley. It is famed as the poison used to execute Socrates and other ancient Greeks; it was mixed with opium and used as a suicide drink for old, frail Roman philosophers. The narcotic drug conium (*see*) comes from the dried, unripe fruit of the hemlock. Herbalists once used it as a sedative, antispasmodic, and an antidote to other poisons. Hemlock is poisonous.

HEMOCCULT II • A diagnostic test for blood in feces.

HEMOCHROMATOSIS • An increased deposit of iron in the tissues, causing scarring and other damage to tissue, and organ failure.

HEMOCYTE • *See* Ferrous Fumarate.

HEMODIALYSIS • Separation of waste materials from blood by passage through a filter.

HEMOFIL M • *See* Antihemophilic Factor.

HEMOLYSIS • Dissolution, breakdown, of red blood cells.

HEMOLYTIC • Pertaining to the disruption of the red blood cell membrane, causing release of hemoglobin.

HEMOPHILUS INFLUENZAE • A bacterial infection that may cause pneumonia in young people affected by viral influenza.

HEMOPTYSIS • Coughing and spitting of blood.

HEMORRHOIDS • Enlarged veins in the anal area.

HEMOSTASIS • The arrest of bleeding.

HEMP (H) • *Cannabis sativa.* **Hashish.** An herb of the nettle family, native to northern India, southern Siberia, and Asia, it has been widely cultivated for its narcotic properties. It was used in folk medicine to stem bleeding, and to treat arthritis, flu, colds, edema, asthma, and diphtheria. It can be habit-forming and has been banned from general therapeutic use.

HEMP DOGBANE • See Dogbane.

HEMP TREE • *See* Chaste Berries.

HEPARIN CALCIUM AND SODIUM (Rx) • **Calciparine. Heparin Lock Flush Solution. Lipo Hepin. Liquaemin Sodium. Normiflo.** An agent that prevents blood coagulation, derived from beef lung or porcine intestinal mucosa. Used to prevent and to treat deep-vein blood clots, blood clots to the lung, and to treat heart attacks. It is used to flush and maintain indwelling catheters. Potential adverse reactions include hemorrhage, irritation, mild pain, and hypersensitivity reactions, including chills, fever, itching, runny nose, burning of feet, red eyes, tearing, joint pain, and hives. Oral anticoagulants and salicylates increase the possibility of bleeding. Contraindicated in active bleeding, blood problems such as hemophilia, liver disease, suspected bleeding into the head, open wounds, ulcers, and ascorbic acid deficiency. Should be used cautiously during menstruation, in mild liver or kidney disease, alcoholism, and in occupations with the risk of physical injury. Two studies reported in 1994 found that high doses of heparin for treating heart attack patients caused about twice the rate of the expected incidence of paralyzing and fatal strokes. The report in the September issue of *Circulation* concluded that low doses of intravenous heparin were relatively safe and effective when given with clot-dissolving drugs.

HEPAR SULPH. (H) • **Hepar Sulphuris. Calcium Sulfide. Liver of Sulfur.** A mixture of potassium and sulfates (*see both*). Used in homeopathic medicine to treat irritability, the common cold, constipation, diarrhea, earache, fever, joint pain, toothache, and night sweats. It is also used by homeopaths and in conventional medicine to treat skin diseases. *See* Tissue Salts.

HEPAR SULPHURIS • *See* Hepar Sulph.

HEPAT-, HEPAR- • Prefixes pertaining to the liver, as in *hepatitis,* inflammation of the liver.

HEPATIC • A term used in herbal medicine to signify a medication that aids the liver and increases the flow of bile. Among these are blue flag and agrimony (*see both*).

HEPATICA (H) • *Anemone hepaticas. Ranunculaceae.* Native to the Americas and parts of Europe, the hepaticas are called liverwort or liver-leaf because they resemble the shape of the lobes of the liver. Used in folk medicine to treat liver ailments. *See* Anemone.

HEPATITIS • Inflammation of the liver.

HEPATITIS A • Among the five viruses that are known to cause hepatitis (*see*), hepatitis A usually causes a flulike malaise, nausea, yellowing of the skin and eyes, and fever. In rare cases it can lead to fatal liver failure. Hepatitis A spreads by contaminated food and water or by person-to-person contact. It has an incubation period of from six to twenty-five weeks. All ages are affected, but it is most common in children and young adults.

HEPATITIS A VACCINE • **Havrix.** A vaccine introduced in 1995 that can protect travelers, food handlers, and others against hepatitis A. Until its introduction, the only protection against hepatitis A (*see*) after exposure was immunoglobulins (*see*).

HEPATITIS B • One of the viruses that causes liver inflammation. It has an incubation period of one to six weeks. May become chronic or a person may become a symptomless carrier of the virus. It is often transmitted by injection, typically by contaminated blood or blood products.

HEPATITIS B IMMUNE GLOBULIN, HUMAN (Rx) • **H-BIG. Hep-B-Gammagee. HyperHep.** An injection that provides passive immunity to hepatitis B if given within seven days after exposure to the virus. It is then repeated twenty-eight days after exposure. Potential adverse reactions include severe allergic reactions. May also cause aches and pains, fever, rash, muscle weakness or numbness, tingling of limbs, and pain or tenderness of the eyes.

HEPATITIS B VACCINE (Rx) • **Engerix-B. Heptavax-B. Recombivax HB.** Promotes active immunity against hepatitis B infection, which is associated with a wide spectrum of liver diseases, including acute hepatitis, chronic hepatitis, liver cancer, and cirrhosis. Potential adverse reactions include a slight fever, malaise, headache, dizziness, nausea, vomiting, flulike symptoms, muscle pain, and inflammation at the injection site.

HEPATITIS C • One of the viruses that cause liver inflammation, it is known to be the culprit in at least 80 percent of posttransfusion hepatitis. May be the cause of many cases of chronic hepatitis. A vaccine for hepatitis C is under development at this writing.

HERBAL ECSTACY (H) • A so-called "natural high" drug promoted to young people. *See* Ma Huang.

HERNIA • An abnormal protrusion of the intestine or other organs through an opening in the abdominal wall.

HEROIN • Has no accepted medical use in the United States.

HERPES SIMPLEX KERATITIS • A viral infection of the cornea of the eye. Causes a foreign-body sensation in the eye, tearing, and redness. Also causes light to hurt the eyes. May lead to chronic inflammation, scarring, and loss of vision.

HERPES SIMPLEX VIRUS I (HSV I) • A virus that causes cold sores or fever blisters on the mouth or around the eyes. It can be transmitted to the genital region. The latent virus can be reactivated by stress, trauma, other infections, or suppression of the immune system.

HERPES SIMPLEX VIRUS II (HSV II) • A virus that causes painful sores of the anus or genitals that may lie dormant in nerve tissue and can be reactivated to produce the sores.

HERPES VARICELLA-ZOSTER VIRUS (HVZ) • **Shingles.** A virus that may appear in adulthood as a result of having had chicken pox as a child. Painful blisters occur on the skin and follow nerve pathways.

HERPLEX • *See* Idoxuridine.

HESPAN • *See* Hetastarch.

HESPERIDIN • A compound found in orange juice that has been found to be an anticancer agent in laboratory experiments.

HETACILLIN • *See* Penicillin.

HETASTARCH (Rx) • **Hespan.** An injection of a starch to expand plasma volume and provide fluid replacement. Potential adverse reactions include headache, peripheral edema of lower extremities, swelling around the eyes, nausea, vomiting, hives, wheezing, and mild fever. Contraindicated in severe bleeding disorders, and with severe heart failure or kidney failure.

HEXA-BETALIN • *See* Vitamin B_6.

HEXACHLOROCYCLOHEXANE • *See* Lindane.

HEXACHLOROPHENE (Rx) • **pHisoHex.** A skin antiseptic. In 1969 scientists reported microscopically visible brain damage in rats from small concentrations of this antibacterial. In December 1971, the FDA curbed the use of hexachlorophene-containing detergents and soaps for total body bathing. The makers of pHisoHex, which contained 3 percent hexachlorophene, sent out further information to doctors saying the product should not be used as a lotion, left on the skin after use, used as a wet soak or compress, or transferred to another container that would allow for misuse. It should always be rinsed thoroughly from the skin after any use. The FDA has limited it up to 0.75 percent. Products containing up to 0.75 percent will continue on the market with the warning "Contains hexachlorophene. For external use only. Rinse thoroughly."

HEXACREST • *See* Vitamin B_6.

HEXADROL • *See* Dexamethasone.

HEXAFLUORENIUM (Rx) • **Mylaxen.** Given by injection to prolong blockage of nerve signals by other compounds such as succinylcholine (*see*).

HEXALEN • *See* Altretamine.

HEXALOL (Rx) • A combination of atropine, hyoscyamine, methenamine, phenylsalicylate, and benzoic acid (*see all*), used to treat urinary tract infections.

HEXAMETHYLMELAMINE • *See* Altretamine.

HEXOCYCLIUM (Rx) • **Tral.** An antispasmodic drug used to treat peptic ulcers and other GI disorders, especially irritable bowel syndrome (*see*).

HEXYLRESORCINOL (OTC) • A pale yellow, heavy liquid that becomes solid upon standing at room temperature. Has a pungent odor and a sharp, astringent taste; has been used medicinally as an antiworm medicine and antiseptic, and in mouthwashes and sunburn creams. Can cause severe gastrointestinal irritation and bowel, liver, and heart damage if ingested. Concentrated solutions can cause burns of the skin and mucous membranes. In 1992, the FDA proposed a ban for the use of hexylresorcinol to treat fever blisters and cold sores, and poison ivy, poison sumac, and poison oak, because it had not been shown to be safe and effective as claimed in OTC products.

H-H-R Tablets (Rx) • A medication for high blood pressure. *See* Hydralazine, Hydrochlorothiazide, and Reserpine.

HIATUS HERNIA • **Hiatal Hernia.** A protrusion of part of the stomach through the diaphragm into the chest cavity.

HIBICLENS • *See* Chlorhexidine Gluconate.

HIBISTAT • *See* Chlorhexidine Gluconate.

HIGH BLOOD PRESSURE DRUGS • *See* Antihypertensives.

HIPBERRIES • *See* Rose Hips Extract.

HIPREX • *See* Methenamine.

HISMANAL • *See* Astemizole.

HISPRIL • *See* Diphenylpyraline.

HISTABID (OTC) • A combination of chlorpheniramine and phenylpropanolamine (*see both*), used to treat upper-respiratory congestion.

HISTAJECT • *See* Brompheniramine.

HISTALET (OTC) • A combination of chlorpheniramine and pseudoephedrine (*see both*), used to treat upper-respiratory congestion.

HISTALOG • *See* Betazole.

HISTAMIC (OTC) • A combination of chlorpheniramine, phenylephrine, phenylpropanolamine, and phenyltoloxamine (*see all*), used to treat the symptoms of allergy.

HISTAMINE • A substance released into the body when an allergic reaction occurs. It may cause itching, sneezing, and even sudden death.

HISTAMINE H2-RECEPTOR ANTAGONIST • A drug that blocks the ability of histamine to induce acid secretion in the stomach.

HISTASPAN-D • *See* Chlorpheniramine.

HISTERONE • *See* Testosterone.

HISTEX • *See* Chlorpheniramine.

HISTOPLASMOSIS • A disease caused by fungal infection that can affect all the organs of the body. Symptoms usually include fever, shortness of breath, cough, weight loss, and physical exhaustion.

HISTOR-D (OTC) • A combination of chlorpheniramine, phenylephrine, and methscopolamine (*see all*) in a sustained-release formulation to treat the symptoms of colds and allergies.

HISTOSAL (OTC) • *See* Acetaminophen, Phenylpropanolamine, Caffeine, and Pyrilamine.

HISTRELIN (Rx) • **Supprelin.** A synthetic hormone introduced in 1992 for the treatment of precocious puberty. It is an orphan drug (*see*). About six thousand American children have this condition, with two thousand new cases diagnosed each year.

HISTREY • *See* Chlorpheniramine.

HIV • **Human Immunodeficiency Virus.** The virus that causes AIDS.

HI-VEGI-LIP • *See* Pancreatin.

HIVES • Popular name for urticaria, an allergic skin reaction characterized by raised wheals or welts. Hives are most often caused by foods or drugs.

HIVID • *See* Zalcitabine.

HIV POSITIVE • Presence of antibodies to the human immunodeficiency virus (the virus that causes AIDS) in the blood.

HMG-COA REDUCTASE INHIBITORS (Rx) • Medications that work by blocking an enzyme that is needed by the body to make cholesterol. Thus, less cholesterol is produced. Those on the market include lovastatin, pravastatin, and simvastatin (*see all*).

HMM • *See* Altretamine.

HMS • *See* Medrysone.

HMS LIQUIFILM OPHTHALMIC • *See* Medrysone.

HOGAPPLE • *See* Mayapple.

HOLLY (H) • *Ilex aquifolium. Ilex opaca.* **American Holly. European Holly.** A small evergreen. The leaves were used to increase perspiration, to treat inflammations of the mucous membranes, and pleurisy, gout, and smallpox. The leaves contain theobromine (*see*). The berries were used to cause vomiting, and as a diuretic to remove excess fluid. The juice of the berries was used to treat jaundice.

HOLY THISTLE (H) • *Cnicus benedictus.* **Blessed Thistle. Cardin.** An annual herb, the plant is a native of the south of Europe and is cultivated in gardens in many parts of the world. Its use in medicine has been recorded since A.D. 100. Once believed to be a panacea, it has been credited with reducing excess fluid, inducing sweating, lowering fever, and easing stomach upset. Still used today to treat indigestion and as an appetite stimulant. Also widely used as an herbal to induce menstruation.

HOMATRINE • *See* Homatropine.

HOMATROPINE (Rx) (OTC) • **Homatrine. Hycodan. I-Homatrine. Isopto Homatropine.** An eye solution that is used to dilate the pupils during diagnosis and to treat certain eye irritations. Potential adverse reactions include eye irritation, blurred vision, sensitivity to light, flushing, dry skin and mouth, fever, rapid heartbeat, awkward movements, irritability, confusion, and sleepiness. Should be used cautiously in infants and elderly people or debilitated patients, children with blond hair and blue eyes, patients with heart disease, or patients with increased pressure in the eyes. Patients who are hypersensitive to atropine will also be allergic to this drug. In 1992, the FDA proposed a ban on homatropine methylbromide in oral menstrual drug products because it had not been shown to be safe and effective as claimed.

HOMEOPATHIC MEDICINES • Remedies based on the belief that "like treats like." Homeopaths regard symptoms of illness as expressions of disharmony within the whole person. For example, a homeopathic allergy medication may contain allium cepa, an onion extract; onions cause tearing and a runny nose, which are also common allergy symptoms. Because of their minute dosages, homeopathic remedies for common, easily self-diagnosed ailments are exempt from the FDA's safety and effectiveness reviews. As such, marketers are free to make advertising claims about the effectiveness of the remedies.

HOMICEBRIN (OTC) • A multivitamin preparation.

HONEY (H) • The common, sweet, viscous material taken from the nectar of flowers and manufactured in the sacs of various kinds of bees. In 1992, the FDA proposed a ban on honey in astringent (*see*) OTC drug products because it had not been shown to be safe and effective as claimed.

HONEYSUCKLE (H) • *Lonicera japonica.* **Caprifolium. Yin Hua.** Tubular flowers filled with honey; used frequently in Chinese detoxifying formulas. Honeysuckle is employed for infectious and inflammatory conditions. It is particularly useful for poison oak and other rashes.

The flowers are considered harmless, but the fruits are toxic when used to excess. Cases of severe but not fatal poisoning have been reported in children as a result of eating berries from this plant. Symptoms of poisoning are drowsiness, dilated pupils, sensitivity to light, and extreme weakness. *See also* Red Clover.

HOP (H) • *Humulus lupulus.* **Silent Night.** Widely cultivated, this plant has been used in folk medicine for its calming effect on the body. Contains an estrogenlike ingredient as well as volatile oil, bitter principle, and tannin. It is used to relieve gas and cramps, and to stimulate appetite. Also used in a poultice to relieve sciatica, arthritis, toothache, and other nerve pain. It has been used to induce sleep and as a tonic in wine. Both Abraham Lincoln and England's King George III reportedly relied on hop to promote a restful calm at bedtime. Hop flowers were listed in the USP (*see*) for ninety years. Contraindicated in depressive illness because it may exacerbate the condition. Excessive doses or chronic use may cause dizziness and intoxication.

HORDEUM VULGARES • *See* Barley.

HOREHOUND (H) • *Ballota nigra* **(Black Horehound) and** *Marrubium vulgare* **(White Horehound). Madweed.** Black horehound was used by the English colonists as a medicine for gout and arthritis. It is occasionally used by herbalists to get rid of lice. When soaked in boiling water, it is applied to the skin to relieve gout and arthritis. It is also used by herbalists to treat chronic hepatitis, cancer, tuberculosis, leukemia, malaria, and hysteria. White horehound, used by ancient Egyptian doctors who dedicated it to the god Horus, and now native to Britain and the United States, is used in cough drops and cold medicines. Tops of young white horehound shoots are still gathered by herbalists to treat upset stomach, jaundice, croup, asthma, and bronchitis.

HORMONE • A chemical substance formed in one gland or part of the body and carried by the blood to another organ, which it stimulates to functional activity.

HORSE CHESTNUT (H) • *Aesculus hippocastanum.* Traditionally used by herbalists to reduce fever, it is also used by modern herbalists to treat varicose veins and hemorrhoids. An extract is used as a sunscreen. The nut reputedly contains narcotic properties. The powdered kernel of the nut causes sneezing. A tincture of the nut is used to treat hemorrhoids. The seeds contain escin, a soapy substance that is used today as a sunburn protective. Escin is also widely used in Europe as an anti-inflammatory agent for a variety of conditions, including varicose veins. Escin has also been found to be a powerful diuretic. Contraindicated during pregnancy and in cases of acute kidney dysfunction. Cases of severe poisoning occur most often in children who have eaten the seeds. Symptoms include vomiting, diarrhea, incoordination, dilated pupils, depression, and even paralysis.

HORSEHOOF • *See* Coltsfoot.

HORSE NETTLE (H) • *Solanum carolinense.* **Ball Nettle. Bull Nettle.** A coarse, prickly weed common in the eastern and southern United States. It has a white or pale purple flower and bright yellow fruit. A member of the nightshade family.

HORSERADISH EXTRACT (H) • *Armoracia lapathifolia.* **Scurvy Grass.** The grated root from the tall, coarse, white-flowered herb native to Europe. Contains vitamin C and acts as an antiseptic, used particularly for this purpose in cosmetics. It is applied by herbalists as a poultice to accelerate the healing of stubborn wounds. Also reputed to be a good diuretic and expectorant. Used for arthritis to relieve pain by stimulating blood flow to inflamed joints. Potential adverse reactions include diarrhea and sweating, if taken internally in large amounts.

HORSETAIL (H) • *Equisetum arvense.* **Equisetum hyemale. Scouring Rush. Shave Grass. Silica.** The American Indians and the Chinese have long used horsetail to accelerate the healing of bones and wounds. Horsetail is rich in minerals the body uses to rebuild injured tissue. It facilitates the absorption of calcium by the body, which nourishes nails, skin, hair, bones, and connective tissue. The herb helps eliminate excess oil from skin and hair. It is a mild diuretic and was used to promote urination in heart failure and kidney dysfunction. In 1992, the FDA issued a notice that horsetail had not been shown to be safe and effective as claimed in OTC digestive-aid products. Contraindicated in acute kidney inflammation, high blood pressure, and heart disease. Because of its direct action, dehydration may occur if used on a daily basis for a long time.

HO SHOU WU • *See* Fo-ti.

HOUND'S-TONGUE (H) • *Cynoglossum officinale.* An erect biennial native to Europe and introduced elsewhere. It is used in homeopathic medicines to treat diarrhea and the common cold. The plant is toxic to the liver and carcinogenic in animals.

HOUSELEEK (H) • *Sempervivum tectorum.* Native to the mountains of Europe and to the Greek islands. Its longevity led to its being named *Sempervivum,* which translated means "ever alive." Houseleek has been used to treat shingles, gout, and to get rid of bugs. Its pulp was applied to the skin for rashes and inflammation, and to remove warts and calluses. The juice was used to reduce fever and to treat insect stings. Houseleek juice mixed with honey was prescribed for thrush (*see*), and an ointment made from the plant was used to treat ulcers, burns, scalds, and inflammation.

HPA • Abbreviation for hypothalamic-pituitary-adrenal axis. The control system involving regulation of cortisol (hydrocortisone), a steroid hormone produced by the adrenal glands.

H.P. ACTHAR GEL • *See* Corticotropin.

HUANG CHI • *See* Skullcap.

HUCKLEBERRY LEAF (H) • *Gaylussacia.* Similar to blueberries but more acidic, the leaves are used by many naturopathic physicians to treat mild diabetes and ailments of the kidney and gallbladder. The huckleberry is related to uva-ursi

(*see*) and contains similar compounds. In 1992, the FDA issued a notice that huckleberry had not been shown to be safe and effective as claimed in OTC digestive-aid products.

HUMALOG • *See* Lispro.

HUMAN CHORIONIC GONADOTROPIN (Rx) • HCG. A.P.L. Glukor. Follutein. Pregnyl. Profasi. Produced by the pituitary gland, it is a hormone that stimulates the ovaries to produce two other hormones, estrogen and progesterone, which are necessary for conception and early growth of the fetus. Since 1939, the hormone, commonly called HCG, has been extracted from the urine of pregnant women for use in the treatment of female infertility. HCG stimulates the ovaries to release eggs so they can be fertilized. Ovulation usually occurs eighteen hours after injection, and intercourse should follow within forty-eight hours. HCG is also given to men to improve sperm production. HCG often produces multiple births. Women who take large doses of the drug may experience abdominal pain or swelling. Other potential adverse reactions include headache, fatigue, moodiness, swollen feet and ankles, and in men, enlarged breasts. Use with alcohol increases fatigue and may reduce fertility. Smoking also decreases fertility.

HUMAN CORTICOTROPIN-RELEASING FACTOR (Rx) • HCRF. A protein compound normally produced by the body, it has long been used as a diagnostic drug to study endocrine function. It is now being tested as a drug to reduce bruising and swelling as well as to speed healing after cosmetic surgery.

HUMAN GROWTH GONADOTROPIN HGH (Rx) • Humatrope. Protropin. Somatrem. Somatropin. Somatrem and somatropin are laboratory-made versions of human growth hormone, naturally produced by the pituitary gland. HGH is necessary to stimulate growth in children. The medications are used in long-term growth failure from lack of adequate self-produced growth hormone. Not used to increase the growth of normally short stature. *See* Growth Hormone.

HUMAN INSULIN (Rx) • Humulin. Novolin. Genetically engineered insulin was introduced in 1982. Insulin is a hormone that helps the body turn food into energy. Diabetes mellitus is a condition where the body does not make enough insulin to meet its needs. The engineered human insulin is preferred by some to beef or pork insulin. All types of insulin must be injected.

HUMATIN • *See* Paromomycin Sulfate.

HUMATROPE • *See* Human Growth Gonadotropin HGH and Somatropin.

HUMECTANT • A substance used to preserve the moisture content of materials. The humectant of glycerin and rose water, in equal amounts, is the earliest-known hand lotion. Glycerin, propylene glycol, and sorbitol (*see all*) are widely used humectants.

HUMEGON • A fertility drug for women approved September 1, 1994, by the FDA. *See* Menotropins.

HUMIBID L.A. • *See* Guaifenesin.

HUMIST • *See* Sodium Chloride.

HUMORAL IMMUNITY • Immune protection provided by soluble factors such as antibodies, which circulate in the body's fluids or "humors," primarily serum and lymph.

HUMORSOL • *See* Demecarium Bromide.

HUMULIN • *See* Human Insulin.

HURRICANE • *See* Benzocaine.

HU SUAN • *See* Garlic.

HYACINTH (Rx) • *See* Topotecan.

HYALURONATE • The salt of hyaluronic acid, a natural protein found in umbilical cords, in sperm, in testes, and in the fluids around the joints. *See* Hyaluronidase.

HYALURONIDASE (Rx) • Wydase. An enzyme used in topical skin preparations to reduce bruising and to increase the absorption of other drugs. Potential adverse reactions include rash, hives, and local irritation. Local anesthetics increase the potential for toxic local reaction. Should be used with caution in patients with blood-clotting abnormalities, and severe kidney or liver disease.

HYBOLIN DECANOATE • *See* Nandrolone.

HYBRID • Plant or animal offspring from parents that have distinctly different genetic make-ups. Using traditional breeding, crossing two different varieties of plants or two purebred lines of animals produces hybrids. Crossbreeding can take place on the molecular level in genetic engineering.

HYCODAN (Rx) • A cough medicine combination containing hydrocodone and homatropine (*see both*).

HYCODAPHEN • *See* Hydrocodone.

HYCOMINE (Rx) • A combination of phenylpropanolamine and hydrocodone (*see both*), used to treat cough.

HYCOTUSS (Rx) • An expectorant containing alcohol, guaifenesin, and hydrocodone (*see all*).

HYDANTOIN • Derived from methanol, an alcohol obtained by distillation of wood. Hydantoin is used commercially as an intermediate in the manufacture of lubricants and resins. A number of drugs are derived from it.

HYDELTRASOL • *See* Prednisolone.

HYDELTRASOL OPHTHALMIC • *See* Prednisolone.

HYDELTRA-T.B.A. • *See* Prednisolone.

HYDERGINE • *See* Ergoloid Mesylates.

HYDEXTRAN • *See* Iron and Dextran.

HYDRALAZINE (Rx) • **Alazine. Apresoline. HHR. Tri-Hydroserpine.** A drug introduced in 1950 that directly relaxes the smooth muscle of the arteries, it is used to lower blood pressure and to treat congestive heart failure in patients with heart valve replacement. It increases the flow of blood and oxygen to the heart, while reducing its workload. Potential adverse reactions include a drop in white blood cells, irritation of the nerves in the arms and legs, headache, dizziness, a drop in blood pressure when rising from a seated or prone position, irregular heartbeat, angina, palpitations, sodium retention, nausea, vomiting, diarrhea, loss of appetite, rash, lupus erythematosus–like syndrome (with high doses), and weight gain. Rare reports of impotence and priapism (*see*) have been made. Hydralazine depletes vitamin B_6, which can result in nerve damage and cause tremors, tingling, and numbness. Diazoxide and other blood-pressure-lowering drugs may cause severe low blood pressure when used with hydralazine. Hydralazine should be used with caution in patients taking MAO inhibitors or NSAIDs (*see both*), especially Anacin. Stimulants, including over-the-counter medications for allergies and colds, make it less effective. Hydralazine should be taken with food.

HYDRANGEA (OTC) (H) • *Saxifragaceae.* **Seven Barks.** Widely distributed shrubs with clusters of showy flowers. The roots contain glycosides, saponins, and resins (*see all*). It is used by herbalists to treat inflamed or enlarged prostate glands, and for urinary stones or gravel associated with infections such as cystitis. In 1992, the FDA proposed a ban on hydrangea extract in OTC oral menstrual drug products because it had not been shown to be safe and effective as claimed.

HYDRASTINE (H) • Found together with berberine (*see*), it is used to stop uterine bleeding and as an antiseptic.

HYDRASTIS CANADENSIS • *See* Goldenseal.

HYDRATE • *See* Dimenhydrinate.

HYDRA-ZIDE • *See* Apresazide.

HYDREA • *See* Hydroxyurea.

HYDREX • *See* Benzthiazide.

HYDRISALIC • *See* Salicylic Acid.

HYDRO-, HYDR- • Prefixes from the Greek word *hydor,* meaning water.

HYDROCET • *See* Acetaminophen and Hydrocodone.

HYDROCHLORIC ACID (OTC) • In 1992, the FDA issued a notice that hydrochloric acid had not been shown to be safe and effective as claimed in OTC digestive-aid products.

HYDROCHLORIDE (HCL) • A compound formed by adding hydrochloric acid to an amine or related substance, such as glutamic acid hydrochloride. It is used to activate or acidify the ingredients in a compound.

HYDROCHLOROTHIAZIDE (Rx) • **Aldoril. Apresoline-Esidrix. Aquazide-H. Capozide. Diaqua. Diuchlor-H. Esidrix. Esimil. HCTZ. HHR. Hydoril. Hydrochlor. HydroDIURIL. Hydromal. Hydroprin. Hydroserpine. Hydro-T. Hydrotensin-50. Hyperetic. Lopressor HCT. Micrin. Mictrin. Oretic. Spironazole. Thiuretic. Timolide. Tri-Hydroserpine. URO. Vaseretic. Zide.** A thiazide diuretic (*see*) introduced in 1959, it increases urine excretion of sodium and water and is used to treat fluid retention, high blood pressure, congestive heart failure, cirrhosis of the liver, kidney dysfunction, and other conditions where it is necessary to rid the body of excess fluid. Potential adverse reactions include nausea, vomiting, pancreatitis, anemia, a drop in blood platelets, a drop in blood pressure when rising from a seated or prone position, impotence, decreased libido, loss of appetite, dehydration, low blood potassium, high blood sugar, fluid and electrolyte imbalances, rash, photosensitivity, and other allergic reactions. Cholestyramine and colestipol make thiazides less effective.

Diazoxide increases its blood-pressure-lowering, blood-sugar, and blood uric-acid effects. NSAIDs (*see*) decrease its effectiveness. Avoid over-the-counter drugs for the treatment of colds, coughs, and allergies because they may have stimulant effects. Use a sunscreen. Contraindicated in absence of urine formation or in those allergic to other thiazides or sulfonamide derivatives. Should be used with caution in patients with severe kidney or liver disease. If you are taking this drug, you may be advised to eat a diet high in potassium, including tomatoes, apricots, dates, and bananas. Hydrochlorothiazide should be taken in the morning to avoid having to urinate during the night.

HYDROCIL • *See* Psyllium.

HYDROCODONE (Rx) • **Anexsia. Bancap HC. Hycodan. Hycomine. Hycotuss. Hydrocet. Hydrogesic. Hy-Phen. Lorcet Plus. Lortab. Norcet 7. Novahistine. Triaminic Expectorant DH. Tussend. Vicodin. Zydone.** A semisynthetic narcotic analgesic and anti-cough medication similar to codeine (*see*). Introduced in 1951, its precise mechanism of action is unknown, although it is believed to relate to the existence of opiate receivers in the brain. In addition to analgesia, narcotics may produce drowsiness, changes in mood, and mental clouding. Serious overdose with hydrocodone is characterized by breathing difficulty, extreme drowsiness to stupor, cold and clammy skin, and sometimes, slow heartbeat and low blood pressure. Long-term use may produce psychological and/or physical dependence, and chronic constipation. In severe overdose, death can occur.

HYDROCORT • *See* Hydrocortisone.

HYDROCORTISONE (Rx) (OTC) • **Cortisol. A-hydroCort. Bactine Hydrocortisone Anti-Itch Cream. CaldeCORT Anti-Itch Hydrocortisone. Cortaid Spray. Cortef. Cortenema. Cortifoam. Hydrocortone. Hydrocortone Acetate. Solu-Cortef. Terra-cortrilopthalmic. Texacort. Acticort. Aeroseb-HC. Carmol HC. Cetacort. Cort-Dome. Cortinal. Cortizone 5. Cortril. Cremesone. Delacort. DermiCort. Der-molate. Durel-Cort. Ecosone HC Cream. FEP Cream. Grecort. Gynecort. H-Cort. HL-Cor-2.5. Heb-Cort. HVC Cream. Hycortole. Hydrocort. Hydromycin. Hydroquin. Hydro-Tex. Hydroxortex. Hysone-A. Hytone. Ivocort. Lanacort. Lexocort. Locoid. Maso-Cort. Microcort. Mity-Ouin. Neo-Cortef. Nutracort. Orabase HCA. Penecort. Proctocort. Rhus Tox HC. Rocort. Squibb-HC. Synacort. Unicort. Dermacort. Epifoam. Hydrocortisone Acetate. MyCort Lotion. Ophthocort. Procto-Foam-HC. Westcort Cream.** An adrenal-gland (*see*) corticosteroid (*see*) hormone introduced in 1952, used to decrease severe inflammation, as an adjunctive treatment of ulcerative colitis and proctitis, for shock, and to treat adrenal insufficiency. Also suppresses the immune response, stimulates bone marrow, and influences protein, fat, and carbohydrate metabolism. Most adverse reactions are the result of dosage or length of time the medication is used. Potential adverse reactions include euphoria, insomnia, psychotic behavior, high blood pressure, swelling, cataracts, glaucoma, peptic ulcer, GI irritation, increased appetite, growth suppression in children, delayed wound healing, acne, skin eruptions, muscle weakness, pancreatitis, hairiness, decreased immunity, and acute adrenal gland insufficiency. When withdrawn, there may be rebound inflammation, fatigue, weakness, joint pain, fever, dizziness, lethargy, depression, fainting, a drop in blood pressure upon rising from a seated or prone position, shortness of breath, loss of appetite, and high blood sugar. Sudden withdrawal may be fatal. Contraindicated in systemic fungal infections. Should be used cautiously in patients with GI ulceration or kidney disease, high blood pressure, diabetes, chicken pox, osteoporosis, Cushing's syndrome, blood-clotting disorders, seizures, myasthenia gravis (*see*), congestive heart failure, tuberculosis, herpes, and emotional instability. When taking hydrocortisone, patients may need low-sodium diets and potassium supplements. Barbiturates, phenytoin, and rifampin (*see all*) increase its effects. Indomethacin and aspirin may increase the risk of GI distress and bleeding. Should be taken with food or milk to reduce GI irritation. Topically, in aerosol, cream, gel, lotion, ointment, or solution, hydrocortisone is used to treat skin inflammation. Potential adverse reactions to these include burning, itching, irritation, dryness, inflammation of the hair follicles, acne, rash around the mouth, spots of pigment loss, hairiness, allergic contact dermatitis, and if covered with a dressing, secondary infection, atrophy, streaks, and blisters. Should be used cautiously in skin problems caused by viruses such as herpes, and in fungal or bacterial skin infections. Should not be used for more than two weeks due to potential absorption into the system, consequently causing an effect on the hypothalamus, and pituitary and adrenal glands. Should not be applied near the eyes or mucous membranes, under the arms, on the face, groin, or under the breast unless medically specified.

HYDROCORTONE • *See* Hydrocortisone.

HYDROCYANIC ACID • **Prussic Acid.** A white liquid with a faint odor of almonds, it occurs naturally in almonds, wild cherry, and other plants. When amygdalin in plums, almonds, and cherries combines with water, it forms hydrocyanic acid. Hydrocyanic acid contributes to the pleasant odor of wild cherry (*see*). It is toxic by ingestion, inhalation, and skin absorption. Used as a pesticide. The cancer treatment laetrile, banned in the United States, but used widely in Mexico, contains amygdalin.

HYDRODIURIL • *See* Hydrochlorothiazide.

HYDROFLUMETHIAZIDE (Rx) • **Saluron.** A thiazide diuretic (*see*) that increases urine excretion of sodium and water and is used to treat edema and high blood pressure. Potential adverse reactions include nausea, vomiting, pancreatitis, anemia, a drop in blood platelets, a drop in blood pressure when rising from a seated or prone position, loss of appetite, dehydration, low blood potassium, high blood sugar, fluid and electrolyte imbalances, rash, photosensitivity, and other allergic reactions. Cholestyramine and colestipol make thiazides less effective. Diazoxide increases hydroflumethiazide's blood-pressure-lowering, blood-sugar, and blood

uric-acid effects. NSAIDs decrease its effectiveness. Take in the morning to avoid having to urinate during the night. Use a sunscreen. Contraindicated in absence of urine formation or in those allergic to other thiazides or sulfonamide derivatives. Should be used with caution in patients with severe kidney or liver disease. If you are taking this drug, you may be advised to eat a diet high in potassium, including tomatoes, apricots, dates, and bananas.

HYDROGEN PEROXIDE (OTC) • H_2O_2. **Peroxyl.** A skin antiseptic used to cleanse wounds, skin ulcers, and local infections, and in the treatment of inflammatory conditions of the external ear canal. Also used in mouthwash gargles. In 1992, the FDA issued a notice that hydrogen peroxide had not been shown to be safe and effective as claimed in OTC poison ivy, poison oak, and poison sumac products.

HYDROGESIC • *See* Hydrocodone and Acetaminophen.

HYDROMAGNESIUM ALUMINATE • *See* Magaldrate.

HYDROMAL • *See* Hydrochlorothiazide.

HYDROMORPHONE (Rx) • A narcotic analgesic that alters both the perception of and emotional reaction to pain. Also suppresses the cough reflex. Used to treat moderate to severe pain. Potential adverse reactions include sedation, sleepiness, lack of alertness, dizziness, euphoria, seizures, low blood pressure, irregular heartbeat, nausea, vomiting, constipation, urine retention, and respiratory depression. Alcohol and central nervous system depressants may have additive effects. Contraindicated in patients with pressure on the brain, severe asthma attacks, respiratory depression, liver or kidney disease, low thyroid, shock, Addison's disease, acute alcoholism, seizures, head injury, brain tumor, lung disease, and in elderly or debilitated patients. May mask or worsen gallbladder pain. Contraindicated in depressed patients, as it may cause or worsen emotional depression. May be addictive.

HYDROMOX • *See* Quinethazone.

HYDROMYCIN (Rx) • *See* Neomycin, Polymyxin B, and Hydrocortisone.

HYDROPHILIC OINTMENT • An oil-in-water emulsion used as a base for skin preparations.

HYDROPHOBIA • *See* Rabies.

HYDROPRES-25 (Rx) • **Hydro-Serp. Hydroserpine. Hydrotensin. Mallopress.** A combination of hydrochlorothiazide and reserpine used to lower blood pressure. Hydrochlorothiazide relaxes the muscles of veins and arteries to reduce volume of blood flow. Reserpine reduces the effect of nerve transmission, lowering blood pressure. Potential adverse reactions include dry mouth, loss of potassium, excessive thirst, weakness, drowsiness, restlessness, muscle pain or cramps, fatigue, difficulty urinating, irregular heartbeat, gastrointestinal distress, sexual impotence, depression, loss of appetite, and gout. The drug-induced depression may last several months after discontinuance. Interaction with digitalis or quinidine may cause irregular heartbeat. Use with lithium may increase lithium's side effects. Over-the-counter cold, cough, or allergy medications contain stimulants that may make it less effective. You may need to increase potassium-containing foods in your diet, such as apricots and bananas, unless your physician has prescribed potassium supplements.

HYDROPRIN (Rx) • *See* Hydrochlorothiazide and Reserpine.

HYDROQUIN (Rx) • *See* Hydrocortisone and Iodochlorhydroxyquin.

HYDROQUINONE (Rx) (OTC) • **Melanex.** Used in strong solution to bleach dark spots on the skin. In weaker solutions, it is used in skin-bleach and freckle creams, and suntan lotions. A white, crystalline phenol that occurs naturally but is usually manufactured in the laboratory. Application to the skin may cause allergic reactions. It can cause depigmentation in a 2 percent solution. Ingestion of as little as one gram (one-thirtieth of an ounce) has caused nausea, vomiting, ringing in the ears, delirium, a sense of suffocation, and collapse. Industrial workers exposed to the chemical have suffered clouding of the eye lens.

HYDROSERPINE (Rx) • A combination of hydrochlorothiazide and reserpine (*see both*).

HYDRO-T • *See* Hydrochlorothiazide.

HYDROTENSIN-5O (Rx) • *See* Hydrochlorothiazide and Reserpine.

HYDRO-TEX (Rx) • *See* Hydrocortisone.

HYDROXACEN (Rx) • *See* Hydroxyzine.

HYDROXIDE • A compound that liberates oxygen and hydrogen upon dissolving in water.

HYDROXOCOBALAMIN • **Alpha Ruvite.** *See* Vitamin B_{12}.

HYDROXYCHLOROQUINE (Rx) • **Plaquenil.** Introduced in 1967, this drug suppresses attacks of malaria. Has also been found to be effective for the treatment of rheumatoid arthritis in patients who have not responded adequately to NSAIDs (*see*). Hydroxychloroquine may cause blood problems, including a drop in white blood cells and platelets, and anemia. May also cause irritability, nightmares, seizures, excitability, toxic psychosis, dizziness, ringing in the ears, nystagmus (*see*), loss of visual acuity, eye damage, bone-marrow toxicity, fatigue, and muscle weakness. It reportedly causes less eye toxicity than chloroquine. Hydroxychloroquine may increase the side effects of penicillamine. Cimetidine may increase the side effects of hydroxychloroquine. Antacids and magnesium salts may decrease its effectiveness. Should be taken with food or milk to prevent stomach irritation.

HYDROXYETHYLCELLULOSE (OTC) • A thickener and bodying agent derived from plants. It is used in artificial-tear (*see*) preparations.

HYDROXYPROGESTERONE (Rx) • Dura-lutin. Gesterol LA. Hy-Gesterone. Hylatin. Hyprogest. Hyproval. Hyroxon. Pro-Depo. Prodrox.

An injectable progestin used to treat menstrual disorders and uterine cancer. It suppresses ovulation, possibly by inhibiting pituitary gonadotropin secretion. Forms a thick cervical mucus. Potential adverse reactions include nausea, vomiting, depression, high blood pressure, dizziness, migraine, libido changes, blood clots, water retention, increased risk of stroke, blood clots to the lung, and heart attack. May also worsen nearsightedness, cause intolerance to contact lenses, and lead to loss of appetite, increased appetite, excessive thirst, pancreatitis, bloating, and abdominal cramps. May cause breakthrough bleeding, altered menstrual flow, painful or absent menstruation, enlargement of benign tumors of the uterus, cervical erosion, abnormal secretions, and vaginal candidiasis. There may be jaundice, high blood sugar, high calcium in the blood, folic acid deficiency, dark spots appearing on the skin, hives, acne, oily skin, and breast tenderness, enlargement, and secretion. Contraindicated in pregnancy, in persons with blood-clot disorders, cancer of the breast, reproductive organs, or genitals, and in those with undiagnosed abnormal genital bleeding. Should be used with caution in high blood pressure, asthma, and mental depression. Effects of progestin injections last seven to fourteen days. Normal menstrual period will not occur usually for two to three months after the drug has been discontinued. Rifampin (*see*) decreases hydroxyprogesterone's effectiveness.

HYDROXYPROPYLCELLULOSE (OTC) • Lacrisert.

A substance derived from plants and used in artificial-tear (*see*) preparations. This medicine can cause blurred vision for a short time after each dose is applied. Also may cause the eyes to become more sensitive to light. Wearing sunglasses and avoiding too much exposure to bright light may help lessen discomfort.

HYDROXYPROPYL METHYLCELLULOSE (Rx) (OTC) • Gonak. Gonisol. Isopto Alkaline. Isopto Tears. Just Tears. Lacril. Moisture Drops. MuroTears.

A substance used in artificial-tear (*see*) preparation. It helps to prevent damage in certain eye diseases. Potential adverse reactions include blurred vision and stickiness of eyelashes. Should not be used for more than three days unless your physician prescribes it.

HYDROXYUREA (Rx) • Hydrea.

An anticancer drug used to treat melanoma, resistant chronic myelocytic leukemia, and recurrent, metastatic, or inoperable ovarian cancer. In 1995, trials to determine hydroxyurea's efficacy in the treatment of sickle-cell anemia (*see*) were halted because the results were so successful. Researchers declared it the first successful treatment for sickle-cell anemia, and the FDA, at this writing, was expected to promptly approve its use for that purpose. Potential adverse reactions include nausea, vomiting, diarrhea, loss of appetite, sore mouth, drowsiness, hallucinations, anemia, bone-marrow suppression, rash, itching, and kidney dysfunction. The doctors involved in the sickle-cell trials advised against its use in women who expected to become pregnant.

HYDROXYZINE (Rx) • Anxanil. Apo-Hydroxyzine. Atarax. Atozine. E-Vista. Hydroxacen. Hy-Pam. Hyzine-50. Marax DF. Orgatrax. Quiess. Theozine. Vistacon. Vistaject. Vistaquel. Vistaril. Vistazine.

A piperazine (*see*) antihistamine introduced in 1953 that depresses the central nervous system at the area of the brain controlling emotions. Used to treat anxiety, tension, restlessness, for emotionally induced allergic conditions, and before or after surgery for anxiety and nausea. Also has been used to treat alcoholism, and for behavior problems in children. Potential side effects include drowsiness, tremors, convulsions, and dry mouth. Should not be used with alcohol and other central nervous system depressants, including other antihistamines. Cimetidine may increase sedation. Contraindicated in shock or coma. May be taken with or without food.

HY-GESTRONE (Rx) • *See* Hydroxyprogesterone.

HYGROTON (Rx) • *See* Chlorthalidone.

HYLAND'S BED WETTING TABLETS (OTC) • *See* Belladonna.

HYLAND'S COLIC TABLETS (OTC) • *See* Chamomile.

HYLAND'S COUGH SYRUP WITH HONEY (OTC) • Contains *Cephaelis ipecacuanha* (ipecac), *Aconitum napellus* (aconite), *Spongia tosta* (sponge), and *Antimonium tartaricum* (potassium tartrate) with honey. A homeopathic combination for the temporary relief of symptoms of simple, dry, tight, or tickling coughs due to colds in children.

HYLAND'S C-PLUS COLD TABLETS (OTC) • *See* Potassium Iodide.

HYLAND'S TEETHING TABLETS (OTC) • *See* Belladonna and Chamomile.

HYLOREL (Rx) • *See* Guanadrel.

HYLUTIN (Rx) • *See* Hydroxyprogesterone.

HYONATAL (Rx) • *See* Hyoscyamine, Atropine Sulfate, Scopolamine, and Phenobarbital.

HYOSCINE (Rx) • *See* Scopolamine.

HYOSCYAMINE (Rx) (OTC) • **Anaspaz. Arco-Lase Plus. Cystospaz-M. Donnagel-PG. Donnatal Tablets. Gastrosed. Haponal. Hexalol. Hyonatal. Hyosophen. Kutrase. Levsin. Levsinex. Pyridium Plus. Relaxadon. Ru-Tuss. Spasmolin. Spasquid. Urised Tablets.** An anticholinergic drug used as an antispasmodic in irritable bowel syndrome (*see*), urinary incontinence, and as an adjunctive therapy in peptic ulcers and other GI disorders. Potential adverse reactions include disorientation, excitability, incoherence, weakness, nervousness, dizziness, headache, palpitations, rapid heartbeat, blurred vision, sensitivity to light, increased eye pressure, difficulty in swallowing, constipation, dry mouth, nausea, vomiting, epigastric distress, urinary retention, impotence, hives, decreased sweating, and fever. Contraindicated in glaucoma, obstructions in the urinary or GI tract, myasthenia gravis (*see*), paralytic ileus (*see*), intestinal flaccidity, unstable cardiovascular status in acute hemorrhage, and toxic megacolon. Should be used with caution in patients with nerve damage, overactive thyroid, coronary artery disease, irregular heartbeat, congestive heart failure, high blood pressure, hiatal hernia, liver or kidney disease, and ulcerative colitis. Should also be used with caution in people over forty years of age due to the possibility of glaucoma. Should be taken thirty minutes to one hour before meals. Use with caution in hot or humid environments. Drug-induced heatstroke can occur. In 1992, the FDA proposed a ban on hyoscyamine sulfate in oral OTC menstrual drug products because it had not been shown to be safe and effective as claimed.

HYOSOPHEN (Rx) • *See* Hyoscyamine, Atropine Sulfate, Scopolamine, and Phenobarbital.

HYP. • The homeopathic abbreviation for hypericum (*see*).

HY-PAM (Rx) • *See* Hydroxyzine.

HYPER- • Prefix from the Greek word for above or over, it means excessive or above the normal.

HYPERACUSIS • Abnormal acuteness of hearing or auditory sensation.

HYPERALDOSTERONISM • Aldosterone is the most potent hormone produced by the adrenal glands lying over the kidneys. It causes sodium retention and potassium loss. When too much aldosterone is released, it causes multiple symptoms, including overloads of salt, fluid retention, weakness, numbness, transient paralysis, and high blood pressure. The cause may be a tumor of the adrenal gland or unknown.

HYPERBILIRUBINEMIA • Raised blood level of bilirubin, a waste product formed from the destruction of red blood cells. Jaundice becomes apparent if the bilirubin level rises to twice the normal level.

HYPERCAL (H) • A homeopathic mixture of calendula and hypericum (*see both*). It is used to treat cold sores, cuts, eye infections, mouth ulcers, and as a mouthwash.

HYPERCALCEMIA • An abnormally high level of calcium in the blood, which can seriously disrupt cell function, particularly in muscles and nerves. Hypercalcemia of malignancy is most commonly caused by metastasis to the bone, which releases calcium in the blood.

HYPERCHOLESTEROLEMIA • An inherited metabolic disorder resulting in an abnormal amount of cholesterol in the blood. It can lead to accelerated atherosclerosis (*see*) and early heart attack.

HYPERESTHESIA • Excessive sensibility to touch, pain, or other stimuli.

HYPERGLYCEMIA • An abnormal amount of sugar (glucose) in the blood.

HYPERICUM (H) • An herb used in homeopathic medicine to treat burns, cuts, insect bites, and sunburn. *See* Saint-John's-Wort.

HYPERLIPIDEMIA • A group of metabolic disorders characterized by high levels of lipids—fatty substances, including cholesterol—in the blood. Hyperlipidemia is a risk factor for accelerated atherosclerosis (*see*) and premature heart attacks.

HYPERPHOSPHATEMIA • Excessive levels of phosphates in the blood that can be caused by chronic kidney problems.

HYPERSENSITIVITY • A condition in persons previously exposed to an antigen in which tissue damage results from an immune reaction to a further dose of the antigen. Classically, four types of hypersensitivity are recognized, but the term is often used to mean the type of allergy associated with hay fever and asthma.

HYPERSTAT • *See* Diazoxide.

HYPERTENSION • High blood pressure, often diagnosed when an adult has readings consistently above $^{140}/_{90}$ mmHg. *See* Antihypertensives.

HYPERTHERMIA • An increase in body temperature above normal.

HY-PHEN (Rx) • *See* Hydrocodone and Acetaminophen.

HYPNO- • Prefix from the Greek word *hypnos,* meaning sleep, as in *hypnosis.*

HYPNOTIC • A drug that induces sleep. The benzodiazepines (*see*) are widely used in prescription sleeping medications. The antihistamines are promoted in OTC sleep-inducing products. Among the herbs used for this purpose are valerian and hop (*see both*).

HYPO- • Prefix from the Greek word *hypo,* meaning under. Denoting deficient or below normal.

HYPOALLERGENIC • A term for a product supposedly devoid of the common allergens that most frequently cause allergic reactions.

HYPOCALCEMIA • Too little calcium in the blood. One cause is insufficient parathyroid hormone. In severe cases, hypocalcemia causes cramplike spasms in the hands, face, and feet due to the effect of low blood calcium on muscle activity.

HYPOCITRATURIA • A condition characterized by a decrease of citric acid in the urine, causing a pH imbalance leading to calcium kidney stones.

HYPOGEUSIA • Diminished ability to taste.

HYPOGLYCEMIA • Low blood sugar.

HYPOGONADISM • Inadequate sex-organ function manifested by deficiencies in sex hormones, atrophy, or deficient development of secondary sexual characteristics.

HYPOSMIA • Diminished ability to smell.

HYPOTEARS (OTC) • *See* Artificial Tears.

HYPOTENSION • Abnormally low blood pressure.

HYPOTHALAMUS • Brain control area involved in emotions, movement, and eating. Less than the size of a peanut and weighing a quarter of an ounce, this small area deep within the brain also oversees appetite, blood pressure, sexual behavior, sleep, and emotions and sends orders to the pituitary gland.

HYPOTHALAMUS-PITUITARY-ADRENAL AXIS • The hypothalamus, a section of the brain, sends hormonal messages to the pituitary gland in the center of the skull behind the nose. The pituitary sends hormonal messages to the adrenal glands above the kidneys. Medicines, particularly adrenocorticoids and corticoptropin, may affect the communication within this system and cause serious side effects, including lowering your resistance to infections.

HYPOTHERMIA • A decrease or drop in body temperature.

HYPROGEST (Rx) • *See* Hydroxyprogesterone.

HYPURIN • *See* Insulin.

HYSKON • *See* Dextran.

HYSONE-A • *See* Hydrocortisone.

HYSSOP (H) • *Hyssopus officinalis.* A perennial herb native to southern Europe and western Asia, it was used to treat cuts and fresh wounds. Herbalists use it today to relieve catarrh (*see*), reduce mucus, clear the chest, and calm the nerves. Used as an herbal tea for gas (flatus). Has been shown to have antiviral properties.

HYTAKEROL • *See* Dihydrotachysterol.

HYTINIC • *See* Iron.

HYTONE (Rx) • *See* Hydrocortisone.

HYTRIN • *See* Terazosin Hydrochloride.

HYTUSS (OTC) • *See* Guaifenesin.

HYZAAR (R) • *See* Losartan Potassium.

HYZINE-50 • *See* Hydroxyzine.

I

-IA • Suffix denoting a condition. Preceded in usage by the organ or system, as in *leukemia,* cancer of the blood.

-IASIS • Suffix indicating a condition, such as *psoriasis.*

IATRO- • Prefix pertaining to a doctor or medicine in general.

IATROGENIC • Caused by a physician.

IBENZMETHYZIN • *See* Procarbazine.

IBERET (OTC) • A multivitamin preparation with iron.

IBEROL (OTC) • A multivitamin preparation with iron.

IBIAMOX • *See* Amoxicillin.

IBIDOMIDE • *See* Labetalol.

IBUPRIN • *See* Ibuprofen.

IBUPROFEN (Rx) (OTC) • **Advil. Aches-N-Pain. Cap-Profen. Cramp End. Dristan Sinus Pain Reliever. Genpril. Haltran. Ibuprin. Iburin. IBU-TAB. Medipren. Menadol. Midol 200. Motrin. Nuprin. Pamprin-IB. Pediaprofen. Rufen. Saleto-200. Trendar. Uni-pro.** Introduced in 1967, this nonsteroidal anti-inflammatory drug (NSAID) works by inhibiting the body's production of hormonelike substances called prostaglandins, which trigger fever, pain, and inflammation. Ibuprofen is used to treat arthritis pain and gout. Also relieves mild to moderate headaches, soft-tissue injuries, and pain following operations. It is especially useful in stopping prostaglandins that cause menstrual cramps. In 1995, the FDA approved an ibuprofen suspension as a nonprescription analgesic to reduce fever and pain in children between the ages of two and eleven years. Ibuprofen has fewer side effects than aspirin, but it can cause itching, rash, upset stomach, blurred vision, ulcers, ringing in the ears, decreased appetite, fluid retention, bleeding, and dizziness. Also may cause menstrual irregularities, and male breast enlargement and tenderness. It is less toxic in large doses than either aspirin or acetaminophen, but may lead to kidney damage when taken in large doses over prolonged periods. Anyone allergic to aspirin or suffering from gout or ulcers should not use ibuprofen. Rare cases of fatal liver toxicity have been reported with the use of ibuprofen. Discontinue ibuprofen's use for at least five hours before visiting your physician because it can mask symptoms and lead to a misdiagnosis. Do not use for at least two weeks before surgery because of its effect on blood clotting. Pregnant or nursing women should not take the drug. Ibuprofen interacts with a wide range of drugs to increase the risk of bleeding and/or peptic ulcer. It increases the blood levels of lithium (*see*), and reduces the effectiveness of some blood-pressure drugs and diuretics. When oral antidiabetics are used with ibuprofen, their effectiveness may be decreased. The OTC brands are 200-mg strength, and it is recommended not to exceed 1.2 g/day and not to self-medicate for extended periods without consulting a physician. Should be taken with milk or meals to avoid stomach distress. *See also* Children's Ibuprofen.

IBURIN • *See* Ibuprofen.

IBU-TAB • *See* Ibuprofen.

IBUTILIDE FUMARATE (Rx) • **Covert.** An injectable medication, introduced in 1995, to treat irregular heartbeat. It rapidly converts atrial fibrillation and atrial flutter, two common causes of irregular contractions of the heart, to normal.

ICELAND MOSS (H) • *Cetraria islandica.* **Iceland Lichen.** So named because Icelanders reputedly were the first to discover its benefits. It is high in mucilage, with some iodine, traces of vitamin A, and usnic acid. Herbalists use the lichen as a gentle laxative, and to treat dysentery, anemia, bronchitis, and upper-respiratory problems associated with degenerative wasting.

I-CHLOR • *See* Chloramphenicol.

ICHTHAMMOL (Rx) • **Ammonium Ichthosulfonate. Medicone Derma-HC. PRID Salve.** A thick, viscous liquid that smells like coal. It has slight bacteria-killing properties and is used in ointments for the treatment of skin disorders. Also a weak skin irritant. Used to relieve minor skin irritations, superficial cuts, scratches, and wounds. Also used to treat acne, boils, and other skin disorders. Should not be covered with a bandage.

IDAMYCIN • *See* Idarubicin.

IDARUBICIN (Rx) • **Idamycin.** Used in combination with other drugs in treatment of chronic myeloid leukemia (CML). *See* Myelogenous Leukemia.

IDIO- • Prefix meaning unusual or peculiar, as in *idiosyncrasy.*

IDIOSYNCRASY • When used in the drug field, the term refers to an abnormal response to a drug by individuals who have a special, often hereditary, defect in their body chemistry. Many people, including 10 percent of American blacks, for example, lack the enzyme G-6-PD, which causes their red blood cells to disintegrate when exposed to drugs such as sulfonamides (*see*). An estimated 5 percent of the American population develop glaucoma with prolonged use of corticosteroids (*see*).

IDOXURIDINE (Rx) • **IDU. IUDR. Herplex. Liquifilm. Stoxil.** An eye ointment introduced in 1963 that is used to treat herpes simplex keratitis (*see*), a viral infection commonly leading to chronic inflammation, scarring, and potentially, loss of vision. Potential adverse reactions include temporary hazy vision, irritation, pain, burning, or inflammation of the eye, light hurting the eye, eye ulcers, slow wound healing, and hypersensitivity. Usually not used for more than three weeks.

IDU • *See* Idoxuridine.

IFEX • *See* Ifosfamide.

IFLRA • A type of interferon (*see*) used to treat hairy-cell leukemia and AIDS-related Kaposi's sarcoma.

IFN • *See* Interferon.

IFOSFAMIDE (Rx) • **IFEX.** An anticancer drug introduced in 1989 that is used to treat testicular cancer. Potential adverse reactions include nausea, vomiting, drowsiness, high blood pressure including a drop in white blood cells, suppression of bone marrow, lethargy, confusion, depressive psychosis, coma, nausea, vomiting, bladder bleeding, kidney damage, liver dysfunction, and loss of hair. Allopurinol, bone-marrow suppressants, and barbiturates may increase ifosfamide's toxic effects. Corticosteroids may make it less effective.

IG • *See* Immune Serum Globulin.

I-GENT • *See* Gentamicin.

IGN • Homeopathic abbreviation for ignatia (*see*).

IGNATIA (H) • **St. Ignatius's Bean.** A homeopathic medicine derived from a small shrub or tree that grows in the Philippines and China. The bean was named by Spanish Jesuits, who brought the tree to Europe. It is used for anxiety, gout, epilepsy, and asthma. The bean is poisonous and large doses can be fatal. Small doses can produce violent headache, loss of appetite, nightmares, trembling, cramps, and perspiration.

I-HOMATRINE • *See* Homatropine.

ILEITIS • *See* Inflammatory Bowel Diseases.

ILEOSTOMY • From the Greek words *ileo,* for the ileum, the lower portion of the intestines, and *stoma,* for mouth. Refers to an artificial opening made in the ileum.

ILETIN • *See* Insulin.

ILEUM • Lowest of the three portions of the small intestine.

ILOPAN • *See* Dexpanthenol.

ILOSONE • *See* Erythromycin.

ILOTYCIN • *See* Erythromycin.

ILOZYME • *See* Pancrelipase.

IL-2 • *See* Interleukins.

IM • Abbreviation for intramuscular, usually referring to an injection of medicine.

IMFERON • *See* Iron.

IMIDAZOLES (Rx) (OTC) • Antifungal medicines that work by killing a fungus or preventing its growth. Vaginal products containing imidazoles are used to treat yeast infections. Among the imidazoles on the market are butoconazole, econazole, and miconazole (*see all*).

IMIGLUCERASE (Rx) • **Cerezyme.** A genetically engineered medication that is injected for long-term enzyme replacement therapy for patients with Gaucher's disease (*see*), which results in anemia, bone disease, and liver and spleen disorders. Introduced in 1994, it was a priority orphan drug (*see*). The FDA approved it after 12.1 months of review. This is reportedly the most complicated biotechnology drug developed to date.

IMIPRAMINE (Rx) • **Janimine. SK-Pramine. Tofranil. Trimipramine.** A tricyclic antidepressant introduced in 1955, it takes up to two weeks to manifest effects. Reportedly causes a lesser increase in heart rate than other tricyclic antidepressants. It is used to treat childhood bedwetting when physical causes have been eliminated. Potential adverse effects include drowsiness, dizziness, excitation, tremor, weakness, confusion, headache, nervousness, a drop in blood pressure when rising from a sitting or prone position, irregular heartbeat, high blood pressure, blurred vision, ringing in the ears, dry mouth, constipation, nausea, vomiting, loss of appetite, intestinal paralysis, urine retention, mania, rash, hives, sweating, decreased or increased libido, impotence, inhibited female orgasm, female breast enlargement with milk production, male breast enlargement, swelling of the testicles, and allergy. Sudden withdrawal of drug may cause nausea, headache, and malaise. Contraindicated soon after a heart attack, in enlarged prostate, and in patients with a history of seizure disorders. Must be used with caution in persons with heart disease, thyroid disease, impaired liver function, blood abnormalities, or elective surgery. Barbiturates decrease imipramine's level. Cimetidine and methylphenidate may increase imipramine's level, causing adverse reaction. Epinephrine and norepinephrine increases its high blood pressure effect. MAO inhibitors (*see*) may cause severe excitation, high fever, or seizures. Alcohol or antidepressants should not be used while taking this drug. Imipramine is most effective when taken on an empty stomach but may be taken with a small amount of food if stomach distress occurs.

IMITREX • *See* Sumatriptan.

IMMUNE COMPROMISED • Refers to persons whose basic medical condition and/or drug therapy has weakened their immune defenses, rendering them highly susceptible to infection.

IMMUNE GLOBULIN • *See* Gamma Globulin.

IMMUNE SERUM GLOBULIN (Rx) • **Gamastan. Gamimune N. Gammagard. Gammar. IG. Sandoglobulin. Venoglobulin-I.** Antibody preparations injected to prevent certain infectious diseases. The serums are made from the concentrated blood serums of people who have survived diseases or poisonous bites. Globulin from the general collection of blood contains antibodies to most common diseases. Specific immune serum globulins against rare diseases or toxins are derived from the blood of specific donors who are likely to have high levels of antibodies to that disease. Because immune serum globulins do not stimulate the body to produce its own antibodies, the effects are not long lasting, and repeated injections may be required. Potential adverse reactions from immune serum globulins are rare. Some people are sensitive to horse glob-ulins and may experience serum sickness with fever, rash, joint swelling, and pain.

IMMUNOGLOBULINS • Family of large protein molecules, also known as antibodies.

IMMUNOMODULATOR • A substance that causes general stimulation of the immune system to fight disease.

IMMUNOSUPPRESSANT • A medicine that reduces the body's natural immunity.

IMMUNOTHERAPY • The use of the immune system or the products of the immune system to control, damage, or destroy malignant cells.

IMODIUM • *See* Loperamide.

IMOVAX • *See* Rabies Vaccine.

IMPATIENS BIFLORA TINCTURE (OTC) (H) • In 1992, the FDA issued a notice that im-patiens tincture had not been shown to be safe and effective as claimed in OTC poison ivy, poison oak, and poison sumac products.

IMPETIGO • An acute skin infection, initially blisterlike in nature, which later becomes crusted after the blisters rupture; painless and often ac-companied by itching.

IMURAN • *See* Azathioprine.

INACTIVE INGREDIENTS • Substances not therapeutically active, such as starches, added to medicines to provide bulk, flavoring, or color.

I-NAPHLINE • *See* Naphazoline.

INDAPAMIDE (Rx) • **Lozol.** A thiazidelike diuretic introduced in 1974 that increases urine excretion of sodium and water and also has a direct blood-vessel-dilating effect. Used to treat edema and high blood pressure, heart failure, and cirrhosis of the liver. Similar in action to the thiazide diuretics (*see*). Potential adverse reactions include headache, irritability, nervousness, nau-sea, pancreatitis, a drop in blood platelets, a drop in blood pressure when rising from a seated or prone position, loss of appetite, dehydration, low blood potassium, fluid and electrolyte imbalances, rash, photosensitivity, and muscle cramps and spasms. Contraindicated in absence of urine for-mation, and in those allergic to thiazides or sul-fonamide derivatives. Should be used with caution in patients with severe kidney or liver disease. Diazoxide and other blood-pressure-lowering drugs increase indapamide's blood-pressure-lowering, blood-sugar, and blood uric-acid effects. NSAIDs (*see*) decrease its effectiveness. Take in the morning after breakfast to avoid having to uri-nate during the night. Use a sunscreen. If you are taking this drug, you may be advised to eat a diet high in potassium, including tomatoes, apricots, dates, and bananas.

INDECAINIDE (Rx) • **Decabid.** An antiar-rhythmic drug for the treatment of life-threatening heartbeat irregularities. Potential adverse reactions include dizziness, nervousness, anxiety, headache, insomnia, new or worsened heart irregularities, blurred vision, abdominal pain, constipation, diar-rhea, heartburn, dry mouth, nausea, shortness of breath, cough, back pain, fever, and numbness. Interacts with other antiarrhythmic drugs and cimetidine (*see*), which increase the blood levels of indecainide.

INDERAL • *See* Propranolol.

INDERIDE (Rx) • A combination of hy-drochlorothiazide and propranolol that is used to treat high blood pressure. The combination of these blood-pressure-lowering compounds dilates the blood vessels and controls the nerve impulses that control blood-vessel dilation. Potential adverse reactions include nausea, vomiting, confusion, exacerbation of heart failure or other heart prob-lems, tingling in the limbs, light-headedness, de-pression, insomnia, weakness, loss of appetite, dizziness, headache, sensitivity to sunlight, muscle spasms, hearing loss, fatigue, GI distress, diarrhea, constipation, allergic reactions, and adverse effects on the blood. Inderide can cause potassium depletion. Contraindicated in those allergic to any of the ingredients or to sulfa drugs, and those with a history of heart failure, asthma, or upper-respiratory disease. Your physician may suggest increasing the intake of high-potassium foods, such as bananas and apricots, but check, because if a potassium supplement has been prescribed, high-potassium foods may pose a problem.

INDIAN ACALYPHA (H) • *Acalypha indica.* An erect plant native to India and Sri Lanka, it is used by homeopaths and in folk medicine as a laxative and to combat worms and in the treatment of cough, bronchitis, and asthma. It irritates the skin and mucous membranes, and used topically may cause skin rash. It is toxic when ingested. Prolonged use can cause a breakdown of blood cells.

INDIAN PINK • *See* Spigelia.

INDIAN TRAGACANTH • *See* Karaya Gum.

INDICATIONS FOR USE • The medical condition for which a medication is intended.

INDIGO • Probably the oldest-known dye. Prepared from various plants of genus *Indigofera* native to Bengal, Java, and Guatemala. Dark blue powder with a coppery luster.

INDIGOWEED • *See* Baptisia.

INDIUM IN-111 PENTREOTIDE • *See* OctreoScan.

INDOCIN • *See* Indomethacin.

INDO-LEMMON • *See* Indomethacin.

INDOLES • Found in cabbage and brussels sprouts and kale, they seem to induce protective enzymes.

INDOMED • *See* Indomethacin.

INDOMETACIN • *See* Indomethacin.

INDOMETH • *See* Indomethacin.

INDOMETHACIN (Rx) • **Indocin. Indo-Lemmon. Indomed. Indometacin. Indometh.** Introduced in 1963, this drug has anti-inflammatory, analgesic, and fever-reducing effects, possibly through inhibition of prostaglandins (*see*). Used to treat severe arthritis, and infants born with the heart problem patent ductus arteriosus. Potential adverse reactions include anemia, headache, dizziness, depression, drowsiness, confusion, peripheral nerve damage, seizures, faintness, high blood pressure, edema, blurred vision, corneal and retinal damage, hearing loss, ringing in the ears, nausea, vomiting, loss of appetite, diarrhea, peptic ulcers, severe GI bleeding, blood in the urine, potassium overload, skin rash, hives, kidney dysfunction, low salt, and low blood sugar. Aspirin may decrease its effectiveness. May produce severe stomach upset and may aggravate emotional problems, Parkinson's disease, or epilepsy. Must be used with great caution in persons with a history of ulcers, bleeding problems, or allergic reaction to aspirin. Alcoholic beverages may increase its side effects. Indomethacin may reduce the effects of high blood pressure medication, may increase lithium toxicity, and may impair response to thiazide diuretics and furosemide (*see both*). Should not use with triamterene because of possible kidney damage. Diflunisal and probenecid may increase indomethacin's toxicity. Serious GI toxicity can occur at any time in long-term NSAID (*see*) use. Causes sodium retention and, thus, weight gain. Should be taken with food to avoid upset stomach.

INERT • A term used to indicate chemical inactivity in an element or compound. However, in drugs, food additives, cosmetics, and other chemical products, the term has come to mean ingredients added to mixtures chiefly for bulk and weight purposes. The chemicals still may have some activity of their own, although not for the product's specific purpose.

INFARCT • Area of tissue death due to local stoppage of blood supply caused by an obstruction.

INFARCTION • Death of an organ or part of an organ due to an interruption of its blood supply.

INFECTROL (Rx) • A combination of neomycin, polymyxin B, and dexamethasone (*see all*).

INFLAMASE FORTE (Rx) • *See* Prednisolone.

INFLAMASE MILD (Rx) • *See* Prednisolone.

INFLAMMATION • Derived from the Latin word *inflammo,* meaning flame, it is an immune reaction to tissue injury and generally involves redness, swelling, pain, and heat. The reddening results from increased blood flowing to the affected part. Many inflammatory conditions are designated by the suffix *-itis,* preceded by the name of the affected tissue. For example, appendicitis, otitis, and arthritis.

INFLAMMATORY BOWEL DISEASES • Two types of inflammatory bowel diseases are as follows:
   Ulcerative Colitis. A chronic inflammatory disease of the lining of the large intestine (colon).
   Chron's Disease (Regional Enteritis, Ileitis). A chronic, recurring inflammatory disease that can affect any part of the gastrointestinal tract, but most often the ileum (small intestine) or colon.

INFLUENZA VACCINE • Protection for people of any age who are at risk of serious consequences from contracting the flu virus. Long-term immunity against influenza is not possible since the virus changes all the time. When the current virus is identified, a vaccine is produced. Protection develops within four weeks of vaccination.

INFUSION • In traditional medicine, it signifies the introduction into a vein of fluid that can be delivered in measured amounts over time. In herbal medicine, it means the steeping in boiled water of the softer parts of plants, such as leaves, flowers, and twigs; also the juice from leaves.

INH • *See* Isoniazid.

INHALATION ANESTHETIC • A drug or combination of drugs given to produce unconsciousness. General anesthesia is usually induced by injection of a drug, such as thiopental (*see*), and maintained by inhalation of a volatile liquid such as halothane or a gas such as nitrous oxide.

INHALER • A device for administering drugs through the mouth or nose. Inhalers are used principally in the treatment of respiratory disorders such as asthma, and upper-respiratory infections related to the common cold.

INHALE THERAPEUTIC SYSTEMS • A method being tested to deliver insulin and anti-blood-clotting medications by nose instead of by injection or other means.

INHIBITOR • A substance that slows down or prevents a process or reaction.

INITIATION • An event that alters the genetic code of a cell or causes some other basic, permanent damage, predisposing that cell to later become a cancer cell. Chemical carcinogens, viruses, radiation, and other factors are thought to be capable of causing initiation.

INK CAP (H) • *Coprinus atramentarius.* A fungus with a white stem native to Europe and introduced to many moderate zones. It is a component of various health food products as a nutrient. It contains disulfiram (*see*), which can cause a severe reaction if taken with alcohol.

INNOVAR • *See* Fentanyl and Droperidol.

INOCOR • *See* Amrinone Lactate.

INOCULATION • The introduction of a disease agent into the body in order to produce a mild form of the disease and provide immunity. Polio vaccine is an example.

INONOTUS (H) • *Iinonotus obliquus.* **Birch Fungus.** A parasitic fungus growing on the common silver birch. It contains steroids and is used as an anti-inflammatory and antiviral remedy. In Eastern Europe and Russia, it is used by doctors to treat terminally ill cancer patients. Its use as an anticancer agent has not been proven.

IN SITU • Carcinoma *in situ,* meaning "on the surface," is tissue cancerous only in the surface cells of an organ, with no sign of spreading to deeper layers.

INSULIN (Rx) • **Antrapid. Humulin. Hypurin. Mixtard. Novolin L, N, R. NPH. Beef Regular Iletin. Lente. Lente Iletin. Pork Regular Iletin. Protamine. Ultralente. Ultralente Purified Beef. Ultratard.** A hormone produced by islet cells of the pancreas gland, essential for metabolism. Insulin is used in the treatment of diabetes. May be obtained from pork, beef, or human cells. Potential adverse reactions include low blood sugar, high blood sugar rebound, hives, high blood fats, swelling, itching, redness, and anaphylaxis. Use with alcohol, beta-blockers (*see*), clofibrate, fenfluramine, MAO inhibitors (*see*), salicylates, and tetracycline causes prolonged low blood sugar effect. Corticosteroids and thiazide diuretics (*see both*) diminish its effectiveness. Cigarette smoking decreases the amount of insulin absorption.

INSULINLIKE GROWTH FACTOR 1 (IGF-1) (Rx) • **Myotropin.** A growth factor that is synthesized by the liver and bone cells and stimulates the production of bone tissue. In 1996, it was made available free to patients with amyotrophic lateral sclerosis (ALS). The FDA's action came seventeen days after an expert advisory committee had recommended it unanimously. Although it does not cure the progressive muscle-paralysis disease, clinical trials in the United States and Europe have shown it can slow down the disease's progression.

INTAL • *See* Cromolyn Sodium.

INTER- • Prefix meaning between.

INTERFERON (IFN) (Rx) • **IFLRA.** In 1957, it was discovered that a protein produced natu-rally by cells could interfere with the ability of a virus to reproduce after it had invaded the body. By the mid-1970s, it appeared that this protein, interferon, might also curtail the spread of certain types of cancer. Genetic engineering enabled the production of sufficient supplies of interferon for experimentation and treatment. One type of leukemia, hairy cell, once invariably fatal, has responded to interferon treatment. The interferons are now being tested against other cancers and viruses. Potential adverse reactions include chest pain, confusion, irregular heartbeat, mental depression, nervousness, numbness or tingling of fingers, toes, and face, insomnia, aches and pains, fever and chills, problems with concentration, blood in urine or stool, and cough or hoarseness.

INTERFERON ALFA-2A and ALFA-2B (Rx) • **Recombinant. Roferon-A. Intron A.** Interferons used to treat hairy cell leukemia and AIDS-related Kaposi's sarcoma (*see*). Approved in 1988 for the treatment of genital warts, in 1991 for non-A and non-B hepatitis, and in 1992 for hepatitis B. In 1995 it was also approved for the treatment of melanoma (*see*). Due to the possibility of severe or even fatal adverse reactions, these interferons must be supervised by physicians experienced in their use. *See also* Interferon.

INTERFERON GAMMA-1B (Rx) • **Actimmune.** An immune-boosting anticancer drug used to treat chronic granulomatous disease, multiple inflammatory tumors. Potential adverse reactions include nausea, vomiting, diarrhea, suppression of bone marrow, headache, chills, fatigue, decreased mental functioning, awkward walking, liver dysfunction, rash, fever, and muscle and joint pain. *See* Interferon.

INTERLEUKINS (Rx) • In the 1960s, it was discovered that interleukin, a natural substance occurring in the body, transmits signals between types of white blood cells. Interleukin-2 has been used to fight cancers, including melanoma, kidney cancer, and non-Hodgkin's lymphoma, and to stimulate immunity in patients with AIDS. Potential adverse reactions include nausea, vomiting, diarrhea, sore mouth, urinary problems, liver dysfunction, fluid retention, weight gain, fever, fatigue, chills, shortness of breath, low blood pressure, headache, confusion, anemia, disorientation, drowsiness, coma, a sensation of pins and needles, psychosis, hallucinations, heart attack, congestive heart failure, rash, itching, and irregular heartbeat. In the March 2, 1995, issue of the *New England Journal of Medicine,* NIH researchers reported IL-2 given intermittently raised immune cells levels lowered by HIV (*see*) to almost normal in ten patients over a significant time.

INTERMITTENT CLAUDICATION • Pain in the calf muscles and limping, occurring while walking, due to inadequate supply of blood to the limb.

INTERSTITIAL CYSTITIS • **IC.** A chronic, painful inflammation of the bladder wall, the causes and cures of which are unknown. It can affect a person of any age. Its symptoms include frequency of urination, a feeling of urgency, and pain. Frequently accompanied by ulcers.

INTERTRIGO • Chafing. Redness, abrasion, and maceration of opposing skin surfaces that rub together.

INTESTINAL OBSTRUCTION • Mechanical or physical blockage of the intestines.

INTESTINEX • *See* Acidophilus.

INTRA- • Prefix meaning within.

INTRADERMAL • Into or within the skin.

INTRAVENOUS • Fluids or medications given by vein.

INTRINSIC FACTOR • A protein released in the gastrointestinal tract that is essential for absorption of vitamin B_{12}. Intrinsic factor preparations may be administered when natural production is impaired.

INTRON A • *See* Interferon Alfa-2A and Alfa-2B.

INTROPIN • *See* Dopamine Hydrochloride.

INTUBATION • The introduction of a tube into a hollow organ such as the larynx, to keep it open.

INULIN (Rx) (OTC) • A sugar from plants. Used by intravenous injection to determine kidney function; also used in bread for diabetics.

INVERSINE • *See* Mecamylamine.

INVIRASE (Rx) • **Saquinavir.** A drug introduced in 1995 to treat HIV infections. It is a protease inhibitor (*see*). It has not been tested in controlled clinical trials but was rushed to market because of the difficulty in treating HIV infections. It has been tried in random studies of 810 patients with advanced HIV infections; in combination with zidovudine (ZVD), it worked better than either drug alone and offers hope that it will keep the virus in control much as diabetes is kept in control by insulin. It can have severe side effects including cyanosis, heart disorders, tooth problems, vomiting, anemia, staggering, facial pain, psychic disorder, and sleepiness. It should be taken after a full meal.

IN VITRO • Outside the body.

IN VIVO • Within the body.

IOBENGUANE SULFATE I-131 (Rx) • A radioactive imaging agent introduced in 1994 for the localization of two rare tumors—pheochromocytoma and neuroblastoma. It has been in use in sixteen countries since 1987.

IODEX • *See* Providone-Iodine.

IODIDE • The negative ion of iodine, made from iodine and water. *See* Iodine Sources.

IODINATED GLYCEROL (Rx) • **Iodur Elixir. Iophen Elixir.** An expectorant, it is used as adjunctive therapy in the management of asthma and bronchitis and other respiratory disorders. It appears to liquefy thick, tenacious sputum. The mode of expectorant action of iodides has not been fully elucidated; whether or not the glycerol molecule contributes to the expectorant effect of iodinated glycerol has not been determined. Hypersensitivity reaction to iodides may occur and may be manifested by large hives, skin swelling, and skin and mucosal hemorrhage, and symptoms resembling serum sickness (*see*). Iodides regularly cross the placenta and may result in abnormal thyroid function and/or goiter in the newborn. Concomitant use of lithium salts and iodides may result in additive or synergistic hypo- and hyperthyroid effects.

IODINE SOURCES (Rx) (OTC) (H) • Calcium Iodate. Cuprous Iodide. Potassium Iodate. Potassium Iodide. Discovered in 1811 and classed among the rarer earth elements, iodine is found in the earth's crust as bluish black scales. Nearly two hundred products, both prescription and over-the-counter medications, contain this element. Iodine is integral to the thyroid hormones, which have important metabolic roles, and is an essential nutrient for humans. Iodine deficiency leads to thyroid enlargement, or goiter. Nutritionists have found that the most efficient way to add iodine to the diet is through the use of iodized salt. The FDA has ordered all table salts to specify whether or not the product contains iodide. However, many commercially prepared food items do not contain iodized salt. Iodized salt contains up to .01 percent iodine; dietary supplements contain .16 percent. Cuprous and potassium iodides are used in table salts, potassium iodide in some drinking water, and potassium iodate in animal feeds. Dietary iodine is absorbed from the intestinal tract; the main human sources are from food and water. Seafood is a good source, and dairy products also, if the cows are fed enriched grain. Adult daily iodine requirement is believed to be 110 to 150 mg. Growing children and pregnant or lactating women may need more. Iodine compounds are used in expectorants and mucous thinners, particularly in the treatment of asthma, and in contrast media for X rays and fluoroscopy. They can produce a diffuse, red, pimply rash, hives, asthma, and some-times anaphylactic shock. Iodine is also used as an antiseptic and germicide in cosmetics. In 1992, the FDA issued a notice that iodine had not been shown to be safe and effective as claimed in OTC digestive-aid products.

IODINE, STRONG • *See* Strong Iodine.

IODO • *See* Clioquinol.

IODOCHLORHYDROXYQUIN (Rx) (OTC) • Clioquinol. Hydroquin. Torofor. Vioform. A cream or ointment to treat fungal infections of the skin, including athlete's foot. Potential adverse reactions include nerve damage with absorption through the skin, altered iodine levels, and possible burning, itching, acne, and allergic reactions of the skin. If corticosteroids are used, it may increase absorption of iodochlorhydroxyquin. Should not be used by persons hypersensitive to iodine, or to treat diaper rash. The drug will stain fabric and hair.

IODO-NIACIN (OTC) • A combination of niacinamide and potassium iodide (*see both*) used as an expectorant.

IODOQUINOL (OTC) • Diiodohydroxyquin. Diodoquin. Moebiquin. Sebaquin. Yodoxin. An iodine derivative used to combat intestinal amebiasis. May cause a drop in white blood cells and be toxic to the nerves, including those in the eye. Gastrointestinal side effects may be manifested as lack of appetite, nausea, vomiting, cramps, diarrhea or constipation, gastritis, and anal irritation. Rash and hives may also occur, as well as discoloration of the hair and nails. Hair loss, thyroid enlargement, fever, chills, and skin infections have also been reported. Should be taken after meals to lessen the chance of stomach upset.

IODOTOPE THERAPEUTIC • *See* Radioactive Iodine.

IODUR ELIXIR • *See* Iodinated Glycerol.

IONAMIN • *See* Phentermine.

IONAX • *See* Benzalkonium Chloride.

I-131 MIBG • *See* Iobenguane Sulfate I-131.

IONIL • *See* Salicylic Acid.

IOPHEN ELIXIR • *See* Iodinated Glycerol.

IOPIDINE • *See* Apraclonidine.

IOPROMIDE (Rx) • **Ultravist.** A new contrast agent, introduced in 1995, for a broad range of X-ray procedures, including the brain and heart.

IOSAT • *See* Potassium Iodide.

IOXILAN (Rx) • **Oxilan.** An imaging agent, introduced in 1995, for use in highlighting blood vessels in patients during X rays.

IP • Homeopathic abbreviation for ipecacuanha root. *See* Ipecac.

IPECAC (Rx) (OTC) (H) • *Cephaelis ipecacuanha.* **Ipecacuanha Root.** From the dried rhizome and roots of a creeping South American plant with drooping flowers. Used by herbalists, homeopaths, and sold in conventional pharmacies, ipecac is primarily used to induce vomiting when ingestion of noncaustic poisons has occurred. It may also be used medicinally to induce expulsion of mucus in lung congestion. Used as a denaturant in alcohol. Fatal dose in humans is as low as twenty milligrams per kilogram of body weight. Irritating when taken internally, but no known toxicity on the skin. Activated charcoal neutralizes its effect. Contraindicated in semicomatose or unconscious patients, those who are drunk, and with seizure, shock, or loss of gag reflex.

IPECACUANHA ROOT • *See* Ipecac.

I-PHRINE • *See* Phenylephrine.

IPOMEA • The resin of a Mexican herbaceous vine. Banned as an ingredient in laxatives, May 1992.

IPRAN • *See* Propranolol.

IPRATROPIUM BROMIDE (Rx) • **Atrovent.** An anticholinergic (*see*) drug introduced in 1975, used in inhalers to treat bronchospasm by increasing air flow in chronic bronchitis. Reportedly produces more bronchodilation than does theophylline in patients with chronic bronchitis and emphysema. The most common side effects reported are cough and dry mouth. Other potential adverse reactions include palpitations, nervousness, dizziness, rash, nausea, gastrointestinal distress, vomiting, tremor, blurred vision, irritation from aerosol, and worsening of symptoms. Contraindicated in those hypersensitive to atropine (*see*) or its derivatives. It is not indicated for the initial treatment of acute episodes of bronchospasm where rapid response is required. Must be used cautiously in patients with glaucoma, enlarged prostate, or bladder-neck obstruction. The drug is not indicated for occasional use, but is said to be most effective if used consistently as prescribed throughout the course of therapy.

IPSATOL (OTC) • A cough-relief preparation containing dextromethorphan, ammonium chloride, and ipecac (*see all*).

IRIGENIN (H) • From the rhizome of *Iris florentia.* The rhizome contains salicylic (*see*) and isophthalic acids, volatile oil, iridin—a glycoside (*see*)—gum, resin, and sterols. Herbalists use it as a cathartic and emetic and to treat liver complaints, swollen glands, hepatitis and jaundice, skin diseases, and loss of appetite. It is promoted in herbal medicines as both relaxing and stimulating.

IRISH MOSS (H) • *Chondrus crispus.* **Carrageenin.** Seaweed used by herbalists for chronic lung and upper-respiratory problems, and diseases associated with wasting. Contains iodine and a number of mucilaginous agents that soothe inflamed and ulcerated surfaces. Used to treat gastric and duodenal ulcers, and as an expectorant. It was banned by the FDA for use in laxatives, May 1992.

IRIS VERSICOLOR • *See* Blue Flag.

IRODEX • *See* Iron Dextran.

IROMIN-G (OTC) • A multivitamin preparation with iron (*see*).

IRON (Rx) (OTC) • **Femiron. Feosol. Feostat. Fergon. Fer-In-Sol. Fer-Iron. Feronim. Ferrous Fumarate. Ferrous Gluconate. Ferrous Sulfate. Hemocyte. Hydextran. Hytinic. Imferon. Iromin-G. Iron Dextran. Iron-polysaccharide. Niferex. NorFeran. Proferdex.** An essential mineral element, it occurs widely in foods, especially organ meats such as liver, red meats, poultry, and leafy vegetables. The principal foods to which iron or iron salts are added are enriched cereals and some beverages, including milk. The recommended daily allowance (RDA) for children and adults is from 0.2 mg to 1.0 mg, and 18 mg per day in pregnancy. Used in the treatment of iron-deficiency anemia. Iron should not be taken with starches, egg yolks, cereals, milk, coffee, tea, or antacids because they will interfere with its absorption. If taken with citrus juices, the side effects of iron may be increased. Iron is potentially toxic in all forms. Most effective when taken on an empty stomach, but may be taken with food to lessen stomach upset.

IRON DEXTRAN (Rx) • **Feronim. Hydextran. Imferon. Irodex. K-Feron. NorFeran. Proferdex.** Injectable iron compound used to treat anemia when oral administration is not appropriate or is ineffective.

IRON OX BILE (OTC) • In 1992, the FDA issued a notice that iron ox bile had not been shown to be safe and effective as claimed in OTC digestive-aid products.

IRON OXIDE (OTC) • A combination of iron and oxygen. In 1992, the FDA issued a notice that iron oxide had not been shown to be safe and effective as claimed in OTC poison ivy, poison oak, and poison sumac products.

IRRITABLE BOWEL SYNDROME • **Spastic Colon.** The coordinated waves of muscular contractions that move food through the intestines become irregular and uncoordinated. The cause of the disorder is not fully known. The symptoms may be either diarrhea or constipation and cramps, usually on one side of the lower abdomen. Nausea and bloating also may be present.

ISCHEMIA • A deficient blood supply due to spasm or obstruction of an artery.

ISCHEMIC BOWEL DISEASE • Tissue damage due to insufficient blood supply to the intestines.

ISD • *See* Isosorbide Dinitrate.

ISMELIN • *See* Guanethidine.

ISMO • *See* Isosorbide Dinitrate.

ISMOTIC • *See* Isosorbide Dinitrate.

ISO- • Greek for "equal." In chemistry, it is a prefix added to the name of one compound to denote another composed of the same kinds and numbers of atoms but different from each other in structural arrangement.

ISO-BID • *See* Isosorbide Dinitrate.

ISOBORNYL THIOCYANOACETATE (OTC) • An insecticide used on cattle. In 1992, the FDA proposed a ban on isobornyl thiocyanoacetate in lice-killing products for humans because it had not been shown to be safe and effective as claimed.

ISOBUTYLBENZOATE • A synthetic fruit flavoring used in pharmaceuticals and foods.

ISOCAINE • *See* Mepivacaine.

ISOCARBOXAZID (Rx) • **Marplan.** An MAO inhibitor (*see*) used to treat depression and nerve pain. Potential adverse effects include dizziness, weakness, headache, overactivity, tremors, muscle twitching, mania, insomnia, confusion, memory impairment, fatigue, a drop in blood pressure when rising from a sitting or prone position, irregular heartbeat, paradoxical high blood pressure, blurred vision, dry mouth, loss of appetite, nausea, diarrhea, constipation, rash, swelling, sweating, weight changes, and altered libido. Use with alcohol, barbiturates, and other sedatives and narcotics may cause unpredictable effects. Amphetamines, antihistamines, ephedrine, levodopa, meperidine, metaraminol, methotrimeprazine, methylphenidate, phenylephrine, and phenylpropanolamine may raise blood pressure when used with isocarboxazid. The drug may also alter the necessary dosage of antidiabetic drugs. Contraindicated in elderly or debilitated patients, and in those with liver or kidney impairment, congestive heart failure, high blood pressure, heart disease, cerebrovascular disease, and severe or frequent headaches. Must also avoid foods containing tryptophan or tyramine, such as herring, cheese, and red wine. Alcohol, caffeine, over-the-counter medications for colds or hay fever, and other depressants should be avoided. Full effect may not be manifested for two to four weeks. Should not be withdrawn suddenly.

ISOCLOR • *See* Chlorpheniramine and Pseudoephedrine.

ISODINE • *See* Providone-Iodine.

ISOETHARINE (Rx) • **Arm-a-Med Isoetharine. Beta-2. Bisorine. Bronkometer. Bronkosol. Dey-Lute Isoetharine. Dispos-a-Med Isoetharine.** An adrenergic bronchodilator used to treat asthma and reversible bronchospasm associated with chronic bronchitis and emphysema. Potential side effects include tremor, nervousness, dizziness, palpitations, increased heart rate, nausea, and vomiting. Propranolol and other beta-blockers (*see*) counteract the effects of isoetharine. Should be used cautiously in patients with overactive thyroid, high blood pressure, or coronary disease, and in those sensitive to stimulants. Excessive use makes it less effective.

ISOFLUROPHATE (Rx) • **Floropryl. Fluostigmin.** An eye ointment used to treat glaucoma. Potential adverse reactions include aching brow, unusual fatigue or weakness, headache, slow or irregular heartbeat, eye pain, retinal detachment, iris cysts, lens opacities, a paradoxical increase in eye pressure, tearing, obstruction of the tear ducts, burning, redness, stinging, irritation, twitching of the eyelids, blurred vision, nausea, vomiting, diarrhea, stomach cramps, and loss of bladder control. Use with anticholinergics and other cholinesterase inhibitors increases the possibility of toxicity. Inhalation or skin absorption of carbamate or organophosphate-type insecticides, local anesthetics, and ophthalmic tetracaine increases the risk of whole-body toxicity. Isofluorphate increases the toxicity risk of cocaine. Contraindicated in patients with bronchial asthma, slow heartbeat or low blood pressure, Down's syndrome, epilepsy, spastic GI disturbances, Parkinson's disease, heart disease, or a history of retinal detachment (*see*). Toxicity is cumulative and symptoms may not appear for weeks or months after the start of therapy.

ISOMETHEPTENE (Rx) • Used in combination with dichloralphenazone and acetaminophen (*see both*) in medications for headaches. It is believed to work by causing certain blood vessels to narrow. Isometheptene is banned for use by athletes and is tested for by the U.S. Olympic Committee and the National Collegiate Athletic Association.

ISONIAZID (Rx) • **INH. DOW-Isoniazid. Isonicotinic Acid. Isotamine. Laniazid. Nydrazid. PMS-Isoniazid. Rimactane INH.** Introduced in 1956, it is the primary treatment against an active case of tuberculosis; also a preventive treatment. Potential side effects include anemia and other blood problems, nerve damage (especially in alcoholics and diabetics), nausea, vomiting, abdominal distress, male breast enlargement, constipation, dryness of the mouth, hepatitis (*see*), high blood sugar, acidosis, and rheumatic symptoms. Aluminum-containing antacids, and laxatives and corticosteroids, may decrease the effectiveness of isoniazid. Used with isoniazid, carbamazepine (*see*) increases the risk of liver damage, and disulfiram (*see*) may cause increased neurologic symptoms, including changes in behavior and coordination. Should be taken with food to avoid stomach upset.

ISONICOTINIC ACID • *See* Isoniazid.

ISONIPECAINE • *See* Meperidine.

ISOPHRIN • *See* Phenylephrine.

ISOPRENALINE • *See* Isoproterenol.

ISOPROPAMIDE (Rx) • **Darbid.** An anticholinergic, antispasmodic drug used to treat irritable bowel syndrome (*see*), and as an adjunctive therapy in peptic ulcers and other GI disorders. Potential adverse reactions include disorientation, irritability, incoherence, weakness, nervousness, drowsiness, dizziness, headache, palpitations, rapid heartbeat, slow heartbeat, blurred vision, sensitivity to light, increased eye pressure, difficulty in swallowing, constipation, dry mouth, nausea, vomiting, epigastric distress, urinary retention, impotence, hives, decreased sweating, and fever. Contraindicated in glaucoma, obstructions in the urinary or GI tract, myasthenia gravis (*see*), paralytic ileus (*see*), sensitivity to iodine, intestinal flaccidity, unstable cardiovascular status in acute hemorrhage, or toxic megacolon. Should be used with caution in patients with nerve damage, overactive thyroid, coronary artery disease, irregular heartbeat, congestive heart failure, high blood pressure, hiatal hernia, liver or kidney disease, and ulcerative colitis. Should also be used with caution in people over forty years of age due to the possibility of glaucoma. Should be taken thirty minutes to one hour before meals. Should be used with caution in hot weather because drug-induced heatstroke may occur.

ISOPROPANOL (OTC) • **Isopropyl Alcohol.** An antibacterial solvent prepared from propylene, which is obtained by cracking petroleum. Used as a rubbing alcohol. Also used in antifreeze compositions and as a solvent for gums, shellac, and essential oils. Ingestion or inhalation of large quantities of the vapor may cause flushing, headache, dizziness, mental depression, nausea, vomiting, narcosis, anesthesia, and coma. In 1992, the FDA issued a notice that isopropyl alcohol had not been shown to be safe and effective as claimed in OTC poison ivy, poison oak, and poison sumac products, as well as in astringent (*see*) drugs.

ISOPROPYL ALCOHOL • *See* Isopropanol.

ISOPROTERENOL (Rx) • **Aerolone. Dey-Dose Isoproterenol. Dispos-a-Med Isoproterenol. Isoprenaline. Isuprel. Medihaler-Iso. Norisodrine Aerotrol. Vapo-Iso.** Used to treat bronchial asthma and reversible bronchospasm. Potential adverse reactions include headache, mild tremor, weakness, dizziness, nervousness, insomnia, palpitations, rapid heartbeat, angina, a rise and then drop in blood pressure, sweating, nausea, vomiting, high blood sugar, and bronchial swelling and inflammation. It may turn sputum pink. Use with epinephrine increases the risk of irregular heartbeat. Propranolol and other betablockers (*see*) make it less effective. Contraindicated in patients with rapid or irregular heartbeat, those having had a recent heart attack, and those with diabetes or overactive thyroids. If the drug causes a feeling of tightness in the chest or shortness of breath, it should be discontinued. If solution contains precipitate or is discolored, it should not be used.

ISOPTIN • *See* Verapamil.

ISOPTO ALKALINE • *See* Artificial Tears.

ISOPTO ATROPINE • *See* Atropine Sulfate.

ISOPTO CARBACHOL • *See* Carbachol.

ISOPTO CARPINE • *See* Pilocarpine.

ISOPTO-CETAMIDE • *See* Sulfacetamide.

ISOPTO FRIN • *See* Phenylephrine.

ISOPTO HYOSCINE • *See* Scopolamine.

ISOPTO P-ES (Rx) • A combination of pilocarpine, physostigmine, and chlorobutanol (*see all*), used to treat glaucoma.

ISORDIL • *See* Isosorbide Dinitrate.

ISORDIL SUBLINGUAL • *See* Isosorbide Dinitrate.

ISOSORBIDE DINITRATE (Rx) • **Dilatrate-SR. ISD. ISMO. Ismotic. Iso-Bid. Isorbid. Isordil. Isordil Sublingual. Isotrate. Sorbitrate.** An antianginal drug introduced in the 1970s to relieve heart and chest pain. It belongs to the family of nitrates. An oral nitrate tablet was introduced in 1991. Isosorbide reduces the heart's need for oxygen and increases blood flow through the collateral coronary vessels. Under-the-tongue or chewable tablets used in the treatment of acute anginal attacks. May lose its effectiveness after several months. It is used as a diuretic for short-term reduction of eye pressure due to glaucoma. The compound ISMO provides antianginal activity for at least twelve hours. Potential adverse reactions to isosorbide include headache, dizziness, weakness, low blood pressure, heartbeat irregularities, swollen ankles, fainting, nausea, vomiting, flushing, sublingual (under-the-tongue) burning, and hypersensitivity reactions. Contraindicated in patients with severe kidney disease, severe dehydration, fluid in the lungs, and hemorrhagic glaucoma. High blood pressure drugs and alcohol may interact with isosorbide to drop blood pressure too low. Over-the-counter medications containing stimulants may counteract its effects. Most effective if taken on an empty stomach.

ISOTAMINE • *See* Isoniazid.

ISOTHIOCYANATES • Found in mustard, horseradish, and radishes, they seem to induce protective enzymes.

ISOTRATE • *See* Isosorbide Dinitrate.

ISOTRETINOIN (Rx) • **Accutane.** Introduced in 1979, it is a derivative of vitamin A that decreases the size of the oil glands and alters the composition of sebum, making it less likely to plug hair outlets. Used to treat severe cystic acne unresponsive to conventional therapy. Potential adverse reactions include nausea, vomiting, anemia, headache, fatigue, pressure on the brain, red eyes, dry eyes, high blood sugar, gum bleeding and inflammation, liver dysfunction, sore lips, rash, dry skin, peeling of palms and toes, skin infection, decreased libido, impotence, decreased vaginal secretions, irregular menstruation, sensitivity to light, high blood fats, muscle and bone pain, and thinning of hair. Contraindicated in women of childbearing age unless the patient has had a negative pregnancy test within two weeks before beginning therapy. It is definitely harmful to the fetus. It must never be taken by a pregnant or likely to be pregnant woman. Also contraindicated in patients with hypersensitivity to parabens, which are used as preservatives. If used with other photosensitivity-causing agents, it may compound the effect. Abrasives, medicated soaps and cleansers, acne preparations containing peeling agents, and topical alcohol preparations (including cosmetics, aftershave, and cologne) may cause increased irritation or excessive drying of the skin. Alcohol ingested increases the risk of high blood fats. Tetracyclines increase the risk of brain pressure. Vitamin A and vitamin supplements containing A increase isotretinoin's toxic effects. Should be taken with or shortly after meals to ensure adequate absorption.

ISOVEX • *See* Ethaverine Hydrochloride.

ISOXSUPRINE (Rx) • **Vasodilan. Vasoprine.** A vasodilator introduced in 1959 that is used for relief of symptoms associated with cerebrovascular insufficiency, peripheral vascular diseases such as arteriosclerosis, and Raynaud's disease. Also used for severe menstrual cramps. Potential adverse effects include irregular heartbeat, low blood pressure, vomiting, abdominal distress, intestinal distension, and severe rash. Should not be discontinued suddenly. Grapefruit juice may cause potentially dangerous, increased levels of this medication in the blood.

ISPAGHULA HUSK • A bulk-forming laxative. *See* Laxative.

ISPID • *See* Sulfacetamide.

ISRADIPINE (Rx) • **DynaCirc.** A calcium channel blocker (*see*) introduced in 1984, it acts to prevent constriction of the blood vessels in order to reduce blood pressure. It reportedly has fewer adverse effects on the heart or kidney than other calcium channel blockers and does not raise blood cholesterol levels or cause a significant drop in blood pressure when rising from a seated or prone position. Potential adverse reactions include dizziness, edema, flushing, palpitations, irregular heartbeat, nausea, diarrhea, decreased libido, impotence, increased urination, rash, and shortness of breath. When used with fentanyl anesthesia, severe low blood pressure may occur. May be taken with food to reduce stomach upset.

I-SULFACET • *See* Sulfacetamide.

ISUPREL • *See* Isoproterenol.

ITCH-X GEL • *See* Benzoyl Peroxide.

ITRACONAZOLE (Rx) • An AIDS drug rushed through the FDA in a little more than two years, it was introduced in 1992. An oral drug for the treatment of fungus infections caused by blastomycosis and histoplasmosis. It has been used in Mexico since 1988. Coadministration of itraconazole with either terfenadine or AZT (*see both*) is contraindicated. The drug was discontinued in 10.5 percent of the trials because of adverse reactions. Nausea was the most common side effect. Other problems included rash, swelling, fatigue, high blood pressure, and liver dysfunction.

I-TROPINE • *See* Atropine Sulfate.

IUDR • *See* Idoxuridine.

IV • Abbreviation for intravenous, medicine administered through the veins.

IVERMECTIN (Rx) • **Mecitzan.** A drug that is used to treat river blindness (onchocerciasis), filariasis, and strongyloidiasis. It was isolated from a substance discovered on a Japanese golf course. It is also effective against some other kinds of worm infections. Potential adverse effects include dizziness, fever, headache, joint and muscle pain, tender, swollen glands, rash, and fatigue.

IVY (H) • **Common Ivy. English Ivy.** A climbing evergreen, *Hedera helix,* it was formerly used to treat gout, arthritis, and liver and gallbladder disorders. It is used externally for skin eruptions and sores. Common ivy has been used in homeopathic medicine to treat hay fever and cataracts. All parts of the plant are poisonous. Contact with the fresh plant can cause skin rash in sensitive individuals.

I-WHITE OPHTHALMIC SOLUTION • *See* Phenylephrine.

J

JAB • Homeopathic abbreviation for jaborandi. *See* Pilocarpine.

JABORANDI • *See* Pilocarpine.

JALAP (H) • *Exogonium purga.* **High John Root.** The plant is a native of Mexico; a powerful cathartic. At one time in the United States, jalap root was administered to treat liver dysfunction, constipation, headache, loss of appetite, and fever. Banned by the FDA as an ingredient in laxatives, May 1992.

JAMAICAN DOGWOOD (H) • *Piscidia erythrina.* The bark is collected from trees grown in Texas, Mexico, and the Caribbean. It contains glycosides, flavonoids, and resin (*see all*). It is used by herbalists as a powerful sedative, a cathartic, and as a fish poison. It is used in the West Indies to treat pain, including that of migraine.

JAMBUL (H) • *Eugenia jambolana. Syzygium cumini.* **Java Plum. Samboo.** The dried fruits of this tree, which grows from India to Australia, contain volatile oil, resin, and tannin (*see all*). Jambul is used to treat diarrhea or any condition where a mild astringent (*see*) is useful. Has been used in folk medicine to treat diabetes.

JANIMINE (Rx) • *See* Imipramine.

JAPANESE GREEN TEA (H) • Scientists at the Cancer Prevention Division of the National Cancer Center Research Institute in Japan are studying the effect of the main constituent of the tea, epigallocatechin gallate (EGCG), on tumor development. They have reported that EGCG was effective in animals in preventing development of tumors in the skin, duodenum, and liver.

JAPANESE TEA FUNGUS • *See* Kombucha.

JAPANESE TURF LILY (H) • *Ophiopogon japonicus.* **Creeping Lily Root. Dwarf Lilyturf.** The bulbs are used by herbalists to treat symptoms associated with dryness and lack of vital body fluids; especially concerned with asthma and dry cough. Herbalists claim that it gives a sense of inner well-being and relieves insomnia and fearfulness.

JAPANESE WHITE OIL • *See* Camphor.

JASMINE (H) • *Jasminum officinale. Gelsemium sempervirens.* **Carolina Jessamine. Gelsemium Root. Yellow Jessamine.** For centuries, the jasmine flower has been brewed in tea to aid relaxation. The rhizomes and roots contain the alkaloid gelsemine, a potent analgesic that is used to treat the severe pain in the face known as tic douloureux or trigeminal neuralgia (*see*). Herbalists claim that jasmine oil rubbed on the body increases sexual interest. Jasmine can be highly toxic and can cause death by respiratory arrest.

JASMINUM OFFICINALE • *See* Jasmine.

JAUNDICE • Yellowish discoloration of the skin and tissues caused by bile pigments in the blood. This symptom indicates that something has happened to cause bile pigments to back up into the blood. Underlying causes of jaundice are numerous. As a drug side effect, it is always considered serious.

JENAMICIN • *See* Gentamicin.

JEN SHANG • *See* Ginseng.

JEQUIRITY (H) • *Abrus precatorius.* **Crab's Eyes. Indian Licorice. Prayer Bean. Precatory Bean. Rosary Pea.** A climbing shrub native to India, it grows in the tropics. The seeds, root, and leaves have been used in folk medicine. Contains abrin, a phytotoxin. Homeopaths use it in dilute solution to treat coughs. The seeds are exceedingly toxic and have been used in India to commit murder. One seed when chewed can kill an adult. Severe poisoning resulted in a person after drinking tea in which one seed had been soaked for fifteen minutes. The leaves and roots of jequirity are safer but may be toxic in large overdose.

JERSEY TEA (H) • *Ceanothus americanus.* **New Jersey Tea.** A shrub with downy stems native to North America that contains up to 10 percent tannins, alkaloids, and resins. It has been used in folk medicine to treat bronchitis, asthma, dysentery, and venereal diseases. It is also used as a sedative. Long-term use in excessive doses can cause an increase in blood clotting. Contraindicated in low blood pressure.

JESUIT'S TEA • *See* Maté Extract.

JIE GENG • *See* Platycodon.

JIMSONWEED (H) • *Datura stramonium.* **Devil's Apple. Jamestown Weed. Mad Apple. Nightshade. Stinkweed. Thornapple.** A weed that belongs to the nightshade family, it is found in gardens, pastures, and roadsides in the Americas and many other parts of the world. Contains belladonna-like alkaloids, and its action is similar to that of belladonna (*see*). It is used to stimulate circulation and respiration, and to overcome spasm of the involuntary muscles. Extracts are known to be antispasmodic and narcotic. Medicinal cigarettes and pipe tobacco are used to treat asthma. Potent; can be highly toxic.

JIN BU HUAN • A Chinese herbal medicine sold as a sedative, sleep aid, and pain reliever, it has caused seven cases of hepatitis (*see*) in the United States in the 1990s, according to the February 1, 1995, issue of the *Journal of the American Medical Association.* The patients had been healthy. Acute hepatitis occurred after a mean of twenty weeks. The FDA says some children who were poisoned by taking jin bu huan had life-threatening rapid heart rate and rapid onset of central nervous system and respiratory depression. The children recovered. FDA researchers, at this writing, were conducting a nationwide search for the herbal product and have banned imports.

JOCK ITCH • *Tinea cruris.* Ringworm of the groin; a fungus infection of the skin of the upper thighs near the genital organs. It is caused by the same group of organisms that causes athlete's foot.

JOE-PYE WEED (H) • *Eupatorium maculatum* and *E. purpureum.* A North American perennial, it is found in moist woods and meadows. It was named after a New England medicine man who was renowned for his cures for typhus and other fevers with his decoctions from this plant. Learning from Indian women, who bathed their ailing children in an infusion of the root, white settlers gathered joe-pye weed for all kinds of medicinal purposes. Its astringent and diuretic (*see both*) properties made it a dependable medicine for arthritis, backache, pain, edema, and urinary problems. It is used by homeopaths to treat aching bones. *See also* Gravelroot.

JOHNSWORT • *See* Saint-John's-Wort.

JUJUBE DATE (H) • *Ziziphus jujuba.* **Da T'sao.** The Chinese jujube date, found dried in most oriental markets, is commonly used in a wide variety of herbal formulas. It is used to enhance the taste and benefits of soups and stews, and to energize the body. Chinese herbalists believe it relieves nervous exhaustion, insomnia, apprehension, forgetfulness, dizziness, and clamminess.

JUNIPER (OTC) (H) • *Juniperus communis.* **Mistletoe. Viscum.** Juniper berries, used by herbalists to treat urinary problems, reportedly act directly on the kidneys, stimulating the flow of urine. Juniper berries and extracts are in several over-the-counter drugstore diuretic and laxative preparations. In fact, gin was created in the 1500s by a Dutch pharmacist using juniper berries, to sell as an inexpensive diuretic. The berries have long been used by herbalists to treat gout caused by high uric acid in the blood. Also recommended to aid digestion and eliminate gas and cramps. The berries are high in vitamin C. Juniper is also used to lower cholesterol and treat arthritis. Large amounts may irritate the kidneys. In 1992, the FDA issued a notice that juniper had not been shown to be safe and effective as claimed in OTC digestive-aid products and oral menstrual drugs. Mistletoe has been reported to be toxic to the liver.

K

KABIKINASE • *See* Streptokinase.

KABOLIN • *See* Nandrolone.

KADAY • *See* Karaya Gum.

KAINAIR • *See* Proparacaine.

KALCINATE • *See* Calcium Gluconate.

KALI-B • Homeopathic abbreviation for kali bichromicum (*see*).

KALI. BICH. (H) • Homeopathic abbreviation for kali bichromicum (*see*).

KALI BICHROMICUM (H) • **Kali-b. Kali. Bich.** A homeopathic (*see*) remedy made up of potassium bichromate for coughs and mucous discharges. It is also used for burns, croup, headache, indigestion, and joint pain. Internally it can be a caustic poison. *See* Tissue Salts.

KALI-C. • Homeopathic abbreviation for kali carbonicum (*see*).

KALI. CARB. • Homeopathic abbreviation for kali carbonicum (*see*).

KALI CARBONICUM (H) • **Kali-c. Kali. Carb. Potassium Carbonate. Salt of Tartar.** A homeopathic medicine (*see*) to treat stitching pains, hacking coughs, and swollen eyes; composed of potassium carbonate. Formerly employed in conventional medicine as a diuretic to reduce body water and as an alkalinizer, it is irritating and caustic to human skin. It is used as an alkali in food processing. *See* Tissue Salts.

KALI-M. • Homeopathic abbreviation for kali muriaticum (*see*).

KALI. MUR. • Homeopathic abbreviation for kali muriaticum (*see*).

KALI MURIATICUM (H) • **Kali-m. Kali. Mur.** A homeopathic (*see*) medicine composed of potassium chloride. A healthy human contains about nine grams of potassium. Most of it is found inside body cells. Potassium plays an important role in maintaining water balance and acid/alkali balance. Chloride is a sterilizing and bleaching agent. The remedy is used to treat the common cold, cough, earache, indigestion, sore throat, and thrush. *See* Tissue Salts.

KALI-P. • Homeopathic abbreviation for kali phosphoricum (*see*).

KALI. PHOS. • Homeopathic abbreviation for kali phosphoricum (*see*).

KALI PHOSPHORICUM (H) • **Kali-p. Kali. Phos.** A homeopathic (*see*) medicine composed of potassium phosphate. A healthy human contains about nine grams of potassium. Most of it is found inside body cells. Potassium plays an important role in maintaining water balance and acid/alkali balance. Phosphate is also needed to maintain the acid/alkali balance. Potassium phosphate has been used through the ages as a urinary acidifier. The homeopathic remedy is used to treat anemia, anxiety, depression, backache, headache, indigestion, and insomnia. *See* Tissue Salts.

KALI-S. • A homeopathic abbreviation for kali sulphuricum (*see*).

KALI. SULPH. • A homeopathic abbreviation for kali sulphuricum (*see*).

KALI SULPHURICUM (H) • **Kali-s. Kali. Sulph.** A homeopathic medicine (*see*) composed of potassium and sulfate. A healthy human contains about nine grams of potassium. Most of it is found inside body cells. Potassium plays an important role in maintaining water balance and acid/alkali balance. Sulfate is the salt of sulfuric acid. It helps control the acid/alkali balance. Kali sulphuricum is used as a homeopathic remedy for discharges, the common cold, cough, earache, headache, and joint pain. *See* Tissue Salts.

KANAMYCIN (Rx) • **Kanasig. Kantres. Kantrex. Klebcil.** An aminoglycoside (*see*) antibiotic given by capsule or injection, it is used to treat serious infections caused by *Escherichia coli, Proteus, Enterobacter aerogenes, Klebsiella, Serratia,* and *Acinetobacter (see all)*. Potential adverse reactions include headache, lethargy, muscle problems, ear problems, kidney dysfunction, dizziness, increased thirst, and allergic reactions. May interact with cephalothin, dimenhydrinate, general and local anesthetics, IV loop diuretics, IV penicillins, cisplatin, and methoxyflurane *(see all)*.

KANASIG • *See* Kanamycin.

KANTRES • *See* Kanamycin.

KANTREX • *See* Kanamycin.

KAOCHLOR • Liquid potassium chloride. *See* Potassium Chloride.

KAOLIN (Rx) (OTC) (H) • **Amogel PG. China Clay. Donnagel. Donnagel-PG. K-C. K-P. K-Pek. Kaopectate. Kao-tin. Kapectolin.** Originally obtained from Kaoling Hill in Kiangsi Province, southeast China, it is essentially an aluminum silicate *(see)*. Kaolin is an absorbent substance used to treat certain types of poisoning and as an antidiarrheal. It is used with pectin *(see)* to decrease the stool's fluid content in mild, nonspecific diarrhea. Also often used with belladonna, opium, or paregoric *(see all)*. Potential adverse reactions include the malabsorption of nutrients, drugs, and enzymes, and fecal impaction or ulceration in infants and in elderly or debilitated patients after chronic use. In large doses it may cause obstructions, perforations, or granuloma (tumor) formation. Contraindicated in suspected obstructive bowel lesions. Central nervous system depressants will add to the sedative effects if belladonna or opium are in the mixture. Should not be used for more than two days. In 1992, the FDA issued a notice that colloidal kaolin had not been shown to be safe and effective as claimed in OTC digestive-aid products.

KAON and KAON LIQUID • *See* Potassium Gluconate.

KAOPECTATE (OTC) • A combination of kaolin, pectin, and attapulgite *(see all)*, used to treat diarrhea.

KAO-TIN • *See* Kaolin.

KAPECTOLIN • *See* Kaolin.

KAPOSI'S SARCOMA • A rare malignant skin tumor that occurs in some AIDS patients.

KARAYA GUM (OTC) (H) • **Indian Tragacanth. Kaday. Katilo. Kullo. Kuterra. Mucara. Sterculia Gum.** The exudate of a tree found in India. The finely ground white powder is used in gelatins and gumdrops. The vegetable gum is used as a bulk-forming laxative. *See* Laxative.

KARELA (H) • *Momordica charantia.* **African Cucumber. Balsam Pear. Bitter guard.** A climbing, thin, round stem native to India and found in tropical regions. Used as a spice. The unripe fruits without seeds are used in homeopathic medicine in dilution. It is used to treat diabetes, high blood pressure, arthritis, and liver ailments. Long-term use may cause a sudden, dangerous drop in blood sugar. Karela is contraindicated in pregnancy and in those suffering from low blood sugar.

KARIDIUM • *See* Fluoride.

KARIGEL • *See* Fluoride.

KASOF • *See* Docusate.

KATILO • *See* Karaya Gum.

KATO POWDER • *See* Potassium Chloride.

KAVA-KAVA (H) • *Piper methysticum.* **Ava. Kawa.** This Polynesian herb's root is used by herbalists as a remedy for insomnia and nervousness. A compound in kava is marketed in Europe as a mild sedative for the elderly. Other agents in kava have been shown in the laboratory to have antiseptic properties. It is also a reputedly potent analgesic and antiseptic that may be taken internally or applied directly to a painful wound.

Chronic use can cause diarrhea, loss of appetite, and apathy. In some cases, disorientation and hallucinations may result. Contraindicated in pregnancy and for young children.

KAWA • *See* Kava-Kava.

KAYBOVITE • *See* Vitamin B$_{12}$.

KAY CIEL • *See* Potassium Chloride.

KAYEXALATE • *See* Sodium Polystyrene Sulfonate.

KAYLIXIR • *See* Potassium Gluconate.

KCl • *See* Potassium Chloride.

K-DUR 20 • *See* Potassium Chloride.

KEFLET • *See* Cephalexin.

KEFLEX • *See* Cephalexin.

KEFLIN • *See* Cephalothin.

KEFTAB • *See* Cephalexin.

KEFUROX • *See* Cefuroxime Axetil and Sodium.

KEFZOL • *See* Cefazolin Sodium.

KELP (H) • Recovered from the giant Pacific marine plant *Macrocystis pyrifera,* kelp is used by herbalists to supply the thyroid gland with iodine, to help regulate the texture of the skin, and to help the body burn off excess fat. In Japan, where kelp is a large part of the diet, thyroid disease is almost unknown. Kelp was banned from over-the-counter diet pills by the FDA, February 10, 1992. Kelp does contain many minerals, and herbalists claim that it has anticancer, antirheumatic, anti-inflammatory, and blood-pressure-lowering properties. Contraindicated in those with overactive thyroids or sensitivity to iodine.

KEMADRIN • *See* Procyclidine.

KENACORT • *See* Triamcinolone.

KENALOG • *See* Triamcinolone.

KERATIN • A tough, fibrous protein that is the main constituent of the outermost layer of skin, nails, and hair.

KERATITIS • Painful inflammation of the cornea of the eye.

KERATOLYTICS • Products that appear to loosen skin flakes and allow them to be more easily washed away. Lotions containing salicylic acid (*see*) are used for this purpose.

KERI LOTION (OTC) • An oil-in-water emulsion used to lubricate dry skin.

KERION • A fungal infection of the beard or scalp.

KERLONE • *See* Betaxolol Hydrochloride.

KETALAR • *See* Ketamine.

KETAMINE (Rx) • **Ketalar.** A nonbarbiturate sedative drug used to induce general anesthesia, especially in short-term diagnostic or surgical procedures. Potential adverse reactions include movement disorders, respiratory depression, increased blood pressure and pulse rate, low blood pressure, slowed heartbeat, inner eye pressure, mild appetite loss, salivation, throat spasms, nausea, vomiting, skin redness, measle-like rash, hallucinations, confusion, excitement, and irrational behavior. Contraindicated in those who have had a stroke or who may be at risk if their blood pressure is raised. Also contraindicated in patients with severe heart problems, in those with a history of alcoholism, and in surgery of the throat or bronchial tree. A potential hallucinogen that produces a feeling of floating, ketamine is a drug of abuse among young people.

KETOCONAZOLE (Rx) • **Nizoral.** Introduced in 1981, it inhibits the growth of fungi and is used to treat systemic candidiasis, chronic mucocandidiasis, oral thrush, candiduria, coccidioidomycosis, histoplasmosis, chromomycosis, and paracoccidioidomycosis—severe skin infections resistant to therapy with topical or oral griseofulvin. Adverse effects include headache, nervousness, dizziness, nausea, enlargement of the male breast, vomiting, stomach pain, diarrhea, constipation, elevated liver enzymes, and fatal liver toxicity. In skin preparations ketoconazole may cause severe irritation, itching, stinging, and localized allergic reactions. If athlete's foot is the problem, the patient should avoid wearing socks made from wool or synthetic materials and, instead, wear clean cotton socks. May interact with many drugs, including antacids, anticholinergics, and some antihistamines. Rifampin and isoniazid may make the antifungal less effective. The medication is a powerful inhibitor of liver enzymes. Coadministration with triazolam (see), for example, inhibits the clearance of the sleep medication. Studies are now under way to detect other such interactions with ketoconazole. May be taken with food to reduce risk of stomach upset. A ketoconazole shampoo is a candidate for OTC status, as of this writing.

KETO-DIASTIX (OTC) • A diagnostic test for urine and ketones in urine.

KETOPROFEN (Rx) (OTC) • **Orudis. Orudis KT. Oruvail.** Produces anti-inflammatory, analgesic, and fever-reducing effects, possibly through inhibition of prostaglandins (see). One of the newer NSAIDs (see), it is used to treat arthritis, mild to moderate pain, and painful menstruation. Potential adverse reactions include prolonged bleeding time, headache, dizziness, excitation or depression, ringing in the ears, visual disturbances, nausea, abdominal pain, diarrhea, constipation, gas, peptic ulcers, loss of appetite, vomiting, sore mouth, decreased libido, impotence, male breast enlargement, irregular menstruation, kidney dysfunction, liver dysfunction, and rash. Contraindicated in patients who are allergic to aspirin or other NSAIDs. Serious GI toxicity can occur at any time with the use of NSAIDs. Medication should be taken thirty minutes before or two hours after a meal, except if GI problems occur; then it should be taken with milk or meals. Approved for OTC use in 1995.

KETOROLAC TROMETHAMINE (Rx) • **Toradol.** An NSAID (see) that acts by inhibiting prostaglandins (see), used for short-term management of pain. Promoted as a nonopiate, nonaddictive, strong painkiller. The most serious risks associated with the injectable form of the drug are ulcerations, bleeding and perforation of the gastrointestinal tract, hemorrhage, and hypersensitivity reactions. The most frequently reported side effects for the oral medication are heartburn, nausea, GI pain, and headache. GI, kidney, and allergic side effects are the most serious. Other potential adverse reactions include drowsiness, dizziness, swelling, water retention, nausea, diarrhea, and pain at the injection site. Ketorolac interacts with lithium (see Lithium Carbonate) or methotrexate (see) to cause increased toxicity of those drugs. Should not be used by patients with nasal polyps or allergy to aspirin. Should be used with caution in those with heart disease, high blood pressure, kidney problems, a history of alcohol abuse, or those taking anticoagulants. Should not be used by nursing mothers. Serious GI toxicity can occur at any time with the use of NSAIDs. Medication should be taken thirty minutes before or two hours after a meal, except if GI problems occur; then it should be taken with milk or meals. Should not be taken for more than five days. Longer use may result in serious adverse effects.

KETOSIS • A condition produced when more fat is eaten than can be burned completely by the body. The unburned fat produces an excess of acid.

KETOSTIX (OTC) • A diagnostic test for acetone in urine.

KEY-PRED • *See* Primaquine.

K-FERON • *See* Iron Dextran.

K-G ELIXIR • *See* Potassium Gluconate.

KHAT (H) • *Catha edulis.* **Catha. Abyssinian Tea.** A shrub or small tree native to Arabia and cultivated in Africa. Contains ephedrine. The fresh twigs and leaves are used in Africa as a cure for malaria and coughs. They are chewed as a stimulant, and to allay hunger and to prevent sleep. Regular use of khat may induce gastrointestinal disorders. Excessive use may cause headaches, irregular heartbeat, elevated blood pressure, excitement, and insomnia. It can also inhibit urination and cause difficulty in concentration. It is banned in some countries.

KI • *See* Potassium Iodide.

K-IDE • *See* Potassium Bicarbonate and Potassium Citrate.

KIE • *See* Ephedrine and Potassium Iodide.

KINO (H) • *Pterocarpus marsupium. Pterocarpus indicus. Pterocarpus echinatus.* **Bibla. Gummi. Narra. Padauk. Prickly Narra.** The exudate from the trunk of this large tree; an astringent (*see*) to treat wounds, scrapes, diarrhea, and skin ulcers. Contains a tanninlike substance. *Pterocarpus angloensis,* bloodwood, is used in Africa as an aphrodisiac.

KLAVIKORDAL • *See* Nitroglycerin.

K-LEASE • *See* Potassium Chloride.

KLEBCIL • *See* Kanamycin.

KLEBSIELLA • A gram-negative bacterium that occurs in soil and water and grain and may cause urinary tract, intestinal, and respiratory infections.

KLONOPIN • *See* Clonazepam.

K-LOR • *See* Potassium Chloride.

KLOR-CON • *See* Potassium Chloride.

KLOR-CON/EF • *See* Potassium Bicarbonate and Potassium Citrate.

KLOROMIN • *See* Chlorpheniramine.

KLORVESS • *See* Potassium Chloride.

KLOTRIX • *See* Potassium Chloride.

K-LYTE • *See* Potassium Bicarbonate and Potassium Citrate.

KNITBONE • *See* Comfrey.

KNOTGRASS (OTC) (H) • In 1992, the FDA issued a notice that knotgrass had not been shown to be safe and effective as claimed in OTC digestive-aid products. Used over a long period of time, it can delete vitamin B_1.

KOATE-HS • *See* Antihemophilic Factor.

KOLANTYL (OTC) • A combination of aluminum hydroxide and magnesium hydroxide (*see both*), used as an antacid.

KOLA NUT (H) • *Cola acuminata.* **Bissy Nut. Cola. Guru Nut.** Collected from a tree that is native to tropical West Africa and is cultivated in South America. The seeds contain caffeine, theobromine, tannin, and volatile oil (*see all*). Kola nut is used for stimulation to counteract fatigue, and as a diuretic. Herbalists use it to treat some types of migraine headache and diarrhea caused by anxiety. Also used to treat emotional depression. Contraindicated in persons with hyperacidity and peptic ulcer. Used chronically, it may slightly increase blood pressure.

KOLYUM (Rx) • A potassium supplement containing potassium gluconate and potassium chloride (*see both*).

KOMBUCHA (H) • **Japanese Tea Fungus.** A mushroom-like culture of yeast and bactria, it is reported by some alternative medicine advocates to improve conditions ranging from cancer to baldness. It has demonstrated antibiotic activity in a Cornell University laboratory study, but the effect may be due to its acid content, according to Cornell researchers. Contamination problems have arisen during consumers' making of the tea, and there was a report of the deaths of two women who had brewed their own teas.

KOMED (Rx) • A combination of sodium thiosulfate, salicylic acid, and isopropyl alcohol (*see all*), used to treat acne.

KONAKION • *See* Phytonadione.

KONDREMUL PLAIN (OTC) • A lubricant laxative containing mineral oil (*see*). *See also* Laxative.

KONSYL (OTC) • *See* Psyllium.

KONYNE-HT (Rx) • *See* Factor IX Complex.

KOOL FOOT • *See* Undecylenic Acid.

KOROMEX FOAM, CREAM, JELLY (OTC) • A spermicide. *See* Nonoxynol-9 and Octoxynol-9.

K-P • *See* Kaolin.

K-PEK • *See* Kaolin.

K-PHEN • *See* Promethazine.

K-PHOS (Rx) • A combination of potassium, sodium, and phosphorus (*see all*), used as a source of potassium and phosphorus in nutritional deficiencies.

KRONOFED-A (OTC) • Antihistamine and decongestant used to treat nasal congestion. A combination of chlorpheniramine and pseudoephedrine (*see both*).

KRONOHIST (OTC) • Antihistamine and decongestant. A combination of chlorpheniramine, phenylpropanolamine, and pyrilamine (*see all*).

K-TAB • *See* Potassium Chloride.

K+ 10 • *See* Potassium Chloride.

KUDROX (OTC) • *See* Aluminum Hydroxide and Magnesium Hydroxide.

KULLO • *See* Karaya Gum.

KUTAJA (H) • *Holarrhena antidysenterica.* **Conessi Bark. Kurchi.** A large shrub native to India. The bark is used in India for the treatment of amebic dysentery and liver ailments. It is toxic in overdose.

KUTERRA • *See* Karaya Gum.

KU-ZYME • *See* Pancrelipase.

KWELL • *See* Lindane.

KWILDANE • *See* Lindane.

KY JELLY (OTC) • A vaginal lubricant.

L

LABETALOL (Rx) • **Ibidomide. Normodyne.** A drug introduced in 1978 that depresses renin secretion and blocks response to alpha and beta stimulation (*see* Beta-Blockers). It is used to treat moderate to severe high blood pressure; used in high blood pressure emergencies. Potential adverse reactions include vivid dreams, fatigue, headache, a drop in blood pressure when rising from a seated or prone position, heart and blood-vessel disease, nasal stuffiness, hypoglycemia, nausea, vomiting, diarrhea, sexual dysfunction, urine retention, rash, shortness of breath, and tingling scalp. Contraindicated in asthmatics and people with severe heart failure and reduced heart rate. Cimetidine may enhance labetalol's effects. Halothane may cause the blood pressure to drop too low. MAO inhibitors (*see*) taken at the same time or within two weeks of this drug may raise the blood pressure dangerously high. Labetalol may cause necessary dosage adjustments of insulin and oral diabetes drugs. May be taken with food, but should be ingested at the same time each day.

LABIA, LABIO- • Lips or liplike organs. *Labia majora* refers to the folds of skin on either side of the entrance of the vulva.

LABID • *See* Theophylline.

LABRADOR TEA EXTRACT (H) • **Hudson's Bay Tea. Marsh Tea.** The extract of the dried flowering plant or young shoots of *Ledum palustre* or *Ledum groenlandicium,* a low-growing, resinous evergreen shrub found in bogs, swamps, and moist meadows. Brewed as tea, it is a pleasing antiscorbutic (*see*) and stimulant. Used by the Indians and settlers as a tonic to purify blood. Was also employed to treat wounds. *Ledum palustre* contains, among other things, tannin and valeric acid (*see both*).

LABURNUM (H) • *Laburnum anagyroides.* **Golden Rain.** A small tree native to Europe and the Mediterranean region, its seeds and flowers are used in homeopathic medicines. It has antispasmodic, diuretic, and emetic effects. It is used in the treatment of depression and intestinal colic. Laburnum yields cytisine, which has been used

as a drug to treat asthma and anxiety. It is highly toxic.

LABYRINTH • The internal ear, comprising the semicircular canals, vestibule, and cochlea.

LACERATION • Refers to a wound caused by the tearing of tissue.

LACH • Homeopathic abbreviation for lachesis (*see*).

LACHESIS (H) • A homeopathic medicine to treat earache, restless sleep, and neck pain. One of the three Fates, it is also the venom from an American pit viper.

LACHNANTHES (H) • *Lachnanthes tinctoria.* **Wool Flower.** A perennial herbaceous plant native to North America and Cuba. It has been used in folk medicine to threat arthritis, cough, and nervous conditions. It is used in homeopathic medicine to reduce fever. It is toxic in excessive doses. Symptoms of poisoning include mental excitement and abnormal behavior followed by headache, dizziness, and death.

LAC-HYDRIN • *See* Propylene Glycol.

LACRIL • *See* Artificial Tears.

LACRI-LUBE • *See* Artificial Tears.

LACRIMAL • Pertaining to tears.

LACRISERT • *See* Artificial Tears.

LACTAID • *See* Lactase.

LACTASE (OTC) • **Beta-D-Galactosidase. Dairy Ease Caplets and Drops. Lactaid. Lactogest. Lactrase. Surelac.** An enzyme that is insufficient in many people, resulting in gastrointestinal disturbances after consumption of the milk sugar lactose. The symptoms include bloating, gas, cramps, and diarrhea. When lactase is given as a supplement, it enables dairy products to be more easily digested. It can also be helpful in digesting other foods containing lactose, such as pizza, hot dogs, pancakes, creamy salad dressings, and soups.

LACTIC ACID (OTC) • Lac-Hydrin. Lacticare. An odorless, colorless, usually syrupy substance normally found in blood and muscle tissue as a by-product of the metabolism of glucose and glycogen (*see both*). Also made by fermentation of some food products such as pickles and sauerkraut. A topical application for skin diseases. Caustic in concentrated solutions when taken internally or applied to the skin. In topical products, it may cause stinging in those who are sensitive to it, particularly in fair-skinned women. In 1992, the FDA issued a notice that lactic acid had not been shown to be safe and effective as claimed in OTC digestive-aid products.

LACTIC ACIDOSIS • An accumulation of excess lactic acid in the blood, which can cause hyperventilation and mental confusion leading to stupor and coma.

LACTICARE (OTC) • An oil-in-water emulsion of lactic acid (*see*) and sodium-PCA. Used as a base for skin-care products.

LACTINEX (OTC) • A medication containing material from bacteria that are naturally present in milk. Used in the treatment of diarrhea. *See* Acidophilus.

LACTOBACILLUS ACIDOPHILUS (OTC) (H) • DDS-Acidophilus. More-Dophilus. Lactobacilli are any of the various rod-shaped bacteria of the genus *Lactobacillus*. These versatile bacteria form lactic acid (*see*). Certain strains reside in the urogenital tract and intestinal tract of healthy people. Yogurt contains lactobacilli. *See* Acidophilus.

LACTOCAL-F (OTC) • A multivitamin preparation.

LACTOFERRIN • A natural antibiotic found in especially high concentrations in tears, sweat, seminal fluid, nasal and genital secretions. Lactoferrin is being produced through bioengineering for use as an antibiotic.

LACTOFLAVIN • *See* Vitamin B_2.

LACTOSE (OTC) • D-Lactose. Milk Sugar. Saccharum Lactin. A slightly sweet-tasting, colorless sugar present in the milk of mammals (humans have 6.7 percent and cows 4.3 percent). Occurs as a white powder or crystalline mass as a by-product of the cheese industry. Produced from whey (*see*). It is inexpensive and is widely used in the food industry as a culture medium, such as in souring milk, and as a humectant (*see*) and nutrient in infants' or debilitated patients' formulas. Also used as a medical laxative or diuretic. Used widely as a base in eye lotions. Generally nontoxic. In 1992, the FDA issued a notice that lactose had not been shown to be safe and effective as claimed in OTC digestive-aid products.

LACTOSE INTOLERANCE • A deficiency of the enzyme lactase (produced in the intestine), which is needed to digest the lactose (*see*) in dairy products.

LACTRASE (OTC) • *See* Lactase.

LACTUCA • *See* Lettuce Extract.

LACTULOSE (Rx) • Cephulac. Cholac. Chronulac. Constilac. Duphalac. Enulose. A substance that acts as a laxative and is also used to treat coma in patients with severe liver disease. Potential adverse reactions include abdominal cramps, belching, diarrhea, gaseous distension, and high sodium. Should be used with caution by diabetics. Certain antibiotics such as neomycin may reduce the effectiveness of lactulose when it is used to treat liver failure.

LADY'S MANTLE EXTRACT (H) • *Alchemilla xanthochlora.* From the dried leaves and flowering shoots of *Achemilla vulgaris*. A common European herb covered with spreading hairs, it has been used for centuries by herbalists to concoct love potions and to treat menstrual problems, diarrhea, and wounds. Contains tannin, glycosides, and salicylic acid (*see all*). Widely used by herbalists throughout Europe, it is prescribed for easing the changes of menopause. May cause constipation.

LADY'S SLIPPER (H) • *Cypripedium pubescens.* The root is used to treat anxiety, stress, insomnia, neurosis, restlessness, tremors, epilepsy, and palpitations. Herbalists claim it is also useful for depression. Contains volatile oils, resins, glucosides, and tannin (*see all*). A large overdose may cause hallucinations.

LAKES, COLOR • A lake is an organic pigment prepared by precipitating a soluble color with a form of aluminum, calcium, barium, potassium, strontium, or zirconium, which makes the colors insoluble. Not all colors are suitable for making lakes.

LAMICTAL • *See* Lamotrigine.

LAMISIL • *See* Terbinafine.

LAMIUM (H) • **Dead Nettle.** An herb of the family Labiatae with showy flowers. Used in homeopathic medications for urinary tract irritation.

LAMIVUDINE (Rx) • **Epivir. 3TC.** A medication, introduced in 1995, for use in combination with zidovudine (Retrovir) (*see both*) for the treatment of HIV infections when therapy is warranted, based on the disease's progression. It was rushed to the market, and there have been no controlled clinical trials evaluating the effect of therapy on the clinical progression of HIV infection, such as the incidence of opportunistic infections on survival. In patients with HIV, the virus became resistant to lamivudine in 12 weeks, but in combination with zidovudine, lamivudine kept the virus from becoming resistant to zidovudine for a longer period of time. Must be used with extreme care in patients who have suffered from pancreatitis or in those with impaired kidney function. Potential adverse effects include headache, fatigue, fever or chills, nausea, diarrhea,

cramps, nerve damage, dizziness, insomnia, and depression.

LAMOTRIGINE (Rx) • **Lamictal.** A medication to treat epileptic seizures that are poorly controlled. Approved in 1993 for the United States market. It had already been approved in more than forty other countries. It is expected to benefit the estimated 30 percent of adult epilepsy patients with seizures that are not helped by other epilepsy drugs. Lamictal is not indicated for absence, atonic, atypical absence, myoclonic, tonic-clonic (primary or secondarily generalized) seizures at this writing, according to the FDA. The only approved indication for this medication is for adjunctive therapy in the treatment of partial seizures in adults with epilepsy.

LAMPRENE • *See* Clofazimine.

LANACORT • *See* Hydrocortisone.

LANIAZID • *See* Isoniazid.

LANOLIN (OTC) • **Lubriderm. Wool Fat. Wool Wax.** A product of the oil glands of sheep that is used as a base for emollient ointments and cosmetics. Used to treat dry skin. A water-absorbing material and a natural emulsifier, it absorbs and holds water to the skin. Chemically, a wax instead of a fat. Lanolin has been found to be a common skin sensitizer, causing allergic contact skin rash. It is usually not used in pure form today because of its allergy-causing potential. Derivatives are less likely to cause allergic reactions. In 1992, the FDA issued a notice that lanolin had not been shown to be safe and effective as claimed in OTC poison ivy, poison oak, and poison sumac products.

LANORINAL (Rx) • A combination of aspirin, butalbital, and caffeine (*see all*), used to relieve pain.

LANOXICAPS • *See* Digoxin.

LANOXIN • *See* Digoxin.

LANSOPRAZOLE • *See* Prevacid.

LANTANA (H) • *Lantana camara.* A shrub native to tropical America, it is used in homeopathic medicine to treat coughs. The plant is highly toxic and may cause miscarriage.

LAPACHO • *See* Pau D'Arco.

LARGON • *See* Propiomazine.

LARIAM • *See* Mefloquine Hydrochloride.

LARKSPUR (H) • *Consolida regalis. Delphinum condolida.* The seeds are used to treat nits and lice on the skin and hair. Larkspur is a poison and should not be taken internally.

LAROBEC (OTC) • A multivitamin preparation.

LARODOPA • *See* Levodopa.

LAROTID • *See* Amoxicillin.

LASAN CREAM • *See* Anthralin.

LASAN HP • *See* Anthralin.

LASIX • *See* Furosemide.

LASSAR'S ZINC PASTE • *See* Zinc Oxide.

LATAMOXEF DISODIUM • *See* Moxalactam Disodium.

LATENCY • The period when a virus is still present within the body, but rests in a harmless state.

LATEX • **Synthetic Rubber.** The milky, usually white juice or exudate of plants obtained by tapping. Used for its coating ability. Any of various gums, resins, fats, or waxes in an emulsion of water and synthetic rubber or plastic are now considered latex. Ingredients of latex compounds can be poisonous, depending upon which plant products are used. Can cause a skin rash.

LAURUS NOBILIS • *See* Bay.

LAVAGE • The washing out of a hollow organ such as the stomach or sinus.

LAVANDULA VERA • *See* Lavender.

LAVENDER (OTC) (H) • *Lavandula vera.* An evergreen of the mint family, it is native to the Mediterranean coast and is cultivated in France, Italy, and England. The name is derived from the Latin word *lavare,* which means to wash. Lavender flower contains a large amount of essential oils that have antispasmodic, antiseptic, and carminative activity. Herbalists use lavender oil to promote relaxation and treat headaches. Lavender tea is used in folk medicine for stomach gas and to relieve anxiety. In 1992, the FDA issued a notice that lavender compound tincture had not been shown to be safe and effective as claimed in OTC digestive-aid products. Contraindicated in patients with gastrointestinal inflammation, peptic ulcer, and liver and kidney disease.

LAXADORON (H) • A homeopathic remedy containing senna leaves and peppermint (*see both*), used as a laxative.

LAXATIVE • An agent that promotes bowel movement by softening or increasing the bulk of the stool, lubricating the intestinal tract, or stimulating muscle contractions of the intestines.

Stimulant Laxatives. Those that agitate or excite intestinal walls, causing the expulsion of fecal matter, include Carter's Little Pills, Castor Oil, Dulcolax, Ex-Lax, Feen-A-Mint, Fletcher's Castoria, and Modane. The following stimulants were banned by the FDA in May 1992: calomel, colocynth, elaterin resin, gamboge, ipomea, jalap, podophyllum resin, aloin, bile salts, bile acids, calcium pantothenate, frangula, ox bile, prune concentrate, prune powder, rhubarb-Chinese, and sodium oleate.

Lubricants. Those that lubricate the intestinal tract to facilitate stool excretion include mineral oil and mineral oil emulsions. Among them are Agoral Plain and Fleet Mineral Oil Enema.

Saline Laxatives. Salines act like sponges to

draw water into the bowel, thereby making passage of stools easier. Loss of body salts is a key risk of long-term use of these products. Among those in this group are milk of magnesia, citrate of magnesia, and Epsom salts. In May 1992, the FDA banned the use of tartaric acid as a saline-laxative ingredient.

Stool Softeners. Emollients that soften hard stools by enabling them to absorb more liquids; often given after childbirth and to patients recovering from surgery. Brands include Colace, Dialose, Regutol, and Surfak. Stool softeners should not be taken within two hours of mineral-oil dose because the combination can result in excessive buildup of mineral oil in the body. In May 1992, the FDA banned Poloxmer 188 as an ingredient in stool softeners.

Hyperosmotics. These laxatives mimic the action of saline laxatives, but pose less risk of salt depletion. Over-the-counter hyperosmotics such as glycerin are available for rectal use only. Oral hyperosmotics must be prescribed by a physician. Overuse of hyperosmotics can cause continuing diarrhea.

Carbon Dioxide–Releasing Agents. These suppositories produce carbon dioxide in the bowels. The gas pushes stubborn stools toward excretion. Suppositories are available over the counter under the brand name Ceo-Two.

Bulk Laxatives. These laxatives absorb water in the intestines and swell stools into easily passed soft masses. Each dose should be taken with an eight-ounce glass of liquid. Although bulk laxatives are generally regarded as the safest form of laxative, they may interfere with the absorption of certain drugs, including aspirin, digitalis, antibiotics, and anticoagulants. The "sugar free" products may contain phenylalanine, which people with the genetic disorder phenylketonuria should avoid. Bulk laxatives include Metamucil and Serutan. The following bulk product ingredients were banned by the FDA in May 1992: carrageenan, agar, and guar gum.

LAX-PILLS • *See* Phenolphthalein.

L-CARNITINE • *See* Levocarnitine.

L.C.D. • *See* Coal Tar.

LCR • *See* Vincristine Sulfate.

L-DEPRENYL HYDROCHLORIDE • *See* Selegiline.

LDL • Abbreviation for low-density lipoprotein, which is believed to collect cholesterol in the blood and deposit it in the cells.

L-DOPA (Rx) • The active form of dopa used to treat Parkinson's disease. *See* Levodopa.

LECITHIN (Rx) (OTC) (H) • From the Greek word *lekithos,* meaning egg yolk. A natural antioxidant and emollient composed of units of choline, phosphoric acid, fatty acids, and glycerin. Commercially isolated from eggs, soybeans, and corn and used as an antioxidant. Used by herbalists and physicians as a nutrient and, experimentally, to lower cholesterol and to help improve mental function in cases of Alzheimer's disease.

LED • The homeopathic abbreviation for ledum (*see*).

LEDERCILLIN VK • *See* Penicillin V.

LEDUM PALUSTRE (H) • A homeopathic remedy to treat insect bites. *See* Labrador Tea Extract.

LEGATRIN • *See* Quinine.

LEGUMES • Plants that include seeds in a pod, such as beans and peas. The Leguminosae family includes over eighteen thousand species. Phytochemicals (*see*) from legumes are being used and tested as anticancer agents.

LEI GONG TANG • *See* Thunder God Vine.

LEMON BALM (H) • *Melissa officinalis.* The leaf of this herb contains essential oils, acids, and tannin (*see*). Herbalists use it to cause sweating and lower fevers. Also used to calm nervous tension and elevate mood. Used like other mints to treat upset stomach and gas. Recently, an ointment has been made with lemon balm leaves to relieve the symptoms of herpes simplex virus (*see*).

LEMON OIL • **Cedro Oil.** A volatile oil expressed from the fresh peel. It is used as a flavoring and scent. It can cause allergic reactions.

LENTE • *See* Insulin.

LEOPARD'S BANE • *See* Arnica.

LEPTANDRA VIRGINICA • *See* Culver's Root.

LEPTIN • A protein product of an obesity gene (*ob*), identified by Rockefeller University researchers in 1994. Researchers are hoping that the discovery will lead to a medication to treat obesity.

LESCOL • *See* Fluvastatin.

LESION • Alteration of tissue or organ function due to injury or disease.

LESPEDEZA (H) • A genus of herbs or shrubby plants of the family Leguminosae widely used for forage. Used in homeopathic medicine to treat urinary tract irritation.

LESSER PERIWINKLE • *See* Periwinkle.

LETTUCE EXTRACT (H) • *Lactuca elongata.* An extract of various species of *Lactuca.* Used in commercial toning lotions and by herbalists to make soothing skin decoctions. During the Middle Ages, lettuce was used as a valuable narcotic, and its milky juice, lactuca, was used with opium to induce sleep. *See* Wild Lettuce.

LEUCOVORIN (Rx) • **Citrovorum Factor. 5-Formyl Tetrahydrofolate. Folinic Acid. Wellcovorin.** An injectable and oral form of folic acid (*see*). Used in the treatment of megaloblastic anemia due to an inborn deficiency of folate in infancy, sprue, or pregnancy. Also given as an antidote to the harmful effects of the cancer and arthritis medication methotrexate (*see*). Potential adverse reactions include rash, hives, itching, and wheezing.

LEUKEMIA • Uncontrolled production of nonfunctional white blood cells in the bone marrow.

LEUKERAN • *See* Chlorambucil.

LEUKINE • *See* Sargramostim.

LEUKO-, LEUK- • Prefixes from the Greek word *leukos,* meaning white.

LEUKOCYTES • White blood cells responsible for combating infections.

LEUKOCYTOSIS • An abnormal increase in the number of white blood cells, often associated with bodily defenses against infection and inflammation.

LEUKODERMA • *See* Vitiligo.

LEUKODYSTROPHY • Destruction of the white matter of the brain.

LEUKOPENIA • Whitish, leathery patches on mucous membranes of the mouth or vulva. May be a precursor to cancer.

LEUKOPLAKIA • Small, whitish patches on the oral mucosa, believed to be premalignant lesions for oral cancer.

LEUKORRHEA • Whitish discharge from the vagina.

LEUKOTRIENES • Substances, produced by cells, that play a part in body reactions, such as inflammation and allergic reactions.

LEUPROLIDE (Rx) • **Leuprorelin. Lupron.** A hormonal anticancer drug used to treat advanced prostate cancer. Potential adverse reactions include nausea, vomiting, dizziness, headache, loss of appetite, swelling and increased tenderness of breasts, hot flashes, blood clots to the lungs, decreased sexual interest, and transient bone pain during the first week of treatment. Similar to diethylstilbestrol in "medical castration" and relief of symptoms, but reportedly has less adverse side effects.

LEUPRORELIN • *See* Leuprolide.

LEUROCRISTINE • *See* Vincristine Sulfate.

LEVAMISOLE (Rx) • **Ergamisol.** A drug that appears to restore depressed immune function and may potentiate the actions of the body's own immune-fighting T-cell responses. Used as an adjuvant (*see*) treatment of Dukes' Stage C colon cancer, after surgical resection. Potential adverse reactions include nausea, vomiting, fatigue, chest pain, dizziness, headache, a feeling of pins and needles, sleepiness, depression, nervousness, insomnia, anxiety, a drop in white blood cells, loss of appetite, abdominal pain, constipation, gas, heartburn, infection, trouble in swallowing, an altered sense of smell, joint and muscle pain, and gallbladder dysfunction. Alcohol may precipitate a disulfiram-like (Antabuse) reaction. Phenytoin levels in the blood may be elevated if administered with levamisole. Contraindicated in patients with a known hypersensitivity to the drug. There was a great deal of controversy over the pricing of this drug in 1992, when it was revealed that as a long-time veterinary drug for sheep parasites, it cost $14, and for human cancer patients, it cost up to $1,500. The company that produces the drug explained that it had backed fourteen hundred studies involving forty thousand patients, and that this was factored into the cost of the drug for humans.

LEVARTERENOL BITARTRATE • *See* Norepinephrine.

LEVATOL • *See* Penbutolol.

LEVLEN • *See* Estradiol.

LEVOBUNOLOL (Rx) • **Betagan.** Beta-blocker (*see*) eyedrops used in the treatment of glaucoma. Potential adverse reactions include nausea, headache, dizziness, hives, depression, low blood pressure, slow heartbeat, faintness, worsening of asthma, and congestive heart failure. Contraindicated in bronchial asthma or serious lung disease, heart problems, chronic lung diseases, diabetes, and overactive thyroid. Propranolol, metoprolol, and other oral beta-blockers increase eye and systemic effects. Reserpine and other catecholamine-depleting drugs add to the drop in blood pressure and slow-heartbeat effects. This medicine may affect blood sugar levels and cover up some signs of low blood sugar.

LEVOCARNITINE (Rx) • **Carnitor. L-carnitine. Vitacarn.** A B vitamin factor found in muscle, liver, and meat extracts. A thyroid inhibitor. Used for patients born with systemic carnitine (*see*) deficiency. It enables fatty acids to produce energy in these persons. Italian researchers reported in 1994 at the European Society of Cardiology meeting in Berlin that L-carnitine has limited left ventricular dilitation of the heart (a risk factor for heart failure and death). Potential adverse reactions include nausea, vomiting, cramps, diarrhea, and body odor. Valproic acid (*see*) increases the requirement for carnitine. Levocarnitine should be taken with or just after meals. If taking the liquid version, drink it slowly. It will be less likely to cause upset stomach.

LEVODOPA (Rx) • **Dopar. Larodopa. Levopa. Parda. Rio-Dopa. Sinemet.** Levodopa, introduced in 1967, counteracts the depletion of the neurotransmitter dopamine in the brain. Used to treat Parkinson's disease (*see*) and parkinsonism resulting from carbon monoxide or manganese intoxication, or associated with hardening of the arteries in the brain. Also used to treat the pain of shingles (herpes zoster). Potential adverse reactions include anemia, involuntary grimacing, awkward or slow movements, jerking, tremor, psychiatric disturbances, memory loss, nervousness, anxiety, bad dreams, euphoria, malaise, fatigue, severe depression, delirium, dementia, hallucinations, a drop in blood pressure upon rising from a seated or prone position, flushing, high blood pressure, phlebitis, spasms of the eyelid, blurred vision, double vision, nasal discharge, nausea, vomiting, loss of appetite, weight loss, stomach pain, hiccups, itching, headache, increased libido, inhibited ejaculation, priapism (*see*), dry mouth, bitter taste, urinary frequency or retention, incontinence, excessive and inappropriate sexual behavior, liver toxicity, hyperventilation, and dark perspiration. Medications for high blood pressure may cause additive low blood pressure effects. Papaverine, phenothiazines and other antipsychotics, and phenytoin may counteract levodopa's beneficial effects. Stimulants may increase the risk of irregular heartbeat. High-protein foods decrease absorption of levodopa. Antacids increase its absorption. Blood pressure medications may cause too much of a drop in blood pressure. Metoclopramide may make it less effective. Levodopa is contraindicated in persons who have glaucoma, melanoma, or undiagnosed skin lesions. Must be used with caution in patients with heart, kidney, liver, or lung disorders, peptic ulcer, asthma, and endocrine disease. Its use may require adjustments in medicine for diabetes. Should not be taken with vitamin preparations that contain B_6 (pyridoxine), which will decrease the effectiveness of levodopa. The drug should be taken, if possible, with carbohydrate and not protein foods, to avoid stomach upset and permit maximum effectiveness. Vitamin B_6, present in some foods and vitamin formulas, reverses the effects of levodopa.

LEVO-DROMORAN • *See* Levorphanol.

LEVOMEPROMAZINE HYDROCHLORIDE • *See* Methotrimeprazine Hydrochloride.

LEVONORGESTREL (Rx) • **Nordette. Norplant System. Triphasil.** A slow release of synthetic progestin into the bloodstream from six capsules implanted under the skin of the upper arm. It suppresses ovulation, possibly by inhibiting pituitary gonadotropin secretion. Forms a thick cervical mucus. Potential adverse reactions include nausea, abdominal discomfort, absence of menstruation, lengthening of menstruation, spotting, irregular onset of menstruation, cervicitis, vaginitis, vaginal discharge, rash, acne, hairiness, scalp hair loss, infection at implant site, enlargement under the arm and of the breast, weight gain, musculoskeletal pain, and breast discharge. Carbamazepine and phenytoin may make levonorgestrel less effective. Contraindicated in pregnancy, and in persons with blood-clotting disorders, cancer of the breast, reproductive organs, or genitals, and those with undiagnosed abnormal genital bleeding. Should be used with caution in persons susceptible to mental depression, which may be worsened by the drug. Should be used cautiously in persons with diabetes or high cholesterol. The implants should be removed if the patient develops blood clots in the veins, jaundice, or if she will be immobilized for a significant length of time due to illness or some other factor. Implant removal may be difficult. If one of the implants falls out, however, the doctor should be contacted, because contraceptive efficiency may be impaired. There have been class action lawsuits against the manufacturer relating to the removal and side effects of this implantable contraceptive.

LEVOPA • *See* Levodopa.

LEVOPHED • *See* Norepinephrine.

LEVOPROME • *See* Methotrimeprazine Hydrochloride.

LEVOROTATORY ALKALOIDS OF BELLADONNA • *See* Belladonna.

LEVORPHAN • *See* Levorphanol.

LEVORPHANOL (Rx) • **Levo-Dromoran. Levorphan.** A narcotic analgesic altering both the perception of and reaction to pain. Used to treat moderate to severe pain. Potential adverse effects include sedation, sleepiness, lack of alertness, dizziness, euphoria, seizures, low blood pressure, a low heartbeat, nausea, vomiting, constipation, urine retention, and respiratory depression. Alcohol and other depressants increase the central nervous system effects of levorphanol. Contraindicated in acute alcoholism, bronchial asthma, increased pressure on the brain, respiratory depression, low thyroid, liver or kidney disease, Addison's disease, seizures, head injury, severe central nervous system depression, brain tumor, chronic lung disease, shock, and in elderly or debilitated patients. May be addictive.

LEVOTHROID • *See* Levothyroxine.

LEVOTHYROXINE (Rx) • **Levothroid. Levoxine. Liotrix. Synthroid. Synthrox. Thyroglobulin.** A synthetic version of thyroxine, the most important hormone of the thyroid (*see*). Levothyroxine stimulates the metabolism of all body tissues by accelerating the rate of cellular oxidation. Used to treat cretinism, myxedema (*see*), and ordinary hypothyroidism in patients of any age or state (including pregnancy), and primary hypothyroidism resulting from functional deficiency, primary atrophy, partial or total absence of the thyroid gland, or the effects of surgery, radiation, or drugs, with or without the presence of goiter. Also used to treat problems with the pituitary gland or hypothalamus. The use of thyroid hormones in the therapy of obesity, alone or combined with other drugs, is unjustified and has been shown to be ineffective. Thyroid hormones should be used with great caution in patients with cardiovascular disease, diabetes, and adrenal cortical insufficiency. Potential adverse reactions include chest pain, increased pulse rate, palpitations, excessive sweating, insomnia, leg cramps, a change in appetite, high blood pressure, heat intolerance, fever, menstrual irregularities, and nervousness. In a study reported in the *Journal of the American Medical Association* in 1994, California researchers documented serious bone loss in the wrists and hips of postmenopausal women taking relatively high doses of thyroid hormone. May increase the effects of anticoagulants and decrease those of insulin or oral hypoglycemics. Cholestyramine impairs absorption of thyroid hormones and therefore should be administered at least four hours before taking levothyroxine. Estrogens tend to increase the need for levothyroxine. Levothyroxine is usually taken as a lifelong replacement therapy. It should be taken at the same time each day, usually in the morning, to prevent insomnia. Most effective on an empty stomach, but may be taken with food.

LEVOXINE • *See* Levothyroxine.

LEVSIN • *See* Hyoscyamine.

LEVSINEX • *See* Hyoscyamine.

LEVULOSE • *See* Fructose.

LEXOCORT • *See* Hydrocortisone.

LHRH (Rx) • Abbreviation for luteinizing hormone-releasing hormone. LHRH stimulates secretion of both luteinizing hormone (LH) and follicle-stimulating hormone (FSH). This stimulates the development of eggs in the ovary and their release.

LIBIDO • Psychic energy in general; commonly used to refer to sexual drive.

LIBRAX (Rx) • **Clindex. Clinoxide. Clipoxide.** A combination of chlordiazepoxide and clidinium (*see*) that is used to treat anxiety and spasms associated with gastrointestinal disease. Librax may be prescribed for gastrointestinal disorders and the management of peptic ulcers, gastritis, irritable bowel syndrome, spastic colon, and mild ulcerative colitis. There are questions about this drug's effectiveness. Potential adverse reactions include drowsiness, dry mouth, difficulty in urination, and constipation, especially in elderly or debilitated people. Other less common adverse reactions include confusion, depression lethargy, tremor, constipation, nausea, changes in sex drive, menstrual irregularity, irregular heartbeat, stuffy nose, fever, heartburn, suppression of lactation in females, bloated feeling, drug allergy, and allergic reactions. The tranquilizer and the atropinelike combination in Librax may interact with alcohol and other drugs that act on the central nervous system, including tranquilizers, narcotics, barbiturates, or antihistamines, causing excessive fatigue and sleepiness. Both Librax ingredients may be increased by MAO inhibitors (*see*). Cimetidine may exaggerate the effects from chlordiazepoxide. Most effective when taken on an empty stomach, but may be taken with a small amount of food to avoid GI symptoms.

LIBRITABS • *See* Chlordiazepoxide.

LIBRIUM • *See* Chlordiazepoxide.

LICE • *Pediculus humanus capitis,* **Head Lice.** *P. humanus corporis,* **Body Lice.** *Phthirus pubis,* **Genital Lice.** The head louse and pubic (crab) louse prefer hairy places; the body louse likes to live in undergarments. Body lice can spread typhus. Crab and head lice are less dangerous but still annoying.

LICE, ENZ FOAM • *See* Piperonyl Butoxide.

LICORICE (OTC) (H) • *Glycyrrhiza glabra.* **Sweet Wood.** A perennial shrub is native to Europe and Asia (China and Mongolia). It was introduced into Britain in the sixteenth century by black friars. A favorite medicine with ancient physicians, it was used in America as a remedy for earache. The black substance is derived from the "sweet root" of the plant, cultured from southern Europe to central Asia. The dried root contains sugars, glycosides (*see*) with adrenocortical-like activity (*see* Adrenocorticoids), flavonoids, coumarins, bitter principle, and estrogen (*see all*). One of its major derivatives, glycyrrhetic acid, has been found to have substantial antiarthritic activity. The leaves were steeped and the liquid used as ear drops. The fresh roots were chewed for toothache, and the boiled roots for fevers. It was also used to treat peptic ulcers. Modern scientists report licorice has an anti-inflammatory action and suppresses coughs as well as codeine does. It stimulates the production of two steroids, cortisone and aldosterone (*see both*). It has also been found to produce sodium and water retention with subsequent loss of potassium in some instances. Scientists in the United States and Japan are studying extracts of licorice to inhibit cancer. Licorice may cause allergic reactions, and it can be toxic if taken in large amounts. It is used by herbalists to treat gastritis and ulcers. It is used in allopathic medicine to treat peptic ulcers. Some people known to have eaten licorice candy regularly and generously have suffered high blood pressure, headaches, and muscle weakness. Licorice reportedly can cause asthma, intestinal upsets, and contact dermatitis. In 1992, the FDA proposed a ban on licorice root in oral menstrual drug products because it had not been shown to be safe and effective for its stated claims.

LIDEX • *See* Fluocinonide.

LIDOCAINE (Rx) (OTC) • **Bactine Antiseptic. Caine-2. Dalcaine. Dilocaine. DuoTrach Kit. LidoPen Auto-Injector. Mycitracin Plus Pain Reliever. Nervocaine. Octocaine. Unguentine Plus First Aid. Xylocaine. Xylocaine Ointment.** Derived from benzene or alcohol, it is a local anesthetic introduced in 1949. It relieves itching, pain, soreness, and discomfort due to rashes, including eczema, and minor burns. It is used to deaden areas subject to minor surgery, dental procedures, and childbirth. Also used to treat heart irregularities. Potential adverse reactions include confusion, tremors, lethargy, sleepiness, stupor, restlessness, slurred speech, euphoria, depression, anxiety, numbness, muscle twitching, seizures, low blood pressure, increase in heart irregularities, ringing in the ears, blurred or double vision, rash, and severe allergic reactions. Interacts with cimetidine and beta-blockers (*see*), both of which may cause lidocaine toxicity. Phenytoin may cause added adverse heart effects. In 1992, the FDA issued a notice that lidocaine had not been shown to be safe and effective as claimed in OTC poison ivy, poison oak, and poison sumac products.

LIDOPEN AUTO-INJECTOR (Rx) • Designed to be used by patients in emergencies. *See* Lidocaine.

LIFE ROOT (H) • *Senecio aureus.* **Golden Ragwort.** The herb contains alkaloids and resins and is used by herbalists as a uterine tonic. Reportedly useful in treating the symptoms of menopause and for delayed or suppressed menstruation. Also used as a general tonic for debilitated states.

LILY OF THE VALLEY (H) • *Convallaria majalis.* **Convallaria. May-Blossom. May Lily.** This wildflower, which grows in woodlands, causes vomiting. The powdered root is used to slow the heartbeat. Also used by herbalists to reduce fluid retention. It has long been used to expel worms from the intestinal tract. The flower was believed to stimulate secretions of the nasal mucous membranes and was employed in the treatment of apoplexy, epilepsy, coma, and dizziness. Contains cardiac glycosides (*see*) similar to those of digitalis (*see*).

LIMBITROL (Rx) • A combination of chlordiazepoxide and amitriptyline (*see*), used to treat moderate to severe anxiety and depression, insomnia, agitation, suicidal thoughts, and appetite loss. The combination is believed to be more effective sooner than either alone. Potential adverse reactions include mild drowsiness, changes in blood pressure, irregular heartbeat, heart attack, hallucinations, confusion, delusions, anxiety, restlessness, lethargy, depression, inactivity, slurred speech, stupor, dizziness, excitement, numbness and tingling, blurred vision, rash, itching, sensitivity to sunlight or bright light, retention of fluids, fever, drug allergy, nausea, vomiting, loss of appetite, stomach upset, diarrhea, breast enlargement, changes in sex drive, and changes in blood sugar. Less common side effects are headache, changes in menstrual cycle, double vision, insomnia, nightmares, a feeling of panic, peculiar taste in the mouth, stomach cramps, black tongue, yellowing of the eyes or skin, changes in the liver, changes in weight, sweating, flushing, loss of hair, and a general feeling of ill health. Should not be taken with MAO inhibitors (*see*), alcohol, sleeping medications, other central nervous system depressant drugs, or with guanethidine. Large doses of vitamin C can reduce the effect of this drug.

LIME (H) • *Tilia cordata*. A small, greenish yellow fruit of a spicy, tropical tree. Its acid pulp yields a juice used as a flavoring agent and antiseptic. It is used to induce sweating, as a sedative, and an antispasmodic in folk medicine. It is used externally as a gargle for sore throats. A source of vitamin C. Ingestion and application to the skin can cause a sensitivity to sunlight.

LIME BLOSSOM (H) • *Tilia europea*. **Linden.** The flowers contain essential oils, mucilage,

flavonoids, coumarin, and vanillin (*see all*). Herbalists use it for relaxation from nervous tension and to lower blood pressure. In 1992, the FDA issued a notice that linden had not been shown to be safe and effective as claimed in OTC digestive-aid products.

LIME WATER (OTC) (H) • An alkaline water solution of calcium hydroxide that absorbs carbon dioxide from the air. Used in medicines, as an antacid, and as an alkali in external washes.

LIMINOIDS • Found in citrus fruits, they seem to induce protective enzymes.

LINCOCIN • *See* Lincomycin.

LINCOMYCIN (Rx) • **Lincocin.** An antibacterial introduced in 1965, it is used to treat respiratory and urinary tract, skin, soft-tissue, and gynecologic infections, and osteomyelitis and blood poisoning caused by streptococci, pneumococci, and staphylococci. Potential adverse reactions may include blood problems, dizziness, headache, low blood pressure, sore tongue, ringing in the ears, nausea, vomiting, severe colitis, persistent diarrhea, abdominal cramps, itching around the anus, vaginitis, jaundice, rash, hives, pain at injection site, and serious allergic reactions. Antidiarrheal medicines reduce oral absorption of lincomycin. Lincomycin may reduce the effectiveness of drugs to treat myasthenia gravis (*see*). Oral lincomycin is best taken on an empty stomach with a full glass of water.

LINDANE (Rx) • **Gamma Benzene Hexachloride. Hexachlorocyclohexane. Bio-Well. GBH. G-well. Kildane. Kwell. Kwildane. Scabene. Thionex.** An insecticide in a cream, lotion, or shampoo introduced in 1952 to treat parasitic infestation such as scabies or lice (*see both*). Lindane is poisonous. Can be absorbed through the skin. Potential adverse reactions include dizziness, seizures, rash, or irritation with repeated use. Contraindicated when skin is raw or inflamed. Should not be applied to open areas, acutely inflamed skin, face, eyes, or mucous membranes. Must be kept away from the mouth because it is poisonous and may be fatal if swallowed.

LINDEN • *See* Lime Blossom.

LINOLEIC ACID • An essential fatty acid (*see*) prepared from edible fats and oils. A major constituent of many vegetable oils—for example, cottonseed and soybean. Used in emulsifiers and vitamins. Large doses can cause nausea and vomiting.

LINOLENIC ACID • Polyunsaturated acid produced in the body as a metabolite of linoleic acid. A nutrient used in the treatment of eczema. Alpha-linolenic acid in the diet of Mediterranean people is believed to be important in the prevention of heart disease.

LIORESAL • *See* Baclofen.

LIOTHYRONINE (Rx) • T$_3$ Triiodothyronine. Cyronine. Cytomel. Liotrix. A thyroid hormone that stimulates the metabolism of all body tissues by accelerating the rate of cellular oxidation. Used to treat cretinism, myxedema (*see*), and ordinary hypothyroidism in patients of any age or state (including pregnancy), primary hypothyroidism resulting from functional deficiency, primary atrophy, partial or total absence of thyroid gland, or the effects of surgery, radiation, or drugs, with or without the presence of goiter. Also used to treat problems with the pituitary gland or the hypothalamus. The use of thyroid hormones in the therapy of obesity, alone or combined with other drugs, is unjustified and has been shown to be ineffective. Thyroid hormones should be used with great caution in patients with cardiovascular disease, diabetes, or adrenal cortical insufficiency. Potential adverse reactions include chest pain, increased pulse rate, palpitations, excessive sweating, insomnia, leg cramps, a change in appetite, high blood pressure, heat intolerance, fever, menstrual irregularities, nervousness, and heart problems, including stoppage. May increase the effects of anticoagulants and decrease the effects of insulin or oral hypo-

glycemics. Cholestyramine impairs absorption of thyroid hormones and should therefore be administered at least four hours before liothyronine is taken. The thyroid drug is usually taken as a lifelong replacement therapy. It is best taken on an empty stomach but may be taken with a small amount of food.

LIOTRIX (Rx) • **Euthroid. Thyrolar.** A combination of the thyroid hormones levothyroxine and liothyronine (*see both*).

LIPANCREATIN • *See* Pancrelipase.

LIPASE (OTC) • An enzyme that breaks down fat, widely distributed in plants and animal tissues, especially in the pancreas. Isolated from castor beans. In 1992, the FDA issued a notice that lipase had not been shown to be safe and effective as claimed in OTC digestive-aid products.

LIPO- • Fat.

LIPOMA • A benign fatty tumor.

LIPOMUL ORAL • *See* Corn Oil.

LIPOTRIAD (OTC) • A multivitamin preparation.

LIQUAEMIN • *See* Heparin.

LIQUI-CHAR • *See* Activated Charcoal.

LIQUID PETROLATUM • *See* Mineral Oil.

LIQUID PRED • *See* Prednisone.

LIQUI-E • *See* Tocophersolan.

LIQUIFILM (OTC) • *See* Artificial Tears.

LIQUIFILM OPHTHALMIC • *See* Fluorometholone.

LIQUIPRIN • *See* Acetaminophen.

LIQUORICE (H) • *See* Licorice.

LISINOPRIL (Rx) • **Prinivil. Zestril.** An ACE inhibitor (*see*) introduced in 1988 to lower blood pressure, it acts on enzymes in the blood to dilate blood vessels. It is expected to be approved for treatment of congestive heart failure. Reportedly has a low incidence of adverse effects, needs be taken only once a day, and does not have an adverse effect on asthma, blood cholesterol, or diabetes. Potential adverse reactions include a low white blood count, dizziness, headache, fatigue, depression, sleepiness, numbness, low blood pressure, chest pain, diarrhea, nausea, heartburn, nasal congestion, impotence, decreased libido, overload of potassium, bad taste in the mouth, rash, cough, muscle cramps, swelling, and decreased libido. Contraindicated in patients who are hypersensitive to the product or who have a history of angioedema (*see*) related to previous treatment with an ACE inhibitor. When used with diuretics or indomethacin, blood pressure may drop too low. Potassium-sparing diuretics, potassium supplements, and potassium-containing salt substitutes may raise blood potassium too high. Over-the-counter diet pills, decongestants, and other such drugs that contain stimulants may counteract lisinopril's effect. Beneficial effects may take several weeks to become apparent. Sudden changes of position should be avoided to minimize orthostatic hypotension (*see*). Strenuous exercise in hot weather should be avoided because it can drop blood pressure too low. Can be taken with food. Best taken on an empty stomach one to two hours before meals.

LISPRO (Rx) • **Humalog.** Approved in 1996, a new form of insulin that is designed to mimic the body's own normal rapid insulin response. Even though health care professionals recommend that injections of regular human insulin be timed at least 30 to 45 minutes before a meal, it has been determined that only 25 percent injected insulin more than 30 minutes before a meal. Diabetics who tested the medication took it within 15 minutes of eating a meal and still effectively controlled blood sugar.

LISTERINE ANTISEPTIC • *See* Eucalyptus.

LISTERMINT WITH FLUORIDE • *See* Sodium Fluoride.

LITH- • Combination form meaning stone, calcification, as in *lithiasis,* stone formation.

LITHANE • *See* Lithium Carbonate.

LITHIUM CARBONATE (Rx) • **Cibalith-S. Eskalith. Lithane. Lithobid. Lithonate. Lithotabs.** A drug introduced in 1949 to prevent relapses of mania in psychiatric patients and to treat cluster headaches. Its exact mechanism of action is unknown. Has a narrow margin of safety. Potential adverse reactions include a drop in white blood cells, tremors, drowsiness, headache, confusion, restlessness, dizziness, slow movements, stupor, lethargy, coma, blackouts, worsened organic brain syndrome, seizures, loss of balance, impaired speech, muscle weakness, incoordination, hyperexcitability, low blood pressure, peripheral circulatory collapse, allergic skin reactions, ankle and wrist swelling, ringing in the ears, impaired vision, nausea, vomiting, a loss of appetite, diarrhea, dry mouth, thirst, metallic taste, frequent urination, decreased libido, impotence, male infertility, female breast swelling with milk production, low thyroid hormone, incontinence, kidney toxicity with long-term use, transient high blood sugar, goiter, low thyroid, low salt in blood, itching, rash, diminished or lost sensation, and drying and thinning of the hair. Interacts with diuretics, which may increase retention of lithium and add to its side effects. Aminophylline, sodium bicarbonate, and sodium chloride may make lithium less effective. Carbamazepine, probenecid, indomethacin, methyldopa, and piroxicam may make it toxic. Haloperidol and thioridazine may cause brain syndrome, including lethargy, tremors, and movement symptoms. Takes one to three weeks to take effect. Should be taken after meals with a lot of water. Fluid intake should be maintained while on this drug.

LITHOBID • *See* Lithium Carbonate.

LITHONATE • *See* Lithium Carbonate.

LITHOSTAT • *See* Acetohydroxamic Acid.

LITHOTABS • *See* Lithium Carbonate.

LIVE-FOREVER (H) • *Sedum telephium.* A sedum, which means to sit, it grows in cool, mountainous regions of Europe. The dried plant is sold in Sicily for use in treating dysentery and diarrhea.

LIVER LILY • *See* Blue Flag.

LIVE YEAST CELL DERIVATIVE (OTC) • **Preparation H. Wyanoids Relief Factor.** Yeast is a one-celled organism that occurs in sugary liquids such as fruit juices or malt liquids. It is used for fermentation by enzymes, which convert sugar and other carbohydrates into carbon dioxide and water in the presence of oxygen, alcohol, carbon dioxide, or lactic acid. Live yeast cell derivative reportedly acts by increasing the oxygen uptake of skin tissue and facilitating the action of collagen (*see*). It is used in preparations for hemorrhoids (*see*).

LIXOLIN • *See* Theophylline.

LMD • *See* Dextran.

LO-AQUA • *See* Furosemide.

LOBELIA (H) • *Lobelia inflata.* **Asthma Weed. Indian Tobacco. Pukeweed.** The leaves and seeds of this bitter common weed contain lobeline, which has an effect similar to nicotine and is used to help break the nicotine habit. It is also used by herbalists as an expectorant, stimulant, an emetic to cause vomiting, and as an antispasmodic. Primarily used to treat asthma, bronchitis, and cough. Externally, it is applied to wounds. Potential adverse reactions include nausea, vomiting, breathing problems, convulsions, and when used in large amounts, even coma and death.

LOCOID • *See* Hydrocortisone.

LODINE • *See* Etodolac.

LODOSYN • *See* Carbidopa-Levodopa.

LODRANE • *See* Theophylline.

LOESTRIN • *See* Estradiol and Norethindrone.

LOFENE (Rx) • *See* Diphenoxylate and Atropine Sulfate. *See also* Lomotil.

LOGEN • *See* Diphenoxylate and Atropine Sulfate.

LOGODERM • *See* Alclometasone.

LOMEFLOXACIN (Rx) • **Maxaquin.** A once-a-day quinolone (*see*) antibiotic introduced in 1992 to treat acute bacterial worsening of chronic bronchitis, and prostate gland and urinary tract infections. Potential adverse reactions include nausea, vomiting, drowsiness, colitis, headache, photosensitivity, dizziness, dry mouth, allergic reactions, gas, swelling of the face, flu-like symptoms, sweating, fatigue, slow heartbeat, irregular heartbeat, heart failure, coma, blood clot to the lung, numbness, cough, yeast infections, genital inflammations, shortness of breath, eczema, taste perversion, difficulty in urinating, gastrointestinal bleeding, back, chest, and stomach pain, and diarrhea. Patients taking this drug should drink fluids liberally. Supplements with iron should not be taken within two hours before or after taking lomefloxacin. Sucralfate or antacids containing magnesium or aluminum should not be taken within four hours before or two hours after taking lomefloxacin. Excessive sunlight should be avoided. May be taken with or without food.

LOMOTIL (Rx) • **Diphenatol. Lofene. Logen. Lomanate. Lonox. Lo-Trol. Low-Quel. Nor-Mil.** A combination of diphenoxylate and atropine sulfate (*see both*) used to treat diarrhea, but not the underlying causes. These drugs should not be used in people with bowel, stomach, or other diseases, who may be harmed by taking antidiarrheal drugs. Contraindicated in those allergic to this medication or any other medication containing atropine sulfate, and in those who are jaundiced or are suffering from diarrhea caused by antibiotics such as clindamycin or lincomycin (*see both*). Potential adverse reactions include dry membranes inside the nose or mouth, flushing or redness of the face, fever, irregular heartbeat, and inability to urinate. Less commonly, people taking Lomotil for extended periods may experience abdominal discomfort, swelling of the gums, interference with normal breathing, a feeling of numbness in the extremities, drowsiness, restlessness, rash, nausea, sedation, vomiting, headache, dizziness, depression, lethargy, loss of appetite, euphoria, itching, and coma. Lomotil, a central nervous system depressant, may cause fatigue or inability to concentrate and may thus increase the effects of sleeping pills, tranquilizers, or alcoholic beverages if used while taking the drug.

LOMUSTINE (Rx) • **CCNU. CeeNU.** An alkylating (*see*) anticancer agent, it is used in the treatment of brain tumors and Hodgkin's disease. Lomustine interferes with the growth of cancer cells, which are eventually destroyed. Since the growth of normal body cells may also be affected, adverse effects may occur such as hair loss. Potential adverse reactions include nausea and vomiting beginning four to five hours after administration and lasting twenty-four hours, a drop in the white blood cell count, sore mouth, and kidney damage.

LONGANBERRY (H) • *Euphoria longana.* **Dragon Eyes. Long Yen Rou.** A red-fruited herb, the berries of which are used by herbalists to make a strong tonic that reputedly strengthens the reproductive organs of women and counteracts anemia, forgetfulness, and hyperactivity. Also an herbal remedy for low blood sugar.

LONG YEN ROU • *See* Longanberry.

LONITEN • *See* Minoxidil.

LONOX • *See* Diphenoxylate and Atropine.

LOOP DIURETICS • Fast-acting, powerful agents that promote excretion of urine by inhibiting reabsorption of sodium and chloride in an area of the kidneys known as Henle's loop. Furosemide and bumetanide are examples (*see both*).

LOOSESTRIFE, PURPLE (H) • *Lythrum salicaria.* A perennial herb grown in many parts of the world in damp, marshy places, it is used as an astringent and tonic. Also used in Europe to treat fevers and in Ireland for diarrhea and the healing of wounds. Used by herbalists in soothing eyedrops and in salves for skin ulcers.

LO/OVRAL (Rx) • An oral contraceptive containing norgestrel and ethinyl estradiol. *See* Oral Contraceptives.

LOPERAMIDE (OTC) • **Imodium. Imodium A-D.** An antibacterial and solvent introduced in 1977, it is derived from isopropanol (*see*). Loperamide acts by slowing intestinal motility and by affecting water and electrolyte (*see*) movement through the bowel. It is widely prescribed for diarrhea. Changed from Rx to OTC in 1988. Potential adverse reactions include stomachache, bloating, or other intestinal discomfort, constipation, dry mouth, dizziness, fatigue, nausea and vomiting, and rash. Contraindicated for acute attacks of ulcerative colitis since it can cause massive dilation and perforation of the bowel. It is also contraindicated in acute diarrhea resulting from toxins until the substances are removed from the intestinal tract. Loperamide should also be used cautiously in persons with an enlarged prostate gland, liver disease, or a history of narcotic dependence. It is prescribed for people who have had colostomies or ileostomies to reduce fluid loss from the outlet. Overdosage of loperamide may result in constipation, central nervous system depression, rash, and nausea. May be taken with or without food.

LOPID • *See* Gemfibrozil.

LOPREMONE • *See* Protirelin.

LOPRESSOR • *See* Metoprolol Tartrate.

LOPROX • *See* Ciclopirox.

LOPURIN • *See* Allopurinol.

LOQUAT (H) • *Eriobotrya japonica.* The leaves and fruit are used by herbalists to treat coughs and lung inflammations. It contains amygdalin (*see*), also found in cherry bark and apricot kernel, both of which are used to treat coughs.

LORABID • *See* Loracarbef.

LORACARBEF (Rx) • **Lorabid.** A synthetic beta-lactam antibiotic introduced in 1992. It is taken orally for the treatment of mild to moderate infections, including those of the sinus, throat, tonsils, skin, urinary tract, and lung. It can cause an allergic reaction in those sensitive to penicillin. Must be used cautiously in persons with impaired kidney function or in those receiving diuretics (*see*). Potential adverse reactions include diarrhea, nausea, rashes, hives, headache, sleepiness, nervousness, dizziness, kidney dysfunction, and vaginal yeast infections.

LORATADINE (Rx) • **Claritin.** A nonsedating seasonal allergy medication approved in 1993. It has been on the market in seventy countries, and in thirteen of those it is sold without prescription. The FDA is not requiring the restrictive labeling it requires for Seldane and Hismanal (*see both*). It may cause sedation in some people, particularly older persons. A candidate for OTC status.

LORAZ • *See* Lorazepam.

LORAZEPAM (Rx) • **Alzapam. Ativan. Loraz.** A benzodiazepine (*see*) antianxiety drug introduced in 1971 that works by depressing the central nervous system at the area of the brain controlling emotions. Used to treat anxiety, tension, agitation, irritability, and inorganically linked anxiety disorders. Should not be used for everyday stress. It is intended for short-term use in treating anxiety or anxiety with depressive symptoms. Potential side effects include drowsiness, lethargy, hangover, fainting, transient low blood pressure, dry mouth, and abdominal discomfort. Contraindicated in glaucoma and psychoses. Should be used cautiously in persons with kidney or liver dysfunction, organic brain syndrome, and myasthenia gravis (*see*). Reportedly has a wide margin of safety with few drug interactions. Should not be used with alcohol and other central nervous system depressants. Cimetidine may increase sedation. It is more quickly processed by the body and thus reportedly has fewer cumulative effects than other benzodiazepines. The drug should not be discontinued abruptly. Best taken on an empty stomach, but may be taken with a small amount of food. May be habit-forming.

LORCET PLUS (Rx) • A combination of acetaminophen and hydrocodone (*see both*). Used as a painkiller.

LORELCO • *See* Probucol.

LOROXIDE-HC • *See* Benzoyl Peroxide.

LORTAB • *See* Hydrocodone and Acetaminophen.

LOSARTAN POTASSIUM (Rx) • **Cozaar. Hyzaar.** Introduced in 1995, Losartan is an angiotensin-II receptor blocker for the treatment of high blood pressure. Hyzaar is combined with hydrochlorothiazide (*see*) and reduces blood pressure reportedly 50 percent more than Cozaar alone. Unlike many other high blood pressure medications, it is claimed Losartan does not raise triglycerides, cholesterol, blood sugar, and uric acid. It also does not cause significant heart rate effects. Neither form of the medication is to be given to pregnant women because of potentially fatal effects on the fetus. Also should not be used in patients with severe congestive heart failure or kidney dysfunction. Other potential adverse effects include upper-respiratory infections, dizziness, and cough. May be taken with or without food.

LOSEC • *See* Omeprazole.

LOTENSIN • *See* Benazepril.

LOTION • Liquid applied to the skin.

LOTREL (Rx) • A combination of amlodipine and benazepril (*see both*), used to treat high blood pressure. Introduced in 1995, it is claimed to be more effective in combination than either drug alone, and has less side effects. It is contraindicated for the initial treatment of high blood pressure, and is not safe for pregnant women because it may harm the fetus.

LOTRIMIN • *See* Clotrimazole.

LOTRISONE (Rx) • A combination of clotrimazole and betamethasone (*see both*), it is a cream used to relieve the symptoms of itching rash, or skin inflammation associated with a severe fungal infection. It may treat the underlying cause of the skin problem by killing the fungus; relieves inflammation that may be associated with the infection. This combination product should only be used on your doctor's prescription. A combination such as this may be less effective than either ingredient alone. Should not be used if you are sensitive or allergic to the ingredients. Potential adverse reactions include stinging, itching, burning, skin peeling, and swelling. Do not apply Lotrisone to the eye or to the ear if the eardrum is perforated, unless specifically directed to do so by your doctor.

LO-TROL • *See* Diphenoxylate and Atropine Sulfate.

LOTUSATE • *See* Talbutal.

LOUSEWORT • *See* Wood Betony.

LOVAGE (H) • *Levesticum officinale. Ligusticum scoticum.* An ingredient in perfumery from an aromatic herb native to southern Europe that has been grown in monastery gardens since the Middle Ages for medicine and food flavoring. It has a hot, sharp, biting taste. The yellow-brown oil is extracted from the root or other parts of the herb. It has a reputation for improving health and inciting love; Czechoslovakian girls reportedly wear lovage in a bag around their necks when dating boys. Added to bathwater for its supposed deodorizing properties. Has been used by herbalists as an eyewash, a cure for colds, and to treat arthritis. Contraindicated in pregnancy and for patients with kidney dysfunction. *See also* OSHA.

LOVASTATIN (Rx) • **Mevacor. Mevinolin. Monacolin K.** A cholesterol-lowering agent isolated from a strain of *Aspergillus terreus,* a fungus, and introduced in 1987. The involvement of low-density lipoprotein (LDL) in clogging of the arteries has been well documented. Epidemiological studies have established that high LDL and low HDL (high-density lipoprotein) cholesterol are both risk factors for coronary heart disease. Lovastatin has been shown to lower both normal and high levels of LDL. A five-year study of the safety and efficacy of lovastatin reported in the *Archives of Internal Medicine,* May 10, 1993, by the Lovastatin Study Groups, concluded that the medication is generally well-tolerated and effective during long-term use. There were no deaths attributable to trauma, suicide, or homicide, and there were fourteen cases of cancer versus twenty-one expected. There was no evidence for an adverse effect on the eye lens. Out of 745 patients in the study, sixteen died of coronary heart disease, fourteen of whom had coronary heart disease when the study began. Potential adverse reactions to Lovastatin include hypersensitivity, constipation, diarrhea, gas, heartburn, abdominal pain, nausea, muscle cramps, dizziness, headache, rash, blurred vision, bad taste in the mouth, liver dysfunction, decreased alertness, opacities of the eye lens, weight gain, and muscle pain. A potentially fatal condition, rhabdomyolysis (*see*), has been associated with lovastatin therapy alone, or when combined with immunosuppressive therapy, and when combined with gemfibrozil (*see*) or lipid-lowering doses of niacin. Lovastatin therapy should be temporarily withheld or discontinued in any patient with an acute, serious condition suggestive of muscle problems, or having risk factors predisposing to the development of kidney failure, including severe acute infection, low blood pressure, major surgery, trauma, severe metabolic, endocrine, and electrolyte disorders, and uncontrolled seizures. Should be taken with the evening meal because cholesterol is made at night. Should be taken with food to avoid GI disturbances. *See* HMG-COA Reductase Inhibitors.

LOVE-IN-WINTER • *See* Pipsissewa Leaves Extract.

LOVE-LIES-BLEEDING • *See* Amaranth.

LOVENOX • *See* Enoxaparin.

LOXAPINE (Rx) • **Loxitane. Oxilapine Succi-nate.** A medication to treat nervous, mental, and emotional conditions. Potential adverse reactions include a drop in white blood cells, extrapyramidal reactions, sedation, tardive dyskinesia (*see*), pseu-doparkinsonism, dizziness, a drop in blood pres-sure when rising from a seated or prone position, irregular heartbeat, blurred vision, dry mouth, con-stipation, urine retention, menstrual irregularities, enlargement of male breast, mild photosensitivity, allergic skin reactions, increased appetite, fever, easy bruising, weight gain, constipation, masklike facial expression, restlessness, and sweating. Con-traindicated in coma, severe central nervous sys-tem depression, or drug-induced depressed states. Should be used with caution in epilepsy, cere-brovascular disorders, glaucoma, enlarged prostate, urine retention, suspected intestinal obstruction, and kidney damage. Use with alcohol and other nervous system depressants increases central ner-vous system depression. Loxapine should be taken with food or a full glass of milk to reduce stomach irritation. The liquid medicine must be mixed with juice to make it easier to swallow.

LOXITANE • *See* Loxapine.

LOZOL • *See* Indapamide.

L-PAM • *See* Melphalan.

L-PCA • *See* L-Pyroglutamic Acid.

L-PHENYLALANINE MUSTARD • *See* Mel-phalan.

L-PYROGLUTAMIC ACID (H) • **L-PCA. Pyroglutamic Acid.** Found in vegetables, fruits, grasses, and molasses, it is being studied as a base for nerve chemical messengers involved in mem-ory storage and recall. Being promoted in health food products for that purpose.

LRA • *See* Gonadorelin.

L.72 (H) • A homeopathic antianxiety formula containing cicuta viros 4x, which is said to reduce anxiety and discontent, asagoetida 3x to relieve restlessness, and ignatia 4x to relieve anger (*see all*). The formula also contains gaultheria, staphysagria, corydalis, sumbulus, valeriana, hyoscyamus, and avena sativa.

LUBRIN • A vaginal lubricant.

LUDIOMIL • *See* Maprotiline.

LUFYLLIN • *See* Dyphylline.

LUGOL'S SOLUTION • *See* Sodium Iodide.

LU HUI • *See* Aloe Vera.

LUMINAL • *See* Phenobarbital.

LUNGWORT (H) • *Pulmonaria officinalis.* **Black Hellebore. Mullein. Virginia Cowslip. Wall Hawkweed.** Any of several plants thought to be helpful in combating lung diseases, coughs, and hoarseness. Lungworts are used by herbalists to treat diarrhea. The leaves contain mucins, sili-cic acid, tannin, saponin, allantoin, quercetin, and vitamin C (*see all*). Externally, this plant is used to heal wounds.

LUPRON • *See* Leuprolide.

LUPUS ERYTHEMATOSUS • A skin or tis-sue disease occurring in two forms, *discoid* and *systemic*. Discoid lupus is a chronic disease of the skin. It is characterized by red, circular, or discoid lesions. Their initial appearance is often preceded by exposure to sunlight. Systemic lupus is one of the connective tissue or collagen (*see*) diseases. It is a deep-seated disease, with symptoms only incidentally manifested in the skin. Among the drugs known to be capable of inducing a lupuslike syndrome are chlorpromazine, clofibrate, hydralazine, isoniazid, oral contraceptives, penicillamine, phenolphthalein, some phenothiazines, phenylbutazone, phenytoin, and procainamide.

LURIDE • *See* Sodium Fluoride.

LU RONG • *See* Deer Antler.

LUSTY GOATHERB • *See* Epimedium.

LUTEINIZING HORMONE–RELEASING HORMONE • A hormone that helps regulate sex hormones. *See* LHRH.

LUTREPULSE • *See* Gonadorelin.

LUVOX • *See* Fluvoxamine.

LYC • Homeopathic abbreviation for *Lycopodium clavatum* (*see*).

LYCHEE (H) • *Litchi chinensis.* **Gay Gee.** The berries are used by herbalists to make a cooling tonic used to reduce fevers and thirst, and to treat bronchial inflammations. Lychee is often prescribed in the treatment of diabetes. The Chinese use it to treat cloudy vision.

LYCOPENE • An antioxidant found in tomatoes and red grapefruit. Seems to be a good antioxidant.

LYCOPODIUM CLAVATUM (H) • A homeopathic medicine used to treat patients with sore throats and flatulence and belching. *See* Club Moss.

LYME DISEASE • A bacterial infection carried by the deer tick. It causes a flulike illness with symptoms such as eye and ear pain, heart flutter, and joint swelling. If untreated, it can be disabling.

LYMPH • A liquid found within the lymphatic vessels, containing white blood cells and some red blood cells. These cells, collected from tissues throughout the body, flow in the lymphatic vessels through the lymph nodes, and eventually into the blood. Lymph is an important part of the body's ability to fight infection and disease.

LYMPHANGITIS • Inflammation of lymph vessels due to the spread of infection.

LYMPHATIC SYSTEM • The network of vessels or channels that make and store cells that fight infection and carry lymphatic fluid through the body to bathe its tissues. The lymphatic system returns fluids from tissue spaces to the circulation, is a filtering system for bacteria and minute foreign particles, and is a vital part of the immune system.

LYMPHATIC VESSELS • A bodywide network of channels, similar to the blood vessels, that transport lymph to the immune organs and into the bloodstream.

LYMPHEDEMA • Swelling of a part of the body, especially the limbs, from fluid retention because of an obstruction or inadequacy of lymphatic drainage.

LYMPH NODES • Small bean-shaped organs of the immune system, distributed widely throughout the body and linked by lymphatic vessels. Lymph nodes are closets for B, T, and other immune cells.

LYMPHOCYTE IMMUNE GLOBULIN (Rx) • **Atgam.** An immunosuppressant used to prevent rejection of kidney transplants. Potential adverse reactions include nausea, vomiting, diarrhea, fever, malaise, seizures, headache, low blood pressure, rapid heartbeat, blood clots, fluid retention, fluid in lungs, high blood sugar, liver dysfunction, a drop in white blood cells, bleeding, chest pain, night sweats, joint pain, and swollen glands.

LYMPHOKINES • Powerful chemicals secreted by the lymphocytes. These soluble molecules help direct and regulate immune responses.

LYMPHOMA • Abnormal multiplication of lymphoid tissue, found mainly in the lymph nodes and spleen. Cancers of the cells of lymphoid tissue multiply unchecked. Lymphomas fall into two categories. One is called Hodgkin's disease, characterized by a particular kind of abnormal cell. All others are called non-Hodgkin's lymphomas, which vary in their malignancy according to the nature and activity of the abnormal cells.

LYPHOCIN • *See* Vancomycin Hydrochloride.

LYSINE ASPIRIN (OTC) • In 1992, the FDA proposed a ban on lysine aspirin in internal analgesic products because it had not been shown to be safe and effective as claimed. *See* Aspirin.

LYSINE HYDROCHLORIDE (OTC) • **Enisyl.** An amino acid used to improve the utilization of vegetable proteins.

LYSODREN • *See* Mitotane.

LYSOZYME • A natural antibacterial substance contained in many bodily secretions, such as tears.

LYTEERS • *See* Artificial Tears.

LYTHRUM SALICARIA • *See* Salicaria Extract.

M

MAALOX (OTC) • *See* Aluminum Hydroxide and Magnesium Hydroxide.

MAC • *See* MAI.

MACROCYSTIS PYRIFERAE • *See* Kelp.

MACRODANTIN • *See* Nitrofurantoin.

MACROLIDES • A class of antibiotics discovered in streptomycetes bacteria. Erythromycin is an example.

MACROPHAGE • A type of white blood cell produced in the bone marrow that destroys bacteria and viruses. It also promotes repair of tissues by removing dead and damaged cells.

MACULE • A flat, discolored spot on the surface of the skin.

MADAGASCAR PERIWINKLE (H) • *See* Periwinkle.

MAD APPLE • *See* Jimsonweed.

MADDER (H) • *Rubia tincorum.* **Dyers' Madder.** A shrub that is a member of the Rubiaceae family, it is widely distributed in Europe. In medicine it is used as a mild tonic and has astringent properties. Was once used for treating edema. The root was boiled in wine or water to treat palsy, jaundice, sciatica, and bruises. The leaves and roots were beaten and applied externally to remove freckles and other skin blemishes. Contraindicated in kidney dysfunction, peptic ulcer, and albuminuria.

MAD WEED • *See* Skullcap.

MAFENIDE (Rx) • **Sulfamylon.** An antibacterial cream applied topically to treat serious burns. Potential adverse reactions include pain, burning sensation, itching, swelling, hives, blisters, redness, swelling of the face, and metabolic acidosis. Should be used with caution in patients with kidney failure or known hypersensitivity to sulfonamides.

MAGALDRATE (OTC) • **Aluminum Magnesium Complex. Hydromagnesium Aluminate. Lowsium. Riopan.** An antacid. Potential adverse reactions include mild constipation or diarrhea. Effects of allopurinol, antibiotics, corticosteroids, diflunisal, digoxin, iron, isoniazid, penicillamine, phenothiazine, and ranitidine may be reduced due to poor absorption caused by magaldrate. Administration times should be separated by at least an hour. Contraindicated in severe kidney dysfunction. Should be used cautiously in the elderly, especially those with slow digestion or who are receiving medicines for diarrhea or taking antispasmodics or anticholinergics. Those who are dehydrated or have mild kidney impairment should also take magaldrate with caution. Good for persons on restricted sodium intake because it is low in sodium. Also contains no sugar. Should not be taken indiscriminately.

MAGAN • *See* Magnesium Salicylate.

MAG-C • Homeopathic abbreviation for magnesia carbonica (*see*).

MAG-CARB (OTC) • A 250-mg magnesium carbonate supplement used widely for transplant patients. *See* Magnesium.

MAGENTA PAINT • *See* Carbol-Fuchsin.

MAG-M • Homeopathic abbreviation for magnesia muriaticum (*see*).

MAGNACEF • *See* Ceftazidime.

MAGNESIA CARBONICA (H) • **Mag-c.** A whitish gray or yellow material that is found in rocks, mainly in southern California, Mexico, and Central America. It is also made commercially. A homeopathic remedy used as a laxative and for headache, indigestion, and toothache. *See* Magnesium.

MAGNESIA MURIATICUM (H) • **Mag-m. Chloride of Magnesium.** Naturally occurring in sea water and in carnallite, it is a by-product of the potash industry. The homeopathic remedy is made from hydrochloric acid, which is neutralized with magnesium (*see*). The homeopathic remedy is used to treat colic, constipation, diarrhea, headache, insomnia, and teething. *See* Magnesium.

MAGNESIA PHOSPHORICA (H) • Mag-p.
Magnesium Phosphate. A homeopathic remedy prepared from magnesium sulfate and sodium phosphate for the treatment of cramps, colic, earache, headache, menstrual problems, sciatica, teething, and toothache. *See* Magnesium.

MAGNESIUM (OTC) • Mag-Ox. Magsal.
Mag-Tab SR. Uro-Mag. A silver-white, light, malleable metal that occurs abundantly in nature and is widely used in combination with various chemicals. Magnesium phosphate, a white, odorless powder, and magnesium sulfate are employed as mineral supplements for food, as antacids, and to treat low blood magnesium and magnesium depletion resulting from malnutrition due to restricted diets, alcoholism, or magnesium-depleting drugs. Magnesium is used for nutrient supplementation during pregnancy. It is also reportedly beneficial for women with premenstrual syndrome (PMS), according to a 1991 study reported in *Obstetrics and Gynecology*. Low magnesium levels have also been reported in chronic fatigue syndrome in the British medical journal *Lancet*. In 1992, it was reported in *Lancet* that injections of magnesium at the time of a heart attack reduced deaths by a fourth in a study of more than 2,300 patients. The recommended daily allowance, according to the National Academy of Sciences, is 40 mg for infants, 100 to 300 mg for children, and 350 mg for adults. Excessive use of magnesium has been shown in animal experiments to cause temporary muscle weakness. *See* Magnesium Carbonate, Magnesium Chloride, Magnesium Citrate, Magnesium Gluconate, Magnesium Hydroxide, Magnesium Lactate, Magnesium Oxide, Magnesium Salicylate, Magnesium Sulfate, and Magnesium Trisilicate.

MAGNESIUM CARBONATE (OTC) •
Gaviscon. Kanalka. Maalox. Marblen. An antacid; very soluble in acid, slightly soluble in water. *See* Magnesium.

MAGNESIUM CHLORIDE (Rx) • Chlor-3.
Slo-Mag. Used to treat low magnesium, and as a magnesium supplement. Replaces and maintains magnesium levels. As an anticonvulsant, reduces muscle contractions by interfering with the release of acetylcholine. Also used to treat preeclampsia and eclampsia (*see both*). Potential adverse reactions include toxicity, weak or absent deep-tendon reflexes, paralysis, low temperature, drowsiness, low calcium, twitching, seizures, slow, weak pulse, irregular heartbeat, low blood pressure, flushing, sweating, and respiratory paralysis. *See* Magnesium.

MAGNESIUM CITRATE (OTC) • Citroma.
Citro-Nesia. A laxative that draws water inside the intestines. Potential adverse reactions include nausea, abdominal cramping, fluid and electrolyte disturbances if used daily, and laxative dependence. Contraindicated in abdominal pain, nausea, vomiting, or other symptoms of appendicitis, heart damage, fecal impaction, rectal fissures, intestinal obstruction or perforation, or kidney disease. Works in three to six hours. Should not be used longer than one week. Oral drugs should not be given within two hours of taking the laxative.

MAGNESIUM GLUCONATE (OTC) • Mag-onate.
A buffering agent used as an antacid and in vitamin tablets. A dietary supplement for treatment of magnesium deficiencies. *See* Magnesium.

MAGNESIUM HYDROXIDE (OTC) • Aludrox. Ascriptin A/D Caplets. Di-Gel Antacid/ Anti-Gas. Fermalox. Gelusil. Haley's M-O. Kolantyl. Kudrox. Maalox. Milk of Magnesia. Mylanta. Silain Gel. WinGel Liquid.
A laxative that draws water inside the intestines. Potential adverse reactions include nausea, abdominal cramping, fluid and electrolyte disturbances if used daily, and laxative dependence. Contraindicated in abdominal pain, nausea, vomiting, or other symptoms of appendicitis, heart damage, fecal impaction, rectal fissures, intestinal obstruction or perforation, or kidney disease. Works in three to six hours. Should not be used longer than one week. Oral drugs should not be given within two hours of taking this laxative. *See* Magnesium.

MAGNESIUM LACTATE (OTC) • **Mag-Tab SR.** A dietary supplement indicated for patients with, or at risk for, magnesium deficiency. Contraindicated in patients with kidney disease, unless prescribed by a physician. *See* Magnesium.

MAGNESIUM OXIDE (Rx) • **Beelith Tablets. Bufferin Analgesic Tablets. Cama Arthritis Pain Reliever. Mag-Ox. Par-Mag. Uro-Mag.** An antacid and laxative. Potential adverse reactions include nausea, abdominal pain, diarrhea, and overload of magnesium. Effects of allopurinol, antibiotics, corticosteroids, diflunisal, digoxin, iron, isoniazid, penicillamine, phenothiazine, and ranitidine may be reduced due to poor absorption due to magnesium oxide. Administration times should be separated by at least an hour. Contraindicated in severe kidney dysfunction. Should be used cautiously in the elderly, especially those with slow digestion or who are receiving medicines for diarrhea or taking antispasmodics or anticholinergics. Those who are dehydrated or have mild kidney impairment should also take magnesium oxide with caution. When used as a laxative, other oral drugs should not be taken within one or two hours. Should not be taken indiscriminately. May cause enteric-coated drugs to be released prematurely in the stomach, so doses should be separated by one hour. *See* Magnesium.

MAGNESIUM PHOSPHATE (OTC) • Made from magnesium oxide and phosphoric acid, it is used as a dentifrice polishing agent, an antacid, a food additive, and a dietary substance.

MAGNESIUM SALICYLATE (OTC) • **Extra-Strength Doan's. Magan. Mobidin. Mobigesic Analgesic Tablets. Original Doan's.** A drug related to aspirin; used to treat rheumatoid arthritis. Produces analgesia by an ill-defined effect on the hypothalamus and by blocking generation of pain impulses. The peripheral action may involve inhibition of prostaglandin synthesis. Relieves fever by acting on the hypothalamic heat-regulating center to produce blood-vessel dilation. This increases peripheral blood flow and promotes sweating, which leads to loss of heat and cooling by evaporation. Potential adverse effects include ringing in the ears and hearing loss, nausea, vomiting, GI distress, abnormal liver function, rash, bruising, and hypersensitivity manifested by asthma or anaphylaxis. Ammonium chloride and other urine acidifiers increase blood levels of salicylates. Antacids in high doses and other urine alkalinizers decrease levels of salicylates. Corticosteroids enhance salicylate elimination and may make magnesium salicylate less effective. Oral anticoagulants and heparin increase the risk of bleeding. Contraindicated in severe chronic kidney dysfunction, GI ulcer, GI bleeding, or aspirin hypersensitivity. Should be used cautiously in patients with vitamin K deficiency and bleeding disorders. Should be taken with food, milk, antacid, or a large glass of water to reduce adverse GI reactions. Unlike aspirin, magnesium salicylate does not inhibit platelet aggregation. *See* Magnesium.

MAGNESIUM SULFATE (OTC) • **Epsom Salts. MG-Plus. Slow-Mag. Vicon-C. Vicon Plus.** A magnesium salt used to treat magnesium deficiency during stress, to decrease the release of certain nerve impulses in the brain to prevent or control seizures in pregnancy (preeclampsia or eclampsia), and to stop hypomagnesemic seizures. Potential adverse reactions include sweating, drowsiness, depressed reflexes, paralysis, low temperature, low blood pressure, flushing, circulatory collapse, depressed heart function, heart block, respiratory paralysis, and low blood calcium. Interacts with neuromuscular-blocking agents, increasing their action. Should be used cautiously in impaired kidney function, heart damage, heart block, and in women in labor; magnesium sulfate can decrease the frequency and force of uterine contractions. Also used as a laxative, drawing water inside the intestines. Potential adverse reactions for that use include nausea, abdominal cramping, fluid and electrolyte disturbances if used daily, and laxative dependence. Contraindicated in abdominal pain, nausea, vomiting, or other symptoms of appendicitis, heart damage, fecal impaction, rectal fissures, intestinal obstruction or perforation, or kidney disease. Works in three to six hours. Should not be used longer than one week. Oral drugs should not be given within two hours of taking the laxative. In 1992, the FDA proposed a ban on magnesium sulfate in oral menstrual drug products because it had not been shown to be safe and effective as claimed. *See* Magnesium.

MAGNESIUM TRISILICATE (OTC) • Gaviscon Antacid Tablets. An antacid. *See* Magnesium.

MAGNOLIA (H) • *Magnolia glauca.* **Beaver Tree. White Bay.** An American tree; the bark is used to reduce the fevers of malaria and other diseases. Used in place of cinchona (*see*), magnolia may be used for longer periods of time with fewer side effects. Also employed to treat rheumatism and as a tonic. The Chinese prize magnolia as an aphrodisiac. In Mexico, the plant is used to treat scorpion stings.

MAGONATE • *See* Magnesium Gluconate.

MAG-OX • *See* Magnesium Oxide.

MAG-P • Homeopathic abbreviation for magnesia phosphorica (*see*).

MAGSAL • *See* Magnesium and Phenyltoloxamine.

MA HUANG (H) • Ultimate Xphoria. Cloud 9. Herbal Ecstacy. This herb, taken with other stimulants or combined with them in a compound, can cause severe adverse reactions, including death. The FDA issued a warning in 1995 that they had received more than one hundred reports of adverse reactions, ranging from heart attacks to hepatitis and even death. Mild side effects include jitters, anxiety, and headache. Among the stimulants that can add to the adverse reactions is caffeine contained in colas and coffee. *See* Ephedra.

MAI • Abbreviation for *Mycobacterium avium intracellulare,* a bacterial infection that can affect internal organs and devastate AIDS patients who have weak immune systems.

MAIDENHAIR FERN (H) • *Adiantum pedatum. Adiantum capillus-veneris.* **Venus' Hair.**

Extract of the leaves of the ornamental fern is used as a flavoring in alcoholic beverages only, and to soothe irritated skin in herbal creams. Also used by herbalists to relieve coughs, nasal congestion, asthma, and to treat dandruff.

MAIGRET-50 • *See* Phenylpropanolamine.

MAIZE OIL • *See* Corn Oil.

MALABSORPTION SYNDROMES • Any condition in which the intestine is unable to absorb food.

MALACIA • Softening of part of an organ.

MALATHION (OTC) • Ovide. An insecticide used to treat head lice infestation. It is absorbed by the skin and inhibits the transmission of nerve signals.

MALIGNANT • Refers to a cancerous growth, indicating that it is likely to penetrate the tissues in which it originated, spread further, and if unchecked, eventually cause death.

MALLAMINT • *See* Calcium Carbonate.

MALLERGAN-VC • *See* Promethazine.

MALLOW (H) • Malva. Malvaceae. An erect European perennial herb with rosy purple flowers. Contains mucilage, essential oil, and a trace of tannin. The herb is used to soothe inflammation in the mouth and throat, and to treat earache. Also used in bathwater or in a compress to heal boils, abscesses, and minor burns.

MALOTUSS • *See* Guaifenesin.

MALT SOUP EXTRACT (OTC) • Maltsupex Liquid, Powder & Tablets. Derived from barley malt, it is a gentle laxative that promotes soft, easily passed stools. Should not be used when abdominal pain, nausea, or vomiting are present. Should be used only under a physician's supervision if kidney disease is present.

MALTSUPEX • *See* Malt Soup Extract.

MALVA (H) • **Malvaceae.** *See* Mallow.

MAMMA-, MAST- • Prefixes meaning pertaining to the breast, as in *mammography* or *mastectomy.*

MANDELAMINE • *See* Methenamine.

MANDOL • *See* Cefamandole Nafate.

MANDRAGORA • *See* Mandrake.

MANDRAKE (H) • *Mandragora officinarum. Podophyllum peltatum.* **Devil's Apple. Mayapple. Podophyllin Resin.** The oldest-known narcotic plant, a native of southern Europe and the Mediterranean, it belongs to the potato family. According to legend, mandrake shrieks when it is pulled out of the ground. It contains agents similar to those in belladonna (*see*). Homeopaths use it for the treatment of cough, asthma, and hay fever. It has been used for chronic constipation, liver dysfunction, and to rid the body of worms. In the Middle Ages, mandrake was believed to be an aphrodisiac. The FDA considers the plant a poisonous narcotic. *See* Podophyllin Resin.

MANGANESE (OTC) • An element first isolated in 1774, it occurs in minerals and in minute quantities in animals, plants, and water. It is used as a nutrient and mineral supplement and is necessary for the development of strong bones.

MANIA • A mood disorder characterized by excessive elation or irritability, hyperactivity, hypersexuality, poor concentration, and accelerated thinking and speaking, resulting in impairment. Mania is seen in major disorders involving disturbance of mood, and in organic mental disorders.

MANIC-DEPRESSIVE DISORDER • *See* Bipolar Disorder.

MANNITOL (Rx) (OTC) • **Osmitrol. Resectisol.** An osmotic diuretic that increases urine flow through pressure of the machinery of the kidney. Also elevates blood plasma passage through tissue, resulting in enhanced flow of water into fluids outside the cells. Used in the treatment of scanty urination, to reduce pressure inside the eye, and to prevent acute kidney failure. Potential adverse reactions include a rebound of pressure in the brain eight to twelve hours after the drug reduces edema, headache, confusion, rapid heartbeat, chest pain, blurred vision, runny nose, thirst, nausea, vomiting, fluid and electrolyte imbalance, water intoxication, and dehydration. Contraindicated in absence of urine formation, severe lung congestion, severe congestive heart disease, severe dehydration, kidney disease, or during active bleeding in the brain. In 1992, the FDA issued a notice that mannitol had not been shown to be safe and effective as claimed in OTC digestive-aid products.

MANTADIL • *See* Chlorcyclizine.

MAO INHIBITORS • *See* Monoamine Oxidase Inhibitors.

MAOIs • *See* Monoamine Oxidase Inhibitors.

MAOLATE • *See* Chlorphenesin.

MAPROTILINE (Rx) • **Ludiomil.** A tricyclic antidepressant (*see*) introduced in 1981, it is reportedly effective in all types of depression. Potential adverse reactions include drowsiness, dizziness, excitation, seizures, tremors, weakness, confusion, headache, nervousness, mania, decreased or increased libido, impotence, male breast enlargement and tenderness, female breast enlargement with milk production, swelling of testicles, a drop in blood pressure when rising from a seated or prone position, irregular heartbeat, high blood pressure, blurred vision, ringing in the ears, dry mouth, constipation, nausea, vomiting, loss of appetite, urine retention, rash, hives, sweating, and allergy. Barbiturates decrease levels of maprotiline in the blood. Cimetidine may increase maprotiline blood levels and lead to increased adverse effects. Epinephrine and norepinephrine increase blood pressure when used with maprotiline. MAO inhibitors may cause severe excitation, high fever, or seizures. Methylphenidate increases maprotiline blood levels. Contraindicated during recovery from heart attack and in enlarged prostate gland. Must be used with caution in patients with cerebrovascular disease, urine retention, glaucoma, thyroid disease, blood abnormalities, and impaired liver function. Also in patients with a history of seizures, and in those who are suicide risks. The drug should not be discontinued suddenly, as this may cause nausea, headache, and malaise. Most effective when taken on an empty stomach, but may be taken with a small amount of food if stomach upset is a problem.

MAP 30 • Abbreviation for *Momordica* anti-HIV protein, derived from the seeds of the bitter melon (*see*).

MARAX (Rx) • **Hydrophen. T.E.H. Compound. Theofedral.** A combination of ephedrine, theophylline, and hydroxyzine (*see all*), it is used to treat asthma and other upper-respiratory disorders. There is some doubt about its effectiveness. Potential adverse reactions include tremor, insomnia, nervousness, rapid heartbeat, irregular heartbeat, chest pains, dizziness, dryness of the nose and throat, headache, sweating, diarrhea, stomach upset, drowsiness, muscle weakness, tics, and excessive urination. Contraindicated in severe kidney or liver dysfunction. Should not be taken with similar medications, alcoholic beverages, erythromycin or similar antibiotics, or with MAO inhibitors (*see*) because side effects may be greatly increased. Marax will make lithium and propranolol less effective. Should be taken with food to avoid stomach upset.

MARAZIDE • *See* Benzthiazide.

MARBAXIN • *See* Methocarbamol.

MARCAINE • *See* Bupivacaine.

MAREZINE • *See* Cyclizine.

MARFLEX • *See* Orphenadrine.

MARGOSA OIL • *See* Neem.

MARIGOLD • *See* Calendula.

MARIJUANA (H) • *Cannabis sativa.* **Bhang. Dagga. Grass. Hash. Pot.** A central nervous system depressant, hallucinogen, and antivomiting drug. It is derived from the leaves and resin of the cannabis plant and has been used medicinally for more than two thousand years. Introduced into Western medicine in the 1800s, marijuana was taken for a variety of conditions, including anxiety, insomnia, rheumatic disorders, migraine, painful menstruation, strychnine poisoning, and opiate withdrawal. Its use is prohibited by the federal government, but in some cases it is permitted for the treatment of pressure within the eye, and for the relief of nausea and vomiting caused by treatment with anticancer drugs. *See* Dronabinol.

MARINOL (H) • *See* Dronabinol.

MARJORAM (H) • *Origanum. Majorana.* A perennial grown in Europe and the United States, it is used in an herbal tea to prevent seasickness, and to treat arthritis, insomnia, edema, toothache, and headache. Its old name was organs, and it was used to stop vomiting, especially at sea.

MARPLAN • *See* Isocarboxazid.

MAR-PRED • *See* Methylprednisolone.

MARSHMALLOW ROOT (H) • *Althaea officinalis.* A demulcent containing up to 35 percent mucilage, it is an old-time remedy for digestive disorders. It soothes mucous membranes, and a respiratory tract irritated by bronchitis, asthma, and cough. Also used as a mouthwash and gargle, and to soothe the pain of teething in infants. Externally, marshmallow has been used for hundreds of years as a wound healer. Marshmallow ointments and creams are used on chapped hands and lips. Internally, it is used to treat inflammation of the genitourinary tract, including painful urination. Also used to treat diarrhea and cholera. Herbalists claim it has a general calming effect on the body. *See also* Althaea Root.

MARSH TEA • *See* Labrador Tea Extract.

MARYLAND PINK • *See* Spigelia.

MASOPROCOL CREAM • **Actinex.** Introduced in 1992 for the treatment of actinic keratosis, a common condition of skin damage resulting from overexposure to the sun. The cream is contraindicated in persons known to be hypersensitive to masoprocol or other ingredients in the formulation. Should be applied carefully near the eyes and mouth. If applied with fingers, hands should be washed immediately after use. The most frequent adverse effect is redness and flaking of the skin. Itching, dryness, and soreness are also potential adverse effects.

MASSÉ BREAST CREAM (OTC) • A combination of glycerin, lanolin, and peanut oil used to soothe nipples in breast-feeding mothers.

MAST CELL • A granulocyte found in tissue. The contents of mast cells, along with those of basophils, are responsible for the symptoms of allergy.

MASTITIS • Inflammation of the breast from bacterial infection or other causes.

MATÉ EXTRACT (H) • **Jesuits' Tea. Maté Tea. Paraguay Tea Extract. St. Bartholomew's Tea.** The extract from small gourds grown in South America where maté is a stimulant beverage. It is used as a generally recognized as safe (GRAS) food additive in the United States. Among its constituents are caffeine, purines, and tannins. The FDA data bank, PAFA, has not yet done a search of the toxicology literature concerning maté. However, it has been reported in the February 1, 1995, issue of the *Journal of the American Medical Association* to be toxic to the liver.

MATERIA MEDICA • A compendium of homeopathic remedies giving indications for their uses.

MATERNA MATERNACAP (OTC) • A multivitamin and mineral preparation for pregnant women.

MATRICARIA CHAMOMILLA • *See* Chamomile.

MATRICARIA EXTRACT and OIL (H) • **Chamomile Oil. Wild Chamomile Extract.** The volatile oil distilled from the dried flower heads or extract of the flower heads of *Matricaria chamomilla.* Used internally as a soothing tea and tonic and externally as a soothing medication for contusions and other inflammation. *See* Tannic Acid and Chamomile.

MATULANE • *See* Procarbazine.

MAXAIR • *See* Pirbuterol.

MAXAQUIN • *See* Lomefloxacin.

MAXIBLOIN • *See* Ethylestrenol.

MAXIDEX • *See* Dexamethasone.

MAXIFLOR • *See* Diflorasone.

MAXITROL • *See* Dexamethasone.

MAXIVATE • *See* Betamethasone.

MAXOLON • *See* Metoclopramide.

MAXZIDE (Rx) • A combination of hydrochlorothiazide and triamterene used to reduce high blood pressure. *See* Thiazide Diuretics.

MAYAPPLE (H) • *Podophyllum peltatum.* **Duck's Foot. Hogapple. Mandrake.** A perennial plant of the barberry family, it is native to North America. It was used by early American settlers as a laxative, and to treat diarrhea, arthritis, and kidney problems. American Indians reportedly used it as a poison to commit suicide. *See* Podophyllin Resin.

MAZANOR • *See* Mazindol.

MAZICON • *See* Flumazenil.

MAZINDOL (Rx) • **Mazanor. Sanorex.** An appetite suppressant similar to the amphetamines, it inhibits the uptake of norepinephrine and dopamine (*see both*). Potential adverse reactions include nervousness, restlessness, euphoria, dizziness, insomnia, discomfort, headache, depression, drowsiness, weakness, tremor, palpitations, irregular heartbeat, dry mouth, nausea, constipation, diarrhea, unpleasant taste, difficulty in urinating, impotence, rash, clamminess, pallor, shivering, excessive sweating, and altered libido. May cause a need to adjust diabetes medications. Use with high blood pressure medications that work on the brain may decrease their blood-pressure-lowering effects. MAO inhibitors taken with mazindol may cause severe high blood pressure. Fatigue may occur when the drug wears off. Caffeinated drinks should be avoided. Should be taken at least six hours before bedtime. Recommended for use for no more than three months as a part of a weight control program under a physician's supervision.

M-CRESYL • Cresylate. Provides an acid medium for use in outer-ear infection caused by bacteria or fungus.

MEADOW BUTTERCUP (H) • *Ranunculus acris*. An erect perennial native to Europe, Asia, and the eastern United States, it is used in homeopathic medicines to treat arthritis, sciatica, and skin disease. All parts of the plant are toxic. It strongly irritates the mucous membrane of the stomach and can also cause severe skin irritation.

MEADOWROOT • *See* Queen-of-the-Meadow and Meadowsweet.

MEADOW SAFFRON (H) • *Colchicum autumnale*. A perennial plant, the leaves of which appear in the spring, and the flowers in the autumn, meadow saffron is a native of the temperate parts of Europe, where it grows wild in meadows. Has been used in home remedies to treat gout, rheumatism, and fluid retention. All parts of the meadow saffron plant contain colchicine (*see*), which is used to treat the pain and inflammation of gout. Meadow saffron can be toxic and may even be fatal.

MEADOWSWEET (H) • *Spiraea ulmaria*. Meadowroot. Queen-of-the-Meadow. A perennial common to Europe, the eastern United States, and Canada, it grows in meadows. It was used to treat diarrhea and stomach upsets. Was also given for gout, arthritis, and flu. It is rich in vitamin C and contains salicylic acid and citric acid (*see both*). May cause constipation.

MEASLES, MUMPS, AND RUBELLA VIRUS VACCINE, LIVE (Rx) • M-M-R11. Promotes immunity to measles, mumps, and rubella virus by inducing production of antibodies. Administered in two doses with the first dose usually given to children at fifteen months. Potential adverse reactions include fever, rash, swollen glands, hives, and severe allergic reaction including anaphylaxis.

MEASLES (RUBEOLA) AND RUBELLA VIRUS VACCINE, LIVE (Rx) • M-R-Vax 11. Promotes immunity to measles and rubella virus by inducing production of antibodies. Usually given to children. Potential adverse reactions include fever, rash, swollen glands, and severe allergic reaction including anaphylaxis.

MEASLES (RUBEOLA) VIRUS VACCINE, LIVE (Rx) • Attenuvax. Promotes immunity to measles virus by inducing production of antibodies. Given in two doses, the first usually at fifteen months and the second at entry into school. Potential adverse reactions include fever, rash, swollen glands, severe allergic reaction, including anaphylaxis, fever seizures in susceptible children, loss of appetite, and a drop in white blood cells.

MEASURIN • *See* Aspirin.

MEBARAL • *See* Mephobarbital.

MEBENDAZOLE (Rx) • Vermox. Used to treat pinworm, roundworm, whipworm, and hookworm. May cause stomach cramps and diarrhea in massive infection and expulsion of worms. Should be taken with meals, which should include fatty items such as whole milk or ice cream.

MECAMYLAMINE (Rx) • Inversine. A high blood pressure medication that blocks the nerve signals that trigger constriction of blood vessels. It is used for moderate to severe essential hypertension and uncomplicated malignant hypertension. Potential adverse effects include numbness, sedation, fatigue, tremor, awkward movement, seizures, psychic changes, dizziness, weakness, headache, a drop in blood pressure when rising from a seated or prone position, dry mouth, sore tongue, dilated pupils, blurred vision, loss of appetite, nausea, vomiting, constipation, diarrhea, urine retention, impotence, and decreased libido. Alcohol and bethanechol may cause excessive low blood pressure when used with mecamylamine. Sodium bicarbonate and acetazolamide may increase the effects of mecamylamine. Contraindicated in recent heart attack patients, and those suffering from uremia or chronic kidney infection. Effects of the drug are increased by high environmental temperature, fever, stress, or severe illness. The drug should not be discontinued suddenly. Should be taken with meals.

MECHLORETHAMINE (Rx) • Nitrogen Mustard. Mustargen. Used in war gas in World War I, it is an anticancer drug used to treat breast, lung, and ovarian cancer, Hodgkin's disease, and non-Hodgkin's lymphomas. Potential adverse reactions include nausea, vomiting, and loss of appetite beginning two to three minutes after administration, and lasting from eight to twenty-four hours. Other reactions may be bone-marrow suppression, mild anemia, headache, ringing in the ears, metallic taste, deafness, high uric acid, rash, loss of hair, herpes zoster, and severe allergic reactions. Use with procarbazine and cyclophosphamide may increase liver toxicity.

**MECLAN • ** *See* Meclocycline.

MECLIZINE (Rx) (OTC) • Antivert. Antrizine. Bonine. Dizmiss. Meclozine Hydrochloride. Meni-D. Motion Cure. Ru-Vert M. A drug introduced in 1951 to prevent and treat nausea and dizziness. Should be taken one hour before travel and repeated daily for duration of journey, if necessary. Potential adverse reactions include drowsiness, fatigue, blurred vision, dry mouth, and urine retention. May mask more serious illnesses such as intestinal obstruction and

brain tumor. Should be used cautiously in glaucoma, GI obstruction, and in elderly males with possibly enlarged prostate. This antihistamine has a slower onset and longer duration of action than other antinausea medications. Should not be taken with tranquilizers, sleeping pills, alcoholic beverages, barbiturates, narcotics, and antihistamines, all of which add to central nervous system depression. May be taken with or without food.

MECLOCYCLINE (Rx) • Meclan. A tetracycline antibiotic used in the topical treatment of inflammatory acne. *See* Tetracyclines.

MECLOFENAMATE (Rx) • Meclomen. Produces anti-inflammatory, analgesic, and fever-reducing effects, probably by inhibiting prostaglandins (*see*). Introduced in 1977, it is used to treat arthritis and mild to moderate pain. Potential adverse reactions include anemia, fatigue, insomnia, dizziness, nervousness, headache, water retention, blurred vision, eye irritation, abdominal pain, gas, peptic ulcer, nausea, vomiting, diarrhea, hemorrhage, painful and/or bloody urine, kidney toxicity, liver toxicity, rash, and hives. Aspirin may decrease blood levels of meclofenamate. Oral blood thinners may increase meclofenamate's blood-thinning effect. Contraindicated in GI ulcers or inflammation, in patients with liver, kidney, or heart disease, blood problems, diabetes, and asthma. Should be taken with meals. Use with other NSAIDs (*see*) or alcohol may increase the danger of gastrointestinal problems.

**MECLOMEN • ** *See* Meclofenamate.

**MECLOZINE HYDROCHLORIDE • ** *See* Meclizine.

**MEDA TAB • ** *See* Acetaminophen.

**MEDICATION • ** A remedy having preventive, relieving, or curative properties.

**MEDICINAL CHARCOAL • ** *See* Charcoal.

**MEDIGESIC (Rx) • ** A combination of acetaminophen, butalbital, and caffeine (*see all*). Used as a painkiller. May be habit-forming.

MEDIHALER-EPI • *See* Epinephrine.

MEDIHALER-ISO • *See* Isoproterenol.

MEDILAX • *See* Phenolphthalein.

MEDIPLAST • *See* Salicylic Acid.

MEDIQUELL • *See* Dextromethorphan.

MEDITRAN • *See* Meprobamate.

MEDI-TUSS • *See* Guaifenesin.

MEDROL • *See* Methylprednisolone.

MEDROL ENPAK • *See* Methylprednisolone.

MEDROL ORAL • *See* Methylprednisolone.

MEDROXYPROGESTERONE (Rx) • **Amen. Curretab. Cycrin. Depo-Provera. Provera.** A progestin that suppresses ovulation, possibly by inhibiting pituitary gonadotropin secretion. Introduced in 1959, it is used to treat abnormal uterine bleeding due to hormonal imbalance, or secondary amenorrhea, and in endometrial or kidney cancer. It forms a thick cervical mucus. Potential adverse reactions include nausea, vomiting, depression, high blood pressure, dizziness, migraine, breakthrough bleeding, painful or absent menstruation, cervical erosion or abnormal secretions, benign tumors in the uterus, vaginal candidiasis, jaundice, high blood sugar, rash, dark spots on the skin, breast tenderness, enlargement or secretion of the breast, and decreased libido. Contraindicated in pregnancy, in persons with blood-clotting disorders, cancer of the breast, reproductive organs, or genitals, and in those with undiagnosed abnormal genital bleeding. Should be used with caution in mental depression, liver dysfunction, heart or kidney disease, migraine, and asthma. Rifampin (*see*) decreases medroxyprogesterone's effectiveness. Medroxyprogesterone may counteract the blood-sugar-lowering effects of insulin. Most effective when taken on an empty stomach, but may be taken with a small amount of food if stomach upset is a problem. *See* Depo-Provera.

MEDRYSONE (Rx) • **HMS Liquifilm Ophthalmic.** A corticosteroid (*see*) drug used mainly in topical eye preparations to treat inflammation caused by allergy. Potential adverse reactions include thinning of the cornea, interference with corneal wound healing, increased susceptibility to viral or fungal corneal infections, and corneal ulceration; with excessive or long-term use, worsening of glaucoma, cataracts, vision problems, optic nerve damage, and systemic effects such as suppression of adrenal gland hormones. Contraindicated if viral or fungal infections are present.

MEFENAMIC ACID (Rx) • **Ponstel.** A NSAID (*see*) introduced in 1967, it produces anti-inflammatory, analgesic, and fever-reducing effects, probably by inhibiting prostaglandins (*see*). It is used to treat arthritis, mild to moderate pain, and painful menstruation. Potential adverse reactions include anemia, drowsiness, dizziness, nervousness, headache, water retention, blurred vision, eye irritation, abdominal pain, gas, peptic ulcer, nausea, vomiting, diarrhea, hemorrhage, painful and/or bloody urine, kidney toxicity, liver toxicity, rash, and hives. Aspirin may decrease blood levels of mefenamic acid. Oral blood thinners may increase mefenamic acid's blood-thinning effects. Contraindicated in GI ulcers or inflammation, and in patients with liver, kidney, or heart disease, blood problems, diabetes, and asthma. Should be taken with meals. Use with other NSAIDs or alcohol may increase the danger of gastrointestinal problems. Should not be taken for more than a week at a time because risk of toxicity increases with time.

MEFLOQUINE HYDROCHLORIDE (Rx) • **Lariam.** A drug introduced in 1989, it is used to treat acute attacks of malaria. May cause dizziness, headache, transient emotional disturbances, irregular heartbeat, tinnitus (*see*), loss of appetite, vomiting, nausea, diarrhea, rash, fatigue, fever, and chills. If it is given with quinine, it may cause seizures. If it is begun with beta-blocking agents, it may cause cardiac arrest. May cause valproic acid to lose its anticonvulsant control. Best taken with food and a full glass of water.

MEFOXIN • *See* Cefoxitin Sodium.

MEGA-, MEGALO- • Huge.

MEGACE • *See* Megestrol.

MEGACOLON • Hirschsprung's Disease. Huge dilation of the large bowel in infants and children due to constriction of the sigmoid colon and the rectum.

MEGESTROL (Rx) • Megace. An anticancer progestin hormone introduced in 1972 that changes the tumor's hormonal environment. Used to treat breast and endometrial cancers. The drug takes about two months to manifest effectiveness. Potential adverse reactions include dysfunctional uterine bleeding when the drug is discontinued. Other adverse reactions may include carpal tunnel syndrome, blood clots, hair loss, loss of appetite, hairiness, and breast tenderness. Most effective when taken on an empty stomach, but may be taken with a small amount of food if stomach upset is a problem.

MELALEUCA LEUCADENDRON • *See* Cajuput.

MELAN- • Prefix meaning black, as in *melanin*.

MELANEX • *See* Hydroquinone.

MELANIN • A black or dark brown pigment occurring naturally in the hair or skin.

MELANOMA • A cancer made up of pigmented skin cells.

MELATONIN (Rx) (OTC) (H) • A hormone secreted in the night by humans. First isolated in the late 1950s, it plays a key role in the transmittal of light information and modulates a variety of endocrinological, neurophysiological, and behavioral functions including the regulation of reproduction, sleep, seasonal disorders, depression and aging, and modulation of retina of the eye. Melatonin has ovulation-inhibitory effects, as well as some activity against certain human breast-cancer cells. Melatonin is available in synthetic tablets from health food suppliers. Sales of melatonin tablets increased after a Massachusetts Institute of Technology study reported in the March 1994 proceedings of the National Academy of Sciences suggested that the hormone works as a sleeping pill. Pharmaceutical companies are working on producing a prescription melatonin sleeping medication. Low doses of melatonin are considered harmless, but the dosage, purity, and usefulness of the OTC preparations are the subject of controversy.

MELFIAT • *See* Phendimetrazine.

MELILOT (H) • *Melilotus officinalis.* **Sweet Flower. Yellow Melilot.** An erect annual or biennial herb native to Europe and northern Asia and introduced into North America. It contains coumarin and tannins (*see both*). Melilot has been used to treat chronic bronchitis, flatulence, arthritis, and to avoid blood clots. The leaves are smoked to treat asthma. It is used in homeopathic medicine to treat migraine. Contraindicated if there is a tendency to bleed or a person is on anticoagulants.

MELISSA OFFICINALIS • *See* Balm.

MELLARIL • *See* Thioridazine.

MELPHALAN (Rx) • Alkeran. L-PAM. L-phenylalanine Mustard. An anticancer drug used to treat multiple myeloma and inoperable ovarian cancer. Potential adverse reactions include a drop in white blood cells, rash, loss of hair, lung dysfunction, and severe allergic reactions. This medicine often causes nausea, vomiting, and loss of appetite. Close medical supervision is, of course, needed.

MEN-, MENO- • Prefixes pertaining to menstruation, as in *menopause*.

MENADIOL (OTC) • Vitamin K_4. A water-soluble vitamin converted to menadione (*see*) after ingestion. It is about half as potent as menadione. *See* Vitamin K.

MENADIONE (Rx) • Menadiol Sodium Diphosphate. Vitamin K₃ Synkayvite. A synthetic with properties of vitamin K. Bright yellow crystals insoluble in water. Used as a dietary supplement and as a preservative in emollients. Also used to prevent blood clotting. Potential adverse reactions include headache, nausea, vomiting, allergic rash, itching, hives, and pain and blood clot at injection site. Should never be used to treat newborns because it can cause hemolytic anemia, high levels of bile in the blood, brain damage, and death. *See* Vitamin K.

MENADOL • *See* Ibuprofen.

MENEST • *See* Estrogens, Esterified.

MENHYL SALICYLATE EXTRACT • *See* Wintergreen Oil.

MENI-D • *See* Meclizine.

MÉNIÈRE'S DISEASE • An increase in fluid in the labyrinth, the part of the ear that controls balance. This distorts and sometimes ruptures the membrane of the labyrinth wall, disturbing the sense of balance. The main symptom of an attack is dizziness, which is often accompanied by noise in the ear and muffled or distorted hearing.

MENINGITIS • An inflammation of the membranes covering the brain and spinal cord.

MENINGITIS VACCINE (Rx) • Menomune-A/C/Y/W-135. Promotes active immunity to meningitis. Potential adverse reactions include headache, malaise, chills, fever, cramps, severe allergic reaction, and pain and swelling at the site of injection.

MENOPAUSE FORMULA (H) • Lachesis Complex. A homeopathic remedy to relieve symptoms of menopause. It contains Lachesis mutus 10x to relieve hot flashes, kali carbonicum 6x to relieve anxiety and nervous tension, and glonoinum 8x to relieve headache and dull head pressure. *See* Lachesis, Kali Carbonicum, and Glonoine.

MENORRHAGIA • Excessive menstrual flow.

MENOTROPINS (Rx) • Pergonal. Humegon. An injection of extract of menopausal urine, containing primarily the follicle-stimulating luteinizing hormone and follicle-stimulating hormone. Introduced in 1970, it mimics the follicle-stimulating hormone, including the development of eggs. Used to treat women who do not ovulate. Also used in men to stimulate the production of sperm. Potential adverse reactions include nausea, vomiting, diarrhea, ovarian enlargement with pain and distension, multiple births, ovarian overstimulation, and fever. Contraindicated in ovarian failure with high urinary gonadotropin levels, thyroid or adrenal dysfunction, pituitary tumor, abnormal uterine bleeding, ovarian cysts or enlargement, and pregnancy. Alcohol and smoking do not interact with menotropins, but reduce the chances of a pregnancy occurring.

MENSTRUAL DRUG PRODUCTS (H) • In 1992, the FDA proposed a ban on the following oral menstrual drugs because they had not been shown to be safe and effective for their stated claims: alcohol, alfalfa leaves, aloes, *Asclepias tuberosa,* asparagus, barosma, bearberry, buchu powdered extract, calcium lactate, calcium pantothenate, capsicum oleoresin, cascara fluid extract, chlorprophenpyridamine maleate, *Cimicifuga, Cnicus benedictus* (blessed thistle), dog grass extract, ethyl nitrite, ferric chloride, ferrous sulfate, *Gentiana lutea* (yellow gentian), *Glycyrrhiza glabra* (licorice root), homatropine, *Hydrastis canadensis* (goldenseal), hyoscyamine sulfate, juniper oil, magnesium sulfate, methapyrilene hydrochloride, methenamine, methylene blue, natural estrogenic hormone, niacinamide, nutmeg oil, oil of erigeron, parsley, peppermint spirit, pepsin (essence), pipsissewa, potassium acetate, potassium nitrate, riboflavin, saw palmetto, *Taraxacum officinale* (dandelion), theobromine sodium salicylate, theophylline, thiamin hydrochloride, triticum, turpentine, turpentine (Venice), and urea.

MENTANE • *See* Velnacrine.

MENTHA • *See* Mint.

MENTHOL (OTC) • **Aurum Analgesic Lotion. Ben-Gay. Cepacol Dry Throat Lozenges. Chloraseptic. Denorex. Dermoplast. Desenex Foot & Sneaker Spray. Eucalyptamint. Feminine Gold Analgesic Lotion. Flex-All 454 Pain Relieving Gel. Halls Mentho-Lyptus. Halls Plus Cough. Icy Hot Balm. Legatrin Rub. Listerine Antiseptic. N'Ice Medicated Sugarless Sore Throat Lozenges. Rhuligel. Robitussin Cough Drops. Selsun Blue Dandruff Shampoo. Soothers Throat Drops. Sucrets. Theragold Analgesic Lotion. Therapeutic Mineral Ice. Vicks Cough Drops.** An alcohol prepared from mint oils or synthetically, it is used as an inhalant and topical anti-itch preparation. Used in body rubs, liniments, and skin fresheners, it gives that "cool" feeling to the skin after use. It is a local anesthetic. Also used as a flavoring agent. Nontoxic in low doses, but in concentrations of 3 percent or more it exerts an irritant action that can, if continued long, induce changes in all layers of the mucous membranes. Can also cause severe abdominal pain, nausea, vomiting, vertigo, and coma when ingested in its concentrated form. In 1992, the FDA issued a notice that menthol had not been shown to be safe and effective as claimed in OTC products, including those to treat fever blisters and cold sores, poison ivy, poison oak, and poison sumac, insect bites and stings, and in astringent (*see*) drugs.

MEOCYTEN • *See* Orphenadrine.

MEPACRINE HYDROCHLORIDE • *See* Quinacrine Hydrochloride.

MEPENZOLATE (Rx) • **Cantil.** An anticholinergic, antispasmodic drug used to treat irritable bowel syndrome (*see*), and as an adjunctive therapy in peptic ulcers and other GI disorders (*see* Adjunct). Potential adverse reactions include disorientation, irritability, incoherence, weakness, nervousness, drowsiness, dizziness, headache, palpitations, rapid heartbeat, slow heartbeat, blurred vision, sensitivity to light, increased eye pressure, difficulty in swallowing, constipation, dry mouth, nausea, vomiting, epigastric distress, urinary retention, impotence, hives, decreased sweating, and fever. Contraindicated in glaucoma, obstructions in the urinary or GI tract, myasthenia gravis (*see*), paralytic ileus (*see*), intestinal flaccidity, unstable cardiovascular status in acute hemorrhage, and toxic megacolon. Should be used with caution in patients with nerve damage, overactive thyroid, coronary artery disease, irregular heartbeat, congestive heart failure, high blood pressure, hiatal hernia, liver or kidney disease, and ulcerative colitis. Should also be used with caution in people over forty years of age due to the possibility of glaucoma. Should be taken thirty minutes to one hour before meals.

MEPERGAN • *See* Meperidine and Promethazine.

MEPERIDINE (Rx) • **Demerol. Isonipecaine. Mepergan. Pethadol.** A narcotic and analgesic introduced in 1939 that alters both the perception of and reaction to pain. Used to treat moderate to severe pain, almost always only in hospitals. Potential adverse effects include sedation, sleepiness, lack of alertness, dizziness, euphoria, seizures, low blood pressure, slow heartbeat, nausea, paradoxical excitement, tremors, vomiting, constipation, urine retention, and respiratory depression. Alcohol and central nervous system depressants are additive. Should not be used within fourteen days of use of MAO inhibitors (*see*). Barbiturates and isoniazid (*see*) increase central nervous system excitation or depression. Phenytoin (*see*) may make meperidine less effective. Contraindicated in acute alcoholism, bronchial asthma, increased pressure on the brain, respiratory depression, low thyroid, liver or kidney disease, Addison's disease, seizures, head injury, severe central nervous system depression, brain tumor, chronic lung disease, shock, and in elderly or debilitated patients. Meperidine's toxicity may be manifested several days after treatment has begun, and therefore it is not recommended for the long-term treatment of pain. May be taken with food to help avoid stomach upset.

MEPHENTERMINE SULFATE (Rx) • **Wyamine.** Stimulates the release of norepinephrine; it is used to treat low blood pressure following spinal anesthesia. Potential adverse reactions include euphoria, nervousness, tremor, incoherence, drowsiness, seizures, irregular heartbeat, and high blood pressure. A number of medications interact with mephentermine, including high blood pressure medications, stimulants, ergot, MAO inhibitors, thyroid hormones, and tricyclic antidepressants (*see all*).

MEPHENYTOIN (Rx) • Mesantoin. Phenantoin. An anticonvulsant that limits seizure activity by controlling the passage of sodium through membranes in the area of the brain that controls movement. Used for generalized tonic-clonic or complex-partial seizures. Potential adverse reactions include potentially fatal destruction of white blood cells, loss of balance, drowsiness, fatigue, irritability, depression, awkward movement, tremor, sleeplessness, dizziness, conjunctivitis (*see*), double vision, swollen gums, water retention, joint pain, swollen glands, arthritis, pulmonary fibrosis, and sensitivity to light. Alcohol and folic acid decrease mephenytoin activity. Heavy use of alcohol may diminish the benefits of the drug. Oral blood thinners, antihistamines, chloramphenicol, cimetidine, diazepam, diazoxide, disulfiram, isoniazid, phenylbutazone, salicylates, sulfamethizole, and valproate may increase mephenytoin levels, leading to toxicity. Contraindicated in hydantoin (*see*) hypersensitivity and should be used cautiously in patients receiving other hydantoin derivatives. Notify your physician if fever, sore throat, bleeding, or rash occur.

MEPHOBARBITAL (Rx) • Mebaral. A barbiturate anticonvulsant that increases the threshold for seizure activity in the area of the brain controlling movement. Used for generalized tonic-clonic or absence seizures. Potential adverse reactions include anemia, dizziness, headache, hangover, confusion, paradoxical excitement, exacerbation of existing pain, drowsiness, low blood pressure, slow heartbeat, nausea, vomiting, epigastric pain, hives, rash, blisters, and allergic reaction. Alcohol and other central nervous system depressants, including narcotic analgesics, may cause excessive central nervous system depression when taken with mephobarbital. The drug decreases the absorption of griseofulvin. MAO inhibitors (*see*) potentiate the barbiturate effect and may depress breathing. Oral blood thinners, oral contraceptives, estrogen, doxycycline, and corticosteroids (*see*) may be less effective when taken with mephobarbital. Rifampin may decrease barbiturate levels, making mephobarbital less effective. Contraindicated in barbiturate hypersensitivity, porphyria (*see*), or respiratory disease with shortness of breath. Should be used cautiously in patients with impaired heart, kidney, or respiratory function, and in myasthenia gravis (*see*) and thyroid disease. The drug should not be withdrawn suddenly. Activities that require alertness and good coordination may have to be avoided until the central nervous system effects of the drug are known. Women using oral contraceptives may have to change to another method of birth control.

**MEPHYTON • ** *See* Phytonadione.

MEPIVACAINE (Rx) • Carbocaine. Cavacaine. Isocaine. Polocaine. A local anesthetic used for pain management. Potential adverse effects include skin reactions, swelling, continuous asthma attacks, severe allergic reactions, anxiety, nervousness, seizures followed by drowsiness, unconsciousness, tremors, twitches, shivering, and respiratory arrest. Other potential reactions include blurred vision, ringing in the ears, nausea, and vomiting. Should be used with extreme caution if MAO inhibitors or tricyclic antidepressants are being taken by the patient. Contraindicated in sensitivity to methylparaben (*see*), in heart block, or for spinal anesthesia.

**MEPRED • ** *See* Methylprednisolone.

MEPROBAMATE (Rx) • Equanil. Meditran. Meprospan. Micrainin. Milpath. Milprem. Miltown. Neuramate. Sedabamate. Tranmep. An antianxiety drug introduced in the 1950s that depresses the central nervous system in the area of the brain controlling emotions. Also a muscle relaxant. Potential adverse reactions include a low white blood cell count, drowsiness, loss of balance, dizziness, slurred speech, headache, palpitation, irregular heartbeat, low blood pressure, loss of appetite, nausea, vomiting, diarrhea, sore mouth, itching, hives, and rash. Contraindicated in patients with hypersensitivity to meprobamate, carisoprodol, mebutamate, or tybamate. Also contraindicated in patients with liver or kidney dysfunction, and in those with suicidal tendencies. Should not be used with alcohol or other central nervous system depressants. Meprobamate may reduce the effect of blood thinners and oral contraceptives. The drug should not be discontinued suddenly. May cause withdrawal symptoms that last from one to four days. Should be taken with meals. Possibility of abuse and addiction with long-term use.

MEPROLONE • *See* Methylprednisolone.

MEPROSPAN • *See* Meprobamate.

MERBROMIN (OTC) • **Mercurochrome.** Derived from dibromofluorescein and mercuric acetate, it is used as a topical antiseptic. Toxic by ingestion. In 1992, the FDA issued a notice that merbromin had not been shown to be safe and effective as claimed in OTC poison ivy, poison oak, and poison sumac products.

MERCAPTOPURINE (Rx) • **Purinethol. 6-Mercaptopurine. 6-MP.** An anticancer drug introduced in 1953 to treat acute lymphoblastic leukemia (in children), acute myeloblastic leukemia, and chronic myelocytic leukemia. Potential adverse reactions include nausea, vomiting, loss of appetite, anemia, painful oral ulcers, liver dysfunction, high uric acid, rash, and dark deposits on the skin. Use of allopurinol (*see*) makes mercaptopurine more toxic. Drugs that are toxic to the liver may enhance this drug's liver toxicity. Warfarin adds to its blood-thinning effects. Mercaptopurine interacts with many drugs; careful medical supervision is vital.

MERC-C • Homeopathic abbreviation for mercurius corrosivus (*see*).

MERC-S • Homeopathic abbreviation for mercurius solubilis (*see*).

MERC. SOL. • Homeopathic abbreviation for mercurius solubilis (*see*).

MERCURIC CHLORIDE (OTC) • A highly toxic mercury that has been used as a topical antiseptic. In 1992, the FDA issued a notice that mercuric chloride had not been shown to be safe and effective as claimed in OTC poison ivy, poison oak, and poison sumac products.

MERCURIC OXIDE (Rx) • **Yellow Mercuric Oxide.** Used to treat minor irritation and infections of the eyelids.

MERCURIUS CORROSIVUS (H) • **Merc-C. Mercuric Chloride.** A mercury-containing homeopathic medicine used to treat delirium, swollen glands, ulcerations of mucous membranes, and diarrhea. It was once used externally by conventional physicians but caused many fatalities because the dosages were too high. Mercury is poisonous. *See* Tissue Salts.

MERCURIUS SOLUBILIS (H) • **Merc-S. Merc. Sol. Ammonionitrate of Mercury.** Mercury is mined from the ore cinnabar. It is the only metal liquid at room temperature. It is extremely toxic. Homeopathic remedies are used to treat bad breath, confusion, abscesses, backache, breast abscess, chicken pox, the common cold, cystitis, diarrhea, earache, exhaustion, eye inflammation, fever, headache, joint pain, mouth ulcers, mumps, sore throat, thrush, and toothache.

MERCUROCHROME • *See* Merbromin.

MERCURY • A poisonous metal, compounds of which are used as skin antiseptics.

MERCURY HERB (H) • *Mercurialis annua.* **American Mercury.** An annual plant with small flowers and rough, hairy fruits. It is native to Europe and contains saponins, volatile oil, and bitter principle (*see all*). Herbalists use it as a diuretic, laxative, emetic, and emmenagogue (*see*). It is used in homeopathic medicine as a treatment for arthritis. It is contraindicated in gastric inflammation and during pregnancy.

MEREPRINE • *See* Doxylamine.

MERITAL • *See* Nomifensine.

MERLENATE • *See* Undecylenic Acid.

MERTHIOLATE • *See* Thimerosal.

MESALAMINE (Rx) • **Fisalamine. Rowasa.** An anti-inflammatory enema preparation used to treat active mild-to-moderate ulcerative colitis, proctitis, or proctosigmoiditis (inflammation of the lower colon). Potential adverse reactions include headache, dizziness, fatigue, abdominal pain, cramps, gas, diarrhea, rectal pain, nausea, itching, inflammation, rash, hives, hair loss, wheezing, allergic reactions, and fever. Contraindicated in patients sensitive to the drug or its components. Some patients sensitive to sulfites may have a reaction because it contains potassium metabisulfite. Patients intolerant of sulfasalazine may also have a reaction. Should be used cautiously in patients with kidney dysfunction.

MESALAZINE • *See* Mesalamine.

MESANTOIN • *See* Mephenytoin.

MESNA (Rx) • **Mesnex.** A medication to reduce the harmful effects on the bladder of some cancer medicines. Given only by or under the immediate supervision of a physician.

MESORIDAZINE BESYLATE (Rx) • **Serentil.** A phenothiazine (*see*) antipsychotic drug used to treat alcoholism, behavioral problems associated with chronic brain syndrome, schizophrenia, and anxiety. Potential adverse reactions include a drop in white blood cells, extrapyramidal reactions, tardive dyskinesia (*see*), sedation, dizziness, a drop in blood pressure when rising from a seated or prone position, enlargement of male breasts, menstrual irregularities, inhibited ejaculation, liver dysfunction, mild photosensitivity, allergic skin reactions, weight gain, increased appetite, fever, irregular heartbeat, and sweating. Use with alcohol and other central nervous system depressants increases central nervous system depression. Antacids inhibit absorption. Barbiturates may decrease the effects of phenothiazine. Contraindicated in coma, bone-marrow depression, brain damage, and with the use of spinal or epidural anesthetics, or adrenergic-blocking agents. Should be used with caution in elderly or debilitated patients, cardiovascular and respiratory disorders, low blood calcium, seizure disorders, severe reactions to insulin, electroshock therapy, glaucoma, and enlarged prostate. Should not be withdrawn suddenly. Sunscreening agents should be worn to avoid photosensitivity (*see*) reactions.

MESTINON • *See* Pyridostigmine.

MESTRANOL (Rx) • **Norethin. Norinyl. Ortho-Novum.** An estrogen (*see*) widely used in combination with progestogen for birth control.

METACORTANDROLONE • *See* Prednisolone.

METAHYDRIN • *See* Trichlormethiazide.

METALONE-TBA • *See* Prednisolone.

METAMUCIL • *See* Psyllium.

METAPROTERENOL (Rx) • **Alupent. Arm-A-Med Metaproterenol. Dey-Dose Metaproterenol. Orciprenaline Sulfate. Prometa.** A bronchodilator introduced in 1964 to treat acute episodes of bronchial asthma and reversible bronchospasm. Potential adverse reactions include nervousness, weakness, drowsiness, vomiting, nausea, bad taste in mouth, tremor, rapid heartbeat, high blood pressure, palpitations, and with excessive use, paradoxical bronchospasm or even cardiac arrest. Propranolol and other beta-blockers (*see*) make it less effective. Some antihistamines, levothyroxine, and MAO inhibitors (*see*) increase its effect and cause a dangerous rise in blood pressure. Contraindicated in those with rapid heartbeat, high blood pressure, coronary artery disease, overactive thyroid, or diabetes.

METARAMINOL BITARTRATE (Rx) • **Aramine.** A stimulant used to treat shock and to prevent a drop in blood pressure. Potential adverse reactions include apprehension, restlessness, dizziness, headache, tremor, weakness, seizures, high blood pressure, low blood pressure, palpitations, irregular heartbeat, nausea, vomiting, decreased urine output, high blood sugar, flushing, pallor, sweating, and respiratory distress. General anesthetics increase the risk of heart problems with metaraminol.

METASTASIS • The spread of cancer cells from the original tumor through the bloodstream and lymphatic system to another part of the body. The term is also used to denote a new tumor caused by this movement of cancer cells.

METATENSIN • *See* Reserpine and Trichlormethiazide.

METAXALONE (Rx) • **Skelaxin.** Used for the relief of muscle pain. Potential adverse effects include fast or slow heartbeat, fainting, mental depression, hives, rash, stinging of the eyes, and stuffy nose; also possible, though rare, are dark stools, cough, and unusual bruising or bleeding.

METED 2 • *See* Salicylic Acid and Sulfur.

METFORMIN (Rx) • **Glucophage.** A drug developed in 1959 and approved in 1994 to treat the noninsulin dependent, Type II, form of diabetes. The FDA warned that some patients who take the drug could suffer lactic acidosis, a life-threatening buildup of lactic acid in the blood, as a side effect.

METFORMIN HCL (Rx) • An oral medication for the treatment of Type II—noninsulin dependent—diabetes or in combination with sulfonylureas (*see*) when sulfonylurea or metformin treatment alone has failed to control high blood sugar. Metformin was introduced in the United States after a fifteen-month review by the FDA. It is used in ninety-three countries and has been on the market in France and Britain since 1959.

METHACHOLINE (Rx) • A bronchoconstrictor for diagnostic purposes only. Administered only by inhalation; severe reduction in respiratory function can result.

METHACYCLINE • *See* Tetracyclines.

METHADONE (Rx) • **Methadose.** A narcotic drug introduced in 1948 as an analgesic, and to treat heroin withdrawal. It alters both the perception of and reaction to pain. Used to treat severe pain. Potential adverse effects include sedation, sleepiness, lack of alertness, dizziness, euphoria, seizures, low blood pressure, low heartbeat, nausea, vomiting, constipation, urine retention, decreased libido, infertility, inhibited female orgasm, sweating, and respiratory depression. Alcohol and central nervous system depressants are additive. Ammonium chloride and other urinary acidifiers and phenytoin (*see*) may lessen methadone's effect. Rifampin may cause withdrawal symptoms and reduce the levels of methadone in the blood. Should be used with extreme caution in elderly or debilitated patients, or in those with acute abdominal conditions, bronchial asthma, increased pressure on the brain, respiratory depression, low thyroid, liver or kidney disease, Addison's disease, seizures, head injury, severe central nervous system depression, enlarged prostate, and chronic lung disease. Addiction may occur. Has a cumulative effect; heavy sedation may occur after repeated doses. May cause physical and emotional dependence. May be taken with food to avoid stomach upset.

METHADOSE • *See* Methadone.

METHAMINODIAZEPOXIDE • *See* Chlordiazepoxide.

METHAMPHETAMINE (Rx) • **Desoxyn.** An amphetamine nervous-system stimulant used to treat attention deficit disorders with hyperactivity and weight loss (banned for this purpose in some states). Potential adverse reactions include restlessness, tremor, hyperactivity, talkativeness, insomnia, irritability, dizziness, headache, chills, overstimulation, palpitations, irregular heartbeat, low blood pressure, high blood pressure, nausea, vomiting, cramps, dry mouth, diarrhea, constipation, metallic taste, loss of appetite, weight loss, hives, impotence, and altered libido. Ammonium chloride, phenothiazines, haloperidol, and vitamin C make it less effective. Antacids, caffeine, sodium bicarbonate, and acetazolamide may increase its effectiveness. MAO inhibitors (*see*) may cause a severe rise in blood pressure. Must be taken at least six hours before bedtime to avoid insomnia. May alter insulin needs. Contraindicated in high blood pressure, overactive thyroid, kidney inflammation, angina or other severe cardiovascular disease, glaucoma, parkinsonism due to hardening of the arteries, agitated states, or a history of drug abuse. Should be used with caution in diabetes mellitus, and in patients who are elderly, debilitated, weak, or psychopathic, or who have a history of suicidal or homicidal tendencies.

METHANOL • Methyl Alcohol. Wood Alcohol. Wood Spirit. A solvent and denaturant obtained by the destructive distillation of wood. Methanol is highly toxic and readily absorbed from all routes of exposure.

METHANTHELINE (Rx) • Banthine. An anticholinergic (*see*), antispasmodic drug used to treat irritable bowel syndrome (*see*), and as an adjunctive therapy in peptic ulcers and other GI disorders (*see* Adjunct). Therapeutic effects appear in thirty to forty-five minutes and persist for up to six hours. Potential adverse reactions include disorientation, irritability, incoherence, weakness, nervousness, drowsiness, dizziness, headache, palpitations, rapid heartbeat, slow heartbeat, blurred vision, sensitivity to light, increased eye pressure, difficulty in swallowing, constipation, dry mouth, nausea, vomiting, epigastric distress, urinary retention, impotence, hives, decreased sweating, and fever. Contraindicated in glaucoma, obstructions in the urinary or GI tract, myasthenia gravis (*see*), paralytic ileus (*see*), intestinal flaccidity, unstable cardiovascular status in acute hemorrhage, and toxic megacolon. Should be used with caution in patients with nerve damage, overactive thyroid, coronary artery disease, irregular heartbeat, congestive heart failure, high blood pressure, hiatal hernia, liver or kidney disease, and ulcerative colitis. Should also be used with caution in people over forty years of age due to the possibility of glaucoma. Should be taken thirty minutes to one hour before meals.

METHAPYRILENE (OTC) • An antihistamine. In 1992, the FDA proposed a ban on the use of methapyrilene hydrochloride to treat fever blisters and cold sores, poison ivy, poison oak, and poison sumac because it had not been shown to be safe and effective as claimed in OTC products. The FDA also banned methapyrilene fumarate for internal pain use and in oral menstrual drugs.

METHARBITAL (Rx) • Gemonil. A barbiturate anticonvulsant used to control grand mal, petit mal, and myoclonic seizures. *See* Barbiturates.

METHAZOLAMIDE (Rx) • Neptazane. An enzyme inhibitor that reduces fluid, it is used primarily to treat glaucoma (*see*).

METHDILAZINE (Rx) • Tacaryl. An antihistamine used to treat stuffy nose due to allergy and itching. Potential adverse reactions include drowsiness (especially in the elderly), dizziness, headache, nausea, dry mouth and throat, urine retention, jaundice, and rash. Use with central nervous system depressants, including alcohol, increases sedation. MAO inhibitors (*see*) may shoot up blood pressure. Contraindicated in acute asthmatic attacks. Should be used cautiously in elderly patients, those with glaucoma, overactive thyroid, heart or kidney disease, high blood pressure, bronchial asthma, enlarged prostate, bladder-neck obstruction, and peptic ulcer. Coffee or tea may reduce drowsiness. Medication should be discontinued four days before taking a skin allergy test because it can lead to inaccurate results.

METHENAMINE, HIPPURATE, MANDELATE (Rx) (OTC) • Hexalol. Hiprex. Mandameth. Mandelamine. Urex. Uro-Phosphate. Drugs used to treat infections of the urinary tract. Potential adverse reactions include nausea, vomiting, diarrhea, urinary-tract irritation, painful urination, urinary frequency, blood in urine, rash, and liver dysfunction. Acetazolamide (*see*) and urine-alkalizing agents make it less effective. Alkaline foods such as vegetables, milk, and peanuts should be limited. Cranberry, plum, and prune juices are useful in aiding acidification of urine. Avoid antacids unless otherwise instructed by your physician. Eating more protein and foods such as cranberries, cranberry juice with vitamin C added, plums, or prunes may also help. In 1992, the FDA proposed a ban on methenamine in oral menstrual drug products because it had not been shown to be safe and effective as claimed.

METHERGINE • *See* Methylergonovine.

METHICILLIN SODIUM (Rx) • **Metin. Sodium Methicillin. Staphcillin.** A penicillin and antibiotic used against systemic infections caused by penicillinase-producing staphylococci (*see*). Potential adverse reactions include anemia, a low white blood cell count, neuropathy, seizures (with high doses), sore throat, kidney inflammation, local vein irritation, and hypersensitivity reactions, including possible fatal anaphylaxis. May also cause an overgrowth of nonsusceptible organisms.

METHIMAZOLE (Rx) • **Tapazole. Thiamazole.** A thyroid-hormone antagonist introduced in 1951 to treat overactive thyroid. Longer-acting than many other drugs in its category, it has the advantage of once-a-day dosing. Its full effects may not be felt for several weeks. Potential adverse reactions include nausea, vomiting, diarrhea, a drop in white blood cells and platelets, headache, drowsiness, dizziness, fever, swollen glands, joint pain, muscle pain, mental depression, cold intolerance, edema, and loss of taste. Should be used cautiously in pregnancy. Over-the-counter medications that contain iodine, shellfish, and iodized salt may cause problems during treatment since this drug inhibits the oxidation of iodine.

METHIONINE (Rx) • **Pedameth.** An essential amino acid (*see*). Used as a nutrient; also in products to treat diaper rash and control odor, skin rash, and ulceration caused by ammoniacal urine.

METHOCARBAMOL (Rx) • **Delaxin. Marbaxin. Robaxin. Robaxisal. Robomol.** A centrally acting skeletal-muscle relaxant introduced in 1957 that reduces transmission of nerve impulses from the spinal cord to the skeletal muscles. It is used as an adjunct (*see*) in acute, painful muscle conditions. Potential adverse reactions include destruction of red blood cells, drowsiness, dizziness, headache, faintness, mild incoordination, seizures, low blood pressure, slow heartbeat, nausea, loss of appetite, GI upset, metallic taste, blood in the urine, blood clots, hives, itching, rash, fever, flushing, and potentially fatal allergic reactions. It may also turn urine green. Use with alcohol and central nervous system depressants increases methocarbamol's central nervous system–depressant effects. Contraindicated in impaired kidney function, myasthenia gravis (*see*), epilepsy, in children under twelve years of age, and in patients receiving anticholinesterase (*see*) agents. May be taken with food to reduce stomach irritation. As of this writing, it is a candidate for OTC status, as a muscle relaxant.

METHOHEXITAL SODIUM (Rx) • **Brevital Sodium.** A barbiturate drug used to induce general anesthesia for short-term procedures such as oral surgery, gynecologic and genitourinary examinations, and reduction of bone fractures. Potential adverse reactions include nausea, vomiting, excessive salivation, twitching, headache, low blood pressure, rapid heartbeat, circulatory depression, throat spasms, respiratory depression, blood clots, hiccups, coughing, and acute allergic reactions. Contraindicated in severe liver dysfunction, hypersensitivity to barbiturates, shock, and in patients for whom general anesthesia would be hazardous.

METHOSARB • *See* Calusterone.

METHOTREXATE (Rx) • **Amethopterin. Folex. Mexate. MTX. Rheumatrex.** The most widely used cytotoxic (*see*) agent in rheumatoid arthritis, it was introduced in the 1950s to treat cancer. Used to treat tumors, hydatidiform mole, acute lymphoblastic and lymphatic leukemia, and meningeal leukemia. Also used in severe psoriasis.

The effects in arthritis may be apparent within four to six weeks of treatment. This drug has a high incidence of serious side effects. Potential adverse reactions include nausea, vomiting, and abdominal pain. Other potential adverse reactions include high uric acid, irregular menses, severe bone-marrow suppression, ulcers, sore mouth, intestinal perforation, and liver, nerve, and kidney damage. Lung problems may also occur. Methotrexate causes birth defects, and pregnancy should be avoided if *either* partner is taking it. Folic acid derivatives make it less effective. Probenecid, phenylbutazone, NSAIDs (*see*), aspirin and other salicylates, and sulfonamides (*see all*) increase methotrexate's toxicity. Deaths have been reported in people taking both methotrexate and NSAIDs. Vaccines should not be given because immunizations may be ineffective or with live viruses may spread infections. Most effective when taken on an empty stomach, but may be taken with a small amount of food if stomach upset is a problem.

METHOTRIMEPRAZINE HYDROCHLO-RIDE (Rx) • Levomepromazine Hydrochloride. Levoprome.

A phenothiazine (*see*) sedative and analgesic, it acts on the limbic system, thalamus, and hypothalamus of the brain to produce hypnotic effects. Potential adverse reactions include blood problems, fainting, weakness, dizziness, confusion, euphoria, headache, slurred speech, palpitations, dry mouth, stuffy nose, difficulty in urinating, and pain and inflammation at injection site. May interact with all blood-pressure-lowering agents, causing a drop in blood pressure when rising from a seated or prone position. Contraindicated in patients receiving high blood pressure drugs, those taking MAO inhibitors (*see*), in persons with seizures, severe heart, liver, or kidney disease, sulfite sensitivity, and in patients with coma or previous overdose of central nervous system depressant. Should be used with extreme caution in elderly or debilitated patients.

METHOXAMINE (Rx) • Vasoxyl.

Used to raise blood pressure when it drops too low during general anesthesia. It is also used to treat rapid heartbeat and shock.

METHOXSALEN (Rx) • 8-Mop. Methoxy-psoralen. Oxsoralen.

A drug introduced in 1953 to induce repigmentation in vitiligo (*see*) and to treat psoriasis. It is used with ultraviolet radiation. Potential adverse reactions include nausea, diarrhea, abdominal discomfort, nervousness, insomnia, depression, dizziness, headache, swelling, redness, blisters, burning, peeling, and itching. Any drug that increases sensitivity to light may increase methoxsalen's toxicity. Contraindicated in liver dysfunction, acute lupus erythematosus (*see*), or persons with sunlight allergy, GI diseases, or chronic infection. Should be taken with meals or milk. The following foods should be avoided while taking this medication: limes, figs, parsley, parsnips, mustard, carrots, and celery.

METHOXYFLURANE (Rx) •

A potent, nonflammable, nonexplosive inhaled anesthetic. Potential adverse effects include kidney dysfunction and increased fluoride in the blood.

METHOXYPHENAMINE (OTC) •

A drug that works on the sympathetic nervous system (*see*). Used for the relief of wheezing and shortness of breath in asthma. Changed from Rx to OTC.

METHOXYPSORALEN • *See* Methoxsalen.

METHSCOPOLAMINE (Rx) • Historal. Histor-D. Pamine.

An anticholinergic, antispasmodic drug used to treat irritable bowel syndrome (*see*).

METHSUXIMIDE (Rx) • Celontin.

An anticonvulsant drug derived from succinimide (*see*) that increases the seizure threshold by depressing nerve transmission in the motor control area of the brain. Potential adverse reactions include destruction of white blood cells, drowsiness, loss of balance, dizziness, irritability, nervousness, headache, insomnia, confusion, depression, aggressiveness, blurred vision, sensitivity to light, swelling around the eyes, nausea, vomiting, loss of appetite, diarrhea, weight loss, abdominal or epigastric pain, hives, itching, and rash. Contraindicated in hypersensitivity to succinimide derivatives. Should be used with caution in liver or kidney disease. The central nervous system–depressant effects of methsuximide are increased by tranquilizers, sleeping pills, narcotics, pain relievers, antihistamines, alcohol, MAO inhibitors (*see*), antidepressants, and other anticonvulsants. Activities that require alertness and good psychomotor coordination should be avoided until the central nervous system effect of methsuximide is known. Should not be withdrawn suddenly. Most effective when taken on an empty stomach, but may be taken with a small amount of food if stomach upset is a problem.

METHYCLOTHIAZIDE (Rx) • Aquatensen. Diutensin-R. Enduron. Enduronyl. Ethon. A thiazide diuretic introduced in 1960 that increases urine excretion of sodium and water. Used to treat edema and high blood pressure. Potential adverse reactions include nausea, vomiting, loss of appetite, dehydration, a drop in blood pressure upon rising from a seated or prone position, liver dysfunction, anemia, a drop in platelets, low potassium, high blood sugar, fluid and electrolyte imbalances, impotence, rash, photosensitivity, and other allergic reactions. Cholestyramine and colestipol (*see both*) make it less effective. Diazoxide increases its blood-pressure-lowering and sugar-raising effects. Contraindicated in kidney and liver diseases, absence of urine formation, or hypersensitivity to other thiazides or sulfonamide-derived drugs. The effects of methyclothiazide are increased by other blood-pressure-lowering drugs. Digitalis and adrenal corticosteroids (*see*) taken with methyclothiazide may increase potentially dangerous body fluid imbalances. Lithium should not be taken while taking this drug. Over-the-counter cough, cold, and allergy medications containing stimulants should be avoided. Methyclothiazide should be taken in the morning to avoid having to urinate during the night. A diet rich in potassium may be recommended. This includes dates, apricots, bananas, and tomatoes. If taking this drug, you should wear sunscreen. Most effective when taken on an empty stomach, but may be taken with a small amount of food if stomach upset is a problem.

METHYLBENZETHONIUM CHLORIDE (OTC) • Diaparene. Puri-Clens. Sween Cream. A skin antiseptic used in diaper rash and ammonia-caused skin rash.

METHYL CATECHOL (OTC) • Prepared from wood, it is a white or slightly yellow mass used as an expectorant in cough medicines. *See* Guaiacol.

METHYL CCNU • *See* Semustine.

METHYLCELLULOSE (OTC) • Cellulose Methyl Ether. Citrucel. Cologel. Murocel. Introduced in 1947, this compound is prepared from wood pulp or chemical cotton by treatment with alcohol. It swells in water and increases the bulk and moisture content of the stool, which encourages bowel movements. It is not absorbed systemically and is nontoxic. Used to treat both chronic and postpartum constipation. Potential adverse reactions include nausea, vomiting, diarrhea, and blockage of the small intestine or colon when the drug is chewed or taken in dry form. Also, abdominal cramps, especially in severe constipation. May involve laxative dependence in long-term or excessive use. Contraindicated in abdominal pain, nausea, vomiting, or other symptoms of appendicitis, heart damage, fecal impaction, rectal fissures, intestinal obstruction or perforation, or kidney disease. Works in twelve to twenty-four hours, or may take up to three days. Oral drugs should not be given within two hours of taking this laxative. *See* Laxative.

METHYLDOPA (Rx) • Aldoclor. Aldomet. Aldoril. Methyldopate. A centrally acting antihypertensive drug introduced in 1963 that targets the brain's mechanism for controlling blood-vessel size. Used for sustained mild to severe hypertension. Potential adverse reactions include anemia, sedation, headache, weakness, dizziness, confusion, involuntary movements, psychic disturbances, depression, nightmares, a drop in blood pressure when rising from a seated or prone position, aggravated angina, heart-muscle irritation, dry mouth, weight gain, nasal stuffiness, decreased libido, diarrhea, pancreatitis, severe liver damage, increased breast size in men, increased female breast with lactation, skin rash, drug-induced fever, and impotence. Levodopa may increase the effect on blood pressure and may possibly increase the central nervous system adverse reactions. Norepinephrine, phenothiazines, tricyclic antidepressants, and amphetamines may possibly increase hypertension when used with methyldopa. The drug is frequently used to treat pregnant women with high blood pressure, apparently without effects on the fetus. Methyldopa increases the effects of other blood-pressure-lowering drugs. Over-the-counter medications containing stimulants such as allergy and cold medications should be avoided. Methyldopa may increase blood sugar, and diabetics may have to have their dosages of antidiabetes medications adjusted. If methyldopa is taken with phenoxybenzamine, it may cause an inability to control urination. The combination of methyldopa and lithium may increase the toxicity of lithium. Methyldopa, when given together with haloperidol, may produce irritability, aggressiveness, assaultive behavior, or other psychiatric symptoms. This drug, especially at first, may impair the ability to perform tasks that require mental alertness. If you are taking the drug, you should rise slowly from a seated or prone position. Most effective when taken on an empty stomach, but may be taken with a small amount of food if stomach upset is a problem.

METHYLENE BLUE (Rx) • **Urolene Blue.** An antiseptic dye used to treat urinary-tract infections, deficient oxygen in the blood, and cyanide poisoning. Potential adverse reactions include anemia (long-term use), nausea, vomiting, diarrhea, pain on urination, bladder irritation, and fever. In 1992, the FDA proposed a ban on methylene blue in oral menstrual drug products because it had not been shown to be safe and effective as claimed.

METHYLERGONOVINE (Rx) • **Methergine.** A uterine stimulant to prevent and treat postpartum hemorrhage caused by uterine problems. Potential adverse reactions include nausea, vomiting, dizziness, high blood pressure, transient chest pain, shortness of breath, headache, sweating, ringing in the ears, and hypersensitivity.

METHYL MORPHINE • *See* Codeine Phosphate and Sulfate.

METHYL NICOTINATE (OTC) • Derived from nicotinic acid. Used as a rubefacient (*see*). In 1992, the FDA proposed a ban for the use of methyl nicotinate to treat fever blisters and cold sores because it had not been shown to be safe and effective as claimed in OTC products.

METHYLONE • *See* Methylprednisolone.

METHYLPARABEN • One of the most widely used preservatives in cosmetics, it has a broad spectrum of antimicrobial activity and is relatively nonirritating, nonsensitizing, and nonpoisonous. Can cause allergic reactions. In 1992, the FDA issued a notice that methylparaben alum had not been shown to be safe and effective as claimed in OTC products.

METHYLPHENIDATE (Rx) • **Ritalin.** A nervous system stimulant introduced in 1956 that promotes nerve impulse transmission by releasing stored norepinephrine (*see*) from nerves in the brain. It is used in attention deficit disorder with hyperactivity in children. It received adverse publicity in the 1980s for this use, but is still regarded by many scientists as the most effective treatment to calm children with attention deficit disorder and focus their attention on tasks that would otherwise be impossible for them. It has a paradoxical sedating effect, although its use is controversial. Also used to treat narcolepsy (*see*). Potential adverse effects include a drop in blood platelets, nervousness, insomnia, dizziness, headache, fidgeting, trouble moving, Tourette's syndrome (*see*), palpitations, angina, irregular heartbeat, changes in blood pressure and pulse rate, blurring of vision, nausea, dry throat, stomach pain, loss of appetite, loss of weight, rash, hives, and growth suppression. May result in toxicity if used with anticonvulsants, tricyclic antidepressants, and oral blood thinners. High blood pressure medications that act on the brain may be less effective. Use with MAO inhibitors (*see*) may cause severe high blood pressure. Contraindicated in some types of heart disease, angina, overactive thyroid, moderate to severe high blood pressure, severe depression, glaucoma, parkinsonism, anxiety or agitation, and in persons with a history of drug abuse. Should also be used with caution in elderly, debilitated, or highly excited patients, and those with a history of cardiovascular disease, diabetes, or seizures. Usually discontinued when children with attention deficit disorder reach puberty. Fatigue may result as the drug's effect wears off. Caffeinated drinks should be avoided, as well as beer, Chianti wine, and vermouth. Foods rich in tyramine (*see*) should also be avoided because they may interact with methylphenidate to greatly increase blood pressure. Should be taken at least six hours before bedtime and after meals to reduce appetite suppression.

METHYLPREDNISOLONE (Rx) • A-Metha-Pred. Mar-Pred. Medrol. Medrol Enpak. Medrol Oral. Mepred. Meprolone. Methylone. Solu-Medrol.
A hormone secreted by the adrenal gland that affects carbohydrate and protein metabolism. It was introduced as a medication in 1957 to treat severe inflammation, for immunosuppression, and to decrease residual damage following spinal cord trauma. Most adverse reactions are the result of dosage or length of time between administration. Potential adverse reactions include euphoria, insomnia, psychotic behavior, high blood pressure, swelling, cataracts, glaucoma, peptic ulcer, GI irritation, increased appetite, high blood sugar, growth suppression in children, delayed wound healing, acne, skin eruptions, muscle weakness, pancreatitis, hairiness, decreased immunity, and acute adrenal gland insufficiency. When withdrawn, there may be rebound inflammation, fatigue, weakness, joint pain, fever, dizziness, lethargy, depression, fainting, a drop in blood pressure upon rising from a seated or prone position, shortness of breath, loss of appetite, and high blood sugar. Sudden withdrawal may be fatal. Contraindicated in systemic fungal infections. Should be used cautiously in patients with GI ulceration, kidney disease, high blood pressure, diabetes, chicken pox, osteoporosis, Cush-

ing's syndrome, blood-clotting disorders, seizures, myasthenia gravis (*see*), congestive heart failure, tuberculosis, herpes, and emotional instability. Barbiturates, phenytoin, and rifampin (*see all*) increase its effects. Indomethacin and aspirin may increase the risk of GI distress and bleeding. When taking the drug, patients may need low-sodium diets and potassium supplements. When taken in pill form, it should be ingested with food or milk to reduce GI irritation. In an ointment, methylprednisolone is used to treat skin inflammation. Potential adverse reactions include burning, itching, irritation, dryness, inflammation of the hair follicles, acne, rash around the mouth, spots of pigment loss, hairiness, allergic contact dermatitis, and if covered with a dressing, secondary infection, atrophy, streaks, and blisters. Should be used cautiously in skin problems caused by viruses such as herpes, and in fungal or bacterial skin infections. Should not be used for more than two weeks due to potential absorption into the system, consequently causing an effect on the hypothalamus, and pituitary and adrenal glands. Should not be applied near the eyes or mucous membranes, under the arms, on the face, groin, or under the breast unless medically specified.

METHYLROSANILINE CHLORIDE CRYSTAL VIOLET • *See* Gentian Violet.

METHYL SALICYLATE (OTC) • Arum Analgesic. Ben-Gay. Ger-O-Foam. Icy Hot Balm. Listerine Antiseptic. Oil of Wintergreen. Salicylic Acid. Theragold Analgesic Lotion.
Found naturally in sweet birch, cassia, and wintergreen, it is used as an analgesic in rubefacient (*see*) preparations to relieve muscle and joint pain. Also used as a counterirritant (*see*), local anesthetic, and disinfectant. Toxic by ingestion. Use in foods is restricted by the FDA. The lethal dose is 30 cc in adults and 10 ml in children. The FDA proposed that liniments and other liquid preparations containing more than 5 percent methyl salicylate be marketed in special child-resistant containers. In 1992, the FDA proposed a ban for the use of methyl salicylate to treat fever blisters and cold sores, and in astringent (*see*) drugs,

because it had not been shown to be safe and effective as claimed in OTC products.

METHYLTESTOSTERONE (Rx) • Android. Metandren. Oreton Methyl. Testred. Virilon. A testosterone drug used to treat breast engorgement of nonnursing mothers, and to treat androgen-deficient males. Potential adverse reactions in women include acne, edema, oily skin, weight gain, hairiness, hoarseness, clitoral enlargement, changes in libido, flushing, sweating, and vaginitis with itching. In prepubescent males, premature epiphyseal closure, priapism (*see*), growth of body and facial hair, phallic enlargement; in post-pubescent males, testicular atrophy, scanty sperm, decreased ejaculatory volume, impotence, breast enlargement, and epididymitis. In both sexes, edema, gastroenteritis, nausea, vomiting, diarrhea, constipation, changes in appetite, bladder irritability, jaundice, liver toxicity, and high levels of calcium in the blood. Contraindicated in women of childbearing potential (may masculinize female infants); in elderly men, who may react adversely to androgen overstimulation; in persons with high calcium levels; in heart, liver, or kidney dysfunction; in prostatic or breast cancer in men; in benign prostatic enlargement or suspected prostate cancer; and in conditions aggravated by fluid retention or high blood pressure. Should also not be used in premature infants. Should be used with caution in persons with heart disease. May cause a drop in blood sugar. Should be taken with food.

METHYPRYLON (Rx) • Noludar. A nonbarbiturate, nonbenzodiazepine sleeping medication that raises the threshold of arousal centers in the brain stem. Used in adults and in children over three months of age. Potential adverse reactions include a drop in blood platelets, anemia, morning hangover, dizziness, headache, paradoxical excitation, low blood pressure, nausea, vomiting, diarrhea, inflamed esophagus, rash, and itching. Alcohol or other central nervous system depressants, including narcotic analgesics, may cause excessive depression of central nervous and respiratory systems. Contraindicated in porphyria (*see*) and to be used cautiously in kidney or liver dysfunction. When the drug is discontinued, increased dreaming may

occur. It is reportedly effective for only a week and has generally been replaced by other medications for the treatment of insomnia.

METHYSERGIDE (Rx) • Sansert. A drug introduced in 1962 that blocks serotonin (*see*) and is used to prevent migraine and vascular headaches. Potential adverse reactions include a drop in white blood cells, insomnia, drowsiness, euphoria, dizziness, loss of balance, hypersensitivity, weakness, hallucinations, thickening of the heart valves and aorta, vasoconstriction causing chest pain, abdominal pain, diminished blood supply to the lower limbs, cold, numb, painful extremities, a drop in blood pressure, rapid heartbeat, edema, heart murmur, nasal stuffiness, nausea, vomiting, diarrhea, constipation, stomach pain, hair loss, rash, sweating, malaise, fatigue, weight gain, backache, low-grade fever, urinary obstruction, thickening of the lungs, shortness of breath, and joint and muscle pain. Contraindicated in severe high blood pressure, blood-vessel and artery diseases, heart disease, and debilitated patients. Should be used with caution in patients with peptic ulcers and those over forty years of age. The drug should not be discontinued suddenly.

METICORTEN • *See* Prednisone.

METIMYD (Rx) • *See* Prednisolone and Sulfacetamide.

METIN • *See* Methicillin Sodium.

METIPRANOLOL (Rx) • OptiPranolol. A drug to lower pressure inside the eye.

METIZOL • *See* Metronidazole.

METOCLOPRAMIDE (Rx) • Clopra. Maxolon. Reclomide. Reglan. A drug introduced in 1973 to counteract the nausea and vomiting induced by anticancer drugs, and in other gastrointestinal problems. Potential adverse reactions include restlessness, anxiety, drowsiness, fatigue, insomnia, headache, dizziness, tardive dyskinesia (*see*), sedation, temporary high blood pressure, nausea, bowel disturbances, rash, fever, and loss of libido. Anticholinergic drugs (see) and narcotic painkillers counteract the effects of metoclopramide. Contraindicated if stimulation of the GI tract may be dangerous, as in hemorrhage, obstruction, or perforation, and in epilepsy. Should be used cautiously in elderly patients. Should be taken thirty minutes before meals and at bedtime.

METOCURINE (Rx) • **Metubine.** A muscle-relaxant drug used in surgical procedures. Potential adverse reactions include low blood pressure, residual muscle weakness, allergic or unusual hypersensitivity reactions, and bronchospasm. Contraindicated in patients who are allergic to iodides.

METOLAZONE (Rx) • **Mykrox. Zaroxolyn.** A thiazidelike diuretic introduced in 1974 to increase urine excretion of sodium and water. It is used to treat edema in heart failure, cirrhosis of the liver, and high blood pressure. Potential adverse reactions include nausea, vomiting, loss of appetite, pancreatitis, dehydration, impotence, a drop in blood pressure upon rising from a seated or prone position, liver dysfunction, anemia, a drop in platelets, low potassium, high blood sugar, fluid and electrolyte imbalances, rash, photosensitivity, and other allergic reactions. Cholestyramine and colestipol (see both) make it less effective. Diazoxide increases its blood-pressure-lowering and sugar-raising effects. NSAIDs (see) decrease its effectiveness. Over-the-counter medications that contain stimulants, such as some cold and allergy medications, may counteract its effectiveness. Contraindicated in kidney and liver diseases, absence of urine formation, or hypersensitivity to other thiazides or sulfonamide-derived drugs. Should be used cautiously in gout. Mykrox tablets are reportedly more rapidly and completely absorbed than other brands. Should be taken in the morning to avoid having to urinate during the night. A diet rich in potassium may be recommended. This includes dates, apricots, bananas, and tomatoes. If taking this drug, you should wear sunscreen. Metolazone may be taken with food.

METOPIRONE • See Metyrapone.

METOPROLOL TARTRATE (Rx) • **Lopressor.** A beta-blocker (see) drug introduced in 1978, it is prescribed for high blood pressure and to prevent a second heart attack. It acts more on the heart than the lungs, so causes fewer problems for asthmatics than other similar drugs. Potential adverse reactions include fatigue, lethargy, dizziness, low blood pressure, decreased libido, impaired erection, chest pain, precipitation of congestive heart failure, nausea, vomiting, diarrhea, rash, shortness of breath, bronchospasm, fever, and joint pain. Barbiturates and rifampin increase the metabolism of metoprolol. It will react with any drug that affects the brain, including MAO inhibitors (see). Use of cardiac glycosides with metoprolol may affect the heart muscle. Chlorpromazine, cimetidine, and verapamil decrease the clearance of metoprolol from the liver. Indomethacin decreases its antihypertensive effects. Metoprolol may cause dosage adjustments of oral diabetic drugs and insulin. Should be taken with food.

METR-, METRO- • Combined form meaning pertaining to the womb, as in *endometrium,* the lining of the womb.

METRA • See Phendimetrazine.

METRETON • See Prednisolone.

METRIC • See Metronidazole.

METRIZAMIDE (Rx) • **Amipaque.** An injected radiopaque (see) agent used to study the blood vessels of the head and neck, the heart, and the spine.

METRODIN • See Urofollitropin.

METROGEL • See Metronidazole.

METROGYL • See Metronidazole.

METRONID • See Metronidazole.

METRONIDAZOLE (Rx) • **Apo-Metronidazole. Femazole. Flagyl. Metizol. Metric. Metro-**

Gel. Metronid. Metrozine. Metryl. Novonidazol. PMS Metronidazole. Protostat. Satric. Introduced in 1960, metronidazole is widely used for the treatment of infections due to parasites, including liver abscesses caused by amoebas. May cause temporary low white blood cell count, headache, dizziness, incoordination, diarrhea, confusion, depression, restlessness, weakness, fatigue, convulsions, insomnia, numbness, and nerve damage. Among other side effects are rash, decreased libido, decreased vaginal secretions, incontinence and other urinary problems, overgrowth of nonsusceptible organisms, especially candida, a metallic taste, fever, and breast enlargement in men. Also may cause sodium retention. Has been shown to cause cancer in animals. In a cream for the skin used to treat acne rosacea, it may cause tearing if applied around the eyes. Oral anticoagulants may potentiate the blood-thinning effects of metronidazole. Contraindicated in persons with a history of blood disease. Alcoholic beverages should be avoided. May cause an Antabuse-like (see Disulfiram) reaction if taken with alcohol. The effect can include facial flushing, a steep rise in blood pressure, and severe nausea and vomiting. Even the amount of alcohol in some cough medicines can cause the interaction effect. May be taken with food to avoid stomach upset.

METROZINE • *See* Metronidazole.

METRYL • *See* Metronidazole.

METUBINE • *See* Metocurine.

METYRAPONE (Rx) • **Metopirone.** Used to test the function of the hypothalamus in the brain and the pituitary gland.

METYROSINE (Rx) • **Demser. OGMT.** An ACE (*see*) inhibitor antihypertensive drug that acts on enzymes in the blood to dilate blood vessels. Potential adverse effects include drowsiness, speech difficulty and disorientation, diarrhea, nausea, vomiting, abdominal pain, blood and crystals in the urine, impotence, and hypersensitivity. Phenothiazines, alcohol, and haloperidol may increase metyrosine's side effects. Intake of fluids should be increased to avoid urinary problems. Insomnia may occur when metyrosine is discontinued.

MEVACOR • *See* Lovastatin.

MEVINOLIN • *See* Lovastatin.

MEXATE • *See* Methotrexate.

MEXILETINE (Rx) • **Mexitil.** Introduced in 1973, mexiletine is chemically similar to lidocaine. It is an antiarrhythmic (*see*) drug that is used to treat both chronic and acute heartbeat irregularities. Potential adverse reactions include tremor, dizziness, blurred vision, double vision, incoordination, confusion, nervousness, headache, decreased libido, low blood pressure, worsened heart function, nausea, vomiting, and rash. Cimetidine (*see*) may increase mexiletine's toxicity. Must be used cautiously in persons with liver dysfunction. Phenytoin, rifampin, and phenobarbital may decrease its effectiveness. Should be taken with food.

MEXITIL • *See* Mexiletine.

MEXSANA MEDICATED (OTC) • A combination of triclosan, zinc oxide, kaolin, eucalyptus oil, camphor, cornstarch, and lemon oil (*see all*), used to treat diaper rash.

MEZLIN • *See* Mezlocillin Sodium.

MEZLOCILLIN SODIUM (Rx) • **Mezlin.** A penicillin antibiotic used to treat systemic infections caused by susceptible strains of gram-positive and especially gram-negative (*see both*) organisms, including *Proteus* and *Pseudomonas aeruginosa* (*see both*). Potential adverse reactions include bleeding, neuromuscular irritability, nausea, diarrhea, low potassium, pain and phlebitis at injection site, hypersensitivity, including a potentially fatal allergic reaction, and overgrowth of nonsusceptible organisms. Should not be taken with aminoglycoside (*see*) antibiotics.

MG-PLUS • *See* Magnesium Sulfate.

MIACALCIN (Rx) • Approved by the FDA in 1994 for the prevention of osteoporosis. *See* Calcitonin and Salcatonin.

MICATIN • *See* Miconazole.

MICONAZOLE (Rx) (OTC) • Micatin. Monistat I.V. Monistat 7. An antifungal used in the treatment of coccidioidomycosis, candidiasis, cryptococcosis, paracoccidioidomycosis, chronic mucocutaneous candidiasis, and fungal meningitis. The vaginal cream is effective in treating vaginal infection caused by yeast only. In creams and sprays, it is also used to control fungal infections of the feet, scalp, and skin. It was changed from Rx to OTC in lower-dose preparations. Adverse reactions may include transient decreases in red blood cells and blood platelets. Also may cause dizziness, drowsiness, nausea, vomiting, diarrhea, a decrease in blood sodium, and rash and phlebitis at injection site. In skin preparations, it may cause irritation, burning, and itching. Miconazole increases the effects of blood thinners, counteracts the effects of oral antidiabetic drugs and amphotericin B, and increases the side effects of phenytoin. *See* Imidazoles.

MICRAININ • *See* Aspirin and Meprobamate.

MICRIN • *See* Hydrochlorothiazide.

MICRO-K • *See* Potassium Chloride.

MICRONASE • *See* Glyburide.

MICRONEFRIN • *See* Epinephrine.

MICRONOR • *See* Norethindrone.

MICROORGANISMS • Tiny organisms that can only be seen under a microscope—such as bacteria and viruses.

MICROSULFON • *See* Sulfadiazine.

MICTRIN • *See* Hydrochlorothiazide.

MIDAMOR • *See* Amiloride.

MIDAZOLAM (Rx) • Versed. A benzodiazepine (*see*) drug used mainly as premedication for surgical or invasive diagnostic procedures and for induction of general anesthesia. Potential adverse reactions include headache, oversedation, involuntary movements, combativeness, variations in blood pressure and pulse rate, nausea, vomiting, hiccups, and decreased respiratory rate. Central neurological system depressants may increase the risk of interrupted breathing. Contraindicated in glaucoma and patients in shock, coma, or acute alcohol intoxication. Must be used cautiously in the elderly, in debilitated patients, and in persons with congestive heart failure or chronic obstructive lung disease.

MI DIE XIANG • *See* Rosemary.

MIDOL 200 (OTC) • Midol contains 32 mg of caffeine. *See* Ibuprofen.

MIDRIN (Rx) • A combination of acetaminophen, dichloralphenazone, and isomethepene (*see all*), used to relieve headaches.

MIFEPRISTONE (Rx) • RU-486. A synthetic steroid used in France, the United Kingdom, and Sweden for more than ten years to induce abortions in the first nine weeks of pregnancy. It has been the object of great controversy in the United States. The National Right-to-Life Committee and other antiabortion groups oppose the use of the drug. The maker of the product, Roussel Uclaf, said in May 1994 that it would donate rights to the drug to the Population Council, a nonprofit research organization, rather than face the protests and boycotts that threatened to accompany the sale of miferpristone in the United States, where it is now being used.

MIGERGOT • *See* Ergotamine Tartrate.

MIGRAINE • An intense headache caused by changes in the blood vessels. It sets in with suddenness on one side of the head, lasts a day or two, and disappears just as suddenly, only to recur periodically. The sudden migraine attack may be accompanied by vomiting and temporary disturbance of vision. Occasionally, speech is affected and the attack may be disabling. The exact cause of migraine is unknown. Drugs are used either to prevent attacks or to relieve them once symptoms occur.

MILFOIL • *See* Yarrow.

MILKINOL (OTC) • A lubricant laxative containing mineral oil. *See* Laxative.

MILK OF MAGNESIA • *See* Magnesium Hydroxide.

MILK SUGAR • *See* Lactose.

MILK THISTLE (H) • *Silybum marianum. Carduus marianus.* **St. Mary's Thistle.** The seeds and stems are used to treat liver problems and mushroom poisoning. Milk thistle is reported by herbalists to lower fat deposits in the liver and to act against cirrhosis, necroses, and hepatitis, conditions affecting the liver. Recent studies have shown that a compound in thistle, sylmarin, increases liver glutathione, a nutritive that plays an important role in the activation of some liver enzymes and in oxygen metabolism. Liver enzymes detoxify many potentially harmful chemicals.

MILONTIN • *See* Phensuximide.

MILOPHENE • *See* Clomiphene Citrate.

MILPREM • *See both* Estrogen and Meprobamate.

MILTOWN • *See* Meprobamate.

MINERAL OIL (OTC) • **Liquid Petrolatum. Agoral Plain. Aqua Care Lotion. Aquaphor. Duolube Eye Ointment. Eucerin Lotion. Fleet Mineral Oil. Haley's M-O. Keri Lotion. Kondremul Plain. Lacri-Lube. Liqui-Doss. Milkinol. Nature's Remedy Enema. Neo-Cultol. Nephrox Suspension. pHisoDerm Skin Cleanser. Refresh. Replens. Ultra Mide. White Mineral Oil. Zymenol.** A mixture of refined liquid hydrocarbons derived from petroleum. Used as an enema or in liquid that acts like a lubricant for the feces. Also used in treatment of constipation and for preparation of bowel studies or surgery. Potential adverse reactions include nausea, abdominal cramping, fluid and electrolyte disturbances, itching, and decreased absorption of nutrients and fat-soluble vitamins. Contraindicated in abdominal pain, nausea, vomiting, or other symptoms of appendicitis, heart damage, fecal impaction, rectal fissures, intestinal obstruction or perforation, and kidney disease. Oral drugs or meals should not be given within two hours of taking this laxative. Should be taken at bedtime. Should not be used for more than one week. Mineral oil is also used as a lubricant in eyedrops and skin preparations. *See* Laxative.

MINERAL SUPPLEMENT (OTC) • A tablet, capsule, or liquid that provides additional inorganic nutrients from sources outside the diet.

MINERAL WAX (OTC) • **Aquaphor Healing Ointment.** Used to soothe dry, cracked skin and minor burns. Also recommended for patients undergoing radiation for follow-up treatment of the skin.

MINIPRESS • *See* Prazosin Hydrochloride.

MINITRAN • *See* Nitroglycerin.

MINIZIDE (Rx) • A combination of prazosin and polythiazide (*see both*) used to treat high blood pressure. There is some reservation about using fixed-dose antihypertensives. Potential adverse reactions include nausea, vomiting, dizziness, weakness, fatigue, heart palpitations, loss of appetite, diarrhea, constipation, upset stomach, swelling of the arms or legs, shortness of breath, fainting, rapid heartbeat, chest pain, muscle spasms, nervousness, depression, tingling in the hands and feet, sensitivity to sunlight, blurred vision, frequent urination, loss of urinary control, impotence, eye redness, ringing in the ears, stuffy nose, sweating, and dry mouth. Anti-inflammatory drugs and pain relievers may make it less effective. Estrogen-containing drugs or drugs with stimulant properties also make it less effective. Minizide's effectiveness is increased when combined with other antihypertensive medications. Should be taken with food.

MINOCIN • *See* Minocycline.

MINOCYCLINE (Rx) • **Minocin.** A tetracycline (*see*) antibiotic introduced in 1970 to treat infections caused by sensitive gram-negative and gram-positive (*see both*) bacterial infections, trachoma, and amebiasis (*see both*). Six clinical centers in the United States tested minocycline against rheumatoid arthritis. The studies, reported in the January 15, 1995, issue of *Annals of Internal Medicine,* concluded that minocycline reduces joint pain and swelling and is safe in patients with mild to moderate disease. Potential adverse reactions to minocycline include a drop in white blood cells, light-headedness, dizziness, inflammation of the heart, sore throat, sore tongue, trouble swallowing, loss of appetite, nausea, vomiting, diarrhea, colitis, anogenital inflammation, skin rash, photosensitivity, increased pigmentation, and hives and other hypersensitivity reactions, as well as blood clots at the site of injection. Antacids, including sodium bicarbonate, and laxatives containing aluminum, magnesium, or calcium may make the drug less effective. Iron also may decrease its effectiveness. Oral contraceptives may be ineffective when taking minocycline. Methoxyflurane (*see*) may cause severe kidney damage when taken with tetracycline (*see*). May be taken with food or milk.

MINODYL • *See* Minoxidil.

MINOXIDIL (Rx) (OTC) • **Loniten. Minodyl. Rogaine.** Introduced in 1972, minoxidil produces a direct effect to relax blood vessels in severe hypertension. In a topical solution, it is used to grow hair. It dilates the blood vessels around the hair follicles. The best results for this use are in patients with balding areas smaller than four inches that occurred within ten years. It takes about four months before any results appear, and only 40 percent of patients will see moderate to dense hair growth in that time. Discontinuing the drug may result in the loss of new hair, which is usually very fine in texture. Potential adverse effects include edema, irregular heartbeat, congestive heart failure, skin rash, hair growth, and breast tenderness. When used topically, it may cause headache, dizziness, faintness, fluid retention, chest pain, increased or decreased blood pressure, palpitations, increased or decreased pulse rate, sinusitis, urinary and upper-respiratory tract infections, kidney stones, inflammation of the urine channel, irritation, allergic contact dermatitis, local scalp redness, itching, dry skin or scalp, flaking, hair loss, back pain, and inflammation of the tendons. Guanethidine may cause severe orthostatic low blood pressure when taken with minoxidil, and those taking the combination must stand up slowly. Topical corticosteroids, topical retinoids, petrolatum, or other drugs that may enhance skin absorption may increase the risk of systemic effects of the topical preparation of minoxidil. Contraindicated in patients with hypersensitivity to any components of the topical solution. During application of the spray, inhalation should be avoided. The oral medication may be taken at any time since it is not affected by food or liquids. An effort by Upjohn to gain FDA approval for an over-the-counter version of minoxidil was turned down in 1994 because it was feared consumers would believe if a little bit helps, a lot may be better and would overtreat their bald heads. It was approved for OTC status in 1996. Generic versions are in the works.

MINT (H) • *Mentha.* Peppermint and spearmint are alike in their actions, but peppermint is the stronger of the two. They are both used as flavorings, and in herbal teas to aid digestion. Peppermint is also used for headaches, vomiting, and insomnia, as a bath additive for general aches and pains, and as a salve for massage. Spearmint is used in folk medicine for "women's complaints."

MINTEZOL • *See* Thiabendazole.

MINT GEL SENSODYNE • *See* Potassium Nitrate.

MINUTE-GEL • *See* Sodium Fluoride.

MIOCHOL • *See* Acetylcholine.

MIOSTAT • *See* Carbachol.

MIOTIC • A drug that constricts or narrows the pupils.

MISOPROSTOL (Rx) • **Cytotec.** A prostaglandin introduced in 1989. Indicated for administration along with nonsteroidal anti-inflammatory drugs, including aspirin, to decrease the chance of developing an NSAID-induced gastric ulcer (*see* NSAIDs), and for other patients with high risk of developing gastric ulceration, such as those with a history of ulcer, the elderly, and the debilitated. Misoprostol has not been shown to prevent duodenal ulcers in patients taking NSAIDs. Contraindicated in pregnant women because it causes miscarriage. Brazilian women use the drug to induce abortions. The most frequent gastrointestinal adverse reactions are diarrhea and abdominal pain. Other potential adverse reactions include nausea, gas, headache, heartburn, vomiting, and constipation. Women who received misoprostol during clinical trials reported spotting, cramps, excessive flow, and painful menstruation. Postmenopausal vaginal bleeding may be related to Misoprostol. It reduces stomach acid and may interfere with absorption of drugs such as diazepam and theophylline (*see both*). Should be taken with food.

MISTLETOE (Rx) (H) • *Viscum album* (**European Mistletoe**). *Phoradendron flavescens* (**American Mistletoe**). A parasitical plant with a root firmly attached to the wood of the tree on which it grows. Mistletoe was sacred to the druids, who reputedly used it to cure sterility and epilepsy, and as an antidote for poisons. Hippocrates and Galen used it as an external remedy and, internally, to treat sleep disorders. Mistletoe is used by herbalists as a purgative, antispasmodic, and emetic. Also used as a sedative. Extracts have been used by physicians to prevent postpartum hemorrhage, treat high blood pressure, and aid in the induction of labor in at-term pregnancy. Should not be taken if MAO inhibitors (*see*) have been taken within two weeks because mistletoe contains a high level of tyramine (*see*), and the combination can cause blood pressure to shoot up to dangerous levels. Mistletoe is reported to be toxic to the liver. It should not be used in pregnancy. *See also* Juniper.

MITHRACIN • *See* Plicamycin.

MITHRAMYCIN • *See* Plicamycin.

MITOMYCIN (Rx) • **Mutamycin.** A cytotoxic (*see*) antibiotic produced by *Streptomyces lavendulae* and used to treat breast, colon, head, neck, lung, pancreatic, and stomach cancers, and malignant melanoma. Potential adverse reactions include nausea, vomiting, loss of appetite, sore mouth, a drop in white blood cells, a sensation of pins and needles in limbs, pain at injection site, reversible hair loss, purple discoloration of nail beds, fever, anemia, kidney failure, and pneumonia. While taking this drug, close supervision by a physician is vital.

MITOSIS • Cell division.

MITOTANE (Rx) • **Lysodren. o,p-DDD.** An anticancer drug that selectively destroys adrenal gland tissue and hinders the use of the adrenal hormone cortisol. Used to treat inoperable cancer of the adrenal gland. Potential adverse reactions include severe nausea, vomiting, drowsiness, dizziness, diarrhea, loss of appetite, adrenal insufficiency, rash, and brain damage. Obese persons may need higher dosages and may have longer-lasting adverse reactions, since the drug distributes mostly to body fat. While taking this drug, close supervision by a physician is vital.

MITOXANTRONE HYDROCHLORIDE (Rx) • **DHAD. Novantrone.** An anticancer drug used for acute nonlymphocytic leukemia (ANL). Potential adverse reactions include nausea, vomiting, diarrhea, sore mouth, abdominal pain, congestive heart failure, irregular heartbeat, fast heartbeat, bleeding, loss of hair, jaundice, fever, seizures, headache, suppression of bone marrow, and high uric acid. While taking this drug, close supervision by a physician is vital.

MITRAL • Pertaining to the valve separating the left atrium from the left ventricle.

MITROLAN • *See* Calcium Polycarbophil.

MIVACRON • *See* Mivacurium.

MIVACURIUM (Rx) • A short-acting muscle relaxant used in surgery, first introduced in 1992.

MIXTARD • *See* Insulin.

MOBAN • *See* Molindone.

MOBIDIN • *See* Magnesium Salicylate.

MOBIGESIC (OTC) • A combination of magnesium salicylate and phenyltoloxamine (*see both*).

MOCLOBEMIDE (Rx) • An MAO inhibitor (*see*) under investigation as an antidepressant and possible anti-Alzheimer's drug. It is believed to have only a mild blood-pressure-raising effect.

MOCTANIN • *See* Monoctanoin.

MODANE • *See* Phenolphthalein.

MODANE BULK • *See* Psyllium.

MODECATE • *See* Fluphenazine Decanoate, Enanthate, or Hydrochloride.

MODICON (Rx) • A combination of ethinyl estradiol and norethindrone (*see both*).

MODRASTANE • *See* Trilostane.

MODURETIC (Rx) • A combination of amiloride and hydrochlorothiazide used as a diuretic to treat high blood pressure or any condition where it is necessary to eliminate excess water from the body. Amiloride spares potassium while producing a diuretic effect. This balances the hydrochlorothiazide's action, which often results in loss of body potassium. Contraindicated in people with diabetes or severe kidney dysfunction, or in those who are allergic to sulfa drugs or any other of the ingredients. The drug may cause abnormally high blood-potassium levels. Potential adverse reactions include nausea, vomiting, headache, weakness, fatigue, dizziness, difficulty in breathing, irregular heartbeat, loss of appetite, rash, itching, leg pain, joint pain, chest and back pain, heart palpitations, constipation, stomach bleeding, stomach upset, a bloated feeling, muscle cramps, tingling in the arms or legs, numbness, stupor, insomnia, nervousness, depression, drowsiness, confusion, visual disturbances, bad taste in the mouth, stuffy nose, sexual impotence, urinary difficulties, blood problems, sugar in the blood or urine, sensitivity to the sun, and restlessness. Moduretic will add to the action of other blood-pressure-lowering drugs. Taking digitalis and adrenal corticosteroids with Moduretic can lead to body fluid imbalances. Lithium carbonate should not be used with this drug, and antidiabetes drug dosages may have to be adjusted. Over-the-counter medications that contain stimulants, such as cough and cold medicines, may cause increased side effects. Moduretic may interfere with oral blood thinners such as warfarin. Should be taken with food.

MOEBIQUIN • *See* Iodoquinol.

MOEX • *See* Moexipril.

MOEXIPRIL (Rx) • **Univase.** A high blood pressure medication introduced in 1995. It is a once-a-day ACE inhibitor (*see*), used alone or in combination with other high blood pressure medications. In some patients, an increase in dosage or twice-daily administration may be necessary because during the end of the dosing interval, the anti–high blood pressure effect may be diminished.

MOI-STIR (OTC) • A saliva substitute.

MOISTURE DROPS • *See* Artificial Tears.

MOISTUREL (OTC) • An oil-in-water emulsion.

MOLECULE • The smallest amount of a specific chemical substance that can exist alone.

MOLINDONE (Rx) • **Moban.** An antipsychotic drug introduced in 1971 for the treatment of acute and chronic schizophrenia. Potential adverse reactions include a drop in white blood cells, extrapyramidal reactions, tardive dyskinesia (*see*), sedation, pseudoparkinsonism, dizziness, a drop in blood pressure when rising from a seated or prone position, blurred vision, dry mouth, urine retention, menstrual irregularities, increased libido, enlargement of male breast, inhibited ejaculation, liver dysfunction, mild photosensitivity, fever, irregular heartbeat, and sweating. Use with alcohol and other central nervous system depressants may increase central nervous system depression. Contraindicated in coma and in central nervous system depression. Should be used with caution when increased physical activity would be harmful, in seizures, and in those who are suicide risks. Should be taken with food or a full glass of water or milk to reduce stomach upset.

MOL IRON • *See* Ferrous Sulfate.

MOMETASONE FUROATE (Rx) • **Elocon.** A corticosteroid ointment or cream used to treat skin inflammation. Potential adverse reactions include burning, itching, irritation, dryness, inflammation of the hair follicles, acne, rash around the mouth, spots of pigment loss, hairiness, allergic contact dermatitis, and if covered with a dressing, secondary infection, atrophy, streaks, and blisters. Should be used cautiously in skin problems caused by viruses such as herpes, and in fungal or bacterial skin infections. Should not be used for more than two weeks due to potential absorption into the system, which may cause an effect on the hypothalamus, and pituitary and adrenal glands. Should not be applied near the eyes or mucous membranes, under the arms, on the face, groin, or under the breast unless medically specified.

MOMORDICA CHARANTIA • *See* Bitter Melon.

MONACOLIN K • *See* Lovastatin.

MONAMINE • Containing one amine group. Amines are derived from ammonia.

MONISTAT • *See* Miconazole.

MONKSHOOD (H) • *Aconitum napellus.* A perennial native to Europe and Asia, it is a member of the buttercup family. The drug aconite radix, which is derived from monkshood, is used internally for fevers and externally to relieve arthritis and pain. Valuable as a painkiller. May be toxic in large amounts. *See* Aconite.

MONK'S PEPPER • *See* Chaste Berries.

MONOAMINE OXIDASE • An enzyme that acts in the nervous system to break down certain types of neurotransmitters (chemical messengers sent between nerve cells) such as dopamine, norepinephrine, and serotonin (*see all*).

MONOAMINE OXIDASE INHIBITORS (MAO INHIBITORS, MAOIs) • A class of antidepressant medications usually prescribed for people who have not responded to tricyclic antidepressants (*see*), or who have certain forms of depression with symptoms including an increase in weight, appetite, or sleep. MAOIs may also be used for cases of mixed anxiety and depression, depression accompanied by pain, panic disorder, post–traumatic stress disorder, and bipolar depression. The drugs raise the level of neurotransmitters by preventing their destruction by enzymes. People taking MAOIs must adhere to a special diet due to the interaction of the medications with certain foods. Foods that contain tyramine (*see*), such as cheeses, yogurt, sour cream, beef or chicken liver, and red wines, should be avoided. The combination of MAOIs and tyramine can cause blood pressure to shoot up to dangerous levels. Potential adverse reactions include headache, increased or decreased heart rate, nausea and vomiting, sweating, fever or cold clammy skin, and chest pain.

MONOAMINERGIC • Nerve cells or fibers that transmit nerve impulses stimulated by the neurotransmitters dopamine, norepinephrine, and serotonin (*see all*).

MONOAZO COLOR • A dye made from diazonium and phenol, both coal tar derivatives. *See* Coal Tar.

MONOBENZONE (Rx) • A topically applied drug used to remove skin pigmentation in the treatment of severe vitiligo (*see*).

MONOCID • *See* Cefonicid Sodium.

MONOCLATE-P • *See* Antihemophilic Factor.

MONOCLONAL ANTIBODIES • Antibodies, large protein molecules produced by white blood cells, seek out and destroy harmful foreign substances (antigens). After the invader has been destroyed, the antibodies remain in the blood, on alert should a similar antigen arrive. Antibodies are also useful in matching donors and recipients in organ transplantation, in blood typing, and in measuring and identifying hormones, toxins, and various antigens in blood and fluids. Monoclonal antibodies are highly specific antibodies that are produced by a single cell and its descendants and that recognize only one type of antigen. A monoclonal antibody "factory" is created when two cells of different origin are fused to make a *hybridoma*. A monoclonal cell carrying a gene that directs production of one specific antibody is fused with an "immortal" cell (a cancer cell), which divides continuously. The result is a hybridoma, which produces copious amounts of a specific, pure antibody.

MONOCTANOIN (Rx) • **Moctanin.** Given by infusion after other nonsurgical methods have failed, it dissolves cholesterol gallstones by rendering them more soluble. Potential adverse reactions include nausea, vomiting, diarrhea, loss of appetite, fever, itching, lethargy, chills, sweating, depression, headache, low blood potassium, allergic reactions, and metabolic acidosis. Contraindicated in jaundice and in those with gallbladder infection or a history of recent duodenal ulcer.

MONO-GESIC • *See* Salsalate.

MONOKINES • Powerful chemical substances secreted by monocytes and macrophages. These soluble molecules help direct and regulate the immune responses.

MONOPRIL • *See* Fosinopril.

MONOTERPENES • Found in parsley, carrots, broccoli, cabbage, cucumbers, squash, yams, tomatoes, eggplant, peppers, mint, basil, and citrus fruits, they have some antioxidant properties. Have been found to inhibit cholesterol production and aid protective enzyme activity.

MORBIDITY • A diseased state. Also the ratio of sick to well in a group.

MORE-DOPHILUS • A medicine to treat uncomplicated diarrhea, particularly that caused by antibiotic therapy. *See* Lactobacillus Acidophilus.

MORICIZINE HYDROCHLORIDE (Rx) • **Ethmozine.** Used to treat life-threatening heartbeat irregularities. Potential adverse reactions include dizziness, headache, fatigue, anxiety, numbness, nervousness, sleep disorders, increased heart irregularities, chest pain, blurred vision, nausea, vomiting, abdominal pain, heartburn, diarrhea, dry mouth, urine retention, rash, shortness of breath, drug fever, sweating, and muscle and bone pain. Cimetidine (*see*) may make it more toxic. Propranolol and digoxin may prolong its effects. Moricizine may make theophylline (*see*) less effective.

MORNING AFTER PILLS • The FDA expert panel recommended that certain oral contraceptives be approved for emergency use after unprotected sex. The use of oral contraceptives for this purpose has been approved in six countries and has proven 75 percent effective. Among the brands targeted for this use are Orval, Lo/Oval, Nordette, Triphasil, Levelen, and Tri-Levelen.

MORPHINE SULFATE or HYDROCHLORIDE (Rx) • **Astramorph/PF. Duramorph.**

MS. MSIR. OMS. Pantopon. RMS. Roxanol. A narcotic analgesic altering both the perception of and reaction to pain. Used to relieve severe pain. Potential adverse effects include sedation, sleepiness, lack of alertness, dizziness, euphoria, seizures, low blood pressure, a low heartbeat, nausea, vomiting, constipation, urine retention, and respiratory depression. Alcohol and central nervous system depressants are additive. Use with extreme caution in head injury, increased pressure on the brain, seizures, asthma, chronic lung disease, alcoholism, enlarged prostate, severe liver or kidney disease, acute abdominal conditions, low thyroid, Addison's disease, narrowing of the tube that carries urine, irregular heartbeat, reduced blood flow, toxic psychosis, and in elderly or debilitated patients. Respiratory depression, low blood pressure, and profound sedation may occur if used with general anesthetics, tranquilizers, sedatives, sleeping medications, alcohol, tricyclic antidepressants, and MAO inhibitors (*see*). May worsen or mask gallbladder pain. May cause dependence.

MORRHUATE (Rx) • **Scleromate.** A mixture of sodium salts of saturated and unsaturated fatty acids. Used in treatment of uncomplicated varicose veins, it causes inflammation of the lining and formation of a blood clot, which blocks the injected vein. Fibrous tissue develops, resulting in the obliteration of the vein. Patients with serious cardiovascular disease are not candidates for this procedure. Potential adverse reactions include hives, sloughing, and death of tissue.

MOTHERWORT (H) • *Leonurus cardiaca.* **Heart Gold. Heart Heal. Heart Wort. Lion's Tail. Mother Herb. Mother Weed.** Used worldwide in folk medicine as a tonic for the uterus, due to its alkaloid (*see*) content, and for the heart, due to its glycoside (*see*) content. The herb is also used to treat diarrhea because it contains tannin (*see*). Motherwort has been used to treat high blood pressure, as a sedative, and as an antispasmodic. Reputedly calms palpitations and generally improves heart function. Also used as a douche for the treatment of vaginitis. Has been employed to induce menstruation. Very large doses may cause drowsiness and impaired concentration.

MOTILIUM • *See* Domperidone.

MOTOR NEURON • A nerve supplying skeletal muscles responsible for movement.

MOTRIN • *See* Ibuprofen.

MOUNTAIN ASH EXTRACT • *Sorbus aucuparia.* The extract from the berries of the European tree. High in vitamin C, the berries have been used by herbalists to cure and prevent scurvy (*see*) and to treat nausea. The extract is used in cosmetics as an antioxidant.

MOUNTAIN GRAPE • *See* Oregon Grape Root.

MOUSE-EAR (H) • *Pilosella officinarum.* **Hawkweed.** Named for the shape of its leaves. Its ingredients include coumarin, flavones, and flavonoids. Used as an antispasmodic, expectorant, and astringent. Also used for respiratory problems where there is inflammation and mucus. Used by herbalists to treat bronchitis and bronchial asthma. Has been used in poultices for wound healing.

MOXALACTAM DISODIUM (Rx) • **Latamoxef Disodium. Moxam.** A cephalosporin (*see*) antibiotic used in the treatment of serious infections of the lower-respiratory and urinary tracts, blood poisoning, and central-nervous-system, gynecologic and abdominal, and skin infections. Potential adverse reactions include anemia, bleeding, headache, malaise, numbness, dizziness, colitis, diarrhea, vomiting, loss of appetite, nausea, heartburn, sore tongue, abdominal cramps, spasm and irritation of the anus, and oral thrush. Also may cause genital moniliasis, rash, hives, pain at the site of injection, hypersensitivity, shortness of breath, and fever. Alcohol should not be drunk even several days after medication has been discontinued. Aspirin and other blood thinners taken with moxalactam may increase the risk of bleeding.

MOXAM • *See* Moxalactam Disodium.

MRI • Abbreviation for magnetic resonance imaging—a scanning technique used to obtain views of the brain or spinal cord. No radiation is involved.

MS • *See* Morphine Sulfate or Hydrochloride.

MSIR • *See* Morphine Sulfate or Hydrochloride.

MTX • *See* Methotrexate.

MUCARA • *See* Karaya Gum.

MUCILAGE • A solution in water of the sticky principles of vegetable substances. Used as a soothing application to the mucous membranes.

MUCIN • A secretion containing carbohydrate-rich proteins. Found in saliva and the lining of the stomach.

MUCOLYTIC • A drug that thins and breaks up mucus.

MUCOMYST • *See* Acetylcysteine.

MUCOSA • *See* Mucous Membranes.

MUCOSOL • *See* Acetylcysteine.

MUCOUS MEMBRANES • Mucosa. The thin layers of tissues that line the respiratory, vaginal, and intestinal tracts and are kept moist by a sticky substance called mucus.

MUCUS • The clear, thick secretion from mucous membranes (*see*).

MUGWORT (H) • *Artemisia vulgaris.* Moxa. St. John's Plant. Hippocrates recommended mugwort to aid in the delivery of the placenta after childbirth. One of the most commonly used herbal preparations to induce menstruation, the extract has been shown to stimulate uterine muscle. The leaves of this plant are used to treat shaking, nervousness, and insomnia. The tea or tincture is used by herbalists for treating liver and stomach disorders. The Chinese dry mugwort and then burn it in a therapeutic technique, moxibustion, to treat a variety of ills. Also used for intestinal complaints, including worms and parasites. Contains bitter principle, volatile oil, tannin, and inulin (*see all*). Contraindicated in pregnancy and for those suffering from acute intestinal inflammation including appendicitis.

MUIRA-PUAMA (H) • *Liriosma ovata.* This Brazilian herb is used primarily to treat impotence, frigidity, and diarrhea.

MUK SHENG • *See* Fu Ling.

MULBERRY (H) • *Morus alba. Morus nigra.* Black Mulberry. White Mulberry. The fruit, leaves, twigs, and root bark are used by herbalists as a tonic to treat coughs, inflammation of the lungs, to reduce fever, and to ease the pain of arthritis. The fruit contains sugars that act as a mild laxative. The syrup has been used to soothe sore throats. The mulberry contains citric acid, vitamin C, carotene, succinic acid, choline, coumarin, and tannin (*see all*), among other constituents.

MULLEIN (H) • *Verbascum thapsus.* A perennial of the figwort family, native to Europe, Asia, Africa, and the United States, it grows wild. Its dried leaves were smoked to treat asthma. The ashes were made into soap to restore gray hair to its former color. The crushed flowers reputedly cured warts, and a cloth dipped in hot mullein tea was used for inflammation. Indians used it for upper-respiratory problems. A high content of mucilage and saponins reportedly make this herb useful to treat coughs. It has also been found to have antibiotic properties. During the Civil War, the Confederates relied on mullein for the treatment of respiratory problems whenever their medical supplies ran out.

MULTIPLE MYELOMA • A malignant condition characterized by the uncontrolled proliferation and disordered function of plasma cells (a type of white blood cell) in the bone marrow. It occurs from middle to old age and leaves patients vulnerable to increased infections and anemia.

MULTIPLE SCLEROSIS (MS) • A progressive disease of the central nervous system in which scattered patches of the covering of nerve fibers (myelin) in the brain and spinal cord are destroyed. Symptoms range from numbness and tingling to paralysis.

MUMPS VIRUS VACCINE, LIVE • **Mumpsvax.** Promotes active immunity to mumps. Given to adults and to children over one year of age. Potential adverse reactions include slight fever, rash, malaise, mild allergic reactions, and rarely, fever seizures.

MUPIROCIN (Rx) • **Bactroban.** An ointment used to treat common bacterial skin infections caused by susceptible bacteria. Used particularly to treat impetigo (*see*). May cause local burning, itching, stinging, and rash.

MURINE EAR DROPS (OTC) • *See* Carbamide Peroxide.

MURINE PLUS (OTC) • *See* Tetrahydrozoline.

MUROCEL • *See* Methylcellulose.

MUROCOLL-2 (Rx) • *See* Phenylephrine.

MUROMONAB-CD3 (Rx) • **Orthoclone OKT3.** An immunosuppressant drug used to prevent organ rejection following transplant surgery. Potential adverse reactions include nausea, vomiting, diarrhea, chest pain, severe fluid in the lungs, fever, chills, tremors, heartburn, and infection.

MURO-128 OINTMENT (Rx) • Removes excess fluid from the cornea. *See* Sodium Chloride.

MURO OPCON-A (OTC) • A combination of naphazoline and pheniramine (*see both*) used to reduce redness of eye irritation.

MURO OPHTHALMIC (OTC) • *See* Sodium Chloride.

MURO TEARS (OTC) • *See* Hydroxypropyl Methylcellulose.

MUSCLE RELAXANT • A pharmaceutical that relaxes muscles that are tense or in spasm. Many tranquilizers have this ability.

MUSCULAR DYSTROPHY • An inherited muscular disorder of unknown cause in which muscle fibers slowly degenerate.

MUSTARD (OTC) (H) • *Brassica hirta. B. alba. Sinapis alba.* **Yellow and White.** The pulverized, dried, ripe seeds of the mustard plant native to southern Europe and western Asia and naturalized in the United States. Used as an emergency emetic to cause vomiting. *See* Mustard, Black.

MUSTARD, BLACK (OTC) (H) • *Brassica nigra.* **Boiss. Koch.** A native of Europe and the Americas, it is cultivated in Holland, Italy, and Germany as a condiment. Mustard seed is used to stimulate appetite. Mustard is used medicinally to treat arthritis, sciatica, and other pain. It is also used as an emetic to counteract ingested poisons. Mustard plasters were a popular treatment for pain and swelling. Mustard is used in footbaths and to treat colds. Mustard is rapidly absorbed and is used as a counterirritant (*see*). It is irritating to the skin, however, and can cause burns that are slow to heal.

MUSTARGEN • *See* Mechlorethamine.

MUTAGENIC • Having the power to cause mutations. A mutation is a sudden change in the character of a gene that is perpetuated in subsequent divisions of the cells in which it occurs. It can be induced by the application of such stimuli as radiation, certain food chemicals, or pesticides. Certain food additives, such as caffeine, have been found to "break" chromosomes.

MUTAMYCIN • *See* Mitomycin.

MUTATION • A permanent change in the genetic material that will be passed on to new generations of cells.

MUXU • *See* Alfalfa.

MY-, MYO- • Prefixes meaning pertaining to muscle, as in *myocardium,* the heart muscle.

MYADEC • A multivitamin and mineral preparation.

MYAMBUTOL • *See* Ethambutol.

MYAPAP • *See* Acetaminophen.

MYASTHENIA GRAVIS • A disease characterized by episodes of muscle weakness, chiefly in muscles that are controlled by the cranial nerves. It is improved by cholinesterase-inhibiting drugs. *See* Cholinesterase.

MYCELEX • *See* Clotrimazole.

MYCIFRADIN • *See* Neomycin.

MYCIGUENT • *See* Neomycin.

MYCITRACIN • *See* Bacitracin and Neomycin.

MYCOBUTIN • *See* Rifabutin.

MYCOLOG • *See* Triamcinolone.

MYCOLOG II • *See* Nystatin and Triamcinolone.

MYCOPHENOLATE MOFETIL (Rx) • **Cellcept.** An oral medication, introduced in 1995, for use in combination with cyclosporine and corticosteroids (*see both*) for the prevention of organ rejection in kidney transplant patients.

MYCOPLASMA • Bacteria that may be found in the human body but that may cause disease under certain conditions.

MYCOSTATIN • *See* Nystatin.

MYCO-TRIACET • A combination of triamcinolone and nystatin.

MYCOZYME • In 1992, the FDA issued a notice that mycozyme had not been shown to be safe and effective as claimed in OTC digestive-aid products.

MYDFRIN • *See* Phenylephrine.

MYDRIACYL • *See* Tropicamide.

MYDRIAFAIR • *See* Tropicamide.

MYDRIASIS • Dilation of the pupil of the eye.

MYDRIATIC • A drug that dilates or widens the pupils.

MYELIN • The protective covering of most nerves.

MYELO- • Prefix meaning pertaining to marrow.

MYELOGENOUS LEUKEMIA • **CGL.** One of the many forms of cancer of the blood-forming organs in the bone marrow.

MYELOID • Referring to or derived from bone marrow.

MYFRIN • *See* Phenylephrine.

MYIDIL • *See* Triprolidine.

MYIDONE • *See* Primidone.

MYKINAC • *See* Nystatin.

MYKROX • *See* Metolazone.

MYLANTA (OTC) • A combination of aluminum hydroxide, magnesium hydroxide, and simethicone (*see all*), used as an antacid and to relieve intestinal gas.

MYLAXEN • *See* Hexafluorenium.

MYLERAN • *See* Busulfan.

MYLICON DROPS • *See* Simethicone.

MYLICON-80 • *See* Simethicone.

MYO- • Prefix meaning related to muscle, as in *myography,* the recording of muscle movements.

MYOCARDIAL INFARCTION • Death of heart muscle tissue due to prolonged inadequate coronary-artery blood flow.

MYOCARDIAL ISCHEMIA • Insufficient blood flow to meet myocardial oxygen needs.

MYOCARDITIS • Inflammation of the myocardium.

MYOCARDIUM • The middle and thickest layer of the heart wall.

MYOCHRYSINE • *See* Aurothioglucose.

MYOCLONUS • Rapid, uncontrollable muscle jerks or spasms that occur at rest or during movement. Can be caused by nerve or muscle disease, epileptic seizures, or brain disorders.

MYOCYTE • A muscle cell.

MYODINE • *See* Iodinated Glycerol.

MYOFLEX ANALGESIC CREAM • *See* Trolamine Salicylate.

MYOGLOBIN • A type of hemoglobin present in muscles. It serves as a short-acting source of oxygen to muscle fibers during contractions.

MYOLIN • *See* Orphenadrine.

MYOPATHY • Any disease of muscle. A usually progressive, degenerative muscle disease, sometimes caused by a chronic immune-system disorder such as AIDS.

MYOSITIS • Inflammation of the muscle.

MYOTONACHOL • *See* Bethanechol.

MYOTROPIN • *See* Insulinlike Growth Factor.

MYPROIC ACID • *See* Valproic Acid.

MYRICACEAE • *See* Bayberry.

MYRICA CERIFERA • *See* Bayberry.

MYRISTICA FRAGRANS • *See* Nutmeg and Mace.

MYROSEMIDE • *See* Furosemide.

MYRRH GUM (H) • *Commiphora molmol* or *myrrha* or *Guggul.* One of the gifts of the Magi, it is a yellowish to reddish brown, aromatic, bitter gum resin that is obtained from various myrrh trees, especially from East Africa and Arabia. The gum resin has been used to break up intestinal gas and as a topical stimulant. The Chinese for centuries used the herb to treat menstrual problems and bleeding. In Asia and Africa, it was used as an antiseptic for mucous membranes. It is also used as a stimulant tonic; some constituents in myrrh stimulate gastric secretions and relax smooth muscles. In modern studies, myrrh has been shown to inhibit grampositive bacteria (*see*) such as *Staphylococcus aureus.* The herb contains volatile oils, including limonene, eugenol, and pinene, which have been found helpful in easing breathing during colds, and increasing circulation. It also contains tannin, which is thought to be the reason that myrrh allays the pain and speeds the healing of mouth ulcers and sore gums. In 1992, the FDA issued a notice that myrrh fluid extract had not been shown to be safe and effective as claimed in OTC digestive-aid products.

MYRRHIS ODORATA • *See* Sweet Cicely.

MYSOLINE • *See* Primidone.

MYSTECLIN-F (Rx) • *See* Amphotericin B and Tetracyclines.

MYTREX • *See* Triamcinolone.

MYTUSSIN • *See* Guaifenesin.

MYXEDEMA • Thyroid deficiency.

N

NABILONE (Rx) • Cesamet. Chemically related to marijuana, it is used to treat nausea caused by anticancer drugs. Potential adverse reactions include drowsiness, vertigo, euphoria, anxiety, depression, disorientation, loss of balance, headache, rapid heartbeat, a sudden drop in blood pressure when rising from a seated or prone position, blurred vision, dry mouth, and increased appetite. Should not be used for nausea and vomiting from any cause other than chemotherapy. Should be used with caution in elderly patients, and those with high blood pressure, heart disease, or psychiatric illness. Alcohol, antihistamines, and other central nervous system depressants may increase adverse effects and will also add to the sedative effects.

NABINOL (Rx) • A synthetic marijuana. *See* Nabilone.

NABUMETONE (Rx) • Relafen. One of a new class of nonsteroidal prostaglandin inhibitors introduced in 1991, it is indicated for the treatment of osteoarthritis and rheumatoid arthritis. It is the first nonacidic NSAID and the first NSAID prodrug (*see both*)—that is, it does not become active as the acidic metabolite until after it passes through the stomach and is processed by the liver. It has anti-inflammatory, analgesic, and fever-lowering properties. Promoted as having fewer GI symptoms than other NSAIDs, including diarrhea, heartburn, and abdominal pain. Also promoted as having a once-a-day dosage. Potential adverse reactions include ulceration and bleeding in patients continuously taking the drug. Must be used with caution in patients with heart failure, high blood pressure, and other conditions predisposing to fluid retention. Must be used with caution when warfarin (*see*) is given because the combination may cause increased blood thinning. Other potential adverse reactions include diarrhea, heartburn, abdominal pain, constipation, gas, nausea, dry mouth, vomiting, dizziness, headache, fatigue, increased sweating, insomnia, nervousness, sleepiness, itching, rash, ringing in the ears, and edema. Rare reactions include loss or increase of appetite, jaundice, duodenal ulcer, gastrointestinal bleeding, hives, depression, agitation, loss of hair, palpitations, abnormal vision, and kidney inflammation. May be taken with or without food.

NADOLOL (Rx) • Corgard. A beta-blocker (*see*) introduced in 1980, it reduces the heart's need for oxygen, high blood pressure, and irregular heartbeat. Also used to treat thyroid gland hyperactivity, and to prevent migraine headaches. When prescribed for hypertension, it is often combined with a diuretic (*see*). One of its advantages over other beta-blockers is that nadolol need be taken only once a day. Potential adverse reactions include fatigue, irregular or slow heartbeat, congestive heart failure, nausea, vomiting, diarrhea, decreased libido, impotence or impaired erection, low blood sugar, rash, and fever. Because it can cause breathing problems, nadolol is not prescribed for asthmatics or persons suffering from chronic bronchitis. Antihypertensive drugs may interact and cause blood pressure to drop too low. Cardiac glycosides and epinephrine (*see both*) may increase heart side effects. Nadolol may alter insulin requirements in diabetics. Will interact with any psychoactive drugs, including MAO inhibitors (*see*) that stimulate the adrenal gland. The drug should not be discontinued suddenly. May be taken with or without food.

NADOPEN-V • *See* Penicillin V.

NADOSTINE • *See* Nystatin.

NAFARELIN ACETATE (Rx) • Synarel. A nasal solution of gonadotropin-releasing hormone (GnRH) (*see*) analog, introduced in 1984, that acts on the pituitary to decrease the release of follicle-stimulating hormone (FSH) and luteinizing hormone (LH). Reportedly causes fewer masculinizing effects than danazol (*see*) and has less of a tendency than danazol to increase blood cholesterol levels. The result is decreased ovarian stimulation, lowered circulating estrogens, and improvement of the symptoms associated with endometriosis (*see*). Potential adverse reactions include headache, emotional instability, insomnia, depression, edema, nasal irritation, vaginal dryness, acne, hairiness, hot flashes, decreased libido, muscle pain, reduced breast size, weight gain or loss, bone loss, and decreased bone density. Contraindicated in patients hypersensitive to GnRH analogs or any component of the formulation (benzalkonium chloride, sorbitol, purified water, glacial acetic acid, hydrochloric acid, and sodium hydroxide). Also contraindicated in the presence of undiagnosed vaginal bleeding, in breast-feeding women, and during pregnancy. Nafarelin may harm the fetus.

NAFAZAIR • *See* Naphazoline.

NAFCIL • *See* Nafcillin.

NAFCILLIN (Rx) • **Nafcil. Nallpen. Sodium Nafcillin. Unipen.** A penicillin antibiotic used to treat systemic infections caused by penicillinase-secreting staphylococci (*see*). Potential adverse reactions include a drop in white blood cells and platelets, nausea, vomiting, diarrhea, vein irritation and clot at site of injection, and hypersensitivity, including potentially fatal anaphylaxis.

NAFTIFINE (Rx) • **Naftin.** A cream to treat fungal infections such as jock itch, athlete's foot, and ringworm. Potential adverse reactions include local burning, dryness, itching, stinging, and irritation. Should not be used around the eyes, nose, or mouth.

NAFTIN • *See* Naftifine.

NALBUPHINE HYDROCHLORIDE (Rx) • **Nubain.** An injectable narcotic analgesic altering both the perception of and reaction to pain. Used to treat moderate to severe pain. Potential adverse effects include sedation, dizziness, euphoria, hostility, unusual dreams, confusion, hallucinations, delusions, cramps, heartburn, vomiting, severe constipation, urinary urgency, itching, burning, hives, a cold, clammy feeling, and respiratory depression. Alcohol and central nervous system depressants are additive. Use with other narcotic analgesics may decrease nalbuphine's analgesic effect. Contraindicated in acute alcoholism, emotional instability, a history of drug abuse, increased pressure on the brain, and respiratory depression.

Should be used cautiously in liver and kidney disease. Also acts as a narcotic antagonist; may cause withdrawal symptoms.

NALDECON CX ADULT LIQUID (OTC) • A combination of phenylpropanolamine, guaifenesin, and codeine (*see all*). It is alcohol free and sugar free. It is used for temporary relief of nasal congestion due to the common cold, hay fever, or other respiratory allergies, or associated with sinusitis. It is also used for dry, hacking coughs. Contraindicated in those allergic to any of the ingredients. Those taking medicine for high blood pressure or depression should consult a physician before taking this drug. Potential adverse effects include constipation. Naldecon may be taken with food.

NALDECON DX ADULT LIQUID (OTC) • Used for dry, hacking coughs, nasal decongestion and expectoration, it contains phenylpropanolamine, guaifenesin, and dextromethorphan (*see all*). It is sugar free. Contraindicated in those allergic to any of the ingredients and must be used with caution in those taking medicines for high blood pressure or depression, and in persons with heart disease, thyroid disease, diabetes, or difficulty urinating. Naldecon may be taken with food.

NALDECON EX CHILDREN'S SYRUP (OTC) • Contains phenylpropanolamine and guaifenesin (*see both*) to treat coughs and stuffy noses. The combination is sugar free. The drug should not be given to a child who is taking a prescription drug for high blood pressure or depression without first checking with the pediatrician. The doctor should also be consulted before giving this medication if the child has heart disease, thyroid problems, or diabetes. Exceeding the recommended dose could cause nervousness, dizziness, or sleeplessness in any child. Naldecon may be taken with food.

NALFON • *See* Fenoprofen.

NALIDIXIC ACID (Rx) • **Nalidixinic Acid. NegGram. Wintomylon.** A quinolone (*see*) introduced in 1963, it is one of the oldest synthetic antibiotics. Used to treat acute and chronic urinary-tract infections caused by susceptible gram-negative (*see*) organisms. Taken by mouth, it does not accumulate in the body tissues, but is concentrated in the urine. Potential adverse effects include lung problems, drowsiness, weakness, headache, dizziness, seizures in epileptics, confusion, hallucinations, sensitivity to light, change in color perception, double vision, blurred vision, abdominal pain, nausea, vomiting, diarrhea, rash, skin photosensitivity, hives, fever, chills, and increased pressure on the brain in infants and children. The drug may give a false high reading of blood sugar level. It increases the effects of blood thinners. Antacids decrease the absorption of nalidixic acid. Most effective when taken with a full glass of water on an empty stomach. If stomach upset is a problem, it may be taken with a small amount of food or milk.

NALIDIXINIC ACID • *See* Nalidixic Acid.

NALLPEN • *See* Nafcillin.

N-ALLYLNOROXYMORPHONE • *See* Naloxone Hydrochloride.

NALMEFENE (Rx) • **Revex.** A newer opiate antagonist (*see*) introduced in 1995. It may cause complete or partial reversal of effects of opiods, including respiratory depression. Unlike naloxone (*see*), which is active for one to two hours in the body, it is active for eight to ten hours.

NALOXONE HYDROCHLORIDE (Rx) • **N-allynoroxymorphone. Narcan.** An antidote for narcotic-induced respiratory depression after surgery or caused by an overdose of narcotics. It is sometimes given to newborns to improve their breathing. Potential adverse reactions include nausea, vomiting, rapid heartbeat, high blood pressure, tremors, and withdrawal symptoms in narcotic-dependent patients.

NALTREXONE (Rx) • **Revia. Trexan.** A drug used in the treatment of narcotic dependence. Not itself a narcotic, it works by blocking the euphoria caused by narcotics. In 1995, it was also approved as a safe and effective adjunct to psychosocial treatments for alcoholism. Potential adverse reactions include nausea, vomiting, loss of appetite, weight gain, itching, headache, swollen glands, insomnia, anxiety, depression, abdominal pain, liver damage, and muscle and joint pain. There is also a risk of liver damage in excessive doses, and the drug is contraindicated in acute hepatitis or liver failure.

NANDROBOLIC LA • *See* Nandrolone.

NANDROLONE (Rx) • **Anabolin. Androlone-D. Deca-Durabolin. Hybolin Decanoate. Kabolin. Nandrobolic LA. Neo-Durabolic.** An anabolic steroid introduced in 1959 that promotes tissue building and reverses loss of tissue. Also stimulates the production of red blood cells. Used to treat severe debility or disease states, and to help control metastatic breast cancer. Potential adverse reactions in women include acne, oily skin, weight gain, hairiness, hoarseness, clitoral enlargement, changes in libido, flushing, sweating, and vaginitis with itching. In prepubescent males, premature epiphyseal closure, priapism (*see*), growth of body and facial hair, and phallic enlargement; in postpubescent males, testicular atrophy, scanty sperm, decreased ejaculatory volume, impotence, breast enlargement, and epididymitis. In both sexes, edema, gastroenteritis, nausea, vomiting, diarrhea, constipation, changes in appetite, bladder irritability, jaundice, liver toxicity, and high levels of calcium in the blood. Contraindicated in men with enlarged or cancerous prostates, carcinoma of the male breast, and in both sexes with high levels of calcium in the blood, and heart, liver, or kidney dysfunction; also, in premature infants. Should be used cautiously in prepubescent males, patients with diabetes or heart disease, and patients taking ACTH, corticosteroids, or anticoagulants. Should be taken with food or meals.

NAPAMIDE • *See* Disopyramide.

NAPHAZOLINE (OTC) • **AK-Con. Albalon. Albalon Liquifilm. Allerest Eye Drops. Allergy Eye Drops. Clear Eyes. Degest-2. Estivin ll.**

4-Way Fast Acting Nasal Spray. I-Naphline. Muro Opcon A. Nafazair. Naphcon. Naphcon-A. Ocu-Zoline. Opcon. Opcon-A. Privine. VasoClear. Vasocon. Introduced in 1942, naphazoline is used in eyedrops to relieve redness due to eye irritation. It constricts the blood vessels in red, irritated, itching eyes. In nose drops or sprays, it is used to treat stuffy nose. Potential adverse reactions to eyedrops include transient stinging, dilation of the pupil, irritation, sensitivity to light, dizziness, headache, increased sweating, nausea, nervousness, and weakness. In nose preparations, it may cause rebound stuffy nose, sneezing, stinging, dryness of mucosa, and in children after prolonged use, marked sedation. Tricyclic antidepressants and MAO inhibitors (*see both*) may increase blood pressure to dangerous levels if used with naphazoline. Contraindicated in glaucoma or hypersensitivity to any ingredients in the naphazoline products. Should be used cautiously in patients with hyperthyroidism, heart disease, high blood pressure, or diabetes. Rebound congestion in the eyes or nose may occur with frequent or prolonged use.

NAPHCON • *See* Naphazoline.

NAPHCON-A • *See* Naphazoline and Pheniramine.

NAPRELAN (Rx) • A once-a-day formulation of naproxen (*see*). Reportedly has less side effects.

NAPROSYN • *See* Naproxen.

NAPROXEN (Rx) (OTC) • **Aleve. Anaprox. Naprosyn.** Introduced in 1974, it produces anti-inflammatory, analgesic, and fever-reducing effects, probably by inhibiting prostaglandins (*see*). It is used to treat arthritis, mild to moderate pain, sprains, strains, acute tendinitis, bursitis, lower-back pain, soft-tissue trauma, and painful menstruation. Naproxen is promoted as a pain reliever that acts within twenty minutes of ingestion. It is nonnarcotic, and its nonsteroidal anti-inflammatory action helps patients return to action faster. Naproxen sodium is more readily absorbed than naproxen alone. The most common side effect is gastrointestinal, such as abdominal pain, gas, peptic ulcer, and nausea. Other potential adverse reactions include a low white blood count, drowsiness, dizziness, shortness of breath, visual disturbances, headache, water retention, hemorrhage, painful and/or bloody urine, kidney toxicity, liver toxicity, rash, and hives. Oral blood thinners or sulfonylureas (*see*) may increase blood toxicity. Contraindicated in asthmatics with nasal polyps. Should be used cautiously in elderly patients, in patients with kidney or heart disease, or GI disorders, and those allergic to NSAIDs (*see*), including aspirin. Should also be used cautiously in patients with ulcers. Use with aspirin, alcohol, or steroids may increase the risk of adverse GI reactions. Should be taken with food, milk, or an antacid to avoid stomach upset. Introduced in weaker form for over-the-counter use in 1994 (*see* Aleve). Also slated to be produced in generic form.

NAPSYLATE • **2-Naphthaleneacetic Acid.** Obtained from coal tar (*see*), used in analgesics. Also used as a plant-growth regulator.

NAPTRATE • *See* Pentaerythritol Tetranitrate.

NAQUA • *See* Trichlormethiazide.

NAQUIVAL • *See* Reserpine and Trichlormethiazide.

NARCAN • *See* Naloxone Hydrochloride.

NARCOLEPSY • Irresistible attacks of sleep, often accompanied by muscle weakness.

NARCOSIS • A state of deep sleep, unconsciousness, and insensibility to pain.

NARCOTICS • Drugs that act on the brain and nerves to relieve pain. Some are used before or during operative procedures as an adjunct to anesthesia. Some, such as codeine and hydrocodone, are included in cough medicine to relieve coughs. Methadone is used to help drug addicts to reduce their need for narcotics. The side effects of narcotics are often related to their effects on the central nervous system, such as confusion, dizziness, drowsiness, nausea, and vomiting. Long-term use of narcotics can cause physical and emotional dependence.

NARDIL • *See* Phenelzine.

NARROW ANGLE GLAUCOMA • Pressure that builds up within the eye because the drainage angle is extremely narrow and then blockage occurs. The outer edge of the iris contracts to enlarge the pupil when light is dim, or when you react to a strong emotion, and the fluid in the eye builds up. When the iris recedes after the light has changed or the emotion has passed, the liquid resumes its normal drainage. If the liquid fails to drain because the outlet is too narrow or blocked, pressure builds up—glaucoma— and if it is not relieved, ultimately sight will be destroyed. Narrow angle glaucoma may occur at any age, but is most common after thirty years. The pupil becomes dilated and fixed and the iris appears muddy. Severe headache and eye ache, blurred vision, seeing halos around lights, general malaise, nausea, and sometimes vomiting result during an acute attack.

NASACORT (Rx) • **Triamcinolone.** A once-a-day nasal anti-inflammatory inhaler for use by asthmatics and persons suffering from nasal allergies. *See* Triamcinolone.

NASAHIST (OTC) • A combination of chlorpheniramine, phenylephrine, and phenylpropanolamine (*see all*) to treat nasal congestion.

NASAHIST B • *See* Brompheniramine.

NASAL ADMINISTRATION OF DRUGS • This route of drug administration is becoming more popular. Although it has been used for a long time for introducing medication for local nasal disease, it offers a number of general advantages. The nose, like the mouth, has a mucosal surface with its multiple blood vessels that is well adapted to the absorption of drugs. This avoids the destruction of drugs by gastrointestinal fluids and by the liver. The rate and extent of absorption and other drug actions can approach those achieved by intravenous administration. A number of drugs are being studied for intranasal sprays and drops. Those already on the market for nasal disease include decongestants, cromolyn sodium, corticosteroids, anticholinergic drugs, saline, propylene glycol, and interferon (*see all*); for nonnasal diseases, desmopressin, oxytocin, insulin, and gentamicin.

NASALCROM • *See* Cromolyn Sodium.

NASAL DECONGESTANT SPRAY • Medicine in spray form used to reduce nasal swelling and congestion and allow the user to breathe more easily.

NASALIDE • *See* Flunisolide.

NASAL MOISTURIZING NASAL SPRAY • *See* Sodium Chloride.

NASTURTIUM (H) • *Tropaeolum majus.* An annual, native to South America and cultivated all over the world. Its name means "trophy," and the plant was said to have arisen from the blood of a Trojan warrior. The extract of the leaves and stems of this member of the mustard family has a pungent taste. It is rich in vitamins A and C and contains vitamins B and B_2 as well. It was used to treat scurvy and as an antiseptic. As a tonic, it was said to benefit the blood and digestive system. It is also used by herbalists to treat bronchitis. It is soothing to the skin and supposedly has blood-thinning factors and increases the flow of urine.

NATABEC • A multivitamin and mineral preparation.

NATACYN • *See* Natamycin.

NATAFORT (OTC) • A multivitamin and mineral preparation.

NATAL CLEFT • The furrow between the buttocks.

NATALINS (OTC) • A multivitamin and mineral preparation.

NATAMYCIN (OTC) • **Myprozine. Natacyn. Pimaricin.** A drug used to treat fungal infections of the eye or eyelid. Potential adverse reactions include swelling around the eyes and "black eyes" from blood gathering there.

NATRA-BIO ACNE (H) • A homeopathic medicine for treating and preventing acne pimples.

NAT-C • Homeopathic abbreviation for natrum carbonicum (*see*).

NAT-M • Homeopathic abbreviation for natrum muriatricum (*see*).

NAT. MUR. • *See* Natrum Muriatricum.

NAT-P • Homeopathic abbreviation for natrum phosphoricum (*see*).

NAT. PHOS. • Homeopathic abbreviation for natrum phosphoricum (*see*).

NATRA-BIO ACNE (H) • A homeopathic medicine for treating and preventing acne pimples.

NATRA-BIO CAFFEINE WITHDRAWAL (H) • A homeopathic medicine for those trying to cut back or discontinue caffeine. The producers claim it helps prevent headaches, nervousness, irritability, or sleeplessness that may occur with normal caffeine withdrawal.

NATRA-BIO COLD TABLETS (H) • A homeopathic medicine for treating all types of colds. The company claims it speeds relief from runny nose, sneezing, sore throat, headache, and itchy, watery eyes.

NATRECOR • *See* Brain Natriuretic Peptide.

NATRUM MURIATRICUM (H) • **Nat-M. Nat. Mur.** A homeopathic medicine (*see*) composed of sodium chloride, common table salt. Sodium chloride is the chief component of blood and other body fluids, and urine. Without sufficient sodium chloride, the human body cannot function. Sodium chloride in solution is used topically to treat inflamed lesions. *See* Tissue Salts.

NATRIUM PHOSPHORICUM (H) • **Nat-P. Nat. Phos.** A homeopathic medicine (*see*) composed of sodium phosphate. Sodium is a metallic element that has many uses. Phosphate is also needed to maintain the acid/alkali balance. Sodium phosphate is used in conventional medicine as a laxative. *See* Tissue Salts.

NATRIUM SULPHURICUM (H) • **Nat-S. Nat. Sulph.** A homeopathic medicine (*see*) composed of sodium and sulfate is the salt of sulfuric acid. It helps control the acid/alkali balance. It is used for anxiety, depression, backache, cough, head injuries, headache, and indigestion. *See* Tissue Salts.

NAT-S • Homeopathic abbreviation for natrium sulphuricum (*see*).

NAT. SULPH. • Homeopathic abbreviation for natrum sulphuricum (*see*).

NATURACIL • *See* Psyllium.

NATURAL ESTROGENIC HORMONE • In 1992, the FDA proposed a ban on natural estrogenic hormone in oral menstrual drug products because it had not been shown to be safe and effective as claimed. *See* Estrogen.

NATURAL KILLER CELLS (NKS) • Large granule-filled lymphocytes that take on tumor cells and infected body cells. They are known as "natural" killers because they attack without first having to recognize specific antigens.

NATURE'S REMEDY • *See* Cascara Sagrada.

NATURETIN • *See* Bendroflumethiazide.

NAVANE • *See* Thiothixene.

NAVELBINE • *See* Vinorelbine Tartrate.

NCI • Abbreviation for National Cancer Institute.

ND-STAT • *See* Brompheniramine.

NEBCIN • *See* Tobramycin.

NEBULIZER • A device that delivers medication through the nose or mouth in spray or mist form.

NEBUPENT • *See* Pentamidine Isethionate.

NECROTIC • Characterized by death of tissue cells.

NEDOCROMIL (Rx) • **Tilade.** A non-steroidal, inhaled anti-inflammatory agent for the preventive management of asthma. Introduced in 1992 in the United States, it has been on the market in the United Kingdom since 1986. It is used for maintenance therapy of mild to moderate bronchial asthma in patients over the age of twelve. Nedocromil is not a bronchodilator and is not used for the reversal of acute bronchospasm, particularly in severe asthma attacks. The medication must be taken regularly to achieve benefit, even during symptom-free periods. Its benefits occur from topical application to the lungs. Nedocromil is contraindicated in those who have shown hypersensitivity to it or to any of the preparations in the inhaler. Potential adverse effects include unpleasant taste, coughing, nose and throat irritation, shortness of breath, nausea, vomiting, heartburn, diarrhea, dizziness, headache, chest pain, fatigue, and bronchospasm.

NEEM TREE (H) • *Azadirachta indica.* **Margosa. Nim.** A native of India and Burma, it is related to mahogany. Materials from the seeds may work like contraceptives. Exploratory trials in male mammals, including monkeys, show that some compounds in neem reduce fertility without inhibiting sperm production. Furthermore, the reduced fertility effects seem to be temporary. The bark, leaves, and seeds are used in India as a treatment for many skin diseases. The extract of the leaves has been shown to have antibacterial and antiviral activity. Neem is also taken internally to eliminate worms. The branches of the tree are chewed and used to clean the teeth and prevent gum inflammation.

Neem oil has been reported to be toxic to the liver.

NEFAZODONE (Rx) • **Serzone.** An oral medication for the treatment of depression. It was approved in 1994 after a 39.6-month review by the FDA. It is closely related to trazodone (*see*). Unlike many recently introduced antidepressants, nefazodone is not a selective serotonin (*see*) uptake inhibitor. It is also chemically unrelated to tricyclic antidepressants and monamine oxidase inhibitors (*see both*). The medication does inhibit serotonin reuptake and also inhibits the uptake of norepinephrine (*see*). The most common adverse reactions reported were nausea, dizziness, and insomnia. About 1.5 percent of the 3,496 patients who received serzone in clinical trials reported some form of sexual dysfunction such as delayed ejaculation, lack of orgasm, or decreased libido. Among other potential adverse reactions reported were nausea, sleepiness, dry mouth, dizziness, light-headedness, constipation, numbness, blurred vision, confusion, and abnormal vision. Approximately 16 percent of the patients discontinued treatment because of adverse experiences, most commonly nausea, dizziness, insomnia, numbness, and agitation. The FDA requires a warning label about potential interactions of nefazodone with triazolam, alprazolam, terfenadine, astemizole, and MAO inhibitors (*see all*).

NEGRAM • *See* Nalidixic Acid.

NEMBUTAL • *See* Pentobarbital.

NEO-CALGLUCON • *See* Calcium Glubionate.

NEO-CORTEF (Rx) • *See* Hydrocortisone and Neomycin.

NEO-CULTOL • *See* Mineral Oil.

NEODECADRON (Rx) • *See* Dexamethasone and Neomycin.

NEO-DURABOLIC • *See* Nandrolone.

NEOFED • *See* Pseudoephedrine.

NEO-FLO • *See* Boric Acid.

NEOLOID • *See* Castor Oil.

NEO-METRIC • *See* Metronidazole.

NEOMYCIN (Rx) (OTC) • **Neomycin Sulfate. Bactine First Aid Antibiotic. Campho-Phenique Triple Antibiotic Ointment. Faille. Hydromycin. Infectrol. Mycifradin. Myciguent. Mycitracin. Mycitracin Plus Pain Reliever. Neo-Cortef. NeoDecadron. Neo-Polycin. Neosporin Ointment. Neosporin Opthalmic Solution. Neosulf. Neo-Synalar. Neo-Tabs. Neotal. Neotricin.** Introduced in 1951, it was one of the first aminoglycoside (*see*) antibiotics. The oral form is used to treat infectious diarrhea caused by *Escherichia coli* (*see*). Potential adverse reactions include headache, lethargy, ear problems, nausea, vomiting, kidney dysfunction, rash, and hypersensitivity reactions. Interacts with cephalothin, dimenhydrinate, oral anticoagulants (decreases vitamin K), IV loop diuretics (*see both*), cisplatin, methoxyflurane, and other aminoglycoside antibiotics. In a cream or ointment it is used to treat skin infections, minor burns, wounds, skin grafts, itching, inflammation of the outer ear, and skin ulcers. Potential adverse skin reactions include rash, contact dermatitis, hives, and possible kidney, ear, and nerve toxicity when absorbed systemically. The skin product should not be used on more than 20 percent of the body surface. It should also not be used without medical advice to treat deep wounds, puncture wounds, or serious burns.

NEOPAP • *See* Acetaminophen.

NEOPLASM • An abnormal growth of tissue, either benign or malignant.

NEO-POLYCIN • *See* Neomycin.

NEOQUESS • *See* Dicyclomine Hydrochloride.

NEORAL (Rx) • Introduced in 1995, it is a new formulation of cyclosporine (*see*), which allows lower dosages of the immunosuppressant and thus reduces adverse side effects associated with the older form of the drug. Clinical studies show that the principal adverse effects of Neoral are similar to those of cyclosporine, including possible kidney dysfunction, tremor, hairiness, high blood pressure, and gum overgrowth.

NEOSAR • *See* Cyclophosphamide.

NEOSPORIN (OTC) • A combination of gramicidin and neomycin (*see both*).

NEOSPORIN OPHTHALMIC SOLUTION (Rx) • A combination of gramicidin, neomycin, and polymyxin B (*see all*). Used to combat eye infections because it has a broad range of antibiotic activity. Prolonged use must be avoided so that sensitivity to the antibiotics does not develop. Potential adverse reaction is eye irritation.

NEOSTIGMINE (Rx) • **Prostigmin.** Introduced in 1931, it inhibits the destruction of acetylcholine (*see*). Used as an antidote for muscle-blocking agents, preoperative abdominal distension, and flaccid urinary bladder. Potential adverse reactions include dizziness, muscle weakness, mental confusion, jitters, sweating, respiratory depression, rash, bronchospasm, muscle cramps, and muscle twitches. Contraindicated in hypersensitivity to cholinergics or to bromide, mechanical obstruction of the intestine or urinary tract, slow heartbeat, and low blood pressure. Should be used with extreme caution in bronchial asthma. Should also be used with care in epileptics, in recent heart attack patients, peritonitis, overactive thyroid, irregular heartbeat, and peptic ulcer. Atropine, anticholinergic drugs, procainamide, aminoglycosides, and quinidine may make neostigmine less effective. Should be taken with milk or food.

NEOSULF • *See* Neomycin.

NEO-SYNALAR • *See* Fluocinolone and Neomycin.

NEO-SYNEPHRINE NASAL SOLUTION • *See* Phenylephrine.

NEO-SYNEPHRINE OPHTHALMIC SO-LUTION • *See* Phenylephrine.

NEO-SYNEPHRINE 12 HOUR • *See* Oxymetazoline.

NEO-TABS • *See* Neomycin.

NEOTAL • *See* Bacitracin, Neomycin, and Polymyxin B.

NEO-TEARS • Hydroxyethylcellulose with thimerosal and edetate disodium (*see all*). *See also* Artificial Tears.

NEOTEP GRANUCAPS • *See* Chlorpheniramine and Phenylephrine.

NEOTHYLLINE • *See* Dyphylline.

NEOTRICIN • A combination of bacitracin, neomycin, and polymyxin B (*see all*), used to treat superficial skin infections.

NEPETA CATARIA • *See* Catmint.

NEPHROCAPS (OTC) • A multivitamin and mineral preparation.

NEPHROX SUSPENSION • *See* Aluminum Hydroxide.

NEPTAZANE • *See* Methazolamide.

NERVE GROWTH FACTOR • **NGF.** Believed to maintain and repair nerves in the brain. These factors are being investigated as a treatment for preventing Alzheimer's disease, and for aiding recovery of function following injury to the central nervous system.

NERVINE • Having a soothing effect on the nerves without numbing them. Among the herbs used for this purpose are damiana and ginseng (*see both*). Approved by the FDA as a sleep aid.

NERVOCAINE • *See* Lidocaine.

NESACAINE • *See* Chloroprocaine.

NESTABS FA (OTC) • A multivitamin and mineral preparation.

NESTREX • *See* Vitamin B_6.

NETILMICIN SULFATE (Rx) • **Netromycin.** An injectable aminoglycoside (*see*) antibiotic introduced in 1983, it is used to treat serious infections caused by *Pseudomonas aeruginosa, Escherichia coli, Porteus, Klebsiella, Serratia, Enterobacter, Citrobacter,* and *Staphylococcus* (*see all*). Potential adverse reactions include headache, lethargy, nerve damage, ear problems, kidney damage, and allergic reactions. Interacts with cephalothin, dimenhydrinate, general and local anesthetics, loop diuretics (*see*), cisplatin, methoxyflurane, and penicillins. Must be used cautiously in persons with kidney dysfunction.

NETROMYCIN • *See* Netilmicin Sulfate.

NETTLE (H) • *Urtica dioica.* **Pellitory-of-the-Wall. Stinging Nettle.** Roman soldiers took nettle seeds to Britain to rub on themselves to keep warm in winter. Nettle is used in a tea to purify the blood and to help relieve hemorrhoids. An infusion of nettles boiled in water reputedly clears the complexion of all blemishes and adds brightness to the eyes. Contains vitamin C, histamine, chlorophyll, and iron. Used by herbalists to treat rheumatism and vaginal infections. Also is said to alleviate stuffy nose, watery eyes, and other symptoms of hay fever. Nettle tea was one of the most popular of all springtime medicines in the 1700s. It was also used to treat consumption. In modern laboratories, it has been shown to have anti-inflammatory activity and to lower sugar levels in the blood. The uncooked plants can cause kidney damage and poisoning. The bristly hairs can be irritating to the skin. In 1992, the FDA issued a notice that nettle had not been shown to be safe and effective as claimed in OTC digestive-aid products.

NEUPOGEN • *See* Filgrastim.

NEURALGIA • Severe pain in a nerve or along its route.

NEURAMATE • *See* Meprobamate.

NEURITIS • Inflammation of the nerve or its parts due to infection, toxins, compression, or trauma.

NEUROLEPTIC MALIGNANT SYNDROME • **NMS.** A potentially fatal symptom complex associated with antipsychotic drugs. Among the manifestations are high fever, muscle rigidity, irregular pulse or blood pressure, irregular heartbeat, sweating, and acute kidney failure.

NEUROLITE • *See* Technerium 99m Bicisate.

NEURON • The basic nerve cell of the central nervous system.

NEUROPATHY • Disease, inflammation, or damage to the peripheral nerves, which connect the central nervous system to the sense organs, muscles, glands, and internal organs.

NEUROPEPTIDES • Any of the molecules composed of amino acids found in brain tissue. Some are both neurotransmitters (*see*) and hormones. They are believed to be involved in carbohydrate craving, as well as in many other physical and emotional functions.

NEUROSIS • An emotional disorder that arises due to unresolved conflicts, anxiety being the chief characteristic. In contrast to psychoses, neuroses do not involve gross distortions of reality.

NEUROSYN • *See* Primidone.

NEUROTENSIN • A peptide of thirteen amino acid derivatives that helps regulate blood sugar by its effects on a number of hormones, including insulin and glucagon. It also is thought to play a part in pain suppression.

NEUROTONIN • *See* Gabapentin.

NEUROTRANSMITTERS • Molecules that carry chemical messages between nerve cells. Neurotransmitters are released from nerve cells, diffuse across the minute distance between two nerve cells (synaptic cleft), and bind to a receptor at another nerve site.

NEUT • *See* Sodium Bicarbonate.

NEUTRA-PHOS • *See* Potassium Phosphate and Sodium Phosphate.

NEUTRA-PHOS-K • *See* Potassium Phosphate.

NEUTREXIN • *See* Trimetrexate Glucuronate.

NEUTROGENA T/GEL • *See* Coal Tar.

NEUTROPENIA • An abnormal deficiency of neutrophils (*see*), infection-fighting white blood cells, in the body.

NEUTROPHIL • Infection-fighting white blood cell.

NEW MOLECULAR ENTITY • **NME.** The FDA classifies a drug as an NME if it has not been previously marketed in any form, including as an ingredient in another compound.

N.G.T. • *See* Nystatin and Triamcinolone.

NIAC • *See* Niacin.

NIACELS • *See* Niacin.

NIACIN (Rx) (OTC) (H) • **Endur-Acin. Nia-Bid. Niac. Niacels. Niacor. Niaplus. Nicobid. Nicolar. Nico-400. Nicotinamide. Nicotinex. Nicotinic Acid. Ni-Span. Slo-Niacin. Span-Niacin. Tega-Span.** Introduced as a nutritional supplement in 1937, it is an essential nutrient that participates in many energy-yielding reactions and aids in the maintenance of a normal nervous system. A component of the vitamin B complex, it releases energy from foods, maintains healthy skin, and helps in the normal functioning of the nervous system and digestive tract. Deficiency symptoms include nervous disorders and skin problems. Recommended daily allowances are newborns to six months, 5 mg; infants six months to one year, 6 mg; children one to three years, 9 mg; four to six years, 12 mg; seven to ten years, 13 mg; males eleven to fourteen years, 17 mg; fifteen to eighteen years, 20 mg; nineteen to fifty years, 19 mg; fifty-one years and over, 15 mg; females eleven to fifty years, 15 mg; fifty-one years and over, 13 mg; pregnant women, 17 mg; lactating women, 20 mg. Niacin is used to treat pellagra, in blood-vessel disease and circulatory disorders, and as an adjunctive treatment of high blood fats, especially with high cholesterol (*see*). Most adverse reactions are dose dependent. Potential adverse reactions include nausea, vomiting, diarrhea, dizziness, headache, possible activation of peptic ulcer, stomach pain, liver dysfunction, high blood sugar, high uric acid, flushing, itching, and dryness. Blood-pressure-lowering drugs may have an additive blood-vessel-dilating effect and cause a drop in blood pressure when rising from a seated or prone position. Contraindicated in liver dysfunction, active peptic ulcer, severe low blood pressure, or bleeding of the arteries. Should be used with caution in patients with gallbladder disease, diabetes, and gout. Most effective when taken on an empty stomach, but may be taken with food to avoid stomach upset.

NIACINAMIDE (OTC) • Nicotinamide. Vitamin B. Geritol Liquid High Potency. Iodo-Niacin. Nicotinex Elixir. Vicon Plus. The biologically active fraction of nicotinic acid. A white or yellow, crystalline, odorless powder used to treat pellagra—a vitamin-deficiency disease—vascular disease, and circulatory disorders, and to help recovery from burns and trauma. In 1992, the FDA proposed a ban on niacinamide in oral menstrual drug products because it had not been shown to be safe and effective as claimed. *See* Niacin.

NIAID • Abbreviation for National Institute of Allergy and Infectious Diseases.

NIAPLUS • *See* Niacin.

NICARDIPINE (Rx) • Cardene. A calcium channel blocker introduced in 1989, it is used to treat chronic stable angina (*see*) and to lower blood pressure. Potential adverse reactions include edema, flushing, dizziness, headache, heartburn, numbness, drowsiness, swelling, angina, irregular or slow heartbeat, nausea, abdominal discomfort, dry mouth, rash, and weakness. Beta-blockers (*see*) may increase nicardipine's blood-pressure-lowering effects and may also increase the depression of heart action. Cimetidine (*see*) may increase nicardipine's side effects. Nicardipine may increase the toxicity of cyclosporine and theophylline. Most effective when taken on an empty stomach at least one hour before or two hours after meals. May be taken with a small amount of food or milk if stomach upset is a problem. Grapefruit juice may cause potentially dangerous, increased levels of this medication in the blood.

NICKEL-PECTIN • In 1992, the FDA issued a notice that nickel-pectin had not been shown to be safe and effective as claimed in OTC digestive-aid products.

NICKEL SULFATE (OTC) • Occurs in the earth's crust as a salt of nickel. Obtained as green or blue crystals. It has a sweet, astringent taste. Used chiefly in nickel plating. Also used in hair dyes and astringents. Used as a mineral supplement, up to 1 mg per day.

NICLOCIDE • *See* Niclosamide.

NICLOSAMIDE (Rx) • Niclocide. Introduced in 1982 to treat tapeworms, it will not work for other types of worm infections. Potential adverse reactions include drowsiness, dizziness, headache, mouth irritation, nausea, vomiting, loss of appetite, rash, and itching around the anus. May be taken with a little food to reduce stomach upset.

NICOBID • *See* Niacin.

NICODERM (Rx) • Nicotine Transdermal System. Provides systemic delivery of nicotine for twenty-four hours following its application to intact skin. The doses are from 7 mg to 21 mg per twenty-four hours. It is indicated as a ten-week weaning program to aid smoking cessation by relieving nicotine withdrawal symptoms. In 1994, there were reports that nicotine delivered via transdermal patch may help improve cognitive function in patients with Alzheimer's disease. Contraindicated in patients with hypersensitivity or allergy to nicotine, or to any of the components of the therapeutic system. Nicotine from any source can be toxic and addictive. The amounts of nicotine that are tolerated by adult smokers can produce symptoms of poisoning and prove fatal if the Nicoderm system is applied to or ingested by children or pets. If patients continue to smoke while using Nicoderm therapy, cardiovascular or other effects attributable to nicotine may increase. The use of Nicoderm beyond three months is not recommended. Nicoderm should be used during pregnancy only if the likelihood of smoking cessation justifies the potential risk of use of nicotine replacement by the patient, who may continue to smoke. Smoking while using Nicoderm can be extremely dangerous. Nicoderm should be used with caution in patients with overactive thyroid, pheochromocytoma, or insulin-dependent diabetes. One double-blind, placebo-controlled trial in 220 smokers treated for eighteen weeks with a sixteen-hour nicotine patch without intensive group counseling found that 25 percent of those who received nicotine were not smoking one year later, compared to 9 percent of those who received placebo. Manufacturers recommend wearing the patches for four to twelve weeks, but the optimal duration of patch use is unknown. Nicotine delays the healing of peptic ulcer and should be used by those with active ulcers only if nicotine replacement therapy outweighs the risks of smoking. Spontaneous abortion during nicotine replacement therapy has been reported; as with smoking, nicotine as a contributing factor cannot be excluded. Although it has been difficult to separate out the effects of nicotine replacement therapy from withdrawal symptoms of smoking cessation, reported probable adverse reactions include diarrhea, heartburn, dry mouth, joint and muscle aches, abnormal dreams, insomnia, nervousness, and sweating. Possible but unproven effects may be weakness, back, chest, or abdominal pain, constipation, nausea, vomiting, dizziness, headache, numbness, increased cough, sore throat, sinusitis, rash, taste perversion, and painful menstruation.

NICO-400 • *See* Niacin.

NICOLAR • *See* Niacin.

NICORETTE • *See* Nicotine Polacrilex.

NICOTINAMIDE • *See* Niacin.

NICOTINE • Obtained from the dried leaves of *Nicotiana tabacum* (Virginia tobacco) and *Nicotiana rustica* (Turkish tobacco). In 1994, there were reports that nicotine delivered via transdermal patch may help improve cognitive function in patients with Alzheimer's disease. This is not yet an approved use. Nicotine is used agriculturally as an insecticide. Nicotine from any source can be toxic and addictive. Smoking causes lung cancer, heart disease, and emphysema and may adversely affect the fetus and the pregnant woman. Tobacco smoke, which has been shown to be harmful to the fetus, contains nicotine, hydrogen cyanide, and carbon monoxide. Nicotine also has been shown, in animal studies, to cause fetal harm. For any smoker, with or without concomitant disease or pregnancy, the risk of nicotine replacement in a smoking cessation program should be weighed against the hazards of continued smoking. Symptoms of nicotine overdose include extreme nausea, vomiting, evacuation of bowel and bladder, mental confusion, twitching, and convulsions. It is readily absorbed through the skin.

NICOTINE POLACRILEX (OTC) • **Nicorette. Nicotine Resin Complex.** A chewing gum used as a temporary aid to the cigarette smoker trying to quit. One piece of this gum, which contains 2 mg of nicotine, is supposed to be chewed slowly for thirty minutes whenever the urge to smoke occurs. Most people require approximately ten pieces of gum daily during the first month, but should not exceed thirty pieces daily. Potential adverse reactions include dizziness, light-headedness, irregular heartbeat, throat soreness, jaw muscle ache from chewing, nausea, vomiting, indigestion, gas, and hiccups. Contraindicated in nonsmokers, right after a heart attack, in life-threatening irregular heartbeat, severe or worsening angina, and active temporomandibular joint disease (see). Use of nicotine gum is not recommended for more than six months at a stretch. It was changed from Rx status to OTC status in 1996.

NICOTINE TRANSDERMAL SYSTEM • See Nicoderm.

NICOTINEX • See Niacin.

NICOTINIC ACID • See Niacin.

NICOTROL (Rx) • A nicotine patch worn to help break the smoking habit; introduced in 1992. It is the first patch worn only during waking hours. The Nicotrol treatment period, using three different patch strengths, enables the body to gradually withdraw from nicotine. The dosages range from 5 mg to 15 mg per twenty-four hours. It is, as of this writing, the least expensive of the nicotine patches. Contraindicated in patients with known hypersensitivity or allergy to nicotine. Nicotine from any source can be toxic and addictive. Smoking causes lung cancer, heart disease, and emphysema and may adversely affect the fetus and the pregnant woman. Potential adverse reactions include mild redness of the skin, dizziness, joint pain, rash, and sweating. Smoking while wearing a nicotine patch may be extremely dangerous. One double-blind, placebo-controlled trial in 220 smokers treated for eighteen weeks with a sixteen-hour nicotine patch without intensive group counseling found that 25 percent of those who received nicotine were not smoking one year later, compared to 9 percent of those who received placebo. Manufacturers recommend wearing the patches for four to twelve weeks, but the optimal duration of patch use is unknown. In 1994, there were reports that nicotine delivered

via transdermal patch may help improve cognitive function in patients with Alzheimer's disease. A candidate for OTC status. See Nicotine.

NICOTROL NS (Rx) • A nasal spray expected to be approved by the FDA soon as an aid in breaking the smoking habit. It will be sold only by prescription to adults. Addiction is not expected to be a problem since the spray carries a "stinging" sensation. See Nicotrol.

NICO-VERT • See Dimenhydrinate.

NIDRYL • See Diphenhydramine.

NIFEDIPINE (Rx) • **Adalat. Novo-Nifedin. Procardia.** A calcium channel blocker (see) introduced in 1982, it is used to treat angina by reversing coronary artery spasm, and Raynaud's disease by reducing artery spasms in the hands and feet. The most common side effect is edema. Other potential adverse reactions include headache, fatigue, dizziness, constipation, nausea, insomnia, nervousness, numbness, sleepiness, itching, rash, leg cramps, joint pain, shortness of breath, abdominal pain, diarrhea, dry mouth, heartburn, gas, hot flashes, malaise, loss of balance, decreased libido, weight gain, respiratory-tract infection, sinusitis, tearing, bloody nose, taste perversion, ringing in the ears, breast pain, painful and/or bloody urination, irregular menstruation, and heart problems. Use with cimetidine and ranitidine (see both) decreases its effectiveness. Should not be used in patients with sick sinus syndrome, heart block (except if a pacemaker has been inserted), those with low blood pressure, acute heart attack, and lung congestion. The FDA has recommended that the use of short-acting nifedipine be discouraged for high blood pressure and angina, because the short-acting version has been reported to increase the risk of heart attack. Propranolol and other beta-blockers (see) may cause a severe drop in blood pressure and heart failure. Blood levels of digoxin (see) may be increased when it is taken with nifedipine. May be taken with food to reduce stomach upset. Grapefruit juice may cause potentially dangerous, increased levels of this medication in the blood. The short-acting version was linked to cancer in 1996, although the results were controversial.

NIFEREX (OTC) • A multivitamin and mineral preparation.

NIGHT-BLOOMING CEREUS (H) • *Selenicereus grandiflorus.* The flowers and young, tender stems of this cactus are used by homeopaths to treat heart palpitations, anxiety, rapid heartbeat, chest pain, inflamed heart, irregular heartbeat, and other heart and lung problems. Potential adverse effects may include gastric irritation, mental confusion, irregular heartbeat, and hallucinations.

NIGHTSHADE, BLACK (H) • *Solanum nigrum.* **Common Nightshade. Garden Nightshade. Morelle.** An annual plant, the leaves were used by North American Indians as a treatment for TB and to expel worms. Many cultures have used the plant to induce sleep. Ancient Greek and Arab physicians used the leaves to treat burns, itching, hemorrhoids, and arthritis. The leaves and berries are poisonous, especially in the unripe state.

NILORIC • *See* Ergoloid Mesylates.

NILSTAT • *See* Nystatin.

NILUTAMIDE (Rx) • **Anandron.** Recommended for approval by an FDA advisory committee in 1995, this medication is used to treat metastatic prostate cancer. It is used in combination with surgical or chemical castration for the palliative treatment of previously untreated metastatic prostate cancer. The drug was first launched in France in 1987. Patients treated with nilutamide reportedly had reduced metastasis-related bone pain, and in one study, 41 percent had regression of the disease. The drug is contraindicated in patients with severe breathing difficulties or known hypersensitivity to the drug. Lung and liver complications may also be severe.

NIMH • Abbreviation for National Institute of Mental Health.

NIMODIPINE (Rx) • **Nimotop.** A calcium channel blocker (*see*) introduced in 1989, it decreases heart contractions and oxygen demand and dilates coronary arteries and arterioles. It is used to improve neurologic deficits after a stroke. Potential adverse reactions include headache, decreased blood pressure, dizziness, swelling of the arms or legs, heart failure, diarrhea, abnormal blood clotting, psychosis, hallucinations, anemia, breathing difficulty, stomach cramps, liver dysfunction, sexual difficulties, vomiting, itching, acne, rash, anemia, flushing, and edema. Antihypertensives may cause blood pressure to drop too low when used with nimodipine. Calcium channel blockers may cause bleeding when taken alone or together with aspirin. Cimetidine may increase nimodipine's effects. Nimodipine, when taken with a beta-blocking drug, may lead to heart failure in those who are susceptible. Most effective when taken on an empty stomach, but may be taken with a small amount of food or milk if stomach distress is a problem. Grapefruit juice may cause potentially dangerous, increased levels of this medication in the blood.

NIMOTOP • *See* Nimodipine.

NIONG • *See* Nitroglycerin.

NIPENT • *See* Pentostatin.

NIPRIDE • *See* Nitroprusside.

NISCORT • *See* Primaquine Phosphate.

NISOLDIPINE (Rx) • **Sular. Nisocor.** An antihypertensive, this long-acting calcium channel blocker was introduced in 1995. In clinical studies, once daily administration at doses ranging from 10 mg to 60 mg produced sustained reductions in blood pressure over twenty-four hours in both supine and standing positions. Efficacy was not influenced by race or gender, according to reports. The label carries a warning concerning its use in patients with severe obstructive coronary artery disease, severe angina, or acute heart attack. The most frequent adverse effects reported were swelling in the extremities, headache, dizziness, pharyngitis, sinusitis, palpitation, chest pain, nausea, and rash. Grapefruit juice may cause potentially dangerous, increased levels of this medication in the blood.

NIT-AC • Homeopathic abbreviation for nitricum acidum (*see*).

NITOMAN • *See* Tetrabenazine.

NITRATES (Rx) • **Isordil. Nitro-Bid. Nitrodisc. Nitrodur. Nitroglycerin. Nitroglyn. Nitrostat. Peritrate. PETN. Transderm Nitro.** A class of drugs used to treat heart attack. They dilate coronary arteries and peripheral arteries and veins, thereby increasing blood flow to the myocardium (*see*) and decreasing circulating blood volume. They reduce the amount of oxygen demanded by the heart. Should not be taken with alcoholic beverages because the combination may cause blood pressure to drop too low.

NITREX • *See* Nitrofurantoin.

NITRIC OXIDE • **NO.** A molecule with many functions in the body, it is believed that it might be used by the immune system to fight viral infections. The gaseous molecule regulates blood pressure and causes penile erections by dilating blood vessels, transmits messages between nerve cells, kills certain parasites and other microorganisms, and may play a part in learning and memory. The National Institutes of Health are hard at work, as of this writing, to design compounds that release nitric oxide to fight infections. Such medications will probably first be developed to treat cold sores and other skin viruses.

NITRICUM ACIDUM (H) • **Aqua Fortis. Nitric Acid.** A homeopathic remedy made from a mineral acid. It is used for bad breath, anger, anxiety, the common cold, earache, joint pain, insomnia, headache, gas, eye inflammation, sore throat, piles, and thrush. *See* Nitrates.

NITRO- • Prefix denoting one atom of nitrogen and two of oxygen.

NITRO-BID • *See* Nitroglycerin.

NITRODISC (Rx) • A transdermal (*see*) infusion system. *See* Nitroglycerin.

NITRO-DUR (Rx) • A transdermal (*see*) infusion system. *See* Nitroglycerin.

NITROFAN • *See* Nitrofurantoin.

NITROFURAL • *See* Nitrofurazone.

NITROFURANTOIN (Rx); MACROCRYSTALS, MICROCRYSTALS • **Furacin. Furadantin. Furalan. Furan. Furanite. Macrodantin. Nitrex. Nitrofan.** Introduced in 1953, it is a fast-acting antibacterial used to treat pyelonephritis, pyelitis, and cystitis due to *Escherichia coli, Staphylococcus aureus, Enterococcus, Klebsiella, Proteus,* and *Enterobacter.* Potential adverse effects include bleeding, nerve damage, headache, dizziness, drowsiness, kidney dysfunction, loss of appetite, nausea, vomiting, abdominal pain, diarrhea, hepatitis, skin eruptions, asthmatic attacks and other serious allergic reactions, hair loss, drug fever, overgrowth of nonsusceptible organisms in the urinary tract, cough, chest pains, fever, chills, and difficulty in breathing. Magnesium-containing antacids diminish its absorption, as do nalidixic acid and norfloxacin. Probenecid and sulfinpyrazone may increase the toxicity of nitrofurantoin. Nalidixic acid (*see*) reduces nitrofurantoin's antibacterial effect. Eating citrus fruits and milk products should be avoided while taking nitrofurantoin. These can change the acidity of urine and affect the drug's action. Nitrofurantoin may be taken with food to reduce stomach upset, loss of appetite, nausea, or other gastrointestinal problems. Most effective when taken with food, to aid absorption.

NITROFURAZONE (Rx) • **Furacin. Nitrofural.** An antibacterial cream or ointment used to treat second- and third-degree burns and to prevent skin-graft rejection. Potential adverse reactions include kidney toxicity, redness, itching, burning, water retention, severe blistering, and allergic rash. Should be used cautiously in patients with kidney dysfunction.

NITROGARD • *See* Nitroglycerin.

NITROGEN MUSTARD • *See* Mechlorethamine.

NITROGLYCERIN[E] (Rx) • **Glyceryl Trinitrate. Deponit. Klavikordal. Minitran. Niong. Nitro-Bid. Nitrocap. Nitrocine. Nitrodisc. Nitro-Dur. Nitrogard. Nitroglyn. Nitrol. Nitrolin. Nitrolingual Spray. Nitrol TSAR. Nitronet. Nitrong. Nitrospan. Nitrostat. NTG. NTS. Transderm-Nitro. Tridil.** A coronary vasodilator introduced in the 1800s, it is one of the oldest drugs in continual use. It is used to relieve the pain of angina (*see*) attacks by decreasing the heart's demand for oxygen. Also increases blood flow through the collateral coronary vessels. Nitroglycerin acts quickly, but for a short time only. Potential adverse reactions include headache, weakness, a severe drop in blood pressure when rising, irregular heartbeat, flushing, fainting, nausea, vomiting, under-the-tongue burning, and hypersensitivity reactions. Nitroglycerin is best taken for the first time when sitting down because it can drop the blood pressure and may cause fainting. Drugs for high blood pressure may increase this drop in blood pressure. Alcohol should also be avoided with nitroglycerin because the combination may drop the blood pressure too low. Drugs that stimulate the nervous system may reduce the effects of nitroglycerin. Do not use any oral nitroglycerin with food or gum in your mouth. Nitroglycerin pills are most effective when taken on an empty stomach. Nitroglycerin patches for heart disease therapy are between four and six times the price of controlled-release capsules taken twice a day, and twice the price of nitroglycerin ointment when dispensed in one-gram pouches applied three times a day.

NITROGLYN • *See* Nitroglycerin.

NITROL • *See* Nitroglycerin.

NITROLIN • *See* Nitroglycerin.

NITROLINGUAL SPRAY • *See* Nitroglycerin.

NITRONET • *See* Nitroglycerin.

NITRONG • *See* Nitroglycerin.

NITROPRESS • *See* Nitroprusside.

NITROPRUSSIDE (Rx) • **Nipride. Nitropress. Sodium Nitroferri Cyanide.** A medication that dilates blood vessels and relaxes the smooth muscles of veins, it is used to lower blood pressure quickly in hypertensive emergencies, and to control pressure in heart failure or heart shock. Potential side effects include headache, dizziness, loss of balance, loss of consciousness, weak pulse, absent reflexes, widely dilated pupils, restlessness, muscle twitching, sweating, palpitations, shortness of breath, vomiting, nausea, abdominal pain, and acidosis. Must be used cautiously in persons with hypothyroidism, liver or kidney dysfunction, or in those receiving other antihypertensive medications.

NITROSPAN • *See* Nitroglycerin.

NITROSTAT • *See* Nitroglycerin.

NITROUS OXIDE (Rx) • **Laughing Gas.** A gas used to induce anesthesia. Can be narcotic in high concentrations.

NIX • *See* Permethrin.

NIZATIDINE (Rx) (OTC) • **Axid.** An antiulcer drug introduced in 1986 that blocks the action of histamine in the stomach, decreasing gastric acid secretion. Used to treat active ulcers and to prevent ulcers from recurring. Has an advantage of once-a-day dosage. It reportedly does not cause confusion or sexual impotence or reduce sperm count, effects that some other antiulcer drugs may produce. Potential adverse reactions include a drop in the number of platelets, which could cause bleeding, sleepiness, irregular heartbeat, sweating, rash, hives, liver damage, increased uric acid, and enlargement of the male breast. The side effects of aspirin may become more likely if taken with nizatidine. Contraindicated in patients with hypersensitivity to H_2 (histamine) receptor antagonists. Dosages should be reduced in patients with impaired kidney function. Cigarette smoking increases gastric acid secretion and will counteract the benefits of antiulcer drugs. The drug should not be discontinued abruptly. Most effective when taken with food. OTC status was approved in 1996.

NIZORAL • *See* Ketoconazole.

NME • Abbreviation for new molecular entity (*see*).

NO • *See* Nitric Oxide.

NOBELITIN • A substance found in citrus fruit that has been found to have anticancer properties in laboratory studies.

NOCTEC • *See* Chloral Hydrate.

NO DOZ MAXIMUM STRENGTH CAPLETS (OTC) • Contains 200 mg of caffeine (*see*).

NOLAHIST • *See* Phenindamine.

NOLAMINE (OTC) • A combination of chlorpheniramine, phenylpropanolamine, and phenindamine (*see all*), used to relieve the symptoms of upper-respiratory and nasal congestion.

NOLUDAR • *See* Methyprylon.

NOLVADEX • *See* Tamoxifen Citrate.

NOMIFENSINE (Rx) • An antidepressant not related to the tricyclics and tetracyclics.

NONCOMPLIANCE • Accidental or deliberate failure to follow instructions for medical therapy.

NONOXYNOL-9 (OTC) • **Because. Conceptrol Contraceptive Gel. Delfen Contraceptive Foam. Encare Vaginal Contraceptive. Gynol II. Koromex Foam, Cream, Jelly. Ramses. Semicid. Shur-Seal. Today Vaginal Contraceptive Sponge.** A spermicide used in contraceptive foams, creams, and gels. It is a detergent-dispersing agent. May cause occasional burning and/or irritation of the vagina or penis. Should not be taken orally.

NONPRESCRIPTION MEDICINE • Medicine available over the counter without a doctor's prescription.

NONSEDATING • Not containing ingredients that may cause drowsiness.

NONSTEROIDAL ANTI-INFLAMMATORY DRUGS (Rx) (OTC) • NSAIDs. Aspirin was the first fever-reducing, painkilling, nonsteroidal anti-inflammatory drug. The first nonaspirin NSAID was introduced in 1964. Today these include diclofenac, etodolac, ibuprofen, indomethacin, naproxen, piroxicam, sulindac, and nabumetone. They inhibit arachidonic acid, a fatty-acid precursor of leukotrienes, prostaglandins, and thromboxanes, all involved in inflammation. NSAIDs are now widely used to treat the pain of arthritis, menstruation, post-surgery, and many other aches. Nonaspirin NSAIDs are used instead of aspirin because, on the whole, they may be better tolerated than aspirin and more convenient in dosage. The chief side effects of NSAIDs are gastrointestinal ulcers and upper-GI bleeding and perforation. Used daily by 13 million Americans, NSAIDs result in 2,600 deaths in the United States each year. A study in the Medicaid population has shown that 29 percent of GI-related deaths among the elderly are due to NSAID use. According to the FDA, 2–5 percent of patients will experience ulceration or hemorrhage during one year's NSAID treatment, and the risk for individual patients accumulates with time. Nonaspirin NSAIDs do not have an anticoagulant effect, but can cause the same hypersensitivity reactions. In a few susceptible patients, NSAIDs have provoked reversible acute kidney failure and chronic kidney dysfunction.

NORADEX • *See* Orphenadrine.

NORADRENALINE • *See* Norepinephrine.

NORCET 7 • *See* Acetaminophen and Hydrocodone.

NORCURON • *See* Vecuronium.

NORDETTE • *See* Estradiol and Levonorgestrel.

NOREPINEPHRINE (Rx) • **Levarterenol Bitartrate. Levophed. Noradrenaline.** A hormone released by the adrenal gland, possessing the ability to stimulate, as does epinephrine, but with minimal inhibitory effects. It has little effect on the lungs' smooth muscles and metabolic processes and differs from epinephrine in its effect on the heart and blood vessels. Given to treat shock because it contracts the muscle tissue of capillaries and arteries, consequently raising blood pressure. Potential adverse reactions include headache, anxiety, weakness, dizziness, tremor, restlessness, insomnia, slow heartbeat, severe high blood pressure, decreased cardiac output, irregular heartbeat, decreased urine output, high blood sugar, fever, and respiratory difficulty. Contraindicated in persons with tendency to blood clots, pregnant women, profound oxygen deficiency, and low blood pressure due to loss of blood volume. Must be used cautiously in persons with high blood pressure, overactive thyroid, severe cardiac disease, and sensitivity to sulfites. Must be used with extreme caution in patients receiving MAO inhibitors or tricyclic antidepressants (*see both*).

NORETHINDRONE (Rx) • **Aygestin. Genora. Loestrin. Micronor. Modicon. Norinyl. Norlestrin. Norlutate. Norlutin. Nor-Q D.** A progestin drug that suppresses ovulation, possibly by inhibiting pituitary gonadotropin secretion. It forms a thick cervical mucus. Used to treat absent menstruation or abnormal uterine bleeding. Potential adverse reactions include nausea, vomiting, depression, high blood pressure, dizziness, migraine, lethargy, blood clots, swelling, bloating, and abdominal cramps. May cause breakthrough bleeding, altered menstrual flow, painful or absent menstruation, enlargement of benign tumors of the uterus, cervical erosion, abnormal secretions, and vaginal candidiasis. There may be jaundice, high blood sugar, dark spots appearing on the skin, breast tenderness, enlargement, and secretion, and decreased libido. Contraindicated in persons with blood-clot disorders, cancer of the breast, undiagnosed abnormal vaginal bleeding, and in pregnancy. Should be used with caution in high blood pressure, seizures, migraine, and mental depression. Rifampin (*see*) decreases norethindrone's effectiveness.

NORETHYNODREL • *See* Progestins.

NORFERAN • *See* Iron.

NORFLEX • *See* Orphenadrine.

NORFLOXACIN (Rx) • **Chibroxin. Noroxin.** A quinolone (*see*) introduced in 1986 for the treatment of urinary tract infections caused by susceptible strains of *Escherichia coli, Klebsiella, Enterobacter, Proteus, Pseudomonas, Citrobacter, Staphylococcus aureus,* and *Streptococcus* (*see all*). Potential adverse reactions include fatigue, sleepiness, headache, dizziness, nausea, constipation, flatulence, heartburn, dry mouth, and rash. Antacids hinder absorption. A broad-spectrum antibacterial drug, norfloxacin was relabeled after introduction when it was found to cause inflammation of the small intestine and colon. Should not be used with probenecid (*see*) because it may increase side effects. Should not be used by persons sensitive to other quinolones. Persons taking this medication should drink at least eight glasses of water a day to ward off side effects. It also is recommended that this drug be taken with a full glass of water on an empty stomach, one or two hours after eating. Antacids should not be ingested for two hours after taking this drug.

NORGESIC FORTE (Rx) • A combination of aspirin, orphenadrine, and caffeine (*see all*). A muscle relaxant used to treat muscle spasms. The primary ingredient, orphenadrine, is a derivative of the antihistamine diphenhydramine (Benadryl). The aspirin is in the compound for pain relief.

Contraindicated in glaucoma, and in persons with a history of stomach ulcer, intestinal obstruction, difficulty in passing urine, or known sensitivity or allergy to any of the drug's ingredients. The aspirin in the compound may increase the effect of blood-thinning drugs, and probenecid, and may increase the blood-sugar-lowering effects of oral antidiabetes drugs. Interaction of Norgesic with propoxyphene (Darvon) may cause confusion, anxiety, or tremors. Alcohol may increase side effects. Norgesic should be taken with food to avoid stomach upset.

NORGESTREL (Rx) • **Ovrette.** A progestin drug that suppresses ovulation, possibly by inhibiting pituitary gonadotropin secretion. It forms a thick cervical mucus. Used as a progestin-only contraceptive. Potential adverse reactions include nausea, vomiting, depression, high blood pressure, dizziness, migraine, lethargy, blood clots, swelling, bloating, and abdominal cramps. May cause breakthrough bleeding, altered menstrual flow, painful or absent menstruation, enlargement of benign tumors of the uterus, cervical erosion, abnormal secretions, and vaginal candidiasis. There may be jaundice, high blood sugar, dark spots appearing on the skin, breast tenderness, enlargement, and secretion, and decreased libido. Contraindicated in persons with blood-clot disorders, cancer of the breast, undiagnosed abnormal vaginal bleeding, and in pregnancy. Should be used with caution in high blood pressure, seizures, migraine, and mental depression. The risks are marked in women over thirty-five years of age. Rifampin (*see*) decreases Norgestrel's effectiveness. The pill should be taken every day, even if menstruating.

NORINYL • *See* Mestranol, Ethinyl Estradiol, and Norethindrone.

NORISODRINE AEROTROL • *See* Isoproterenol.

NORLESTRIN (Rx) • *See* Ethinyl Estradiol and Norethindrone.

NORLUTATE • *See* Norethindrone.

NORLUTIN • *See* Norethindrone.

NORMIFLO • *See* Heparin.

NOR-MIL (Rx) • *See* Diphenoxylate and Atropine.

NORMODYNE • *See* Labetalol.

NOROXIN • *See* Norfloxacin.

NORPACE • *See* Disopyramide.

NORPACE CR • *See* Disopyramide.

NORPANTH • *See* Propantheline.

NORPLANT SYSTEM • *See* Levonorgestrel.

NORPRAMIN • *See* Desipramine.

NOR-PRED • *See* Prednisolone.

NOR-Q D • *See* Norethindrone.

NOR-TET • *See* Tetracycline.

NORTRIPTYLINE (Rx) • **Aventyl. Pamelor.** A tricyclic antidepressant (*see*). Potential adverse side effects include drowsiness, dizziness, excitation, seizures, tremors, weakness, confusion, headache, nervousness, irregular heartbeat, high blood pressure, blurred vision, ringing in the ears, dry mouth, constipation, nausea, vomiting, changes in libido, male impotence, inhibited female orgasm, breast enlargement, swelling of the testicles, loss of appetite, intestinal paralysis, urine retention, rash, hives, sweating, and allergy. Sudden discontinuation may cause nausea, headache, and malaise. Barbiturates decrease its effectiveness. Cimetidine and methylphenidate may increase its effects. Epinephrine and norepinephrine may increase nortriptyline's blood-pressure-raising effect. MAO inhibitors (*see*) may cause severe excitation, high fever, or seizures. Contraindicated during recovery from a heart attack, in prostate enlargement, in patients with cardiovascular disease, urine retention, glaucoma, thyroid disease, impaired liver function or blood abnormalities, and in patients who are suicidal or undergoing elective surgery. Other drugs, including OTC, should not be used with nortriptyline without consulting a physician. Most effective when taken on an empty stomach, but may be taken with a small amount of food if stomach upset is a problem.

NORTUSSIN • *See* Guaifenesin.

NORVASC • *See* Amlodipine Besylate.

NOSCAPINE (Rx) • **Narcompren. Narcotussin. Nipaxon.** An opium alkaloid from the plant *Papaver somniferum*. It is used in cough medicine.

NOSOCOMIAL INFECTION • Hospital-acquired infection.

NOSTRIL • *See* Phenylephrine.

NOSTRILLA LONG ACTING NASAL SOLUTION • *See* Oxymetazoline.

NOVAFED • *See* Pseudoephedrine.

NOVAFED A (OTC) • A combination of chlorpheniramine and pseudoephedrine (*see both*).

NOVAHISTINE DMX (OTC) • A combination of dextromethorphan, pseudoephedrine, and guaifenesin (*see all*), used for the temporary relief of coughs and nasal congestion. *See also* Novahistine Expectorant.

NOVAHISTINE EXPECTORANT (OTC) • **Alamine Expectorant. Deproist Expectorant. Dihistine Expectorant. Histor-D. Myhistine Expectorant. Phenhist Expectorant. Mytussine DAC. Robitussin-DAC.** These medications contain a combination of pseudoephedrine, codeine, and guaifenesin (*see all*). They are used for the relief of cough, nasal congestion, runny nose, and other symptoms associated with the common cold, viruses, and other upper respiratory diseases. The drug may also be used to treat allergies, asthma, ear infections, or sinus infections. Poten-tial adverse reactions include anxiety, insomnia, blurred vision, difficulty passing urine, headache, palpitations, constipation, dizziness, and restlessness. Contraindicated in persons with glaucoma, diabetes, heart disease, high blood pressure, thyroid disease, or a prostate condition. Should be taken with food and a full glass of water to reduce stomach upset. May be addicting.

NOVAMOXIN • *See* Amoxicillin.

NOVANTRONE • *See* Mitoxantrone.

NOVIR • *See* Ritonavir.

NOVO AMPICILLIN • *See* Ampicillin.

NOVOCAIN • *See* Procaine.

NOVOCLOXIN • *See* Cloxacillin Sodium.

NOVOCOLCHICINE • *See* Colchicine.

NOVOFOLACID • *See* Folic Acid.

NOVOLEXIN • *See* Cephalexin Monohydrate.

NOVOLIN L, N, R • *See* Insulin.

NOVONIDAZOL • *See* Metronidazole.

NOVO-NIFEDIN • *See* Nifedipine.

NOVOPEN-VK • *See* Penicillin V.

NOVO-PREDNISONE • *See* Prednisone.

NPH • *See* Insulin.

NP-27 • *See* Tolnaftate.

NSAIDs • Abbreviation for nonsteroidal anti-inflammatory drugs (*see*).

NTG • *See* Nitroglycerin.

NTZ LONG ACTING NASAL SPRAY • *See* Oxymetazoline.

NUBAIN • *See* Nalbuphine Hydrochloride.

NUCLEIC ACIDS • Large, naturally occurring molecules composed of chemical building blocks known as nucleotides. There are two kinds of nucleic acids, DNA and RNA.

NUCOFED (Rx) • *See* Pseudoephedrine, Codeine Phosphate, and Sulfate.

NUMORPHAN • *See* Oxymorphone.

NUPERCAINAL • *See* Dibucaine.

NUPRIN • *See* Ibuprofen.

NUTMEG and MACE (H) • *Myristica fragrans.* The tree that produces both nutmeg and mace is native to the Banda islands and Molucca islands of the Malay archipelago, India, the West Indies, and Brazil. Both nutmeg and mace are used for flatulence, nausea, and vomiting. They are mildly narcotic. They are used to flavor medicines. In 1992, the FDA proposed a ban on nutmeg oil in oral menstrual drug products because it had not been shown to be safe and effective as claimed. Nutmeg taken in large doses causes hallucinations and has become a drug of abuse in recent years. It is harmless in small doses as a spice. When used as a medicine, it may cause nausea and vomiting.

NUTRACEUTICAL • A product between a drug and a food; any substance that may be considered a food or part of a food and provides medical or health benefits, including the prevention and treatment of disease. An example is L-carnitine, which is sold over the counter as a dietary supplement and as the drug Carnitor, to treat an inborn error of metabolism.

NUTRACORT • *See* Hydrocortisone.

NUTRAMAX (OTC) • A high-calorie liquid nutrition product that is lactose free. *See* Lactose.

NUTRAPLUS • *See* Urea.

NUX-V • Homeopathic abbreviation for nux vomica (*see*).

NUX VOMICA (OTC) (H) • **Nux-v. Poison Nut.** Derived from *Strychnos nux-vomica,* a small evergreen tree native to India, Sri Lanka, and Malaysia. The seeds, which contain strychnine, the poison, are used for a homeopathic (*see*) medication for indigestion. In 1992, the FDA issued a notice that nux vomica extract had not been shown to be safe and effective as claimed in OTC digestive-aid products.

NYDRAZID • *See* Isoniazid.

NYSTAGMUS • Involuntary rapid eye movement.

NYSTATIN (Rx) • **Mycolog II. Mycostatin. Myco-Triacet. Mykinac. Nadostine. N.G.T. Nilstat. Nystex. Nyst-Olone II. O-V Statin.** An antifungal medication introduced in 1954 to treat oral, vaginal, and intestinal infections caused by *Candida albicans* (*Monilia*) and other *Candida* species. In a cream or ointment, it is used to treat infant eczema, itching around the anus or vagina, and localized forms of candidiasis. Potential adverse reactions include nausea, vomiting, and diarrhea. Skin application may cause occasional contact dermatitis from preservatives in some formulations. It is a candidate for OTC status.

NYSTEX • *See* Nystatin.

NYST-OLONE II • *See* Nystatin and Triamcinolone.

NYTILAX • *See* Senna.

NYTOL (OTC) • Approved by the FDA as a sleep aid. *See* Diphenhydramine.

O

OAK BARK EXTRACT (H) • *Quercus alba.* **Oak Chip Extract. Stone Oak. White Oak.** The extract from the white oak, used in flavorings. Contains tannic acid (*see*) and is exceedingly astringent. In a wash, the Indians used it for sore eyes and as a tonic. Used in astringents and to treat hemorrhoids. It has been used in a gargle to treat sore throats and in homeopathic medicine to treat spleen and liver ailments. May cause constipation and decrease the absorption of some nutrients.

OAK CHIP EXTRACT • *See* Oak Bark Extract.

OAT FIBER (H) • *Avena sativa.* An extract is used by herbalists to treat anxiety and aid digestion. It is rich in silicic acid, mucin, and calcium (*see all*). The grain has been found by modern scientists to be effective in lowering cholesterol. Oat fiber also is used by herbalists to treat general debility and exhaustion.

OAT FLOUR (OTC) (H) • Flour from the cereal grain that is an important crop grown in the temperate regions. Light yellow or brown to weak green powder. Slight odor; starchy taste. Makes a bland ointment to soothe skin irritation; is used in powdery form for soothing baths to treat skin irritation, rash, and hemorrhoids.

OBALAN • *See* Phendimetrazine.

OBE-NIX • *See* Phentermine.

OBEPHEN • *See* Phentermine.

OBERMINE • *See* Phentermine.

OBESTIN-30 • *See* Phentermine.

OBEVAL • *See* Phendimetrazine.

OBSESSIVE-COMPULSIVE DISORDER • A type of anxiety disorder marked by the persistent intrusion of unwanted and uncontrollable thoughts. This condition may cause someone to perform repeated, senseless rituals in an attempt to reduce anxiety. While compulsive behavior is almost always preceded by obsessive thoughts, some people have obsessive thoughts but do not ritualize. An estimated 5 million Americans suffer from this disorder.

OBY-TRIM • *See* Phentermine.

OCCIPUT • The back part of the head.

OCCLUSAL • *See* Salicylic Acid.

OCCLUSION • Blockage.

OCCULT • Hidden, not evident to the naked eye.

OCEAN NASAL MIST (OTC) • *See* Sodium Chloride.

OCIMUM BASILICUM • *See* Basil.

OCTOCAINE • *See* Lidocaine.

OCTOXYNOL-9 (Rx) • **Koromex Foam, Cream, Jelly. Koromex Water-Jel Sterile Burn Dressings. Massengill Liquid Concentrate. Ortho-Gynol Contraceptive Jelly. pHisoDerm For Baby. pHisoDerm Skin Cleanser.** Waxlike emulsifiers, dispersing agents, and detergents derived from phenol. Used as a bactericide and spermicide in cleansing products and douches, and as a dispersing agent in vaginal contraceptive creams.

OCTREOSCAN (Rx) • A kit for the preparation of indium In-111 pentreotide, a radiopharmaceutical imaging agent for the localization of metastatic neuroendocrine tumors. Introduced in 1994 after a 19.3-month priority review, the agent allows for the diagnoses of tumors without surgical biopsy.

OCTREOTIDE (Rx) • **Sandostatin.** An injectable antidiarrheal drug introduced in 1989. Used to treat diarrhea associated with carcinoid tumors. It does not cure the tumor, but helps the patient live a more normal life.

OCTYL DIMETHYL PABA (OTC) • Herpecin-L Cold Sore Lip Balm. A sunscreen that also relieves dryness and chapping by providing a fat barrier to help restore normal moisture balance to the lips. *See* Para-Aminobenzoic Acid.

OCTYL METHOXYCINNAMATE (OTC) • Aquaderm Combination Treatment. Neutrogena Moisture. PreSun Active. A sunblock derived from balsam of Peru, cinnamon leaves, or coca leaves. May be isolated from wood-rotting fungus.

OCU-DROP (OTC) • *See* Tetrahydrozoline.

OCUFEN • *See* Flurbiprofen.

OCUL-, OCULO- • Prefixes meaning pertaining to the eye.

OCULAR • Pertaining to the eye.

OCULAR LUBRICANT • *See* Artificial Tears.

OCULINUM • *See* Botulinum Toxin Type A.

OCU-PENTOLATE • *See* Cyclopentolate.

OCU-PHRIN OPHTHALMIC SOLUTION • *See* Phenylephrine.

OCU-PRED • *See* Prednisolone.

OCUSERT PILO • *See* Pilocarpine.

OCU-TROPIC • *See* Tropicamide.

OCU-TROPINE • *See* Atropine Sulfate.

OCU-ZOLINE • *See* Naphazoline.

O-FLEX • *See* Orphenadrine.

OFLOXACIN (Rx) • Floxin. One of the broad-spectrum quinoline (*see*) antibacterials introduced in 1991, it is used to treat pneumonia, chronic bronchitis, urinary tract infections, bacterial prostatitis due to *Escherichia coli,* sexually transmitted diseases (not proven in syphilis), and skin infections. Potential adverse reactions include headache, dizziness, fatigue, lethargy, drowsiness, sleep disorders, nervousness, light-headedness, seizures, chest pain, nausea, abdominal pain, diarrhea, vomiting, dry mouth, flatulence, vaginitis, painful menstruation, genital itching, rash, photosensitivity, visual disturbances, bad taste in the mouth, loss of appetite, and fever. Antacids containing aluminum or magnesium hydroxide, iron salts, sucralfate, products containing zinc, and some anticancer drugs interfere with the absorption of ofloxacin. The drug increases the effects of blood thinners. Some quinolones may increase the side effects of theophylline (*see*). Contraindicated in persons with a history of hypersensitivity to ofloxacin or the quinolone group of antibacterial agents. Serious and occasionally fatal hypersensitivity reactions, some following the first dose, have been reported in patients receiving quinolones. When taking this drug, you should use sunscreen and protective clothing when outside. The drug should not be taken with food, but on an empty stomach. Antacids should be avoided for one hour before or two hours after taking the drug. Fluids should be ingested liberally during the entire course of treatment.

OGEN • *See* Estrogen.

OGMT • *See* Metyrosine.

-OID • Suffix meaning like, as in *carcinoid,* which is like cancer but not as malignant.

OIL OF MELALEUCA ALTERNIFOLIA (OTC) (H) • Honeymyrtle. Koromex Water-Jel Burn Dressings. Tea Tree. The oil of an Australian or East Indian shrub of the family *Myrtaceae* used by herbalists to treat burns. The gel is a proprietary formulation of natural gums and oils in a preserved, sterile base. It reportedly cools the burn area and protects the covered wound from contamination. *See also* Cajuput.

OIL OF WINTERGREEN • *See* Methyl Salicylate.

OINTMENT • A semisolid preparation or salve, applied externally, usually containing a drug.

OLANZAPINE (Rx) • **Zyprex.** Expected to be introduced on the market soon, this drug for the treatment of schizophrenia was more effective than haloperidol (*see*) and reportedly has fewer side effects than other schizophrenia drugs in use.

OLEOVITAMIN A • *See* Vitamin A.

OLEUM RICINI • *See* Castor Oil.

OLEYL ALCOHOL • **Ocenol.** Found in fish oil. Chiefly used in the manufacture of detergents and wetting agents and as an antifoam agent and as a carrier for medications. No known toxicity.

OLIG-, OLIGO- • Prefix meaning scanty, as in *oligospermia,* abnormally small amount of sperm in the ejaculate.

OLIGURIA • Scanty secretion of urine.

OLIVE (H) • *Olea europaea.* The oil is used as a laxative. The leaves have been used to reduce fever, and as a mild tranquilizer. Externally, the oil has been used to soothe insect bites, itching, and bruises. It has been found by modern scientists to help reduce the "bad" cholesterol, the LDLs (low-density lipoproteins), while not affecting the "good" cholesterol, the HDLs (high-density lipoproteins).

OLSALAZINE SODIUM (Rx) • **Dipentum.** A local anti-inflammatory agent used to maintain remission of ulcerative colitis (*see*) in patients intolerant of sulfasalazine (*see*). Potential adverse reactions include nausea, headache, diarrhea, abdominal pain, depression, dizziness, rash, itching, heartburn, and joint pain. Contraindicated in patients hypersensitive to salicylates (*see*). Should be used cautiously in patients with kidney dysfunction. Should be taken with food to reduce stomach upset and diarrhea.

-OMA • Suffix meaning pertaining to a tumor.

OMEGA-3 FATTY ACIDS • Found in fish oils. Reported to lower fats in the blood and thus reduce the risk of coronary artery disease.

OMEPRAZOLE (Rx) • **Prilosec (formerly Losec).** A once-a-day drug introduced in 1989, it is the first of a new class of drugs called acid pump inhibitors (*see*). It is used to relieve symptoms of certain acid-related gastrointestinal ailments such as gastroesophageal reflux disease (GERD) (*see*) and erosive esophagitis. It is also approved for treatment of Zollinger-Ellison syndrome, a rare condition marked by chronic and unusually high levels of stomach acid secretion and recurrent ulcers. After oral administration, the onset of the antisecretory effect occurs within one hour, with the maximum effect occurring within two hours. Potential adverse reactions include abdominal pain, chest pain, constipation, diarrhea, dizziness, gas, headache, heartburn, muscle pain, nausea and vomiting, rash or itching, fever, weight gain, cough, back pain, dry mouth, taste perversion, urinary tract infection, and unusual sleepiness and fatigue. The FDA advisory committee recommended that omeprazole be used for maintenance therapy as well as for acute treatment. Before, omeprazole's use was restricted to four to eight weeks. The European Committee for Proprietary Medicinal Products labeled omeprazole as safe, but the German regulatory authority suspended the license for two intravenous preparations and ordered the manufacturer to undertake studies that would be specified at a later date. The German agency insisted further on labeling changes to alert doctors to rare visual and auditory adverse reactions even with the oral form. Diazepam, warfarin, and phenytoin increase omeprazole's levels in the body. Ketoconazole, iron derivatives, and ampicillin may be less effective if taken with omeprazole. Inform your physician if you are taking or plan to take over-the-counter or prescription medications because of possible interaction with omeprazole. It should be taken immediately before eating, preferably before breakfast.

OMNIFLOX • *See* Temafloxacin.

OMNIPEN • *See* Ampicillin.

OMNIPEN-N • *See* Ampicillin.

OMS • *See* Morphine Sulfate or Hydrochloride.

ONCASPAR 7 • *See* Pegaspargase.

ONCOSCINT (Rx) • The first monoclonal-antibody-based cancer imaging agent (*see* Monoclonal Antibody) was approved for marketing in 1992 for detecting colorectal and ovarian cancers. It is used in conjunction with CAT scans and other existing diagnostic tools. The patient is scanned forty-eight hours after OncoScint is injected to determine if there are any "hot spots" of cancer in the body.

ONCOVIN • *See* Vincristine Sulfate.

ONDANSETRON (Rx) • **Zofran.** A drug introduced in 1991, it raises serotonin levels in the brain. It is injected to prevent nausea and vomiting associated with cancer chemotherapy. Potential adverse reactions include headache, diarrhea, constipation, rash, and rarely, bronchospasm. Contraindicated in patients hypersensitive to the drug.

ONION (H) • *Allium cepa.* A syrup made from onion juice has been used by herbalists for centuries to treat congestion caused by colds. According to ancient folklore, onion also aids sexual potency. It has also long been used to treat indigestion, and the roasted onion has been used as a poultice for earache. Modern scientists have found that onion can lower overall cholesterol and blood pressure and help to prevent blood clots. A study by the National Cancer Institute showed that people with diets high in allium vegetables, such as onion and garlic (*Allium sativum*), suffer from fewer incidences of stomach cancer. The sulfur content in the onion probably explains its action as a strong disinfectant. Onions are diuretic.

ONYCH-, ONYCHO- • Prefixes meaning pertaining to the nails.

ONYCHIA • Inflammation of the nail bed.

OO- • Denotes an egg, as in *oophorectomy*, removal of the ovary.

OP • Homeopathic abbreviation for opium.

OP-CCK • *See* Sincalide.

OPCON • *See* Naphazoline.

OPCON-A • *See* Naphazoline and Pheniramine.

o,p-DDD • *See* Mitotane.

OPHIOGLOSSUM VULGATUM • *See* Adder's-Tongue.

OPHIOPOGON JAPONICUS • *See* Japanese Turf Lily.

OPHTHAINE • *See* Proparacaine.

OPHTHALGAN • *See* Glycerin.

OPHTHALMIC PRODUCTS • Medicines for the eyes. Those available over the counter are used in treating minor ailments such as tear insufficiency, sties, or mild conjunctivitis.

OPHTHALMO- • Prefix meaning pertaining to the eye.

OPHTHETIC • *See* Proparacaine.

OPHTHOCHLOR OPHTHALMIC • *See* Chloramphenicol.

OPHTHOCORT (Rx) • A combination of chloramphenicol, hydrocortisone, and polymyxin B.

OPIUM (Rx) (H) • *Papaver somniferum.* **Camphorated Opium. Laudanum. Opium Poppy. Pantopon. Paregoric.** A natural substance derived from the opium poppy, containing morphine. Opium was formerly used in many medications. Highly addictive, opium itself is now little used, but its derivatives and synthetic versions of these (narcotics) are used as analgesics, cough suppressants, and antidiarrheal drugs. Homeopathic remedies are made from opium dissolved in alcohol. As an antidiarrheal medication, opium inhibits motility and propulsion and diminishes secretions in the GI tract. Potential adverse reactions include nausea, vomiting, bloating, convulsions, confusion, dizziness, drowsiness, low blood pressure, nervousness, slow heartbeat, irregular breathing, weakness, rash, and dependence after long-term use. Contraindicated in acute diarrhea resulting from poison (until toxic material is removed from GI tract) and diarrhea caused by organisms that penetrate intestinal mucosa. Should be used cautiously in asthma, enlarged prostate, liver disease, or those with a history of narcotic dependence. Risk of physical dependence increases with long-term use. Should not be used for more than two days.

OPPORTUNISTIC INFECTIONS • Infections occurring in patients with a defective immune system.

OPTI-CLEAN • A contact lens cleaning solution.

OPTICROM • *See* Cromolyn Sodium.

OPTIGENE-3 • *See* Tetrahydrozoline.

OPTILETS-M-500 (OTC) • A multivitamin and mineral preparation.

OPTIMINE • *See* Azatadine Maleate.

OPTIMYD (Rx) • An anti-infectant for the eyes. *See* Prednisolone and Sulfacetamide.

OPTIPRANOLOL • *See* Metipranolol.

ORABASE HCA • *See* Hydrocortisone.

ORACIT • *See* Sodium Citrate and Citric Acid.

ORAJEL • *See* Benzocaine.

ORAL CONTRACEPTIVES (Rx) • **Brevicon. Demulen. Enovid. Levlen. Loestrin. Lo/Ovral.** **Micronor (progestin only). Modicon. Nelova. Norcept-E. Nordette. Norethin. Norinyl. Norlestrin. Nor-Q D. Ortho Cyclen. Ortho-Novum. Ovcon. Ovral. Ovrette (progestin only). Tri-Levlen. Tri-Norinyl. Triphasil.** Introduced in 1956, products that enabled women to be effectively "immune" to pregnancy brought one of the major behavioral changes to modern society. Most oral contraceptives today consist of a combination of the female hormones estrogen and progestin. Some contain only a minimum dose of one component, a progestin. While used primarily to prevent pregnancy, oral contraceptives are sometimes used to treat menstrual irregularity, excessively heavy menstrual flow, and endometriosis (*see*). Contraindicated in those who have had an allergic reaction to any dosage form, a history of blood clots, heart attack, stroke, breast cancer, liver disease, abnormal vaginal bleeding, sickle cell disease, or are pregnant. Must be used with caution in those with the following conditions: fibrocystic breast disease, fibroid tumors of the uterus, endometriosis, migrainelike headaches, epilepsy, asthma, heart disease, high blood pressure, gallbladder disease, diabetes, porphyria (*see*), or previous cancer. Also, regular smokers are at higher risk. Potential adverse reactions include nausea, vomiting, drowsiness, high blood pressure, allergic reactions, bloating, diarrhea, tannish pigmentation of the face, reduced tolerance to contact lenses, impaired color vision, joint and muscle pain, emotional depression, eye changes, gallbladder disease, benign liver tumors, jaundice, erosion of the cervix, enlargement of uterine fibroid tumors, cystitislike syndrome, blood clots, stroke, heart attack, and blood clot in abdominal artery. Also decreased libido, irregular menstruation, breast enlargement with tenderness. Temporary infertility after stopping the pill may occur. In a well-controlled study in the Netherlands reported in 1994 in *Lancet* (September 26), as well as in other meta-analyses, long-term use of oral contraceptives, either early or late in life, may be associated with an increased risk of breast cancer. Taken concurrently with antidiabetic drugs, tricyclic antidepressants, troleandomycin, or warfarin, the effects of these medications may be unpredictable, and their adverse effects may be increased. Estrogens taken during pregnancy can predispose the female child to later development of vaginal or cervical cancer following puberty. Oral contraceptives may increase the effects of some benzodiazepines (*see*) and cause excessive sedation. They also may increase the effects of metoprolol, prednisolone, prednisone, and theophylline, increasing the risk of side effects. The following drugs may decrease the effectiveness of oral contraceptives: barbiturates, carbamazepine, griseofulvin, penicillins, phenytoin, primidone, rifampin, and tetracyclines (*see all*). Oral contraceptives need to be taken on schedule for maximum protection against pregnancy. A missed pill can allow pregnancy to occur. Excessive use of salt should be avoided if fluid retention occurs. *See also* Estrogen and Depo-Provera.

ORAL TOLERIZATION • A treatment that seeks to turn off patients' rejection of their own tissue by feeding them small amounts of a protein directly or indirectly attacked by their immune system. The approach was derived from the well-established fact that people rarely mount an immune response to food. For example, patients with diabetes would be given insulin, which is produced by the pancreas; those with multiple sclerosis are already being given a protein from the coverings of the nerves in the brain and spinal cord. Patients with arthritis are being given the joint protein, collagen. The first two are administered in powdered form and the collagen is a liquid given in orange juice. In early tests on human patients, oral tolerization has enabled some to stop taking steroids or other powerful immunosuppressant drugs.

ORAMIDE • *See* Tolbutamide.

ORAP • *See* Pimozide.

ORAPHEN-PD • *See* Acetaminophen.

ORASONE • *See* Prednisone.

ORA-TESTRYL • *See* Fluoxymesterone.

ORAZINC • *See* Zinc.

ORBENIN • *See* Cloxacillin Sodium.

ORCH- • Prefix meaning pertaining to the testicles.

ORCHITIS • Inflammation of the testicles.

ORCIPRENALINE SULFATE • *See* Metaproterenol.

OREGON GRAPE ROOT (H) • *Berberis aquifolium. Berberis. Mountain Grape. Rocky Mountain Grape. Trailing Mahonia. Wild Oregon Grape.* Employed by early American physicians to treat skin diseases or other illnesses that dried out the skin or produced sores, including syphilis and chronic hepatitis. Oregon grape root contains hydrastine, used to stop uterine bleeding, and berberine (*see both*), used today as an antiseptic and decongestant in eye lotions. Modern studies have found that Oregon grape also contains oxyacanthine chloride and columbine chloride, both of which show antibacterial properties. Herbalists have also used the root to treat hepatitis, arthritis, cancer, and heart problems. *See also* Barberry.

ORETIC • *See* Hydrochlorothiazide.

ORETICYL (Rx) • *See* Hydrochlorothiazide and Reserpine.

ORETON METHYL • *See* Methyltestosterone.

OREX (OTC) • A saliva substitute.

ORFLAGEN • *See* Orphenadrine.

ORGANIC • There are no federal standards for the term, but *organic* usually means produce grown without pesticides, herbicides, or synthetic fertilizers, on land that has been free of such chemicals from one to seven years.

ORGANIC MENTAL DISORDER • A temporary or permanent impairment of the brain caused by physiological disturbance of brain tissue at any level of organization—structural, hormonal, or biochemical. Causes are aging, toxic substances, and a variety of physical disorders.

ORGANIDIN • *See* Guaifenesin.

ORG NC 45 • *See* Vecuronium.

ORIGANUM • *See* Marjoram.

ORIGINAL DOAN'S • *See* Magnesium Salicylate.

ORINASE • *See* Tolbutamide.

ORMAZINE • *See* Chlorpromazine.

ORNADE (OTC) • *See* Chlorpheniramine and Phenylpropanolamine.

ORNEX (OTC) • *See* Acetaminophen and Phenylpropanolamine.

ORNIDYL • *See* Eflornithine.

ORO-, OS- • Prefixes meaning mouth or opening.

ORPHAN DRUG • A pharmaceutical for a rare disease. Under the Orphan Drug Act of 1983, the FDA has granted nearly five hundred orphan drug designations. Such status, granted before the drug is approved for marketing by the FDA, entitles sponsors to certain incentives to develop drugs for rare diseases. The most important of these incentives is seven years of market exclusivity following FDA approval of the drug. This helps sponsors recover the large sums spent on research and development, which would be difficult to do otherwise, because orphan status is granted to drugs that treat diseases with a patient population of two hundred thousand or less. In March 1992, congressional hearings were held on the Orphan Drug Act because some companies had received orphan drug status for medications that required little development cost and had considerable market potential. During the Senate hearings, a proposal was put forth to revise the act by rescinding on a product the designation of orphan drug if it earns a company more than $200 million.

ORPHENADRINE (Rx) • **Banflex. Disipal. Flexagin. Flexoject. Flexon. K-Flex. Marflex. Myolin. Myotrol. Noradex. Norflex. Norgesic Forte. O-Flex. Orflagen. Orphenate. Tega-Flex. X-OTAG.** A muscle relaxant that reduces transmission of impulses from the spinal cord to skeletal muscles. Used to treat painful, acute musculoskeletal conditions. Potential adverse reactions include anemia, disorientation, restlessness, irritability, weakness, drowsiness, headache, dizziness, palpitations, rapid heartbeat, blurred vision, difficulty in swallowing, constipation, dry mouth, nausea, vomiting, intestinal stoppage, urine retention, and stomach pain. Alcohol and other central nervous system depressants increase the central nervous system–depressant effects of orphenadrine. Contraindicated in glaucoma, enlarged prostate, duodenal, bowel, or bladder-neck obstructions, myasthenia gravis (*see*), rapid heartbeat, severe liver or kidney dysfunction, and ulcerative colitis. Should be used cautiously in elderly or debilitated patients with heart disease or sulfite sensitivity, and those exposed to high temperatures. Anticholinergic (*see*) drugs may increase the relaxation of the muscles too much. Propoxyphene (*see*) taken with orphenadrine may cause confusion, anxiety, and tremors. Orphenadrine may be taken with food to reduce stomach irritation.

ORPHENATE • *See* Orphenadrine.

ORTHO- • Prefix meaning straight, correct, normal.

ORTHOCLONE OKT3 • *See* Muromonab-CD3.

ORTHO-CYCLEN (Rx) • An oral contraceptive introduced in 1992, it contains a synthetic version of the female hormone progesterone (*see*).

ORTHO-NOVUM (Rx) • A combination of estradiol and norethindrone.

ORTHOPHOSPHORIC ACID • In 1992, the FDA issued a notice that orthophosphoric acid had not been shown to be safe and effective as claimed in OTC digestive-aid products.

ORTHOPNEA • Difficulty in breathing when lying flat.

ORTHOSTATIC • Standing position.

ORTHOSTATIC HYPOTENSION • Low blood pressure causing dizziness or fainting after abruptly standing or sitting up.

OR-TYL • *See* Dicyclomine.

ORUDIS • *See* Ketoprofen.

ORUVAIL • *See* Ketoprofen.

OS-, OSTE-, OSTEO- • Prefixes meaning pertaining to bone.

OS-CAL (OTC) • A combination of calcium and vitamin D (*see both*).

OSCILLOCOCCINUM (H) • Introduced in the United States in 1983, it is an official homeopathic medicine prepared from *Anas barbariae hepatis,* a perennial herb, and *Cordis extractum,* natural substances from a perennial herb and a tree. It is used to treat symptoms of flu, including fever, chills, and aches and pains. Oscillococcinum's active ingredient is diluted homeopathically two hundred times before being impregnated on tiny sugar pellets enclosed in a tube. The pellets are placed under the tongue. No adverse effects have been reported.

OSHA (H) • *Ligusticum porteri.* An herb used by western American Indians to treat colds, flu, and upper-respiratory infections. Osha is reputed to build immunity. It is related to lovage (*see*).

-OSIS • Suffix meaning pertaining to a condition of production or increase, such as *leukocytosis,* the multiplication of white blood cells.

OSMITROL • *See* Mannitol.

OSMOGLYN • *See* Glycerin.

OSTEITIS DEFORMANS • *See* Paget's Disease.

OSTEOMA • A benign tumor of bone.

OSTEOMYELITIS • Infection of bone and marrow due to the growth of germs within the bone.

OSTEOPOROSIS • A condition characterized by low bone mass and an increased susceptibility to bone fractures.

OSTOMY • **Colostomy. Ileostomy.** A surgical diversion of the intestine to manage waste discharge after removal of some or all of the colon.

OTC • Abbreviation for over-the-counter, referring to nonprescription medicine.

OTIC HC (Rx) • A combination of hydrocortisone, chloroxylenol, and pramoxine hydrochloride (*see all*).

OTIC SOLUTION • Ear drops. Used to relieve minor ear discomfort by softening earwax.

OTI-SONE (Rx) • A combination of neomycin, polymyxin B, and hydrocortisone (*see all*), used to treat skin infections and inflammations.

OTO • *See* Auralgan.

OTOBIOTIC (Rx) • A combination of hydrocortisone and polymixin B (*see both*).

OTOCORT (Rx) • A combination of hydrocortisone and neomycin (*see both*).

OTO EAR DROPS • *See* Antipyrine and Benzocaine.

OTOMYCIN-HPN (Rx) • A combination of neomycin, polymyxin B, and hydrocortisone (*see all*).

OTRIVIN (OTC) • *See* Xylometazoline.

OUABAIN • *See* Digitalis.

OUTGRO SOLUTION (OTC) • A combination of chlorobutanol and tannic acid (*see both*) used to provide temporary relief of pain, swelling, and inflammation accompanying ingrown toenails. Daily use is supposed to toughen tender skin, allowing the nail to be cut. For external use only. Should not be used for more than a week unless directed by a doctor. Contraindicated in diabetes and poor circulation, or if there is swelling of the toe or discharge around the nails.

OVCON • *See* Estradiol and Norethindrone.

OVER-THE-COUNTER MEDICINE (OTC) • Medicine available without a doctor's prescription. Used for the temporary relief, prevention, or cure of self-recognizable conditions.

OVIDE • *See* Malathion.

OVRAL • *See* Estradiol.

OVRETTE • *See* Norgestrel.

O-V STATIN • *See* Nystatin.

OVULEN (Rx) • *See both* Ethynodiol and Mestranol.

OVUSTICK (OTC) • A diagnostic test for ovulation.

OXACILLIN SODIUM (Rx) • **Bactocill. Prostaphlin. Sodium Oxacillin.** A penicillin antibiotic used to treat systemic infections caused by penicillinase-producing staphylococci (*see*). Potential adverse reactions include anemia, neuropathy, neuromuscular irritation, seizures, oral lesions, kidney dysfunction, hepatitis, blood clot at site of injection, and hypersensitivity, including potentially fatal allergic reactions. Also, overgrowth of nonsusceptible organisms. Should be taken on an empty stomach.

OXALIC ACID • Occurs naturally in many plants and vegetables, particularly in the *Oxalis* genus; also in many molds. Some plants such as rhubarb, spinach, and *Amaranthus* are high in it. Oxalic acid has the ability to bind some metals such as calcium and magnesium and has therefore been suspected of interfering with the metabolism of these minerals.

OXALID • *See* Oxyphenbutazone.

OXAMNIQUINE (Rx) • **Vansil.** Used to treat schistosomiasis, an intestinal worm infection. Side effects may include seizures, dizziness, drowsiness, headache, nausea, vomiting, abdominal pain, loss of appetite, and hives. Should be taken after meals to reduce side effects, unless directed otherwise by your physician.

OXANDROLONE (Rx) • **Anavar.** An anabolic steroid introduced in 1964 to promote tissue building and reverse the loss of tissue. Used to combat the loss of tissue related to corticosteroid therapy, osteoporosis, prolonged immobilization, and debilitated states. Continuous therapy should be limited to three months. Potential adverse reactions in women include acne, oily skin, weight gain, hairiness, hoarseness, clitoral enlargement, changes in libido, flushing, sweating, and vaginitis with itching. In prepubescent males, premature epiphyseal closure, priapism (*see*), growth of body and facial hair, phallic enlargement; in postpubescent males, testicular atrophy, scanty sperm, decreased ejaculatory volume, impotence, breast enlargement, and epididymitis. In both sexes, edema, gastroenteritis, nausea, vomiting, diarrhea, constipation, changes in appetite, bladder irritability, jaundice, liver toxicity, and high levels of calcium in the blood. Contraindicated in men with enlarged or cancerous prostates, carcinoma of the male breast, high levels of calcium in the blood, or heart, liver, or kidney dysfunction, and in premature infants. Should be used cautiously in prepubescent males, patients with diabetes or heart disease, and those taking ACTH, corticosteroids, or anticoagulants. Should be taken with food.

OXAPROZIN (Rx) • **Daypro.** A nonsteroidal anti-inflammatory drug (*see* NSAIDs) approved in 1993 for once-daily treatment of rheumatoid arthritis and osteoarthritis. Controlled clinical trials in patients with arthritis have found oxaprozin, 1,200 mg once-a-day, to be at least as effective as other NSAIDs. Potential adverse effects include abdominal pain, heartburn, nausea and vomiting, kidney and liver toxicity, and prolonged bleeding. The long-acting drug may provide relief of arthritis symptoms with one dose per day, but when adverse effects occur, they may persist longer than with other NSAIDs.

OXAZEPAM (Rx) • **Serax.** An antianxiety drug introduced in 1965 that depresses the central nervous system at the area of the brain that controls emotion. Used to treat alcohol withdrawal, and moderate to severe anxiety. Potential side effects include drowsiness, lethargy, irregular menstruation, hangover, fainting, transient low blood pressure, nausea, vomiting, abdominal discomfort, and liver dysfunction. Should not be used with alcohol or other central nervous system depressants. Contraindicated in psychoses. Should be used cautiously in persons with convulsive disorders, drug allergy, blood problems, kidney disease, and depression. Has the possibility of abuse and addiction. The use of some OTC drugs that contain antihistamines may cause excessive sedation in some people. Heavy smoking may decrease the effectiveness of this drug. Intake of caffeine-containing beverages may make it less effective. Oxazepam increases the effects of digoxin and phenytoin and decreases the effectiveness of levodopa. Oral contraceptives and theophylline make oxazepam less effective. Oxazepam should not be discontinued suddenly. May be taken with or without food.

OX BILE • Banned as an ingredient in laxatives by the FDA, May 1992.

OXICONAZOLE NITRATE (Rx) • **Oxistat.** A medication introduced in 1989 for the treatment of fungus infections of the skin such as athlete's foot, jock itch, and ringworm of the body. Potential adverse reactions include itching, burning, irritation, swelling, cracking, and redness of the skin. Do not use this product near the eyes.

OXILAN (Rx) • *See* Ioxilan.

OXILAPINE SUCCINATE • *See* Loxapine.

OXIPOR VHC • *See* Benzocaine.

OXISTAT • *See* Oxiconazole Nitrate.

OXLYR • *See* Oxycodone.

OXPENTIFYLLINE • *See* Pentoxifylline.

OXPRENOLOL (Rx) • **Slow-Trasicor. Trasicor.** A beta-blocker (*see*) used to treat angina (*see*), high blood pressure, irregular heartbeat, anxiety, tremors, overactive thyroid gland, and mitral valve prolapse. Also used to prevent heart attacks in people who have already experienced one. Potential adverse reactions include nausea, vomiting, gastrointestinal disturbances, tingling of the scalp, taste distortion, fatigue, sweating, male impotence, urinary difficulty, diarrhea, bile duct blockage, breathing difficulty, bronchial spasms, muscle weakness, cramps, dry eyes, blurred vision, rash, hair loss, facial swelling, mental depression, confusion, short-term memory loss, and emotional instability. In rare instances, oxprenolol can aggravate lupus erythematosus (*see*) or cause a stuffy nose, chest pains, back and joint pains, colitis, allergy, and unusual bleeding or bruising. It also may aggravate angina and may be contraindicated in persons with liver dysfunction. Should be used cautiously in persons with asthma, severe heart failure, slow heart rate, and heart block because the drug can worsen these conditions. Beta-blockers may interact with surgical anesthesia, increasing the risk of heart problems during surgery. Oxprenolol may interfere with oral antidiabetes medications and with tests for diabetes. Taking oxprenolol with aspirin-containing drugs, indomethacin, sulfinpyrazone, or estrogen can interfere with its blood-pressure-lowering effects. Oxprenolol may interfere with the effectiveness of some drugs taken for asthma, especially ephedrine and isoproterenol, and with theophylline or aminophylline (*see all*). If taken with phenytoin or digitalis, the result may be an excessive slowing of the heart and possible heart block. Oxprenolol should not be discontinued abruptly. May be taken with food to avoid gastrointestinal upset.

OXSORALEN • *See* Methoxsalen.

OXTRIPHYLLINE (Rx) • **Choledyl Theophyllinate. Choline Theophyllinate.** A xanthine (*see*) bronchodilator introduced in 1954 to relieve acute bronchial asthma and reversible bronchospasm associated with chronic bronchitis and emphysema. Potential adverse reactions include nausea, vomiting, irritability, insomnia, excitability, low blood pressure, restlessness, dizziness, headache, light-headedness, seizures, muscle spasms, heart palpitations, irregular heartbeat, rapid heartbeat, flushing, an increase in respiratory rate, loss of appetite, bitter aftertaste, fever, dehydration, local irritation, heartburn, and hives. Contraindicated in hypersensitivity to xanthines such as caffeine and theobromine, and in irregular heartbeat or ulcers. Some colorings (*see*) are xanthine derivatives. Barbiturates, phenytoin, and rifampin decrease its effectiveness. Beta-blockers (*see*) may cause bronchospasms in sensitive patients. Erythromycin, troleandomycin, cimetidine, flu vaccine, and oral contraceptives may cause an increase in toxic effects. When given with ephedrine, excessive nerve stimulation may occur. Charcoal-broiled food and cigarette smoke decrease oxtriphylline's effectiveness. Oxtriphylline should be taken on an empty stomach.

OXYBENZONE (OTC) • **Aquaderm Combination Treatment. Chap Stick. Petroleum Jelly Plus with Sunblock. PreSun for Kids. Vaseline Intensive Care Moisturizing Sunblock Lotion.** Derived from isopropanol (*see*), it is used as a sunscreening agent. Sunscreens may irritate the skin or cause an allergic rash.

OXYBUTYNIN (Rx) • **Ditropan.** An anticholinergic (*see*) drug used to treat incontinence. It has a direct antispasmodic effect and increases urinary bladder capacity plus provides some local painkilling. Potential adverse reactions include nausea, vomiting, drowsiness, dizziness, insomnia, dry mouth, flushing, palpitations, rapid heartbeat, blurred vision, constipation, a bloated feeling, impotence, urinary hesitancy or retention, hives, and severe allergic reactions in patients sensitive to anticholinergics. Also may cause decreased sweating (hot weather may lead to fever or heatstroke) and suppression of lactation. Contraindicated in those with intestinal or urinary obstructions, ulcerative colitis, myasthenia gravis (*see*), and in elderly or debilitated patients. Should be used cautiously in those with kidney or liver dysfunction. Should not be used with alcohol or other central nervous system depressants, including antihistamines. Most effective on an empty stomach, but may be taken with a small amount of food if stomach upset is a problem.

OXYCHLOROSENE (Rx) • **Clorpactin.** A topical antiseptic used to treat localized infections.

OXYCODONE HYDROCHLORIDE or PECTINATE (Rx) • **Percocet. Roxicet. Roxicodone. Roxiprin. Tylox.** A narcotic analgesic introduced in 1950 that alters both the perception of and reaction to pain. Used to treat moderate to severe pain. Potential adverse effects include sedation, sleepiness, lack of alertness, dizziness, euphoria, seizures, low blood pressure, slow heartbeat, nausea, vomiting, constipation, urine retention, and respiratory depression. Alcohol and central nervous system depressants are additive. Anticoagulants used with oxycodone products containing aspirin may increase blood-thinning effects. Should be used with extreme caution in head injury, bronchial asthma, increased pressure on the brain, respiratory depression, alcoholism, enlarged prostate, severe liver or kidney disease, acute abdominal conditions, low thyroid, Addison's disease, irregular heartbeat, narrowing of the tube that carries urine, reduced blood flow, toxic psychosis, and in elderly or debilitated patients. May be addictive. May worsen gallbladder pain. May be taken with food to reduce stomach upset.

OXYCONTIN (Rx) • A controlled pain medication. *See* Oxycodone.

OXYDESS II • *See* Dextroamphetamine.

OXY-5 • *See* Benzoyl Peroxide.

OXYMETA-12 NASAL SOLUTION • *See* Oxymetazoline.

OXYMETAZOLINE (OTC) • **Afrin. Allerest 12 Hour Nasal. Chlorphen-LA. Coricidin Nasal Mist. Dristan Long Lasting. Drixine Nasal. Duramist Plus. 4-Way Long-Acting Nasal. General Nasal Solution. Neo-Synephrine 12 Hour. Nostrilla Long Acting Nasal Decongestant. NTZ Long Acting Nasal Spray. Oxymeta-12 Nasal Solution. Sinex Long-Acting. Twice-A-Day Nasal. Vicks Sinex. Visine.** Used in nose drops that produce constriction of blood vessels to reduce blood flow and nasal congestion. In eyedrops, it is used for the relief of eye redness due to minor irritations. It was changed from Rx to OTC. Potential adverse reactions include headache, drowsiness, dizziness, insomnia, possible sedation, heart palpitations, low blood pressure, high blood pressure, rebound nasal congestion or irritation with excessive or long-term use, dryness of nose and throat, increased nasal discharge, stinging, and sneezing. In children, with excessive or long-term use, sedation. Should be used cautiously in people with overactive thyroid, heart disease, high blood pressure, or diabetes since it can be absorbed systemically. Should not be used by persons taking MAO inhibitors (*see*) or high blood pressure medications.

OXYMETHOLONE (Rx) • **Anadrol-50.** An anabolic steroid (*see*) that promotes tissue-building processes and reverses loss of tissue. Also stimulates the manufacture of red blood cells. Used to treat aplastic anemia, osteoporosis, and wasting conditions. Potential adverse reactions in women include acne, oily skin, weight gain, hairiness, hoarseness, clitoral enlargement, changes in libido, flushing, sweating, and vaginitis with itching. In prepubescent males, premature epiphyseal closure, priapism (*see*), growth of body and facial hair, phallic enlargement; in postpubescent males, testicular atrophy, scanty sperm, decreased ejaculatory volume, impotence, enlargement of breasts, and inflammation of the testes. In both sexes, edema, gastroenteritis, nausea, vomiting, diarrhea, constipation, changes in appetite, bladder irritability, jaundice, liver toxicity, and high levels of calcium in the blood. Can cause liver and splenic blood-filled cysts and liver failure. Contraindicated in men with enlarged or cancerous prostates, carcinoma of the male breast, high levels of calcium in the blood, and heart, liver, or kidney dysfunction, and in premature infants. Should be used cautiously in prepubescent males, patients with diabetes or heart disease, and those taking ACTH, corticosteroids, or anticoagulants. Should be taken with food to reduce stomach upset.

OXYMORPHONE (Rx) • **Numorphan.** A narcotic analgesic used to treat moderate to severe pain. Used preoperatively as a sedative and a supplement to anesthesia.

OXYPHENBUTAZONE (Rx) • **Oxalid. Tandeasil.** A nonsteroidal anti-inflammatory drug that is analgesic and lowers fever, probably through inhibition of prostaglandins (*see*). Used to treat pain, inflammation in arthritis, bursitis, and superficial blood clots in the veins. Potential adverse reactions include potentially fatal bone-marrow suppression, anemia, restlessness, confusion, lethargy, high blood pressure, inflammation of the heart, heart failure, inflammation of the optic nerve, blurred vision, retinal hemorrhage or detachment, hearing loss, nausea, vomiting, diarrhea, peptic ulcer, occult blood loss, blood in the urine and kidney failure, hepatitis, goiter, respiratory problems, metabolic acidosis, and severe rash. Oxyphenbutazone enhances the blood-sugar-lowering effect of antidiabetic drugs and, when used with oral blood thinners, may induce bleeding. Phenytoin and lithium increase levels of oxyphenbutazone in the blood. Contraindicated in children under fourteen years of age, and in patients with senility, GI ulcer, blood problems, and kidney, heart, liver, or thyroid diseases. Should be used only if less toxic alternatives are ineffective or contraindicated. Should be taken with milk, food, or antacid.

OXYPHENCYCLIMINE (Rx) • Daricon. An anticholinergic, antispasmodic drug used to treat irritable bowel syndrome (*see*) and as an adjunctive therapy in peptic ulcers and other GI disorders (*see* Adjunct). May have less atropine-like adverse reactions (*see* Atropine). Potential adverse reactions include disorientation, irritability, incoherence, weakness, nervousness, drowsiness, dizziness, headache, heart palpitations, rapid heartbeat, slow heartbeat, blurred vision, sensitivity to light, increased eye pressure, difficulty in swallowing, constipation, dry mouth, nausea, vomiting, epigastric distress, urinary retention, impotence, hives, decreased sweating, and fever. Contraindicated in glaucoma, obstructions in the urinary or GI tract, myasthenia gravis (*see*), paralytic ileus (*see*), intestinal flaccidity, unstable cardiovascular status in acute hemorrhage, and toxic megacolon. Should be used with caution in patients with nerve damage, overactive thyroid, coronary artery disease, irregular heartbeat, congestive heart failure, high blood pressure, hiatal hernia, liver or kidney disease, and ulcerative colitis. Should also be used with caution in people over forty years of age due to the possibility of glaucoma. Should be taken thirty minutes to one hour before meals.

OXYPHENONIUM (Rx) • Antrenyl. An anticholinergic, antispasmodic drug used to treat irritable bowel syndrome (*see*), and as an adjunctive therapy in peptic ulcers and other GI disorders (*see* Adjunct). Potential adverse reactions include disorientation, irritability, incoherence, weakness, nervousness, drowsiness, dizziness, headache, heart palpitations, rapid heartbeat, slow heartbeat, blurred vision, sensitivity to light, increased eye pressure, difficulty in swallowing, constipation, dry mouth, nausea, vomiting, epigastric distress, urinary retention, impotence, hives, decreased sweating, and fever. Contraindicated in glaucoma, obstructions in the urinary or GI tract, myasthenia gravis (*see*), paralytic ileus (*see*), intestinal flaccidity, unstable cardiovascular status in acute hemorrhage, and toxic megacolon. Should be used with caution in patients with nerve damage, overactive thyroid, coronary artery disease, irregular heartbeat, congestive heart failure, high blood pressure, hiatal hernia, liver or kidney disease, and ulcerative colitis. Should also be used with caution in people over forty years of age due to the possibility of glaucoma. Should be taken thirty minutes to one hour before meals.

OXYQUINOLINE • A white, crystalline powder used as a fungistat, and for creating reddish orange colors when combined with bismuth. Used internally as a disinfectant. Has caused cancer in animals both orally and when injected. In 1992, the FDA issued a notice that oxyquinoline and oxyquinoline sulfate had not been shown to be safe and effective as claimed in OTC products, including astringent (*see*) drugs.

OXYSTEARIN • A mixture of the glycerides of partially oxidized stearic acids and other fatty acids (*see all*). Occurs in animal fat and is used chiefly in the manufacture of soap, candles, cosmetics, suppositories, and pill coatings.

OXYTETRACYCLINE (Rx) • E.P. Mycin. Terramycin. Uri-Tet. A tetracycline (*see*) antibiotic introduced in 1950, it is used to treat gram-negative and gram-positive (*see both*) organisms, trachoma, rickettsiae, brucellosis, pneumonia, syphilis, gonorrhea, and for the long-term treatment of acne. It is one of the most widely prescribed antibiotics. Potential adverse reactions include a drop in white blood cells, pressure on the brain, inflammation of the heart, sore throat, sore tongue, trouble in swallowing, loss of appetite, nausea, vomiting, diarrhea, colitis, anogenital inflammation, rash, photosensitivity, increased pigmentation, hives and other hypersensitivity reactions, as well as irritation at the site of injection. Not prescribed for people with poor kidney function because it can worsen the condition. Antacids, including sodium bicarbonate, and laxatives containing aluminum, magnesium, or calcium, may make oxytetracycline less effective. Iron, zinc, and phenobarbital also decrease its effects. Oral contraceptives may be ineffective when taking oxytetracycline. Oxytetracycline should be taken at least an hour before or two hours after meals. Incidentally, oxytetracycline is used in feed to increase growth and is found in edible tissue of chickens and turkeys. The birds are permitted up to .0007 percent. There is a question about how much of the drug is left in poultry and whether it can cause a reaction or create resistance to the antibiotic when it is given medically.

OXYTOCIC • A substance that stimulates the contraction of the uterus and aids in childbirth. The drug oxytocin (*see*) is used for this purpose.

Herbs that are reputed to induce childbirth include squawvine and blue cohosh (*see both*).

OXYTOCIN (Rx) • **Pitocin.** A pituitary hormone that, when injected, stimulates muscle contractions. Used to induce or stimulate labor. Potential adverse reactions for the mother include increased bleeding, nausea, vomiting, high blood pressure, low blood pressure, irregular heartbeat, hypersensitivity, and severe allergic reaction. For the baby, they include an increase in bile, slow or fast heartbeat, and lack of oxygen. In a nasal solution, oxytocin is used to promote initial milk ejection and to relieve postpartum breast engorgement. May cause nasal irritation, runny nose, or tearing of the eyes.

P

PABA • *See* Para-Aminobenzoic Acid.

PABALATE (OTC) • A combination of sodium aminobenzoate and sodium salicylate.

PACLITAXEL (Rx) • **Taxol.** A drug derived from the Pacific yew tree, *Taxus brevifolia,* native to old-growth forests of the Pacific Northwest. It is also found in bark and needles of related species throughout the world. It was approved in 1992, a little more than five months after application was made to the FDA, for the treatment of ovarian cancer after other therapies have failed. One of the problems with the drug has been the large amount of the bark—equivalent of three or more trees—needed to treat a single patient. Scientists first began clinical studies of Taxol in 1983, and by 1988, preliminary results showed it was active against ovarian cancer. Taxol has been the focus of great scientific interest because of its unique mode of action and its potential to treat a number of cancers, including breast cancer. Like other cancer drugs, Taxol has unpleasant side effects and occasional severe toxicity, but the adverse effects are generally thought to be worth it because of Taxol's benefits. Bristol-Meyers Squibb Company signed an agreement with the federal government to develop and provide Taxol without charge to patients who were not insured, were ineligible for government assistance, or who lacked the ability to pay. In 1993, Bristol-Meyers said it would provide the drug to those who could not pay, continue to supply researchers with the drug free, and to charge those patients who could pay $986 for each cycle of therapy.

PADIMATE O (OTC) • **Dimethylaminobenzoic Acid. Chap Stick Lip Balm. Filteray Broad Spectrum Sunscreen Lotion.** Esters used as sunscreening agents. *See* Aminobenzoic Acid.

PAGET'S DISEASE • **Osteitis Deformans.** A bone disorder of unknown cause in which the normal process of bone formation is disrupted and calcium is lost, causing bones to weaken, thicken, and become deformed. It usually affects the pelvis, skull, spine, and long bones of the leg.

PAI SHU (H) • *Atractylodis macrocephala* or *A. alba.* The root is used by Chinese herbalists to increase the energy of the body by eliminating excess sodium. This process is reputedly done without interfering with kidney function. It is given for diarrhea, indigestion, fluid retention, abdominal distension, and vomiting.

PALLIATIVE TREATMENT • A treatment that relieves symptoms but does not cure.

PALMA CHRISTI • *See* Castor Oil.

PALMITIC ACID • A mixture of solid organic acids obtained from fats. Palmitic acid occurs naturally in allspice, anise, calamus oil, cascarilla bark, celery seed, butter acids, coffee, tea, and many animal fats and plant oils. It forms 40 percent of cow's milk.

PAMABROM (OTC) • **Midol. Pamprin Cramp Relief. Premsyn PMS.** A weak diuretic (*see*), often combined with an analgesic to relieve premenstrual syndrome.

PAMA NO. 1 • *See* Calcium Carbonate.

PAMELOR • *See* Nortriptyline.

PAMIDRONATE (Rx) • **Aredia.** Introduced in 1991 for the treatment of hypercalcemia (*see*) of malignancy. It inhibits bone resorption. Potential adverse reactions include fatigue, fever, fluid overload, abdominal pain, nausea, upper-respiratory infections, and low phosphate, calcium, and potassium. Given by injection.

PAMINE • *See* Methscopolamine.

PAMISYL • *See* Aminosalicylic Acid.

PAMOATE • *See* Pyrantel, Embolate, and Pamoate.

PAMPRIN-IB • *See* Ibuprofen.

PANADOL • *See* Acetaminophen.

PANASOL-S • *See* Prednisone.

PANAX GINSENG • *See* Ginseng.

PANAX QUINQUEFOLIA • *See* Ginseng.

PANCREASE • *See* Pancrelipase.

PANCREATIN (Rx) (OTC) • **Creon. Dizymes. Hi-Vegi-Lip. Pancreatin Enseals.** A preparation of pancreatic hormones used in disorders of the pancreas to aid digestion of starches, fats, and proteins. Potential adverse reactions include nausea and diarrhea. Antacids may negate pancreatin's beneficial effects. Should be used cautiously in patients who are allergic to pork.

PANCREATITIS • An inflammation of the pancreas that may be acute (of short duration) or chronic.

PANCRELIPASE (Rx) • **Cotazym. Creon. Entolase-HP. Festal. Ilozyme. Ku-Zyme. Lipancreatin. Pancrease. Viokase. Zymase.** A preparation of hog pancreatic extract used in disorders of the pancreas to aid digestion of starches, fats, and proteins. Used to treat cystic fibrosis (*see*). Potential adverse reactions include nausea and diarrhea. Antacids may negate pancrelipase's beneficial effects. Should be used cautiously in patients who are allergic to pork.

PANCURONIUM (Rx) • **Pavulon.** A muscle-relaxant drug used as an adjunct (*see*) to anesthesia. Potential adverse reactions include rapid heartbeat, high blood pressure, rash, excessive sweating and salivation, respiratory problems, residual muscle weakness, and allergic or unusual hypersensitivity reactions. Contraindicated in hypersensitivity to bromides and in patients with rapid heartbeat.

PANEX • *See* Acetaminophen.

PANHEMATIN • *See* Hemin.

PANIC DISORDER • A type of anxiety disorder in which a person suffers intense, overwhelming terror, suddenly and for no apparent reason. The fear is accompanied by such physical symptoms as shortness of breath, heart palpitations, chest discomfort, choking or smothering sensations, unsteadiness, a feeling of unreality, tingling, hot or cold flashes, sweating, faintness, trembling, and fear of losing control, dying, or going crazy.

PANMYCIN • *See* Tetracyclines.

PANOXYL • *See* Benzoyl Peroxide.

PANSY, WILD (H) • *Viola tricolor.* **Heart's Ease. Johnny-Jump-Up. Violet.** Widely grown for its large, attractive flowers, the herb contains mucilaginous material that is used as a soothing lotion for boils, swellings, and skin diseases. Also contains salicylates, saponins, alkaloids, flavonoids, and tannins (*see all*). Pansy also is used as a gentle laxative, and to treat kidney diseases. The root is both emetic and cathartic.

PANTHENOL (Rx) (OTC) • **Albee. Dexpanthenol. Geritol Liquid. Vitamin B Complex Factor. Sigtab.** A viscous, slightly bitter liquid used as a supplement in foods, medicinally, to aid digestion, and in liquid vitamins. Panthenol helps to metabolize protein, fat, and carbohydrates, and to form nerve-regulating substances and hormones. Deficiency symptoms include restlessness, stomach and digestive problems, and increased susceptibility to infection. In 1992, the FDA proposed a ban on the use of panthenol to treat insect bites and stings, and poison ivy, poison sumac, and poison oak because it had not been shown to be safe and effective as claimed in OTC products.

PANTOPON (Rx) • A combination of morphine sulfate or hydrochloride and opium (*see both*), used to treat severe pain.

PANTOTHENAMIDE (OTC) • **B Complex Vitamin. Vitamin B$_5$.** Made synthetically from the jelly of the queen bee, yeast, and molasses. Cleared for use as a source of pantothenic acid activity in foods for special dietary use. Pantothenic acid (common sources are liver, rice, bran, and molasses) is essential for metabolism of carbohydrates, fats, and other important substances. It helps release energy from carbohydrates in the breakdown of fats. Nerve damage has been observed in patients with low pantothenic acid. Children and adults need from 5 to 10 mg per day. *See* Calcium Pantothenate.

PANTOTHENIC ACID (OTC) • **Vitamin B₅. Dexol T.D. Z-Bec Tablet S.** Deficiencies of this vitamin are reportedly rare. Found in foods such as peas, whole-grain cereals, lean meat, and poultry. There is some controversy over claims that pantothenic acid is effective for treatment of nerve damage, breathing problems, itching and other skin problems, and to prevent gray hair, arthritis, allergies, and other ills. *See* Panthenol.

PANTOTHENYL ALCOHOL • *See* Panthenol.

PANWARFIN • *See* Warfarin.

PAPAIN (Rx) (H) • **Panafil Ointment.** An enzyme prepared from papaya (*see*), a fruit grown in tropical countries. Papain is a potent digestant of dead protein matter, but is harmless to live tissue. The same extract is used in meat tenderizer. Papain is used medically to prevent adhesions and treat varicose veins, ulcers, burns, and postoperative wounds. May cause allergic reactions or a slight burning when applied to the skin. *See* Papaya.

PAPAVERINE HYDROCHLORIDE (Rx) • **Cerespan. Genabid. Pavabid. Pavagen. Pavasule. Pavatab. Pavatine. Pavatym. Paverolan Lanacaps. Plateau Caps.** A vasodilator that directly relaxes smooth muscle, it is used to relieve the lack of blood flow associated with spasms of the arteries. Also used to treat angina pectoris (*see*), the aftermath of a blood clot to the lungs or elsewhere in the body, visceral spasms, and certain brain-artery spasms. Papaverine has also been used to treat impotence due to vascular problems. Potential adverse reactions include headache, increased heart rate, increased blood pressure, irregular heartbeat, low blood pressure, priapism (*see*), loss of appetite, constipation, nausea, sweating, flushing, malaise, liver damage, and increased depth of respiration. Papaverine may interfere with the therapeutic effects of levodopa in Parkinson patients. Most effective when given early in the course of a disorder.

PAPAW • *See* Papaya.

PAPAYA (H) • *Carica papaya.* **Fan Muc Gua. Melon-Tree. Papaw.** The fruit, seeds, and leaves of this tree are used by herbalists to aid digestion. The leaf contains the powerful protein-digesting enzymes papain and chymopapain (*see both*). These agents are chemically similar to pepsin, an enzyme that helps digest protein in the body. They may be found in many commercial digestive aids. Recent studies have reported that papaya can ease menstrual problems such as cramps. It is widely used by South Africans to treat wounds. In the Fiji islands, a filtrate of the inner bark is used to treat toothache, while the fresh, milky, white sap is applied directly on boils and to treat wounds. In 1992, researchers at Purdue University announced they had isolated a powerful anticancer drug from the pawpaw tree. In animals, it proved to be many times as potent as the widely used cancer drug Adriamycin. In 1992, the FDA issued a notice that natural papaya had not been shown to be safe and effective as claimed in OTC digestive-aid products. *See also* Papain.

PAPILLEDEMA • Swelling of the optic nerve in the back of the eye.

PAPILLOMA • A benign tumor derived from epithelial tissue.

PAPILLOMAVIRUS • The viral agent of warts.

PARA- • Prefix meaning alongside, near, or abnormal.

PARA-AMINOBENZOIC ACID (OTC) • **4-Aminobenzoic Acid. Mega-B. Paba. p-Aminobenzoic Acid.** The colorless or yellowish acid found in the vitamin B complex, sold under a wide variety of names. It is used to treat depletion of B vitamins due to stress and during prolonged convalescence. Can cause allergic eczema and sensitivity to light in those who are susceptible. In 1992, the FDA proposed a ban on sodium para-aminobenzoic acid in internal analgesic products because it had not been shown to be safe and effective as claimed.

PARABENS • The parabens, methyl-, propyl-, and parahydroxybenzoate, are the most commonly used preservatives in the United States. The parabens have a broad spectrum of antimicrobial activity, are safe to use—relatively nonirritating, nonsensitizing, and nonpoisonous—are stable over the pH range, and are sufficiently soluble in water to be effective in liquids.

PARABROMDYLAMINE • *See* Brompheniramine.

PARACETALDEHYDE • *See* Paraldehyde.

PARACETAMOL • *See* Acetaminophen.

PARACHLOROMETAXYLENOL (OTC) • **Metasep. PCMX. Unguentine Plus First Aid.** An aid in the relief of dandruff and associated conditions.

PARADIONE • *See* Paramethadione.

PARADOXICAL REACTION • An unexpected drug response that is not consistent with the known pharmacology of the drug and may actually be the opposite of the intended response.

PARAFLEX • *See* Chlorzoxazone.

PARAFON FORTE (Rx) • **Blanex. Chlorofon-F. Chlorozone Forte. Flexaphen. Lobac. Mus-Lax. Paracet Forte. Polyflex. Skelex. Soma. Zoxaphen.** A combination of acetaminophen and chlorzoxazone (*see both*) used for the treatment of pain and spasm of lower-back problems, and muscle strains, sprains, and trauma. Chlorzoxazone acts primarily at the spinal-cord level and on areas of the brain. It does not directly relax tense muscle. Potential adverse reactions include nausea, vomiting, drowsiness, stomach bleeding, dizziness, light-headedness, malaise,

liver dysfunction, and overstimulation. Should not be taken with alcohol or other central nervous system depressants. Should be taken with food.

PARAGUAY TEA • *See* Maté Extract.

PARAL • *See* Paraldehyde.

PARALDEHYDE (Rx) • **Paracetaldehyde. Paral.** An anticonvulsant drug, the action of which is unknown. It is used to treat hard-to-control generalized tonic-clonic seizures and continuous seizures (status epilepticus). Also used as a sedative and sleeping medication, and to treat alcohol withdrawal syndrome. Potential adverse reactions include confusion, tremor, weakness, irritability, dizziness, irritation, bad breath, kidney damage, rash, and respiratory depression. When given intravenously, may have severe side effects such as hemorrhage, fluid in the lung, circulatory collapse, and enlargement of the heart. Alcohol increases its central nervous system depression. Disulfiram increases paraldehyde levels in the blood and may cause toxic reactions to both drugs. Contraindicated in gastric ulcers and should be used cautiously in impaired liver function, asthma, and other lung diseases. May cause drug dependence and severe withdrawal symptoms. Oral or rectal administration of decomposed paraldehyde may cause severe corrosion of the stomach or rectum. Do not use a plastic spoon or cup to take this medication since paraldehyde interacts with the plastic. Use metal or glass instead. Paraldehyde in oral form may be mixed with a glass of milk or cold fruit juice to improve the taste and odor, and to lessen stomach upset.

PARALLEL STUDY • Patient uses one of several products in a study to evaluate a pharmaceutical by comparison.

PARALYTIC ILEUS • Obstruction of the bowel due to paralysis of the bowel wall. May be accompanied by severe colicky pain, abdominal distension, vomiting, absence of passage of stool, and often, fever and dehydration.

PARAMETHAD • *See* Paramethadione.

PARAMETHADIONE (Rx) • **Paradione. Paramethad.** An anticonvulsant drug that raises the threshold for seizures but does not modify seizure pattern. Used for difficult-to-treat absence seizures (*see*). Potential adverse reactions include anemia, drowsiness, fatigue, dizziness, headache, numbness, irritability, high or low blood pressure, sensitivity to light, double vision, eye hemorrhage, nausea, vomiting, abdominal pain, weight loss, bleeding gums, vaginal bleeding, kidney dysfunction, liver dysfunction, acne, rash, hair loss, swollen glands, and lupus erythematosus (*see*). Contraindicated in kidney and liver dysfunction or severe blood abnormalities. Should be used cautiously in retinal or optic-nerve diseases. The drug should not be withdrawn suddenly. People taking this drug may have to wear dark glasses because of sensitivity to light. They should report sore throat, fever, malaise, bruises, or blood blisters to their physician.

PARAMETHASONE (Rx) • **Haldrone. Stemex.** A hormone secreted by the adrenal gland that affects carbohydrate and protein metabolism. It is used as an anti-inflammatory drug in the treatment of acute arthritis, collagen diseases, inflammations of the eyes and skin, and allergic reactions. Most adverse reactions are the result of dose or length of time between administration of dosages. Potential adverse reactions include euphoria, insomnia, psychotic behavior, high blood pressure, swelling, cataracts, glaucoma, peptic ulcer, GI irritation, increased appetite, high blood sugar, growth suppression in children, delayed wound healing, acne, skin eruptions, muscle weakness, pancreatitis (*see*), hairiness, decreased immunity, and acute adrenal gland insufficiency. When withdrawn, there may be rebound inflammation, fatigue, weakness, joint pain, fever, dizziness, lethargy, depression, fainting, a drop in blood pressure upon rising from a seated or prone position, shortness of breath, loss of appetite, and high blood sugar. Sudden withdrawal may be fatal. Contraindicated in systemic fungal infections. Should be used cautiously in patients with GI ulceration, kidney disease, high blood pressure, diabetes, chicken pox, osteoporosis, Cushing's syndrome, blood-clotting disorders, seizures, myasthenia gravis (*see*), congestive heart failure, tuberculosis, herpes, and emotional instability. Barbiturates, phenytoin, and rifampin (*see all*) increase its effects. Indomethacin and aspirin may increase the risk of GI distress and bleeding. When taking the drug, patients may need low-sodium diets and potassium supplements. Should be taken with food or milk to reduce GI irritation.

PARANOIA • A rare condition characterized by the gradual development of an intricate, complex, and elaborate system of thinking based on misinterpretations of an actual event. Persons with paranoia often consider themselves endowed with unique and superior abilities.

PARAPHENYLENE DIAMINE • A coal tar dye used in hair coloring. Found to be carcinogenic in animals and is believed to be a potential cancer-causing agent in humans.

PARAPLATIN • *See* Carboplatin.

PARAPLEGIA • Paralysis of the lower part of the body, including the legs.

PARASYMPATHETIC NERVOUS SYSTEM • A part of the autonomic nervous system (*see*), it is made up of a group of nerve fibers that extend from the brain and spinal cord to nerve cell clusters (ganglia) at specific sites. From there they contact blood vessels, glands, and other internal organs. Parasympathetic nerves are involved in the heart rate, in stimulating digestion, contracting bronchioles (in the lungs), pupils (in the eyes), and the esophagus. The parasympathetic nervous system works in conjunction with the sympathetic nervous system (*see*).

PARATHAR • *See* Teriparatide.

PARATHYROID GLAND • At the four corners of the thyroid (*see*) gland, these pearl-sized glands produce parathyroid hormones, which work with calcitonin, a hormone from the thyroid gland, to control calcium in the blood. Calcium not only has a role in developing bones and teeth, but also is involved in blood clotting, and nerve and muscle function.

PARATHYROID HORMONE • PTH. A hormone secreted by the parathyroid gland in the neck that activates the bone resorption process.

PARDA • *See* Levodopa.

PAREDRINE • *See* Amphetamine.

PAREGORIC (Rx) • **Camphorated Opium Tincture.** A derivative of opium (*see*) used for short-term treatment of diarrhea. Potential adverse reactions include nausea, drowsiness, inability to concentrate, dizziness, sedation, vomiting, difficulty in breathing, and light-headedness. Drugs that depress the central nervous system, including alcohol, should not be taken with paregoric. May be taken with food or juice.

PAREIRA BRAVA (H) • **False Pareira. White Pareira. Yellow Pareira.** The root of a South American vine, *Chondodendron tomentosum,* that is used as a diuretic by herbalists and homeopaths.

PARENTAL • The administration of drugs or other substances by any route other than via the gastrointestinal tract. *Parental* commonly refers to substances given by injection or infusion instead of by mouth.

PAREPECTOLIN (Rx) • A combination of kaolin, pectin, and opium (*see all*), used to treat diarrhea.

PARESTHESIA • A sensation of numbness, prickling, or tingling.

PARETHOXYCAINE HYDROCHLORIDE (OTC) • **Maxicaine.** A local anesthetic. In 1992, the FDA issued a notice that parethoxycaine had not been shown to be safe and effective as claimed in OTC poison ivy, poison oak, and poison sumac products.

PARGYLINE (Rx) • **Eutonyl.** Used to treat moderate to severe high blood pressure, it is a monoamine oxidase (MAO) inhibitor (*see*). Potential adverse reactions include constipation, drowsiness, dizziness, dryness of mouth, fatigue, weakness, weight gain, increased sensitivity to sunlight, restlessness, headache, insomnia, and swelling. Foods that are high in tyramine (*see*) content such as cheeses, yeast, or meat extracts may cause a dangerous rise in blood pressure if taken with pargyline. Also interacts with many other drugs including antidiabetics, antidepressants, anticholinergics, cocaine, and antihypertensives (*see*). Those taking pargyline should not eat or drink anything containing alcohol, large amounts of caffeine, or take over-the-counter medications containing stimulants.

PARKINSON'S DISEASE • A chronic neurologic disease of unknown cause, characterized by tremors, rigidity, and an abnormal gait. There is a deficiency of the brain chemical dopamine (*see*). The most common form is paralysis agitans. Postencephalitic parkinsonism is the diseaselike state occurring after brain inflammation.

PARLODEL • *See* Bromocriptine.

PAR-MAG • *See* Magnesium Oxide.

PARNATE • *See* Tranylcypromine Sulfate.

PAROMOMYCIN SULFATE (Rx) • **Humatin.** Acts as an intestinal amebicide. It is used to treat acute and chronic intestinal infections of tapeworms and other parasites. Side effects include headache, dizziness, heartburn, abdominal cramps, diarrhea, constipation, itching around the anus, and malabsorption syndrome (*see*). Also may cause blood in the urine, kidney damage, and overgrowth of nonsusceptible organisms.

PAROXETINE (Rx) • **Paxil.** A once-a-day oral medication for the treatment of depression, introduced in 1992. It is contraindicated for patients taking MAIOs (*see*) or those with a history of seizures. Concomitant use of this drug with tryptophan is not recommended and it should be used cautiously in patients taking warfarin (*see*). In rats, there was evidence of an increase in cancers. The most common adverse reactions observed in humans were weakness, sweating, nausea, decreased appetite, somnolence, dizziness, insomnia, tremor, nervousness, and ejaculatory disturbance and other male genital disorders. Twenty-one percent of Paxil patients surveyed worldwide in clinical trials discontinued treatment due to side effects.

PAROXYSMAL • Tending to occur in sudden, acute episodes.

PARSLEY (H) • *Petroselinum crispum. Petroselinum sativum.* A perennial of the carrot family, it is native to southern Europe, especially to Sardinia, where it is believed to have originated. Parsley is given in a tea to colicky infants and to settle the stomachs of adults after a meal. A tea was also used for urinary infections, insect bites, and swollen glands. The oil is used to induce menstruation. The crushed seeds were made into an eyewash. Parsley is rich in vitamins C and A. Ancient herbalists maintained that it would grow hair if it were rubbed into the scalp. It is a source of chlorophyll, nature's breath freshener. It also contains vitamin B, potassium, protein, apiol—an anti-inflammatory in parsley oil—and myristicin, another oil. In 1992, the FDA proposed a ban on parsley in oral menstrual drug products because it had not been shown to be safe and effective as claimed. In excessive doses, parsley can cause uterine contractions and should therefore be avoided as an herbal medicine during pregnancy. Parsley oil can cause liver damage and a drastic fall in blood pressure.

P.A.S. • *See* Aminosalicylic Acid.

PASQUEFLOWER (H) • *Anemone pulsatilla.* A low, perennial herb with white or purple flowers, it is used by herbalists to treat insomnia and other tension-induced conditions. Also used to treat painful menstrual periods and painful conditions of the testes. The antibacterial effects are used by herbalists to treat skin infections and asthma.

PASSIFLORA INCARNATA • *See* Passionflower.

PASSIONFLOWER (OTC) (H) • *Passiflora incarnata.* **Hyland's Calms Forte Tablets.** An extract of the various species of *Passiflora incarnata.* American Indians used passionflower for swellings, sore eyes, and to induce vomiting. It is also used as a flavoring. An extremely popular herb in Europe, where it is often used to induce relaxation and sleep. It has been shown that an extract of the plant depresses the motor nerves of the spinal cord. One of the ingredients in passionflower is serotonin (*see*), a neurotransmitter (*see*) that is low in persons who are depressed. Hyland's Calms Forte Tablets are promoted for temporary relief of simple nervous tension and insomnia. An excessive dose can cause headache and temporary visual disturbance.

PATH-, PATHO- PATHY- • Prefixes denoting feeling, suffering, disease, as in *pathology,* the specialty concerned with all aspects of disease.

PATHIBAMATE • *See* Meprobamate.

PATHILON • *See* Tridihexethyl Chloride.

PATHOCIL • *See* Dicloxacillin Sodium.

PATHOGEN • Any microorganism causing disease.

PAU D'ARCO (H) • *Tabecuia heptaphylla* or *impetiginosa.* **Lapacho.** The inner bark of a tree in the forests of Brazil, it was used by Brazilian Indians for the treatment of cancer. Contains quinones and lapachol. It also is used to treat fungal and parasitic infections, and to aid digestion. Also reportedly lowers blood sugar. Pau d'arco is now being studied in Brazil to treat cancers, including leukemia.

PAVABID • *See* Papaverine Hydrochloride.

PAVAGEN • *See* Papaverine Hydrochloride.

PAVASULE • *See* Papaverine Hydrochloride.

PAVATAB • *See* Papaverine Hydrochloride.

PAVATYM • *See* Papaverine Hydrochloride.

PAVERAL • *See* Codeine Phosphate and Sulfate.

PAVEROLAN LANACAPS • *See* Papaverine Hydrochloride.

PAVULON • *See* Pancuronium.

PAWPAW • **Papaw. Papaya, Melon Tree.** A small tree native to the Americas. It has been used by folk medicine practitioners to treat indigestion and externally to remove warts. It is also used to treat eczema and other skin problems. It is being studied by Purdue University researchers for a compound contained in its bark, asimicin, that has pesticidal properties. The compound has also shown anticancer effects and is being explored by pharmaceutical companies.

PAWPAW TREE • *See* Papaya.

PAXIL • *See* Paroxetine.

PAXIPAM • *See* Halazepam.

PAZO HEMORRHOID OINTMENT & SUP-POSITORIES • *See* Camphor and Ephedrine.

PBR-12 • *See* Phenobarbital.

PBZ • *See* Tripelennamine.

PCE • *See* Erythromycin.

PCMX (OTC) • Used to treat dandruff and associated conditions. *See* Parachlorometaxylenol.

PCP • Abbreviation for *Pneumocystis carinii* pneumonia, a severe lung infection eventually affecting nearly 80 percent of all AIDS patients, and a major cause of death.

PE • *See* Pilocarpine and Epinephrine.

PEACH (H) • *Prunus persica.* The leaves or bark from young trees native to China, but widely cultivated, are used by herbalists to make sedatives, diuretics, expectorants, and soothing compounds.

PEANUT • *Arachis hypogaea.* **Ground Nut. Earth Nut.** An annual plant widely used as a foodstuff. Refined peanut (arachis) oil is widely used in pharmaceutical preparations.

PEARL ASH • *See* Potassium Carbonate.

PECAN SHELL POWDER (H) • Used by the American Indians for medicinal purposes, it is the nut from a hickory tree. Also used as a coloring in cosmetics.

PECTIN (OTC) (H) • **Kaopectate.** Found in roots, stems, and fruits, this soluble fiber forms an integral part of such plant structures. The richest sources of pectin are lemon and orange rind, which contain about 30 percent of this polysaccharide. Used in antidiarrheal medications. In the late 1950s, researchers reported that dietary pectin increased the excretion of fats, cholesterol, and bile acids. It is believed that pectins work by binding with bile acids, thereby decreasing cholesterol and fat absorption. Another group of researchers found that adding pectin to a meal lowered blood-sugar levels in nondiabetic as well as non-insulin-requiring patients. In 1992, the FDA issued a notice that pectin had not been shown to be safe and effective as claimed in OTC digestive-aid products, or to treat fever blisters and cold sores.

PECTORAL • A term used in herbal medicine to signify herbs that have a general strengthening and healing effect on the respiratory system. Among such reputed herbs are pleurisy root and horehound (*see both*).

PED- • The Latin root means foot, as in *pedal.* The Greek root refers to children, as in *pediatrics.*

PEDAMETH • *See* Methionine.

PEDIACARE • *See* Pseudoephedrine.

PEDIACARE 1 • *See* Dextromethorphan.

PEDIACARE ORAL • *See* Pseudoephedrine and Codeine Phosphate and Sulphate.

PEDIACOF (Rx) • A combination of chlorpheniramine, codeine phosphate and sulfate, phenylephrine, and potassium iodide (*see all*). Used to treat coughs.

PEDIAFLOR • *See* Sodium Fluoride.

PEDIAMYCIN • *See* Erythromycin.

PEDIAPRED • *See* Prednisolone.

PEDIAPROFEN • *See* Ibuprofen.

PEDIAZOLE (Rx) • A combination of erythromycin and sulfisoxazole used to treat ear and sinus infections in children. The combination of an antibiotic and a sulfa drug was specifically formulated to kill *Hemophilus influenzae* organisms responsible for many cases of hard-to-treat middle-ear infections in children. Potential adverse reactions include nausea, vomiting, sensitivity to sunlight, cramps, drug allergy, and rash. Pediazole may increase the effects of digoxin, tolbutamide, chlorpropamide, methotrexate, and theophylline. Theophylline, warfarin, phenylbutazone, aspirin or other salicylates, carbamazepine, phenytoin, and probenecid may cause an increased incidence of the side effects of Pediazole. Most effective when taken on an empty stomach, but may be taken with food if stomach upset is a problem. The intake of fluids should be increased while Pediazole is being used.

PEDI-BORO • *See* Aluminum Acetate.

PEDICULICIDE • Medicine that kills lice.

PEDI-DRI • *See* Undecylenic Acid.

PEDIOTIC (Rx) • A combination of neomycin, polymyxin B, and hydrocortisone (*see all*), used to treat eye infections.

PEDRIC WAFERS • *See* Acetaminophen.

PEG • Abbreviation for polyethylene glycol.

PEG-ADA • *See* Pegademase.

PEGADEMASE (Rx) • **Adagen. PEG-ADA.** A drug that contains the enzyme adenosine deaminase (ADA), used to treat children who do not have a properly developed immune system due to lack of ADA in the body. Given only with a doctor's immediate supervision.

PEGANONE • *See* Ethotoin.

PEGASPARGASE • **Oncaspar 7.** A modification of the enzyme L-asparaginase, it is combined with chemotherapy to treat lymphoblastic leukemia in patients who are hypersensitive to L-asparaginase. It is not used alone. It should be given only under the supervision of specially trained cancer specialists.

PEGNOLOGY • A patented drug delivery technology that reduces the quantity and frequency of doses and lowers allergic reactions to proteins used as therapeutic agents.

PELLITORY-OF-THE-WALL • *See* Nettle.

PELVIC INFLAMMATORY DISEASE • **PID.** An infection of the fallopian tubes, ovaries, uterus, and surrounding tissues that causes abdominal pain.

PEMOLINE (Rx) • **Cylert. Phenylisohydantoin. PIO.** A nervous system stimulant that promotes nerve impulse transmission by releasing stored norepinephrine (*see*) from nerves in the brain. Though structurally unlike amphetamines or methylphenidate, it has similar adverse reactions. It is used to treat attention deficit disorder with hyperactivity. Potential adverse reactions include insomnia, seizures, malaise, irritability, fatigue, mild depression, dizziness, headache, drowsiness, hallucinations, nervousness, Tourette's syndrome (*see*), psychosis, irregular heartbeat, loss of appetite, stomach pain, nausea, diarrhea, liver dysfunction, and rash. Pemoline may alter requirements for antidiabetes drugs. Contraindicated in patients with liver dysfunction and in children under six years of age. Should be used with caution in patients with kidney dysfunction. May cause drug dependence. Therapeutic effects may not be manifest for more than a month. Should be taken on an empty stomach at least six hours before bedtime.

PENAMP • *See* Ampicillin.

PENAPAR VK • *See* Penicillin V.

PENBRITIN • *See* Ampicillin.

PENBUTOLOL (Rx) • **Levatol.** A beta-blocker (*see*) introduced in 1989 that reduces the force of the heartbeat, it is used in the treatment of mild to moderate high blood pressure. It is a once-a-day medication. Potential adverse reactions include faintness, dizziness, headache, fatigue, mental depression, numbness, lethargy, anxiety, diminished concentration, sleep disturbances, nightmares, sedation, hallucinations, alteration of time perception, chest pain, congestive heart failure, dry mouth, worsening of angina, heart palpitations, heart block, gastric pain, flatulence, nausea, constipation, heartburn, vomiting, taste alteration, impotence, urine retention, raised or lowered blood sugar, sore throat, respiratory distress, pallor, flushing, rash, allergic reactions, eye discomfort, decreased libido, memory loss, and emotional mood swings. When given with clonidine, penbutolol may cause paradoxical high blood pressure or rebound hypertension when clonidine is discontinued. NSAIDs (*see*) may decrease penbutolol's effects. Isoproterenol, dopamine, dobutamine, and norepinephrine may decrease the blood-pressure-lowering effects of penbutolol. Penbutolol may decrease the effects of the bronchodilator theophylline. Contraindicated in patients allergic to penbutolol, other beta-blockers (*see*), and those with chronic bronchitis or emphysema. The drug should not be withdrawn suddenly. May be taken with food.

PENECORT • *See* Hydrocortisone.

PENETREX • *See* Enoxacin.

PEN G • *See* Penicillin G.

-PENIA • Suffix meaning scarcity, deficiency, as in *erythropenia,* deficiency of red blood cells.

PENICILLAMINE (Rx) • **Cuprimine. Depen.** A metabolite of penicillin. When penicillamine was introduced in 1963, it was first used to treat Wilson's disease, where copper is deposited in organs and tissues, and in heavy metal poisoning; penicillamine binds to copper and heavy metals, but not to gold. It is also now used to treat severe, active, or progressive rheumatoid arthritis. It takes eight to twelve weeks at the earliest to work. When a response occurs, there is a reduction in morning stiffness duration, and a reduction in joint swelling, tenderness, and pain. The usefulness of penicillamine is compromised by a high incidence of adverse reactions. The most common side effect is rash. The most serious side effect is a drop in white blood cells. Treatment with penicillamine has also been associated with the development of a number of autoimmune (*see*) syndromes including myasthenia gravis and systemic lupus erythematosus (*see both*). Other potential adverse reactions include loss of taste, loss of appetite, nausea, and skin problems such as wrinkling, redness, hives, blood spots, and breaks. Rash and fever are important signs of toxicity and should be reported to a physician at once. Antacids and oral iron decrease penicillamine's effectiveness and should be given at least two hours before or after. Contraindicated in pregnant women with kidney problems. Should be used cautiously in patients allergic to penicillin.

PENICILLIN G (Rx) • **Benzylpenicillin Potassium. Peng. Pentids. Permapen. Wycillin.** An antibiotic used to treat susceptible infections, including moderate to severe systemic upper-respiratory-tract, lower-respiratory-tract, and skin infections. Potential adverse reactions include anemia, nerve damage, seizures, severe potassium poisoning with high doses, blood clots at site of injection, hypersensitivity, rash, chills, fever, water retention, potentially fatal allergic reactions, and overgrowth of nonsusceptible organisms. Contraindicated in patients with a history of hypersensitivity to any penicillin. Should be used with caution in any persons with a history of allergies and/or asthma. Bacteriostatic antibiotics such as chloramphenicol, erythromycins, sulfonamides, or tetracyclines may interfere with its effectiveness. Probenecid may increase its effects. Penicillin G is most effective when taken on an empty stomach.

PENICILLINS • Amdinocillin. Amoxicillin. Ampicillin. Azlocillin. Bacampicillin. Carbenicillin. Cloxacillin Sodium. Dicloxacillin Sodium. Hetacillin. Methicillin Sodium. Mezlocillin Sodium. Nafcillin Sodium. Oxacillin Sodium. Penicillin G. Penicillin V. Piperacillin. Ticarcillin Disodium. A group of beta-lactam (*see*) antibiotics produced by several species of mold and/or semisynthetically. There are many kinds, and they offer a broad clinical spectrum of activity. They inhibit bacterial enzymes that help make cell walls. Penicillins should not be taken with acidic fruits or juices, wines, syrups, or aged cheeses because these make penicillins less effective.

PENICILLIN V (Rx) • Phenoxymethyl Penicillin. Penicillin VK. Wincillin-VK Potassium. Beepen-VK. Betapen-VK. Ledercillin VK. Nadopen-V. Penapar VK. Pen Vee. Pen•Vee K. Pen VK. Pfizerpen VK. PVK. Robicillin VK. V-Cillin K. VC-K. Veetids. An antibiotic used to prevent and treat mild to moderate upper-respiratory infections. Potential adverse reactions include anemia, nerve damage, abdominal distress, vomiting, diarrhea, nausea, hypersensitivity including potentially fatal allergic reactions, and overgrowth of nonsusceptible organisms. Should be used with caution in persons who have histories of significant allergies and/or asthma. Bacteriostatic antibiotics such as chloramphenicol, erythromycins, sulfonamides, and tetracyclines may interfere with its effectiveness. May make oral contraceptives less effective. Aspirin and phenylbutazone may increase the level of penicillin in the blood. Penicillin V is most effective when taken on an empty stomach.

PENICILLIN VK • *See* Penicillin V.

PENNTUSS • *See* Codeine Phosphate and Sulfate.

PENNYROYAL OIL (H) • *Hedeoma pulegioides. Mentha pulegium.* **Hedeoma. Squaw-** **mint. Tickweed.** An extract of the flowering herb *Mentha pulegium.* Used since ancient days as a medicine, scent, flavoring, and food. Obtained from the dried flower tops and leaves, pennyroyal oil contains tannin (*see*), which is soothing to the skin. It is a gentle stimulant. Used by herbalists in an infusion as an aromatic perspirant, to stimulate menstrual flow, for flatulence, as an abortifacient (*see*), and as a counteractant for painful menstruation. The oil is applied externally to repel flying insects, but must not be taken internally. Brain damage has been reported following doses of less than one teaspoon. Nausea, vomiting, bleeding, circulatory collapse, confusion, restlessness, and delirium have been reported with large doses. In 1996, the death of a 24-year-old woman who had ingested a pennyroyal herbal potion for two weeks was reported.

PENTAERYTHRITOL TETRANITRATE (Rx) • Dilar. Duotrate. Naptrate. Pentritol. Pentylan. Peritrate. PETN. A nitrate drug that reduces the heart's need for oxygen and increases blood flow through the collateral coronary vessels. It is used to prevent anginal attacks. Potential adverse reactions include headache, weakness, low blood pressure when standing, flushing, heart palpitations, fainting, nausea, vomiting, and hypersensitivity reactions.

PENTAMIDINE ISETHIONATE (Rx) • NebuPent. Pentam 300. Used in the treatment of *Pneumocystis carinii* pneumonia in high-risk individuals, especially those who are infected with the AIDS virus. May cause anemia, confusion, hallucinations, low blood pressure, irregular heartbeat, low or high blood sugar, low calcium, nausea, anorexia, metallic taste, renal toxicity, elevated liver enzymes, rash, and fever.

PENTAM 300 • *See* Pentamidine Isethionate.

PENTAZINE • *See* Promethazine.

PENTAZOCINE HYDROCHLORIDE or LACTATE (Rx) • Talacen. Talwin. A narcotic analgesic introduced in 1967 that alters both the perception of and reaction to pain. Used to treat moderate to severe pain. Potential adverse effects include sedation, sleepiness, visual disturbances, lack of alertness, dizziness, euphoria, seizures, low blood pressure, nausea, vomiting, dry mouth, constipation, urine retention, and respiratory depression. Central nervous system drugs including alcohol and sleeping pills may increase its sedative or depressive effects. Narcotic analgesics may decrease the painkilling effect. Contraindicated in acute alcoholism, drug abuse, head injury, and increased pressure on the brain. It is a narcotic antagonist and may cause withdrawal symptoms. Should be used cautiously in liver or kidney disease. May be addictive. May be taken with food to reduce stomach upset.

PENTHRANE • *See* Methoxyflurane.

PENTIDS • *See* Penicillin G.

PENTOBARBITAL (Rx) • **Nembutal.** A barbiturate sleeping drug for adults and children that probably interferes with transmission of impulses from the thalamus to the cortex of the brain. Potential adverse reactions include drowsiness, lethargy, hangover, paradoxical excitement in elderly patients, nausea, vomiting, rash, hives, swelling, and exacerbation of porphyria (*see*). Alcohol or other central nervous system depressants, including narcotic analgesics, can lead to excessive central nervous system and respiratory system depression. Pentobarbital decreases the absorption of griseofulvin. MAO inhibitors (*see*) inhibit metabolism of barbiturates and may cause prolonged central nervous system depression. Pentobarbital may make less effective oral blood thinners, estrogens, oral contraceptives, doxycycline, and corticosteroids. Use with rifampin may decrease barbiturate levels. Elderly patients are more sensitive to the drug's adverse effects. Contraindicated in uncontrolled severe pain, respiratory disease, hypersensitivity to barbiturates, previous addiction to sedatives, or porphyria. Used with caution in liver or kidney impairment. When the drug is discontinued, increased dreaming may occur. Most effective when taken on an empty stomach, but may be taken with some food if upset stomach is a problem.

PENTOSTATIN (Rx) • **Nipent.** An anticancer drug introduced in 1991, it is used to treat patients with hairy cell leukemia who have not responded to interferon. Pentostatin may compromise the patient's ability to handle infections.

PENTOTHAL • *See* Thiopental.

PENTOXIFYLLINE (Rx) • **Trental.** A drug that improves blood flow. It is used in the treatment of intermittent claudication—pain in the calf muscle while walking caused by inadequate blood supply. Potential adverse reactions include headache, dizziness, heartburn, nausea, and vomiting. Anticoagulants increase its blood-thinning effect. High blood pressure medications increase its blood-pressure-lowering effect. Contraindicated in patients who are intolerant to methylxanthines such as caffeine, theophylline, and theobromine. Smoking should be avoided because it constricts arteries and will impair the effectiveness of pentoxifylline. Most effective on an empty stomach, but may be taken with a small amount of food if stomach upset is a problem. Pentoxifylline is now being studied for its potential in the treatment of the common cold. The medication has an inhibitory effect on the lung's production of the cytokine (*see*), interleukin-8, which is involved in immunity to the common cold.

PENTRAX • *See* Coal Tar.

PENTYLAN • *See* Pentaerythritol Tetranitrate.

PEN VEE • *See* Penicillin V.

PEN•VEE K • *See* Penicillin V.

PEN VK • *See* Penicillin V.

PEONY (H) • *Paeonia lactiflora.* **Shao-yao.** The root is used by herbalists as a liver tonic. Also used to treat all female "complaints," especially menstrual irregularity and abdominal pains associated with the menstrual cycle. It is also used to treat gallstones and liver complaints. Externally, it has been used to treat wounds and skin growths. Peony is toxic when used internally in excessive doses. Potential adverse effects from herbal use include colic, nausea, and diarrhea. It may also produce uterine contractions. Contraindicated in pregnancy.

PEPCID • *See* Famotidine.

PEPPER, BLACK (H) • *Piper nigrum.* **Fan Jia.** There are more than fifty species of plants called pepper, many unrelated. The Greeks and Romans used pepper as both a medicine and condiment. In medicine it was used to treat gout, arthritis, smallpox, scarlet fever, dysentery, typhus, cholera, and bubonic plague. It was also used to stop bleeding and as an antiseptic. Pepper is used to treat digestive upsets, including flatulence and nausea. It is a stimulant.

PEPPERMINT (H) • *Mentha piperita.* **Brandy Mint.** The oil made from the dried leaves and tops of a plant common to Asian, European, and American gardens. Peppermint is used as a flavoring in many products. In medicine, it has been used as far back as recorded history to treat indigestion and calm spasm of the bowel. It relaxes the stomach muscles, herbalists say, and promotes burping. Modern researchers have found that peppermint contains antiulcer, anti-inflammatory, and liver-bile-stimulating agents. Peppermint can also inhibit the growth of many kinds of germs. It can, however, cause allergic reactions such as hay fever and rash. In 1992, the FDA issued a notice that peppermint and peppermint spirit have not been shown to be safe and effective as claimed in OTC digestive-aid products, insect bite and sting drug products, oral menstrual drug products, and in astringent (*see*) drugs.

PEPSIN (OTC) • A digestive enzyme found in gastric juice that helps break down protein. The product used to aid digestion is obtained from the glandular layer of the fresh stomach of a hog. Slightly acid taste and a mild odor. No known toxicity. In 1992, the FDA proposed a ban on pepsin in oral menstrual drug products because it had not been shown to be safe and effective as claimed.

PEPTIDE • Two or more amino acids chained together in head-to-tail links. Generally larger than simple amino acids or the monoamines, the largest peptides discovered thus far have forty-four amino acids. Neuropeptides signal the body's endocrine glands to balance salt and water. Opiate peptides can help control pain and anxiety. The peptides work with amino acids. A peptide is present at two ten-thousandths of its partner amino acid or a hundredth the amount of a monoamine.

PEPTO-BISMOL • *See* Bismuth.

PEPTO DIARRHEA CONTROL (OTC) • *See* Bismuth and Loperamide.

PERCOCET (Rx) • **Roxicet. Tylox.** A combination of acetaminophen and oxycodone (*see both*) used to treat mild to moderate pain. May be taken by people allergic to aspirin. Should be used with caution in persons suffering from asthma or other respiratory problems. Potential adverse reactions include euphoria, weakness, insomnia, headache, agitation, incoordination, minor hallucinations, confusion, visual disturbances, dry mouth, loss of appetite, constipation, flushing of the face, rapid heartbeat, heart palpitations, faintness, urinary difficulties, reduced sex drive and/or impotence, itching, rash, anemia, low blood sugar, and convulsions. Should not be taken with central nervous system depressants, including sleeping pills, alcohol, and tranquilizers, because such a combination may affect breathing. Best taken with food or a glass of water to prevent stomach upset.

PERCODAN (Rx) • **Roxiprin. Oxycodone with Aspirin. Percodan-Demi.** A combination of aspirin and oxycodone, it is used to treat mild to moderate pain. Potential adverse reactions include nausea, vomiting, drowsiness, light-headedness, euphoria, weakness, headache, agitation, incoordination, dry mouth, loss of appetite, constipation, flushing, rapid heartbeat, heart palpitations, faintness, urinary difficulties, reduced sex drive and/or impotence, low blood sugar, convulsions, sweating, and difficulty breathing. Contraindicated in persons known to be allergic to any of its components, or those with asthma or other breathing problems. Central nervous system depressants such as alcohol, tranquilizers, or barbiturates may seriously increase the depressant effects of Percodan. The aspirin component may increase the effect of blood thinners. Interaction with adrenal corticosteroids, phenylbutazone, or alcohol can cause severe stomach problems, including bleeding. Should be taken with food or a glass of water to prevent stomach upset.

PERCOGESIC (Rx) • A combination of acetaminophen and phenyltoloxamine (*see both*) for the temporary relief of minor aches and pains associated with headache, muscle aches, toothache, backache, and premenstrual periods, as well as the common cold, flu, and arthritis. Potential adverse reactions include excitability, especially in children. Central nervous system depressants, including alcohol and sleeping pills, may increase the sedative effects of this drug and affect breathing. Contraindicated in those with asthma, glaucoma, emphysema, chronic lung disease, shortness of breath, or difficulty urinating.

PERCORTEN • *See* Corticosterone.

PERCUTANEOUS • Movement through or into the skin.

PERDIEM • *See* Psyllium.

PERFUSION • The passage of blood through the vessels supplying an organ or tissue.

PERGOLIDE (Rx) • **Permax.** An ergot-derived (*see* Ergot) anti-Parkinson drug introduced in 1980 that directly stimulates dopamine receptors and is an adjunctive treatment to carbidopa-levodopa (*see*). Dopamine is a neurotransmitter (*see*) that is involved in movement. Potential adverse reactions include headache, weakness, trouble moving, confusion, sleepiness, insomnia, anxiety, depression, tremor, abnormal dreams, personality disorder, psychosis, abnormal gait, impotence, changed libido, breast pain, priapism (*see*), incoordination, numbness, pain, speech

disorder, a drop in blood pressure upon rising from a sitting or prone position, heart palpitations, faintness, high blood pressure, irregular heartbeat, heart attack, stuffy nose, bloody nose, abnormal vision, abdominal pain, nausea, constipation, diarrhea, heartburn, loss of appetite, vomiting, dry mouth, taste alteration, urinary frequency, urinary-tract infection, rash, sweating, flulike symptoms, chest pain, back pain, chills, swelling, weight gain, joint pain, muscle pain, and twitching. Contraindicated in patients allergic to the drug or to ergot, or those with severe artery and blood-vessel disease. Phenothiazines, butyrophenones, thioxanthenes, metoclopramide, and other drugs that are dopamine antagonists may make pergolide less effective. May be taken with food or milk to decrease stomach upset.

PERGONAL • *See* Menotropins.

PERI- • Prefix meaning around or surrounding, as in *pericardium,* surrounding the heart.

PERIACTIN • *See* Cyproheptadine.

PERICARDIAL • Referring to the membranous and fibrous sac enclosing the heart.

PERICARDITIS • Inflammation of the pericardium, the sac encircling the heart.

PERI-COLACE (OTC) • **Dialose Plus. Diocto-C. Diolax. Diothron. Disanthrol. Di-Sosul Forte. D-S-S Plus. Genasoft-Plus. Peri-Dos. Pro-Sof Plus. Regulace.** All of the above have a similar formula of casanthranol and docusate (*see both*). They are used as a laxative and stool softener. Potential adverse reactions include nausea, vomiting, diarrhea, and stomach cramps. Contraindicated in patients with abdominal pain, nausea, vomiting, or symptoms of appendicitis. These drugs should be taken on an empty stomach. *See also* Laxative.

PERIPHERAL NERVOUS SYSTEM • **PNS.** The nerves that branch out from the brain and spinal cord to the farthest tips of the body. Some of the nerves, such as those for the eyes and nose, attach directly to the brain and are called cranial nerves. The others connect to the spinal cord and are the spinal nerves. Two types of messages are telegraphed along the PNS. Sensory nerve cells transmit to your brain what you sense from your environment, such as smelling bread baking or seeing a dangerous situation. The motor neurons transmit instructions from your brain to your body parts that must react to what you have sensed, such as telling your legs to jump out of the way. Connecting nerve cells provide crossovers between the sensory (afferent) and motor (efferent) pathways.

PERIPHERAL NEURITIS • Inflammation of the nerve tissues in the arms and legs.

PERIPHERAL VASCULAR DISEASE • The narrowing or blocking of the arterial, venous, and/or lymph vessels that supply blood to the extremities.

PERITONEUM • The sac that contains the liver, stomach, and intestines.

PERITRATE • *See* Pentaerythritol Tetranitrate and Nitrates.

PERIWINKLE (H) • *Catharanthus roseus. Vinca rosea.* An everblooming perennial herb or small shrub, it is popular in gardens. The tropical periwinkle is an example of a folk medicine that made its way into modern medicine. In 1953, at the Pacific Science Congress, Dr. Faustino Garcia reported that periwinkle is used as a folk medicine in the Philippines, taken orally for diabetes. Researchers at the Eli Lilly Company screened the plant and found that it revealed good anticancer activity in test animals. The result was the discovery of two alkaloids that are useful in treating cancer. (*See* Vincristine and Vinblastine.) Periwinkle has also been found to be useful in treating diabetes. It has been found to stop external hemorrhages and is assumed to do so because it contains tannins (*see*). Its effectiveness in controlling menstrual hemorrhaging may be due to vincamine, a substance in periwinkle that dilates blood vessels.

PERMANENT LISTING • Signifies that the FDA is convinced that a dye is safe to use as it is now employed in food, drug(s), and/or cosmetic(s). Some colorings that have been permanently listed in the past have been removed from the market because they cause cancer or unfavorable reactions.

PERMAPEN • *See* Penicillin G.

PERMAX • *See* Pergolide.

PERMETHRIN (OTC) • **Elimite. Nix.** A drug used in preparations for the treatment of head lice and nits that was changed from Rx to OTC in 1990. It is used after hair has been washed with shampoo, rinsed with water, and towel-dried. Potential adverse reactions include itching, burning, stinging, tingling, numbness or scalp discomfort, and mild redness or rash on the scalp. Contraindicated in patients hypersensitive to pyrethrins or chrysanthemums. Do not use on infants because their skin is more absorbent than that of children or adults.

PERMITIL • *See* Fluphenazine Hydrochloride, Decanoate, or Enanthate.

PERNOX • *See* Sulfur and Salicylic Acid.

PEROXIDE • *See* Hydrogen Peroxide.

PEROXYL • *See* Hydrogen Peroxide.

PERPHENAZINE (Rx) • **Etrafon. Trilafon.** An antipsychotic and antiemetic (to stop vomiting) drug introduced in 1957, it is used to treat hospitalized psychiatric patients, acute alcoholism, nausea, vomiting, and hiccups. Potential adverse reactions include a low white blood cell count, tardive dyskinesia (*see*), sedation, pseudoparkinsonism, dizziness, a drop in blood pressure when rising from a seated or prone position, eye changes, dry mouth, constipation, urine retention, menstrual irregularities, enlargement of male breast, liver dysfunction, inhibited ejaculation, false positive pregnancy test results, mild photosensitivity, allergic skin reactions, weight gain, increased appetite, fever, irregular heartbeat, sweating, headache, and insomnia. The drug can increase the risk of low body temperature in the elderly. Contraindicated in coma, central nervous system depression, bone-marrow suppression, brain damage, and the use of spinal or epidural anesthetic, or adrenergic-blocking agents (*see*). Should be used cautiously with other central nervous system depressants, anticholinergics, in elderly or debilitated patients, acutely ill or dehydrated children, in liver disease, hardening of the arteries or cardiovascular disease, respiratory disorders, low blood calcium, seizure disorders, electroshock therapy, intestinal obstruction, glaucoma, and enlarged prostate. Riboflavin (vitamin B_2) supplementation should be taken with long-term use of perphenazine. Perphenazine should not be withdrawn suddenly. May be taken with food.

PERSA-GEL • *See* Benzoyl Peroxide.

PERSANTINE • *See* Dipyridamole.

PERTOFRANE • *See* Desipramine.

PERTUSSIN • *See* Dextromethorphan.

PERTUSSIS • **Whooping Cough.** An acute infectious disease characterized by inflammation of the throat and lungs, producing recurrent bouts of spasmodic coughing that continue until the breath is exhausted, and ending in a noisy inhalation called a whoop, caused by a windpipe spasm.

PERTUSSIS VACCINE (Rx) • **DPT.** The vaccine given to children to prevent whooping cough, combined with diphtheria and tetanus vaccine. DPT shots are administered between two months and six years of age. The new pertussis vaccine approved in 1991 reportedly has fewer side effects than the older version, which caused some concern among physicians and parents.

PERUVIAN BALSAM (OTC) (H) • **Balmex Baby Powder** and **Ointment.** A dark brown, thick liquid with a pleasant, lingering odor, it is obtained in Central America near the Pacific Coast. An ingredient of topical treatments for hemorrhoids, and anti-inflammatory ointments and powders. It is mildly antiseptic. May be irritating to the skin and cause contact dermatitis, and a stuffy nose. One of the most common sensitizers, it may cross-react with benzoin, benzoic acid, rosin, cinnamic acid, orange peel, and wood tars, among others.

PETECHIAE • Minute blood spots in the skin.

PETHADOL • *See* Meperidine.

PETIT MAL EPILEPSY • *See* Absence Seizure.

PETN • Abbreviation for pentaerythritol tetranitrate (*see*). *See also* Nitrates.

PETROGALAR (OTC) • A lubricant laxative preparation. *See* Laxative.

PETROLATUM (OTC) • **Crude** or **Mineral Oil. Paraffin Jelly. Petroleum Jelly. A & D Ointment. Aqua Care Cream. Aquaphor. Chap Stick. Desitin. Eucerin Dry Skin Care. Extra Strength Vaseline. Keri Lotion. Moisturel Cream. pHisoDerm for Baby. Preparation H. Vaseline.** A purified mixture of semisolid hydrocarbons from petroleum. Yellowish to light amber or white, semisolid, unctuous mass, practically odorless and tasteless, almost insoluble in water. Helps to soften and smooth the skin in the same way as any other emollient, but is less expensive. The oily film helps prevent evaporation of moisture from the skin and protects it from irritation. However, petrolatum does cause allergic skin reactions in those who are sensitive to it. When ingested, it produces a mild laxative effect. Not absorbed, but may inhibit digestion. It is generally nontoxic.

PERTROPIN SOLUCAP E • *See* Vitamin E.

PETROSELINUM CRISPUM • *See* Parsley.

PEYRONIE'S DISEASE • A permanent deformity of the penis caused by scarlike tissue within the system of penile vessels that become engorged with blood during erection. During sexual arousal, the fibrous tissue causes a bowing of the penis that hampers or precludes sexual intercourse. Peyronie's disease has sometimes been a side effect of drugs, including phenytoin and beta-blockers (*see both*).

PFEIFFER'S ALLERGY • *See* Chlorpheniramine.

PFIZERPEN-AS • *See* Penicillin G.

PFIZERPEN VK • *See* Penicillin V.

PGA • *See* Prostaglandins.

PGB • *See* Prostaglandins.

PGC • *See* Prostaglandins.

PGD • *See* Prostaglandins.

PGE₁ • *See* Alprostadil.

PGE₂ • *See* Dinoprostone.

pH • The scale used to measure acidity and alkalinity. pH is the hydrogen (H) ion concentration of a solution. The p stands for the *power* of the hydrogen ion. The pH of a solution is measured on a scale of 14. A truly neutral solution, neither acidic nor alkaline, such as water, is 7. The pH of blood is 7.3; vinegar is 2.3; lemon juice is 8.2; and lye is 13. Skin and hair are naturally acidic. Soap and detergents are alkaline.

PHAG-, -PHAGY • Prefix and suffix meaning pertaining to eating, as in *esophagus,* the food channel.

PHAGOCYTE • A type of immune cell that surrounds, engulfs, and digests invading microorganisms and cellular debris.

PHARMACOKINETICS • The study of the movement of drugs in the body, including distribution, metabolism, and excretion of drugs.

PHARYNGITIS • An infection or inflammation of the mucous membranes that line the pharynx (throat); characterized by a sore throat, swelling of the pharynx, and pus covering the throat surface.

PHASE I • Safety testing and pharmacological profiling of a new drug in humans.

PHASE II • Effectiveness testing of a new drug in humans.

PHASE III • Extensive clinical trials in humans.

PHAZYME • *See* Simethicone.

PHENACEMIDE (Rx) • **Phenacetylcarbamide. Phenurone.** An anticonvulsant drug that regulates the flow of sodium through the cell membranes in the area of the brain that controls movement. Used to treat complex, generalized, tonic-clonic, absence, and atypical absence epileptic seizures. Potential adverse reactions include anemia, drowsiness, dizziness, insomnia, headaches, numbness, depression, suicidal tendencies, aggressiveness, loss of appetite, weight loss, kidney dysfunction, liver dysfunction, and rash. Anticonvulsants increase the risk of toxicity. Ethotoin (*see*) used with phenacemide may cause paranoia. Contraindicated in patients with personality disturbances or in patients achieving good seizure control without anticonvulsants. Should be used with caution in patients with liver dysfunction or a history of allergy; also when a hydantoin (*see*) derivative is used concurrently. Patients should report a sore throat or fever to their physicians immediately. The drug should never be withdrawn suddenly.

PHENACETIN • A nonnarcotic analgesic no longer used because of its adverse effects. Phenacetin is converted in the body to acetaminophen (*see*). In 1992, the FDA issued a notice that phenacetin had not been shown to be safe and effective as claimed in OTC digestive-aid products, internal painkillers, and oral menstrual drugs.

PHENAMETH • *See* Promethazine.

PHENANTOIN • *See* Mephenytoin.

PHENAPHEN • *See* Acetaminophen.

PHENAPHEN WITH CODEINE • *See* Acetaminophen and Codeine.

PHENAZINE • *See* Promethazine.

PHENAZODINE • *See* Phenazopyridine.

PHENAZOPYRIDINE HYDROCHLORIDE (Rx) (OTC) • **Azo-Gantanol. Azo-Standard. Baridium. Di-Azo. Eridium. Geridium. Phenazodine. Pyrazodine. Pyridiate. Pyridin. Pyridium. Sprx-105. Urodine. Urogesic. Viridium.** An analgesic introduced in 1927 that exerts its effect on urinary mucosa through an unknown mechanism and relieves pain and discomfort. It is not very effective in curing infection. Usually combined with a sulfa drug. Potential adverse effects include headache, vertigo, nausea, drug-induced hepatitis, and rash. Contraindicated in kidney insufficiency and liver disease. Colors urine red or orange and may stain fabrics. Taking the drug with meals may minimize GI distress. Should be discontinued if the skin or white of the eye becomes yellow-tinged, which may indicate accumulation caused by impaired kidney excretion.

PHENDIMETRAZINE (Rx) • **Adipost. Adphen. Anorex. Bacarate. Bontril. Dyrexan. Hydrex. Melfiat. Metra. Obalan. Obeval. Phenazine 35. Plegine. Prelu-2. Slyn-LL. Sprx-105. Statobex. Trimstat. Trimtabs. Wehless. Weightrol. X-Trozine.** An appetite suppressant that promotes nerve impulse transmission by releasing stored norepinephrine (*see*) from the nerves in the brain. Used for short-term weight loss. Potential adverse reactions include nervousness, euphoria, dizziness, insomnia, tremor, headache, irregular heartbeat, heart palpitations, a rise in blood pressure, blurred vision, dry mouth, nausea, abdominal cramps, diarrhea, constipation, and painful urination. Ammonium chloride and ascorbic acid (vitamin C) decrease its effectiveness. Antacids, sodium bicarbonate, and acetazolamide enhance its effects. MAO inhibitors (*see*) may cause severe high blood pressure. Phendimetrazine should not be taken with any other stimulants or antidepressants, including those stimulants found in cold and allergy medications. Contraindicated in patients with overactive thyroid, high blood pressure, glaucoma, angina, or other severe cardiovascular disorders. Should be used with caution in highly excited states, or with a history of drug abuse. Tolerance or dependence can develop. Fatigue may result as drug effects wear off. Caffeinated drinks should be avoided. Should be taken before meals, but at least six hours before bedtime.

PHENELZINE (Rx) • **Nardil.** An MAO inhibitor (*see*) for the treatment of depression, introduced in 1961. It is reportedly beneficial in some depressions that do not respond to other treatments. Potential adverse side effects include drowsiness, dizziness, excitation, tremors, muscle twitching, confusion, mania, memory impairment, fatigue, high blood pressure, a drop in blood pressure when rising from a sitting or prone position, dry mouth, irregular heartbeat, constipation, decreased libido, impaired erection, inhibited ejaculation, inhibited orgasm, swelling, nausea, loss of appetite, intestinal paralysis, urine retention, liver dysfunction, rash, hives, sweating, and weight changes. Alcohol, barbiturates and other sedatives, narcotics, dextromethorphan, and tricyclic antidepressants, when taken with phenelzine, may have unpredictable side effects. Amphetamines, antihistamines, ephedrine, levodopa, meperidine, metaraminol, methotrimeprazine, methylphenidate, phenylephrine, and phenylpropanolamine enhance phenelzine's blood-pressure-raising effects. Dosages of diabetes medicine may have to be adjusted. Contraindicated in elderly or debilitated patients, in those with liver dysfunction, congestive heart failure, high blood pressure, heart or cerebrovascular disease, and severe or frequent headaches. Also contraindicated with foods containing tryptophan (broad beans) or tyramine (cheese, herring, and wine). Should not be used within ten days of MAO inhibitor use, and within ten days of elective surgery or local anesthetic. Combining the drug with alcohol or cocaine should be avoided. Effects may not be manifested for two weeks. Precautions should be continued ten days after discontinuation of the drug because effects are long-lasting. May be taken with or without food, but it should not be taken late in the evening because it can interfere with sleep.

PHENERGAN (Rx) • *See* Promethazine.

PHENERGAN D (Rx) • A combination of promethazine and pseudoephedrine (*see both*).

PHENERGAN VC (Rx) • A combination of phenylephrine and promethazine (*see both*).

PHENETRON • *See* Chlorpheniramine.

PHENINDAMINE (RX) • **Nolahist. Nolamine.** An antihistamine used for the temporary relief of runny nose, sneezing, itching of the nose or throat, and itchy, watery eyes due to hay fever or other upper-respiratory allergies, and the common cold. May cause excitability, especially in children. Contraindicated in individuals with asthma, glaucoma, emphysema, chronic lung disease, shortness of breath, difficulty in breathing, and difficulty in urination due to enlargement of the prostate gland, unless directed by a physician. May cause drowsiness; alcohol may increase this effect. May cause nervousness and insomnia in some people. In 1992, the FDA proposed a ban on phenindamine tartrate in oral menstrual drug products because it had not been shown to be safe and effective as claimed.

PHENIRAMINE (OTC) • **Dristan Menthol Nasal Spray. Dristan Nasal Spray. Fiogesic. Muro Opcon A. Opcon A.** Crystals from amyl alcohol. Used as an antihistamine for the relief of nasal congestion due to colds, sinusitis, hay fever congestion, and other upper-respiratory allergies. In 1992, the FDA proposed a ban on pheniramine maleate in internal analgesic products because it had not been shown to be safe and effective as claimed.

PHENMETRAZINE (Rx) • **Preludin.** An appetite suppressant that promotes nerve impulse transmission by releasing stored norepinephrine (*see*) from the nerves in the brain. Used for short-term weight loss. Potential adverse reactions include nervousness, dizziness, insomnia, tremor, headache, irregular heartbeat, heart palpitations, a rise in blood pressure, blurred vision, dry mouth, nausea, abdominal cramps, diarrhea, constipation, and painful urination. Ammonium chloride and ascorbic acid (vitamin C) decrease its effectiveness. Antacids, sodium bicarbonate, and acetazolamide enhance its effects. MAO inhibitors (*see*) may cause severe high blood pressure. Contraindicated in patients with overactive thyroid, high blood pressure, glaucoma, angina, or other severe cardiovascular disorders. Should be used with caution in highly excited states and with a history of drug abuse. Tolerance or dependence can develop. Fatigue may result as drug effects wear off. Caffeinated drinks should be avoided. Should be taken at least six hours before bedtime on an empty stomach.

PHENOBARBITAL (Rx) • **Barbidonna. Bellergal Spacetabs. Bronkolixir. Chardonna-2. Dilantin. Donnatal. Donnazyme. Phenobarbitone. Phenylethylmalonyurea. Barbita. Bronkotabs. Haponal. Hyonatal. Hyosophen. Kanalka. Kinesed. Luminal. PBR-12. Solfoton. Spasmolin. Spasquid.** A barbiturate sedative and anticonvulsant drug introduced in 1912, it increases the threshold for seizures in the area of the brain controlling movement and probably interferes with transmission of impulses from the thalamus to the cortex of the brain. Used to treat all forms of epilepsy, seizures in children due to high fever, continuous seizures (status epilepticus), sedation, insomnia, and liver and gallbladder problems. Potential adverse effects include drowsiness, lethargy, hangover, paradoxical excitement in elderly patients, nausea, vomiting, liver dysfunction, decreased libido, impotence, decreased effectiveness of oral contraceptives, rash, hives, pain, and swelling. Use with alcohol and other central nervous system depressants, including narcotics, may cause dangerous central nervous system depression. Should be used cautiously with diazepam (*see*) because diazepam increases the effects of both drugs. Phenobarbital decreases the effectiveness of griseofulvin, oral blood thinners, estrogens, oral contraceptives, doxycycline, and corticosteroids. MAO inhibitors (*see*), valproic acid, and primidone increase its effects and may result in dangerous central nervous system depression. Rifampin may make phenobarbital less effective. Contraindicated in those sensitive to barbiturates, in porphyria (*see*), liver dysfunction, respiratory disease with shortness of breath, kidney disease, and in women who are breast-feeding. Should be used cautiously in those with overactive thyroid, diabetes, anemia, and in elderly or debilitated patients. It may cause physical and psychological dependence. Should not be discontinued suddenly. Most effective when taken on an empty stomach, but may be taken with a small amount of food to avoid gastrointestinal distress.

PHENOBARBITONE • *See* Phenobarbital.

PHENOJECT-50 • *See* Promethazine.

PHENOL (OTC) • **Anbesol Gel. Baker's P&S. Campho-Phenique Cold Sore Gel. Carbolic Acid. Cepastat. Cepastat Cherry Flavor Sore Throat Lozenges. Cheracol Sore Throat Spray. Chloraseptic. Phenolate Sodium. Phenyl Pelargonate. PRID Salve.** Obtained from coal tar. Occurs in urine and has the characteristic odor present in coal tar and wood. Phenol compounds are found in many plants such as willow bark and wintergreen. It is a general disinfectant and anesthetic for the skin. Ingestion of even small amounts may cause nausea, vomiting, and greenish urine, as well as necrosis of the mouth and gastrointestinal tract. Also, circulatory collapse, paralysis, convulsions, coma, and death resulting from respiratory failure. Fatalities have been reported from ingestion of as little as 1.5 grams (thirty grams to the ounce). Fatal poisoning can occur through skin absorption. Although there have been many poisonings from phenolic solutions, it continues to be used in commercial products such as disinfectants and shaving creams. Swelling, pimples, hives, and other rashes following application to the skin have been widely reported. A concentration of 2 percent causes burning and numbness. In 1992, the FDA issued a notice that phenol had not been shown to be safe and effective as claimed in OTC products, including astringent (*see*) drugs and those for insect bites and stings.

PHENOLATE SODIUM • *See* Phenol.

PHENOLAX WAFERS • *See* Phenolphthalein.

PHENOLIC ACIDS (TANNINS) • Found in parsley, carrots, broccoli, cabbage, tomatoes, eggplant, peppers, citrus fruits, whole grains and berries, they have antioxidant properties, inhibit formation of nitrosamine, a cancer-causing agent, and affect enzyme activity.

PHENOLPHTHALEIN (OTC) • **Agoral. Alophen Pills. Correctol Laxative. Dialose. Evac-U-Gen. Evac-U-Lax. Ex-Lax. Feen-A-Mint. Lax-Pills. Medilax. Modane. Phenolax Wafers. Phillips' Lax Caps. Prulet.** A stimulant laxative used for constipation. Potential adverse reactions include nausea, vomiting, diarrhea, colic when taken in large doses, loss of normal bowel function in excessive use, abdominal cramps, malabsorption of nutrients, colitis, rash, itching, pigmentation, and dependence in long-term use. Contraindicated in abdominal pain, nausea, vomiting, and other symptoms of appendicitis or acute abdomen, fecal impaction, and intestinal obstruction or perforation. Takes six to eight hours to work. Yellow phenolphthalein is twice as potent as the white variety. *See* Laxative.

PHENOTHIAZINE • A compound obtained from coal tar derivatives, it was formerly used for the treatment of intestinal worms in animals. Phenothiazine serves as the parent compound of a wide range of antipsychotic drugs including chlorpromazine, thioridazine, and fluphenazine. Contraindicated in severe central nervous system depression or coma from any cause, in severe high or low blood pressure, and heart disease.

PHENOTYPE • The physical characteristics or visible traits of an organism.

PHENOXYACETIC ACID • A synthetic fruit and honey flavoring agent. Also used as a fungicide to soften calluses, corns, and other hard surfaces. A mild irritant.

PHENOXYBENZAMINE (Rx) • **Dibenzyline.** A vasodilator used to treat high blood pressure and sweating as a result of pheochromocytoma (*see*), and to control Raynaud's disease (*see*), frostbite, and acrocyanosis (*see*). Potential adverse effects include lethargy, drowsiness, a drop in blood pressure when rising from a sitting or prone position, nasal stuffiness, irregular heartbeat, dry mouth, vomiting, abdominal distress, impotence, and inhibition of ejaculation. When given with other antihypertensives, it may cause a dangerous drop in blood pressure. Rising rapidly from a sitting or prone position should be avoided.

PHENSUXIMIDE (Rx) • **Milontin.** An anticonvulsant derived from succinimide (*see*), it acts by depressing the transmission of nerve signals in the area of the brain controlling movement. Used for absence seizures (*see*). Potential adverse reactions include a drop in white blood cells, nausea, vomiting, loss of appetite, muscular weakness, drowsiness, dizziness, loss of balance, headache, urinary frequency, kidney damage, itching, rash, and lupuslike syndrome. Contraindicated in hypersensitivity to succinimide derivatives. Should be used cautiously in patients with kidney or liver dysfunction. The central nervous system effects of phensuximide are increased by tranquilizers, sleeping pills, narcotic pain relievers, alcohol, antihistamines, MAO inhibitors, antidepressants, and other anticonvulsants. Phensuximide may increase the action of phenytoin by increasing the levels of that drug in the blood. Should not be withdrawn suddenly. Most effective when taken on an empty stomach, but may be taken with a small amount of food to avoid upset stomach.

PHENTERMINE (Rx) • **Adipex-P. Dapex. Fastin. Ionamin. Obe-Nix. Obephen. Obermine. Obestin-30. Oby-Trim. Paramine. Parmine. Phentride. Phentrol. Span R/D. T-Diet. Teramine. Unifast. Wilpowr.** An appetite suppressant that promotes nerve impulse transmission by releasing stored norepinephrine (*see*) from the nerves in the brain. Similar to amphetamines. Used for short-term weight loss. Potential adverse reactions include nervousness, dizziness, insomnia, tremor, headache, irregular heartbeat, heart palpitations, a rise in blood pressure, euphoria, blurred vision, dry mouth, nausea, abdominal cramps, diarrhea, constipation, and difficult and/or painful urination. Ammonium chloride and ascorbic acid (vitamin C) decrease its effectiveness. Antacids, sodium bicarbonate, and acetazolamide enhance its effects. MAO inhibitors (*see*) may cause severe high blood pressure. Stimulants, including those in over-the-counter medications for colds and allergies, may increase phentermine's side effects. Contraindicated in patients with overactive thyroid, high blood pressure, glaucoma, angina, or other severe cardiovascular disorders. Should be used with caution in highly excited states and with a history of drug abuse. Tolerance or dependence can develop. Fatigue may result as drug effects wear off. Caffeinated drinks should be avoided. Should be taken before meals, and at least six hours before bedtime.

PHENTOLAMINE MESYLATE (Rx) • **Regitine.** An antihypertensive drug that is used to aid in the diagnosis of the adrenal tumor pheochromocytoma (*see*) and to prevent hypertension before or during surgery to remove the tumor. Potential adverse reactions include dizziness, weakness, flushing, low blood pressure, shock, irregular heartbeat, palpitations, angina, diarrhea, abdominal pain, nausea, vomiting, nasal stuffiness, and low blood sugar. Should not be used with epinephrine because together they may cause excessive low blood pressure. Contraindicated in persons with angina, coronary artery disease, and a history of heart attack. Should be used cautiously in gastritis or peptic ulcer and in patients receiving other high blood pressure medications.

PHENTRIDE • *See* Phentermine.

PHENTROL • *See* Phentermine.

PHENURONE • *See* Phenacemide.

PHENYLEPHRINE (Rx) (OTC) • **AK-Dilate. AK-Nefrin. Alconefrin-25. Anusol-HC Hemorrhoidal Suppositories. Cerose-DM. Congespirin for Children. Dimetane. Doktors. Dristan Cold Nasal Decongestant/Antihistamine. Duration. 4-Way Fast Acting Nasal Spray. Guaiahist. Histamic. Histor-D. I-Phrine. I-White Ophthalmic Solution. Isophrin. Isopto Frin. Murocoli-2. Murocoll-2. Myfrin. Mydfrin. Nasahist. Neo-**

Synephrine. Neotep Granucaps. Nostril. Nostril Nasal Decongestant. Novahistine. Ocu-Phrin Ophthalmic Solution. Prefrin. Prefrin Liquifilm. Rhinall. Robitussin Night Relief. Sinarest Nasal Solution. Sinex. St. Joseph Measured Dose Nasal Decongestant. Vicks Sinex Decongestant. A blood-vessel constrictor, it is the injectable used in low blood pressure emergencies during spinal anesthesia. Also used to treat mild to moderate low blood pressure, in certain cases of rapid heartbeat, in shock, and to prolong spinal anesthesia. In an eye solution, it is used to dilate the pupil and to remove redness. In nasal jellies or drops, it is used to treat nasal congestion. It was changed from Rx to OTC for relief of anal itching and pain. Potential adverse reactions include headache, restlessness, light-headedness, weakness, heart palpitations, slow heartbeat, irregular heartbeat, high blood pressure, angina, blurred vision, goose bumps, and a feeling of coolness. In eye preparations, it may cause headache, aching brow, high blood pressure, rapid heartbeat, heart palpitations, transient burning or stinging on instillation, blurred vision, redness, floaters, glaucoma, and rash. In nose drops it may cause nausea, heart palpitations, fast heartbeat, transient burning, stinging, dryness of nasal mucosa, and rebound nasal congestion. Contraindicated in glaucoma, low blood pressure, rapid heartbeat, severe coronary disease, heart disease, and in patients who are taking MAO inhibitors or tricyclic antidepressants (*see both*). Should be used with extreme caution in persons with overactive thyroid, diabetes, severe atherosclerosis (*see*), slow heartbeat, sulfite sensitivity, and in elderly patients. Causes little or no central nervous system stimulation. Guanethidine increases phenylephrine's pupil-dilating and high blood pressure effects. Levodopa makes it less effective.

PHENYLETHYLMALONYLUREA • *See* Phenobarbital.

PHENYLISOHYDANTOIN • *See* Pemoline.

PHENYL PELARGONATE • A liquid, insoluble in water. Used in flavors, perfumes, bactericides, and fungicides. *See* Phenol.

PHENYLPROPANOLAMINE (OTC) • Acutrim. Allerest. A.R.M. Allergy Relief Medicine. BC Cold Powder. Cheracol. Contac. Control. Coricidin. Dex-A-Diet. Dexatrim. Dl-norephedrine Hydrochloride. Diet Gum. Dimetapp. Fiogesic. 4-Way Cold Tablets. Histabid. Histamic. Histosal. Hycomine. Kronohist. Maigret-50. Naldecon CX. Nasahist. Nolamine. Orthoxicol. PPA. Precision Release. Prolamine. Propadrine. Propagest. Pyrroxate. Rhindecon. Sine-Off Sinus Medicine. Sinubid. Sinulin. St. Joseph Cold Tablets for Children. Stay Trim. Tavist-D. Triaminic. Tylenol Cold Medication. Westrim LA. A blood-vessel constrictor used as a nasal decongestant and bronchodilator. Also used to reduce appetite. Used in combination with caffeine and a low-calorie regimen, it reportedly helps people lose weight, although its use is controversial. Changed from Rx to OTC. High doses may be associated with anxiety, nausea, dizziness, and with a rise in blood pressure, causing heart palpitations, headache, and breathlessness. MAO inhibitors (*see*) increase the risk of adverse blood pressure effects. Phenylpropanolamine makes high blood pressure drugs less effective. Contraindicated in those with high blood pressure, heart problems, glaucoma, overactive thyroid gland, diabetes, and urinary difficulties. Should be used with caution if you are taking other medicines.

PHENYL SALICYLATE (OTC) • Derived from phenol and salicylic acid (*see*), it is used externally as a disinfectant and internally as an intestinal antiseptic and fever reducer. In 1992, the FDA issued a notice that phenyl salicylate had not been shown to be safe and effective as claimed in OTC products, including those used for oral menstrual drugs.

PHENYLTOLOXAMINE (Rx) (OTC) • Histamic. Magsal. Mobigesic Analgesic Tablets. Momentum Muscular Backache Formula. Percogesic Analgesic Tablets. Sinubid. Sinutab. An antihistamine for temporary relief of minor aches and pains associated with menstrual periods, colds, flu, toothache, and arthritis. May cause excitability, especially in children. Should not be taken in those with asthma, glaucoma, emphysema, chronic pulmonary disease, shortness of breath, or difficulty in urination due to enlargement of the prostate gland, unless directed by a doctor. May cause drowsiness. In 1992, the FDA issued a notice that phenyltoloxamine had not been shown to be safe and effective as claimed in OTC poison ivy, poison oak, and poison sumac products.

PHENYTOIN (Rx) • **Dilantin. Diphenylan Sodium. Diphenylhydantoin.** An anticonvulsant and antiarrhythmic hydantoin (*see*) drug introduced in 1938. By stabilizing the passage of sodium through cell membranes in the area of the brain controlling movement, phenytoin controls the following types of seizures: generalized tonic-clonic, continuous (status epilepticus), and nonepileptic (Reye's syndrome and post–head trauma). Potential adverse effects include anemia, low blood pressure, impotence, decreased libido, decreased effectiveness of oral contraceptives, irregular heartbeat, jerky eye movements, double vision, blurred vision, nausea, vomiting, swollen gums, slurred speech, irritability, weight gain, hepatitis, rash, hairiness, sensitivity to light, and swollen glands. It may also leach calcium from the bone and lead to osteoporosis (*see*). Alcohol, dexamethasone, and folic acid (*see all*) may decrease phenytoin's activity. Oral blood thinners, antihistamines, amiodarone, chloramphenicol, cimetidine, cycloserine, diazepam, diazoxide, disulfiram, influenza vaccine, isoniazid, phenylbutazone, salicylates, sulfamethizole, and valproate (*see all*) may increase phenytoin's activity and toxicity. Contraindicated in phenacemide or hydantoin hypersensitivity, and slow heartbeat and other heart irregularities. Should be used cautiously in liver or kidney dysfunction, low blood pressure, respiratory problems, in the elderly, and in patients receiving other hydantoin (*see*) derivatives. Heavy use of alcohol may diminish the effects of the drug. If you develop a rash while using phenytoin, notify your physician. Good dental hygiene is also recommended to minimize the development of gum complications. The drug should not be discontinued abruptly. May be taken with meals to reduce upset stomach.

Skip the vanilla pudding, however, since it has been found to cause blood levels of this medication to drop by half.

PHEOCHROMOCYTOMA • A tumor usually arising in the inner part of the adrenal gland (above the kidney), that secretes excessive amounts of hormones, producing such symptoms as tremor, cramps, heart palpitations, headache, nausea, and high blood pressure.

PHERAZINE VC • *See* Promethazine and Phenylephrine.

PHILLIPS' MILK OF MAGNESIA • *See* Magnesium Hydroxide.

PHISOAC-BP • *See* Benzoyl Peroxide.

PHISOHEX • *See* Hexachlorophene.

PHOBIA • An obsessive, persistent, unrealistic fear of an object or situation.

PHOS • Homeopathic abbreviation for phosphorus.

PHOS-AC • Homeopathic abbreviation for phosphoric acid (*see*).

PHOSCHOL (OTC) • **Phosphatidylcholine.** A highly purified lecithin that aids the transport of choline to the brain. Choline reportedly aids nerve cells that make a biochemical, acetylcholine, which is in turn released by nerve cells as a neurotransmitter (*see*). Acetylcholine is depleted or ineffective in brain disorders such as Alzheimer's disease (*see*). No major side effects have been reported. Potential adverse reactions include minor stomach upsets and salivation. Should be taken with meals or immediately afterward.

PHOS-EX • *See* Calcium Acetate.

PHOS-FLUR • *See* Sodium Fluoride.

PHOSLO • *See* Calcium Acetate.

PHOSPHALJEL • *See* Aluminum Phosphate.

PHOSPHOLINE • *See* Iodide.

PHOSPHORIC ACID (H) • **Phos-ac.** A colorless, odorless solution made from phosphate rock. Mixes with water and alcohol. The homeopathic remedy is made from pulverized phosphate rock dissolved in sulphuric acid and then diluted. It is used for fatigue, forgetfulness, cough, diarrhea, hair loss, headache, insomnia, and shock.

PHOSPHORUS (OTC) (H) • **K-Phos. Phos. One-A-Day Maximum Formula Vitamins.** A mineral supplement. Also used as a homeopathic medicine (*see*) for hemorrhages, headaches, and hoarseness. *See* Tissue Salts.

PHOTOAGING • **Dermatoheliosis.** Refers to skin damage due to sun exposure. Wrinkling, mottling, and lesions can be caused or made worse by photodamage.

PHOTOFRIN • *See* Porfimer.

PHOTOSENSITIVITY • A condition in which the application or ingestion of certain chemicals, such as propylparaben (*see*), causes skin problems, including rash, hyperpigmentation, and swelling, when the skin is exposed to sunlight.

PHOTOTOXICITY • A reaction to sunlight or ultraviolet light resulting in inflammation.

PHRENILIN • *See* Acetaminophen and Butalbital Compounds.

PHTHALIC ANHYDRIDE • Prepared from naphthalene by oxidation, it consists of lustrous white needles. It is used in the manufacture of dyes and resins. It is moderately irritating to the skin and mucous membranes.

PHYLLOCONTIN • *See* Aminophylline.

PHYLLOQUINONE • *See* Phytonadione.

PHYSIC ROOT • *See* Culver's Root.

PHYSOSTIGMINE (Rx) (H) • **Antilirium. Eserine. Isopto Pes.** Obtained from the dried, ripe seed (calabar bean) of *Physostigma venenosum.* Used topically to produce contraction of the pupil and decrease pressure inside the eye in glaucoma. Also used to inhibit the destruction of acetylcholine (*see*), treat central nervous system toxicity associated with tricyclic antidepressant and anticholinergic poisonings, and experimentally, to treat Alzheimer's disease. Should be used cautiously in persons with intestinal or urinary-tract obstruction, in bronchial asthma, gangrene, diabetes, cardiovascular disease, slow heartbeat, low blood pressure, epilepsy, Parkinson's disease, overactive thyroid, and peptic ulcer. Potential adverse reactions include seizures, hallucinations, muscular twitching, muscle weakness, loss of balance, restlessness, excitability, sweating, irregular heartbeat, heart palpitations, nausea, vomiting, epigastric pain, diarrhea, excessive salivation, bronchospasm, and shortness of breath.

PHYT • Homeopathic abbreviation for phytolacca (*see*).

PHYTOCHEMICAL • *Phyto* is from the Greek meaning "to bring forth" and is used as a prefix to designate from "a plant." Hence *phytochemical* means a chemical from a plant. Epidemiological studies have shown that diets containing large quantities of vegetables and, to a lesser extent, fruits are associated with lowering risks of certain cancers.

PHYTOESTROGENS • The female hormone in plants.

PHYTOLACCA (H) • **Phyt. Americana. Decandra.** A perennial that grows in moist ground along roadsides in the United States, North Africa, and China, it is also common in Mediterranean countries. Phytolacca has a high potassium content. It has been used in folk medicine to treat cancerous growths and by Indians as a purgative. A remedy from the fresh root is used by homeopaths to treat cracked nipples, mumps, sore throat, teething pain, and bad breath. *See* Pokeweed.

PHYTOMENADIONE • *See* Phytonadione.

PHYTONADIONE (Rx) • **Vitamin K. AquaMephyton. Konakion. Mephyton. Phylloquinone. Phytomenadione.** Promotes liver formation of blood-clotting factors. Found in leafy green vegetables; produced by bacteria in the intestine, and necessary for blood clotting. Used in the prevention and treatment of bleeding disorders caused by vitamin K deficiency due to drug therapy or excessive vitamin A. Also used to prevent bleeding in newborns. It can reverse bleeding induced by oral blood thinners such as warfarin and dicumarol (*see both*). It is stronger, faster acting, and longer lasting than other vitamin K preparations and is used for long-term therapy. Potential adverse reactions usually are mild and may include flushing, dizziness, bad taste in the mouth, chest pain, and heart palpitations. Other potential adverse reactions include nausea, vomiting, seizures, low blood pressure, rapid and weak pulse, heart irregularities, sweating, redness, bronchospasms, shortness of breath, cramps, and severe allergic reactions. Should be used with caution in persons who have impaired liver or kidney function or heart problems.

PICRIS • **Bitter Lettuce. Ox Tongue.** A weedy herb with leafy stems and large yellow flowers. It has a bitter taste and is used in homeopathic medicines as a stimulant.

PICROTOXIN (OTC) • Bitter principle (*see*) isolated from the seed of *Anamirta cocculus*. Very poisonous. Used as a central nervous system and respiratory stimulant. In 1992, the FDA proposed a ban on picrotoxin in lice-killing products because it had not been shown to be safe and effective as claimed.

PID • Abbreviation for pelvic inflammatory disease.

PILAGAN • *See* Pilocarpine.

PILEWORT (H) • *Ranunculus ficaria.* **Buttercup. Lesser Celandine.** A starry, little, yellow blossom, it is widely found under hedges. It has astringent qualities, and the herb is considered specific for piles—hence its name. A green pilewort ointment is sold by many herbalists. The plant is toxic if used internally.

PILOCAR • *See* Pilocarpine.

PILOCARPINE (Rx) • **Adsorbocarpine. Akarpine. Isopto Carpine. Isopto Pes. Ocu-Carpine. Ocusert Pilo. Piligan. Pilocar. Pilocel. Pilomiotin. Pilopine HS Gel. Pilostat. PV Carpine. P.V. Carpine Liquifilm. Spectro-Pilo.** An eye solution or gel introduced in 1875 to treat glaucoma. It is absorbed through the eye. Potential adverse reactions include nausea, vomiting, drowsiness, high blood pressure, headache, nearsightedness, blurred vision, brow pain, diarrhea, salivation, bronchial spasms, fluid in the lungs, and allergic reactions. Carbachol and echothiophate increase pilocarpine's effects. Belladonna derivatives and cyclopentolate decrease its effectiveness. Should be used cautiously in asthmatics, and those with liver dysfunction and/or high blood pressure.

PILOCEL • *See* Pilocarpine.

PILOPINE HS GEL • *See* Pilocarpine.

PILOSTAT • *See* Pilocarpine.

PIMA • *See* Potassium Iodide.

PIMARICIN • *See* Natamycin.

PIMENTA • *Pimenta officinalis.* **Allspice. Jamaican Pepper. Pimento.** An evergreen tree whose unripe fruits have been used in herbal medicine to treat dyspepsia. The oil is occasionally taken internally to relieve gas and to improve digestion. Should not be used in cases of inflammation of the gastrointestinal tract.

PIMOZIDE (Rx) • **Orap.** An antipsychotic drug used to treat movement disorders, including Tourette's syndrome (*see*). Potential adverse reactions include parkinsonism-like symptoms and other movement disorders, tardive dyskinesia (*see*), sedation, low blood pressure, visual disturbances, dry mouth, constipation, impotence, fever, irregular heartbeat, sweating, and muscle tightness. Use with alcohol and other central nervous system depressants may increase central nervous system depression. Contraindicated in persons with a history of irregular heartbeat, severe toxic central nervous system depression, or in coma. Should be used cautiously in liver or kidney dysfunction, glaucoma, and enlarged prostate. Should not be discontinued suddenly.

PIMPERNEL, SCARLET (H) • *Anagallis arvensis.* A small annual of the primrose family that grows in temperate regions of the world, the scarlet pimpernel flourishes on sunny banks and in fields. It has been used by herbalists to treat many ailments, including mental diseases, epilepsy, jaundice, and tuberculosis.

PIMPINELLA ANISUM • *See* Aniseed.

PINDOLOL (Rx) • **Visken.** A beta-blocker (*see*) drug introduced in 1972 to lower blood pressure (*see* Antihypertensives). Potential adverse reactions include insomnia, fatigue, dizziness, nervousness, vivid dreams, hallucinations, lethargy, water retention, congestive heart failure, low blood pressure, visual disturbances, nausea, vomiting, diarrhea, low blood sugar, decreased libido, impaired erection, rash, shortness of breath, and muscle, joint, or chest pain. Contraindicated in diabetics, asthmatics, and those with allergic rhinitis (stuffy nose). Must be used with caution in patients with heart disease, liver dysfunction, and those taking other antihypertensive medications. Interaction with cardiac glycosides may adversely affect heart action. When used with epinephrine, severe constriction of the blood vessels may occur. Indomethacin decreases pindolol's effectiveness. Pindolol may cause a need for dosage adjustments in diabetes medications. Should not be discontinued abruptly. May be taken with or without meals. A generic version was approved in 1995.

PINE, SCOTS (H) • *Pinus sylvestris.* The needles and young buds of this pine tree and other pines contain tannin, resins, essential oils, and terpenes (*see all*). Herbalists use pine to treat upper-respiratory infections, arthritis, fatigue, nervous debility, and sleeplessness. They also use pine preparations to aid healing of cuts and to soothe skin irritation.

PINE TAR (OTC) (H) • A product obtained by distillation of pinewood. A blackish brown, viscous liquid, slightly soluble in water. Used as an antiseptic in skin diseases. May be irritating to the skin.

P-I-N FORTE • *See* Isoniazid and Pyridoxine Hydrochloride.

PINKROOT (H) • *Spigelia marilandica.* **Star-Bloom. Worm Grass. Wormweed.** An herbaceous plant native to the southern United States, it grows in rich soils on the edge of woods. It is usually prescribed by herbalists with calomel, senna, or some other cathartic. Used primarily as a worm medicine, particularly for roundworms. The roots contain spigeline, which is similar to nicotine. It is toxic, and an overdose can be fatal. *See* Spigelia.

PIO • *See* Pemoline.

PIPERACILLIN (Rx) • **Pipracil.** A penicillin antibiotic used to treat systemic infections caused by gram-positive and especially gram-negative (*see*) organisms including *Proteus* and *Pseudomonas aeruginosa.* Potential adverse reactions include a high incidence of allergic reactions and in some instances, anaphylactic (*see*) shock. Other adverse effects may be bleeding, decrease in white blood cells and platelets, neuromuscular irritability, seizures, headache, dizziness, nausea, diarrhea, pain at injection site, low potassium, and overgrowth of nonsusceptible organisms. Interacts adversely with aminoglycoside antibiotics (*see*).

PIPERAZINE (Rx) • **Antepar. Bryrel. Entacyl. Helmizin. Pin-Tega Tabs. Pipril. Ta-Verm. Vermirex. Vermizine.** An anthelmintic agent that paralyzes worms, causing their expulsion by normal movement of the human intestines. Adverse reactions include incoordination, numbness, seizures, memory problems, headache, dizziness, eye problems, nausea, vomiting, diarrhea, abdominal cramps, hives, rash, joint pain, fever, bronchospasm, and anemia.

PIPER CUBEBA • *See* Cubeb Berries.

PIPER METHYSTICUM • *See* Kava-Kava.

PIPER NIGRUM • *See* Pepper, Black.

PIPERONYL BUTOXIDE (OTC) • **A-200 Pediculicide Shampoo. Lice Enz Foam. Pronto Lice Killing Shampoo. R&C Shampoo. Rid Lice Killing Shampoo.** A compound derived from petroleum used in combination with pyrethrins to treat skin parasites. For external use only. Should not be inhaled or used on irritated, infected, or broken skin. Should not be used by persons sensitive to ragweed. Harmful if swallowed.

PIPOBROMAN (Rx) • **Vercyte.** Used to treat polycythemia and chronic myelocytic leukemia.

PIPRACIL • *See* Piperacillin.

PIPSISSEWA LEAVES EXTRACT (H) • *Chimaphila umbellata.* **Ground Holly. King's Cure. Love-in-Winter. Prince's Pine. Winter Rheumatism Weed.** Extracted from the leaves of an evergreen shrub, it is used in many commercial flavorings. Its leaves have been used as an astringent, diuretic, and tonic. The Cree word *pipisisikweu* means to break up—bladder stones, that is. It has properties similar to uva-ursi (*see*). Also used as a treatment for arthritis. In 1992, the FDA proposed a ban on pipsissewa in oral menstrual drug products because it had not been shown to be safe and effective as claimed.

PIRBUTEROL (Rx) • **Maxair.** A bronchodilator introduced in 1983 that prevents and reverses bronchospasm in asthma. Potential adverse reactions include insomnia, tremors, nervousness, headache, rapid heartbeat, high blood pressure, and dry throat. Propranolol and other beta-blockers (*see*) decrease its effectiveness. Contra-

indicated in hypersensitivity to pirbuterol or other adrenergics (*see*), and in patients with irregular heartbeat. Since it is taken only by spray, food is unrelated to dosing.

PIROXICAM (Rx) • **Feldene.** Introduced in 1982, this drug produces anti-inflammatory, analgesic, and fever-reducing effects, probably by inhibiting prostaglandins (*see*). It is used to treat arthritis. It was the first NSAID (*see*) approved by the FDA for once-daily dosing and lasts longer in the body than other similar drugs. Potential adverse reactions include prolonged bleeding time, anemia, dizziness, drowsiness, water retention, abdominal pain, gas, peptic ulcer, nausea, occult blood loss, kidney toxicity, liver toxicity, and sensitivity to light. It is more likely to cause a rash than other NSAIDs. Aspirin may decrease blood levels of piroxicam. Oral blood thinners may increase its blood-thinning effects. Oral diabetes drugs may have to be adjusted due to Piroxicam's lowering of blood sugar. Contraindicated in asthmatics with nasal polyps. Must be used cautiously in patients with GI ulcers or inflammation, in patients with liver, kidney, or heart disease, blood problems, diabetes, and asthma or allergy to other NSAIDs. Piroxicam raises the levels of lithium in the blood. Use with other NSAIDs or alcohol may increase the danger of GI problems. Should be taken with meals to reduce the risk of stomach upset. A candidate for OTC status.

PISCIDIA ERYTHRINA • In 1992, the FDA proposed a ban on *Piscidia erythrina* in oral menstrual drug products because it had not been shown to be safe and effective as claimed. *See* Dogwood.

PIT • *See* Oxytocin.

PITOCIN • *See* Oxytocin.

PITRESSIN • *See* Vasopressin.

PITUITARY GLAND • The pea-sized gland situated at the base of the brain, once thought to be the master gland that gave "orders" to other glands. It is now known that the pituitary gland takes its orders from the hypothalamus (*see*). The pituitary then sends out orders to the other glands in the body. The frontal lobe of the gland produces growth hormone, which regulates growth; prolactin, which stimulates the breasts and has other functions as yet not clearly understood; and hormones that stimulate the thyroid, adrenals, ovaries, and testes. The back lobe of the pituitary produces antidiuretic hormone, which acts on the kidneys and regulates urine output, and oxytocin, which stimulates the contractions of the womb during childbirth.

PITUITARY HORMONES, POSTERIOR (Rx) • *See* Pituitrin.

PITUITRIN (Rx) • A medication from the back of the pituitary gland used to stop bleeding from the uterus after childbirth. Also used to stimulate smooth-muscle contractions, to relieve postoperative distension, and to control bed-wetting in diabetes insipidus (*see*). *See also* Pituitary Gland.

PIX CARBONIS • *See* Coal Tar.

PLACEBO • An inert or innocuous substance given in place of medication.

PLACIDYL • *See* Ethchlorvynol.

PLAGUE • An acute feverish disease caused by bacilli. It is primarily a disease of rats and other rodents, which tend to carry the fleas that can transmit the plague to humans.

PLAGUE VACCINE (Rx) • An injection of killed plague bacilli (*Yersinia pestis*), which promotes immunity to plague. Given to adults and to children over ten years of age. Potential adverse reactions include malaise, headache, slight fever, swollen glands, severe allergic reaction, and swelling and redness at the site of injection.

PLANT • Homeopathic abbreviation for plantago (*see*).

PLANTAGO (H) • A homeopathic medicine used to treat earaches and toothaches. *See* Plantain Extract.

PLANTAIN EXTRACT (H) • *Plantago major.* The extract of various species of plantain. The starchy fruit is a staple item of diet throughout the tropics. Used for bladder infections by herbalists. Its seeds contain a large amount of mucilage and will thus have a demulcent and emollient effect externally. It is a natural astringent and antiseptic with soothing and cooling effects on blemishes and burns. Plantain poultices are used for open sores and inflammation. Herbalists also use plantain for asthma, bronchitis, and for digestive problems. It is a mild laxative.

PLANT ESTROGENS • A host of estrogens have been identified in plants. Although they are considerably less active than those in animals, chronic exposure may lead to the accumulation of levels that are active in humans. *See* Genistein.

PLANT STEROLS • Vitamin D precursors found in broccoli, cabbage, cucumbers, squash, yams, tomatoes, eggplant, peppers, soy products, and whole grains. Cause cells to differentiate.

PLAQUE • Buildup on the teeth of a film of acid-forming bacteria and material from saliva. Believed to be a main cause of gingivitis (inflamed gums), the formation of tartar, and dental cavities.

PLAQUENIL • *See* Hydroxychloroquine.

PLASMA • The fluid in which blood cells are bathed.

PLASMID • A small, circular piece of DNA that carries selected genes as well as directions to reproduce itself when put into a host cell. Plasmids cannot survive outside a host cell.

PLASMIN • An enzyme that digests fibrin as well as other substances in surrounding blood.

PLASMINOGEN • A protein found in many tissues and body fluids that is important in preventing fibrin (*see*) clot formation.

PLASMINOGEN ACTIVATOR • A substance that activates a protein called plasminogen (*see*) to produce a substance known as plasmin, which dissolves blood clots.

PLASTER • Herbal materials are placed between two pieces of cloth and applied to the affected area.

PLATEAU CAPS • *See* Papaverine Hydrochloride.

PLATELET • A component of blood that plays an important role in blood coagulation.

PLATINOL • *See* Cisplatin.

PLATYCODON (H) • *Platycodon grandiflorum.* **Jie Geng.** The root is used by Chinese herbalists as a cough medicine, to treat asthma, and to soothe sore throats. A strong expectorant, it helps to clear mucus from the lungs.

-PLEGIA • Derived from the Greek word *plessein,* meaning to strike ("stroke"), it usually denotes paralysis, as in *paraplegia,* both legs paralyzed.

PLEGINE • *See* Phendimetrazine.

PLENDIL • *See* Felodipine.

PLEURA • A special membrane surrounding the lungs from the outside.

PLEURAL EFFUSION • An accumulation of fluid inside the pleura (*see*), compressing the lungs and interfering with their function.

PLEURISY ROOT (H) • *Asclepias tuberosa.* **Butterfly Weed. Canada Root.** The herb is used for ailments involving the lungs and upper respiratory tract. Contains glycosides and essential oils (*see both*). Also good for indigestion and stomach gas, according to herbalists. Native Americans used this root to treat bronchitis, pneumonia, and diarrhea. Herbalists use it to induce sweating and vomiting, and as an expectorant and a laxative. Large doses may cause severe vomiting, diarrhea, depression of the central nervous system, seizures, and kidney and liver damage. Overuse of the plant, because it contains cardiac glycosides, may cause death through heart failure.

PLICAMYCIN (Rx) • **Mithracin. Mithramycin.** An anticancer drug used to treat testicular cancer, and hypercalcemia (abnormally high levels of calcium in the blood) associated with malignancies. Potential adverse reactions include nausea, vomiting, diarrhea, loss of appetite, sore throat, metallic taste, kidney dysfunction, bleeding, facial flushing, decreased calcium and potassium in the blood, liver dysfunction, and paleness around the eyes.

PLUM EXTRACT (H) • The extract of the fruit of the plum tree, *Prunus domestica.* American Indians boiled the wild plum and gargled with it to cure mouth sores.

PMS-ISONIAZID • *See* Isoniazid.

PMS METRONIDAZOLE • *See* Metronidazole.

PMS PYRAZINAMIDE • *See* Pyrazinamide.

PNEUMO- • Pertaining to the lungs.

PNEUMOCOCCAL • Relating to certain bacteria that cause pneumonia.

PNEUMOCOCCAL PERITONITIS • An infection caused by *Pneumococcus* of the membrane that lines the inside of the abdomen.

PNEUMOCOCCAL VACCINE, POLYVALENT (Rx) • **Pneumovax 23. Pnu-Imune 23.** Promotes active immunity to infections caused by *Streptococcus pneumoniae.* Potential adverse reactions include slight fever, severe allergic reactions, and local soreness at the site of vaccination.

PNEUMOCYSTIS CARINII PNEUMONIA • PCP. A severe lung infection caused by a parasite. It is found in nearly 80 percent of all AIDS patients at some time during the disease and is a major cause of death in these patients.

PNS • Abbreviation for peripheral nervous system (*see*).

PODO • Homeopathic abbreviation for podophyllum (*see* Podophyllin and Mayapple).

PODOFILOX (Rx) • **Condylox.** A topical solution used to treat external genital warts. Potential adverse reactions include vomiting, dizziness, insomnia, foreskin retraction, painful or bloody urination, local burning, pain, inflammation, itching, tingling, tenderness, chafing, scarring, blisters, swelling, dryness, and peeling. Contraindicated in patients hypersensitive to or intolerant of any component of the medication.

PODOFIN • *See* Podophyllin Resin.

PODOPHYLLIN (Rx) (H) • *Podophyllum peltatum.* **Podo.** An ingredient in topical medications to treat warts. A few hours after podophyllin is applied to a wart, the growth becomes whitened and, in one to three days, begins to disintegrate. Podophyllin can cause severe irritation of normal skin. Therefore, petrolatum is usually applied on the perimeter of the wart to keep podophyllin from touching healthy tissue. It can be toxic if too much is absorbed into the body, causing confusion, diarrhea, abdominal pain, and convulsions. *See* Podophyllin Resin.

PODOPHYLLIN RESIN (Rx) (H) • **Mandrake. Mayapple. Pod-Ben. Popo-Ben. Pudofin. Verrex–C&M.** Used in the treatment of benign growths, including genital and perianal warts, papillomas, and fibroids. The resin is poisonous and a strong purgative. Banned by the FDA, May 1992, as an ingredient in laxatives. *See* Mandrake and Mayapple.

PODOPHYLLUM PELTATUM • *See* Mayapple.

-POIESIS • Suffix meaning formation of, such as *hematopoiesis,* formation of blood.

POINT-TWO • *See* Sodium Fluoride.

POISON IVY (H) • *Rhus toxicodendron.* **Poison Oak. Poison Vine.** A shrub native to the northeastern United States, it contains urshiols, allergy-causing substances. A homeopathic medicine with highly diluted extract of fresh leaves is used to treat skin diseases and arthritis. Poison ivy is one of the most highly irritating and allergenic plants.

POKEROOT • *See* Pokeweed.

POKEWEED (H) • *Phytolacca americana.* **Coakum. Pokeroot.** Native to the southern United States and the Mediterranean area, the dried roots reduce inflammation and arthritic pain. It has antibiotic, antiviral, and anti-inflammatory properties. Among its constituents are tannin, formic acid, saponins, and alkaloid (*see all*). Prescribed by herbalists for a variety of ailments from swollen glands to weight loss. A member of the bloodberry family, it is an emetic and laxative, with narcotic properties. Both berries and roots contain potentially harmful compounds. Some people are more sensitive to pokeweed's adverse effects than others, and fatalities have occurred.

POLARAMINE • *See* Dexchlorpheniramine.

POLOCAINE • *See* Mepivacaine.

POLOXAMER 188 • Banned by the FDA, May 1992, as an ingredient in laxatives.

POLY- • Prefix meaning many.

POLYARTHRITIS • Inflammation of several joints.

POLYCILLIN (Rx) • *See* Ampicillin.

POLYCILLIN-PRB (Rx) • A combination of ampicillin and probenecid (*see both*) used to combat infections.

POLYCITRA • A combination of potassium, sodium citrate, and citric acid (*see all*).

POLYCYSTIC OVARIAN DISEASE • A condition in which the ovaries contain multiple cysts. Characterized by scant or absent menstruation, infertility, excessive facial hair, and obesity.

POLYCYTHEMIA VERA • A disorder of the bone marrow that causes an increased production of red blood cells.

POLYESTRADIOL (Rx) • **Estradurin.** An estrogen drug used to treat prostrate cancer.

POLYETHYLENE GLYCOL (Rx) (OTC) • **PEG. CoLyte. GoLYTELY. Allergy Drops. Visine Extra Eye Drops.** An emulsifying agent used in skin preparations. It also is used in eyedrops to relieve minor irritation caused by allergens, and in certain preparations for clearing the bowel for GI examination. Potential adverse reactions include nausea, bloating, cramps, and vomiting. Contraindicated in GI obstruction or perforation, gastric retention, toxic colitis, or megacolon (*see*).

POLYETHYLENE GLYCOL (600) DIOLEATE • Polyethylene glycol esters of mixed fatty acids from tall oil; polyethylene glycol (400 through 6,000). An agent in nonnutritive artificial sweeteners; a component of coatings and binders in tablet food. Improves resistance to oxidation and moisture.

POLYGONUM BISTORTA • *See* Bistort.

POLY-HISTINE CS (Rx) • A combination of brompheniramine, codeine phosphate and sulfate, and phenylpropanolamine (*see all*), used to treat coughs.

POLY-HISTINE D (OTC) • A combination of phenylpropanolamine, pheniramine, phenyltoloxamine, and pyrilamine (*see all*).

POLY-HISTINE DM (OTC) • A combination of brompheniramine, dextromethorphan, and phenylpropanolamine (*see all*), used to treat coughs.

POLYMOX • *See* Amoxicillin.

POLYMYXIN B (Rx) (OTC) • **Aerosporin. Aquaphor Antibiotic Ointment. Bactine First Aid Antibiotic. Campho-Phenique Triple Antibiotic Ointment. Foille. Hydromycin. Infectrol. Mycitracin. Neosporin Cream and Ointment. Neosporin Ophthalmic Solution. Neotal. Neotricin. Ophthocort. Polysporin. Pyodicin-Otic. Terramycin Opthalmic Ointment.** An antibacterial drug used topically, for the most part, to treat infections of the skin, eyes, and ears. Used systemically to treat acute urinary-tract infections, or blood poisoning caused by bacteria; also when other antibiotics are ineffective or contraindicated. Potential adverse reactions include irritability, drowsiness, facial flushing, weakness, respiratory paralysis, headache, and irritation of the covering of the brain. Also may cause hives, fever, and possibly, fatal allergic reactions.

POLYMYXIN E • *See* Colistin.

POLYNEURITIS • Inflammation of many nerves simultaneously.

POLYP • Swollen or tumorous tissue that may or may not be cancerous.

POLYPHENOLS • Compounds found in many plants including garlic, green tea, soybeans, cereal grains, cruciferous vegetables such as broccoli, umbelliferous vegetables such as celery, citrus, solanaceous such as potatoes, curcuma such as ginger, licorice root, and flaxseed. Polyphenols have been reported to interfere with tumor promotion by dampening steroid hormones. They are also antioxidants and act as "garbage collectors," disposing of mutagens and cancer-causing agents.

POLYPODY ROOT (H) • *Polypodium vulgare.* **Adder's-Tongue. Boar Fern. Brakeroot. Oak Fern. Rheum-Purging.** A common fern on shady banks and in old, ruined walls, it is used as a tonic and recommended by herbalists for upset stomach, loss of appetite, and rheumatic disorders. Also used to treat coughs. It may cause a rash.

POLY-PRED • *See* Prednisolone, Neomycin, and Polymyxin B.

POLYSPORIN • *See* Bacitracin and Polymyxin B.

POLYTAR • *See* Coal Tar.

POLYTHIAZIDE (Rx) • **Minizide. Renese.** A thiazide diuretic (*see*) that increases urine excretion of sodium and water, it is used to treat edema in heart failure and kidney failure, and high blood pressure. Potential adverse reactions include nausea, vomiting, loss of appetite, pancreatitis, dehydration, a drop in blood pressure upon rising from a seated or prone position, liver dysfunction, anemia, a drop in platelets, low potassium, high blood sugar, fluid and electrolyte imbalances, rash, photosensitivity, and other allergic reactions. Cholestyramine, colestipol, and NSAIDs (*see all*) decrease its effectiveness. Diazoxide increases its blood-pressure-lowering and sugar-raising effects. Contraindicated in kidney and liver diseases, absence of urine formation, and hypersensitivity to other thiazides or sulfonamide-derived drugs. Should be used cautiously in gout. Mykrox tablets are reportedly more rapid and completely absorbed than other brands. Should be taken in the morning to avoid having to urinate during the night. A diet rich in potassium may be recommended. This includes dates, apricots, bananas, and tomatoes. If you are taking this drug, you should wear a sunscreen.

POLY-VI-FLOR • A multivitamin preparation with fluoride and iron (*see both*).

POLYVINYL ALCOHOL (OTC) • **Murine Eye Lubricant. Tears Plus Lubricant.** A synthetic resin prepared from polyvinyl acetates, it is an ingredient of artificial tear (*see*) preparations.

POLY-VI SOL (OTC) • A multivitamin preparation with iron.

POMEGRANATE (H) • *Punica granatum.* **Grenadier.** A small, shrubby tree. The powdered fruit rind was held to be astringent and was utilized to treat diarrhea, excessive perspiration, as a gargle for sore throats, for intermittent fevers, and for vaginal discharge. The rind contains a high level of tannins (*see*). Through the ages, the root bark has been administered to rid the intestines of worms, particularly tapeworm. May cause diarrhea if regularly used.

PONDERAL • *See* Fenfluramine.

PONDERAZ • *See* Fenfluramine.

PONDIMIN • *See* Fenfluramine.

PONSTEL • *See* Mefenamic Acid.

PONTOCAINE • *See* Tetracaine.

POPLAR EXTRACT (H) • **Balm of Gilead.** Extract of the leaves and twigs of *Populus nigra.* In ancient times, the buds were mashed to make a soothing salve that was spread on sunburned areas, scalds, scratches, inflamed skin, and wounds. They were also simmered in lard for use as an ointment and for antiseptic purposes. The leaves and bark were steeped by American colonists to make a soothing tea. Supposedly helped allergies and soothed reddened eyes. No known toxicity.

POPPY (Rx) • *Papaver.* **California Poppy. Opium Poppy. Red Poppy.** Early monasteries grew poppy for use in their hospitals, and the sap was used throughout the Middle Ages during crude surgical operations and after serious battlefield injuries. The exudates from the poppies all contain alkaloids (*see*) with sedative and hypnotic properties. They are generally used as sedatives, narcotics, and analgesics. Used to treat diarrhea, pain, cough, sweating, and insomnia. Poppy seeds, commonly used on bagels and other pastries, can cause a false positive in routine drug screening in the workplace, organized sports, and the military. *See also* Opium.

PORFIMER • Photofrin. A medication for the palliative photodynamic therapy of totally obstructing esophageal cancers, and for certain partially obstructing cancers of the esophagus. The FDA approved it in 1994. Porfimer is a photosensitizer, and after it is injected, the drug is preferentially retained by tumor tissue and, after three days, activated by laser. The light stimulates the production of oxygen radicals from porfimer, which are toxic to cells in which they are produced.

PORPHYRIA • A group of inborn errors-of-metabolism disorders involving excessive excretion of porphyrins, pigments in the blood. Causes dark urine and severe photosensitivity accompanied by anemia.

POSTURE-D (OTC) • A combination of vitamin D and calcium used to help maintain healthy bodies.

POTAGO • *See* Potassium Chloride.

POTASALAN • *See* Potassium Chloride.

POTASSIUM • The healthy body contains about nine grams of potassium. Most of it is found inside body cells. Potassium plays an important role in maintaining water balance and acid-base balance. It participates in the transmission of nerve impulses and in the transfer of messages from nerves to muscles. It also acts as a catalyst in carbohydrate and protein metabolism. Potassium is important for the maintenance of normal kidney function. It has a major effect on the heart and all the muscles of the body. Some diuretics (water pills) commonly used to treat high blood pressure cause potassium to be lost from the body. To compensate, physicians may advise the addition of potassium-rich foods such as bananas, oranges, and dried peas or may prescribe potassium supplements. Potassium replacement has to be carefully monitored, even when it comes to diet. Potential adverse reactions due to potassium tablets include ulcers, compression of the esophagus, nausea, vomiting, diarrhea, and abdominal discomfort. Also, tingling of the hands and feet, listlessness, confusion, weakness, increased blood pressure, and irregular heartbeat. Potassium supplements should not be taken with a diet high in potassium and vice versa. Potassium supplements should not be taken with potassium-sparing diuretics such as spironolactone and triamterene (*see both*). Salt substitutes may contain large amounts of potassium. Should be taken with food or diluted in juice or water and drunk slowly.

POTASSIUM ACETATE (Rx) (OTC) • An injection that replaces and maintains potassium. Potential adverse reactions include nausea, vomiting, tingling and heaviness in the legs, paralysis, a drop in blood pressure, irregular heartbeat, possible cardiac arrest, diarrhea, bowel ulceration, abdominal pain, scanty urine, and cold skin and gray pallor. Contraindicated in severe kidney impairment, untreated Addison's disease (*see*), high blood potassium, and tissue breakdown. In 1992, the FDA proposed a ban on potassium acetate in oral menstrual drug products because it had not been shown to be safe and effective as claimed.

POTASSIUM BICARBONATE (OTC) • Alka-Seltzer Effervescent Antacid. K+ Care. K-Ide. Klor-Con/EF. Klorvess Effervescent Tablets. K-Lyte. Effervescent tablets; antacid preparations; also to replace and maintain potassium. Potential adverse reactions include tingling in the extremities, listlessness, mental confusion, weakness or heaviness of the legs, paralysis, irregular heartbeat, nausea, vomiting, abdominal pain, diarrhea, ulceration, hemorrhage, obstruction, and perforation. Contraindicated in severe kidney impairment and untreated Addison's disease (*see*). The potassium replacement products should be taken with meals and sipped slowly over a five-to-ten-minute period. In 1992, the FDA issued a notice that potassium bicarbonate had not been shown to be safe and effective as claimed in OTC digestive-aid products.

POTASSIUM BROMATE (OTC) • An antiseptic and astringent in toothpaste, mouthwashes, and gargles as a 3–5 percent solution. Colorless or white crystals. Toxic when taken internally. In toothpaste it has been reported to have caused inflammation and bleeding of gums. Burns and skin irritation have been reported from its industrial uses.

POTASSIUM BROMIDE • A preservative used in the washing of fruits and vegetables. Used medicinally as a sedative and antiepileptic. In large doses it can cause central nervous system depression. Prolonged intake may cause bromism, the main symptoms of which are headache, mental inertia, slow heartbeat, gastric distress, rash, acne, muscular weakness, and occasionally, violent delirium. Bromides can cross the placental barrier and have caused rashes in the fetus.

POTASSIUM CARBONATE • Pearl Ash. In 1992, the FDA issued a notice that potassium carbonate had not been shown to be safe and effective as claimed in OTC digestive-aid products.

POTASSIUM CHLORIDE (Rx) • Gen-K. Potago. Potasalan. Salivart. Thermotabs. Kaochlor. Kaon. Kato Powder. Kay Ciel. K+ Care. KCI. K-Dur 20. K-Lease. K-Lor. Klor-Con. Klor-10%. Klorvess. Klotrix. K-Lyte. Kolyum. K-Tab. K+ 10. Micro-K. Micro-K Extencaps. Rum-K. SK-Potassium Chloride. Slow-K. Ten-K. In over-the-counter preparations, it is used to relieve dryness of the mouth or throat, and to prevent muscle cramps and heat prostration due to excessive perspiration. In prescription products, coated tablets and capsules are used to replace and maintain potassium. Potential adverse reactions include high blood potassium, a sensation of pins and needles in the extremities, listlessness, mental confusion, weakness, heaviness of the limbs, and paralysis. Also, peripheral vascular collapse with a fall in blood pressure, irregular heartbeat, possible cardiac arrest, nausea, vomiting, abdominal pain, diarrhea, GI ulceration, obstruction, and absence of urine production. Contraindicated in severe kidney disease and untreated Addison's disease; also in acute dehydration. Should be used with caution in those with heart disease. *See* Potassium.

POTASSIUM CITRATE (OTC) • K-Ide. Klor-Con/EF. K-Lyte. Ricelyte. A transparent or white powder, odorless, with a cool, salty taste. Used as an antacid, urinary alkalizer, and mineral supplement. *See* Potassium.

POTASSIUM CLAVULANATE • A compound added to some penicillin antibiotic products to prevent inactivation and increase antibacterial activity of the antibiotic.

POTASSIUM FERROCYANIDE (OTC) • Yellow prussiate of potash. In 1992, the FDA proposed a ban on potassium ferrocyanide in astringent (*see*) drug products because it had not been shown to be safe and effective as claimed.

POTASSIUM GLUCONATE (Rx) • Duo-K. Glu-K. Kaon. Kaon Liquid. Kaon Tablets. Kaylixir. K-G Elixir. Kolyum. Kolyum Liquid. A potassium salt used to replace and maintain potassium. Potential adverse reactions include high blood potassium, a sensation of pins and needles in the extremities, listlessness, mental confusion, weakness, heaviness of the limbs, and paralysis. Also, peripheral vascular collapse with a fall in blood pressure, irregular heartbeat, possible cardiac arrest, nausea, vomiting, abdominal pain, diarrhea, GI ulceration or obstruction, and absence of urine production. Contraindicated in severe kidney disease and untreated Addison's disease; also in acute dehydration. Should be used with caution in those with heart disease. *See* Potassium.

POTASSIUM GUAIACOLSULFONATE • A mixture of potassium salts and guaicol, it is used as an expectorant in cough medicines. *See* Guaicol.

POTASSIUM IODIDE (Rx) (OTC) • Hyland's C-Plus Cold Tablets. Iodo-Niacin. Iosat. KI. KIE. Pima. SSKI. Thyro-Block. An antifungal drug also used to treat hyperthyroidism and as an expectorant. It increases production of respiratory fluids to help liquefy and reduce the viscosity of thick secretions; also protects the thyroid against nuclear radiation. Potential adverse reactions include nausea, vomiting, stomach pain, metallic taste, goiter, thyroid tumors (with excessive use), collagen-disease-like symptoms, rash, drug fever, and with prolonged use, chronic iodine poisoning, sore mouth, sneezing, and swelling of the eyelids. Contraindicated in iodine hypersensitivity, tuberculosis, high potassium, acute bronchitis, and swollen glands. When used to reduce thyroid hormone, stuffy nose, swollen glands, swelling around the eyes, frontal headache, tooth discoloration, and fever may occur. Should not be discontinued suddenly. If rash appears, a physician should be contacted. A physician should also be asked about using iodized salt and eating shellfish since these products may interfere with the effects of the medication. Incompatible with calomel and tartaric acid. Lithium carbonate may cause too large a drop in thyroid hormone. *See* Potassium and Iodine.

POTASSIUM NITRATE (OTC) • Niter. Salt Peter. Denquel Sensitive Teeth Toothpaste. Mint Gel Sensodyne Toothpaste. Promise Toothpaste. A white, crystalline powder that absorbs water; has a salty taste. Used in toothpastes to relieve tooth sensitivity. It takes at least two weeks of use before relief occurs. The theory is that potassium nitrate has an effect on nerve transmission, interrupting the signal that would otherwise result in the sensation of pain. In 1992, the FDA proposed a ban on potassium nitrate in oral menstrual drug products because it had not been shown to be safe and effective as claimed.

POTASSIUM PERSULFATE • White crystals, soluble in water or alcohol. Derived from potassium sulfate. Used as an antiseptic. Strong irritant.

POTASSIUM PHOSPHATE • Neutra-Phos. Neutra-Phos-K. Used as a source of potassium and phosphorus (*see both*).

POTASSIUM TARTRATE • Rochelle Salt. Used in the manufacture of baking powder and mouthwashes. No known toxicity.

POTATO STARCH • A flour prepared from potatoes ground to a pulp and washed of fibers. Swells in hot water to form a gel on cooling. Combined with glycerin, it forms a soothing, protective application to treat eczema, rash, and chapped skin. May cause allergic skin reactions and stuffy nose in those who are hypersensitive.

POTENCY • Term referring to the relative strength of a drug.

POULTICE • A warm mass of powdered herbs applied directly to the skin to reduce swelling.

POVIDONE (OTC) • Murine Eye Lubricant. Tears Plus Lubricant. A faintly yellow solid resembling albumin, it is a polyvinyl polymer. Used to lubricate the eyes.

POVIDONE-IODINE (OTC) • Massengill Medicated Disposable Douche and Liquid. A polyvinyl polymer used as a skin antiseptic; changed from Rx to OTC. It is used to cleanse the vaginal area.

POVIDONE-VINYLACETATE COPOLYMERS • In 1992, the FDA issued a notice that povidone-vinylacetate copolymers had not been shown to be safe and effective as claimed in OTC poison ivy, poison oak, and poison sumac products.

PPA • *See* Phenylpropanolamine.

PPL • *See* Benzylpenicilloyl-polylysine.

PPM • Abbreviation for parts per million.

PRAGMATAR (OTC) • A combination of coal tar, sulfur, and salicylic acid (*see all*), used to treat psoriasis and other chronic skin disorders.

PRALIDOXIME (Rx) • Pyridine-2-Aldoxime Methochloride. Protopam. 2-PAM. An antidote used in cases of poisoning by organophosphate pesticides. Potential adverse reactions include nausea, dizziness, headache, drowsiness, excitement, manic behavior, rapid heartbeat, blurred vision, double vision, throat spasm, muscle weakness or stiffness, and rapid breathing. Contraindicated in poisoning with Sevin, a carbamate insecticide, because it will increase the drug's toxicity. Should be used with caution in kidney dysfunction or myasthenia gravis (*see*), asthma, and peptic ulcer.

PRAMET (OTC) • A multivitamin and mineral preparation.

PRAMILET (OTC) • A multivitamin and mineral preparation.

PRAMOSONE (Rx) • A combination of hydrocortisone and pramoxine hydrochloride (*see both*), used to treat skin inflammation and itching.

PRAMOXINE HYDROCHLORIDE (Rx) (OTC) • **Anusol Ointment. Aveeno Anti-Itch Concentrated Lotion. Epifoam. FEP Cream. Fleet Relief. Itch-X Gel. Pramosone. Prax. ProctoFoam HC. Rhulicream. Tronolane Anesthetic Cream for Hemorrhoids. Tronothane.** A topical anesthetic that reportedly produces analgesia up to five hours. Patients who are sensitized to the "-caine " anesthetics may be able to use this.

PRAVACHOL • *See* Pravastatin.

PRAVASTATIN (Rx) • **Pravachol.** One of a new class of lipid-lowering compounds introduced in 1991, it inhibits the key enzyme that controls cholesterol, HMG-COA reductase. Pravastatin reduces the level of LDL cholesterol (*see*) by an average of 22–34 percent and total cholesterol by an average of 16–25 percent. It also raises HDL cholesterol by an average of 2–12 percent and decreases triglycerides by an average of 11–24 percent. The effects of a dose are seen in about four weeks. Potential adverse reactions include liver dysfunction, kidney dysfunction, muscle damage, chest pain, nausea, vomiting, diarrhea, abdominal pain, constipation, flatulence, heartburn, fatigue, influenza, headache, dizziness, urinary abnormality, common cold, stuffy nose, and cough. Animal studies reported central nervous system lesions, swelling, and liver tumors. Contraindicated in patients with active liver disease. Must be used with caution if there is heavy ingestion of alcohol or a history of alcohol abuse. Pravastatin should be taken at bedtime without food. The lipid-lowering effects of pravastatin are enhanced when combined with a bile-acid-binding resin, such as cholestyramine or colestipol (*see both*). Pravastatin should be given either one hour or more before the resin or at least four hours following the resin. *See* HMG-COA Reductase Inhibitors.

PRAX • *See* Pramoxine Hydrochloride.

PRAZEPAM (Rx) • **Centrax.** An antianxiety drug introduced in 1969 that depresses the central nervous system at the area that controls emotions. It should not be used for everyday stress. Potential adverse reactions include drowsiness, lethargy, hangover, confusion, headache, slurred speech, insomnia, changes in sex drive, dizziness, loss of balance, fainting, transient low blood pressure, dry mouth, nausea, vomiting, abdominal discomfort, inability to control urine, and rash. Should not be used with alcohol, MAO inhibitors (*see*), and other central nervous system depressants. Cimetidine (*see*) may increase sedation. Contraindicated in narrow angle glaucoma and psychoses. Should be used cautiously in persons with kidney or liver dysfunction. There is a possibility of abuse and addiction. The drug should not be discontinued abruptly. Most effective when taken on an empty stomach, but may be taken with some food if stomach upset is a problem.

PRAZIQUANTEL (Rx) • **Biltricide. Cysticide.** A drug to combat *Schistosoma mekongi,* a species of intestinal worms, tapeworms, and liver flukes found in the Mekong delta in southern Vietnam. Introduced in the United States in 1983, it is primarily used to treat beef, fish, pork, and dwarf tapeworm infections. Ingested by the parasites, praziquantel causes them to undergo muscle paralysis, disintegration of the outer skin, and death. It is not indicated for use with ocular cysticercosis, in which tapeworm larvae invade the eye, because destruction of the parasite in that location may cause permanent eye damage. Related to benzodiazepine (*see*) tranquilizers, it may produce drowsiness and vomiting.

PRAZOSIN HYDROCHLORIDE (Rx) • **Furazosin. Minipress. Minizide.** A beta-blocker (*see*) antihypertensive medication introduced in 1970 that relaxes both artery and vein smooth muscles. Used to treat mild to moderate high blood pressure, alone or in combination with a diuretic or other antihypertensive drug. Also used to decrease the work of the heart in congestive heart failure and to treat Raynaud's disease (*see*). It need be taken only once a day. Potential adverse effects include dizziness, headache, drowsiness, weakness, a drop in blood pressure when rising from a sitting or prone position, heart palpitations, blurred vision, dry mouth, vomiting, diarrhea, abdominal cramps, constipation, nausea, priapism (*see*), decreased libido, and impotence. Its use with propranolol and other beta-blockers may cause a loss of consciousness. Elderly patients may be more sensitive to the drug's effect. NSAIDs (*see*), especially indomethacin, may lessen prazosin's effectiveness. Tobacco smoking and the use of estrogens and stimulants, including over-the-counter medications for colds and allergies, may decrease its effects. Prazosin's effectiveness is increased when combined with other medications for high blood pressure. Should be taken with food.

PRECEF • *See* Ceforanide.

PRECOSE (Rx) • *See* Acarbose.

PRECURSOR • A biologic process in which a substance turns into another active or more mature substance. Beta-carotene is a precursor of vitamin A because the body can use it to make vitamin A.

PREDAIR • *See* Prednisolone.

PREDAJECT • *See* Prednisolone.

PREDALONE • *See* Prednisolone.

PREDALONE TBA • *See* Prednisolone.

PREDATE • *See* Prednisolone.

PREDCOR • *See* Prednisolone.

PRED FORTE, PRED MILD • *See* Prednisolone.

PREDICORT • *See* Prednisolone.

PREDNICEN-M • *See* Prednisolone.

PREDNISOLONE (Rx) • AK-Pred. Articulose. Codesol. Cortalone. Delta-Cortef. Econopred Ophthalmic. Hydeltrasol. Hydeltrasol Ophthalmic. Hydeltra-T.B.A. Inflamase Forte. Inflamase Mild. Key-Pred. Metacortandrolone. Metalone-TBA. Metimyd. Metreton. Niscort. Nor-Pred. Ocu-Pred. Pediapred. Predair. Predaject. Predalone. Predalone TBA. Predate. Predate-S. Predcor. Pred Forte. Predicot. Pred Mild Ophthalmic. Prednicen-M. Predsol Eye Drops. Prelone. Sintisone. Sulphrin. Introduced in 1955, prednisolone is related chemically to cortisol (*see*), and is used in tablet, syrup, liquid, salve, suppository, enema, and injection form. It is used to treat severe inflammation, and as an immunosuppressant, and in the treatment of ulcerative colitis and proctitis (*see both*). Most adverse reactions are the result of dosage or length of time between administration of doses. Should be taken with food or milk to reduce GI irritation. Potential adverse reactions include euphoria, insomnia, psychotic behavior, high blood pressure, swelling, cataracts, glaucoma, peptic ulcer, GI irritation, increased appetite, high blood sugar, growth suppression in children, delayed wound healing, skin eruptions, muscle weakness, pancreatitis, hairiness, decreased immunity, and acute adrenal gland insufficiency. When withdrawn, there may be rebound inflammation, fatigue, weakness, joint pain, fever, dizziness, lethargy, depression, fainting, a drop in blood pressure upon rising from a seated or prone position, shortness of breath, loss of appetite, and high blood sugar. Sudden withdrawal may be fatal. Contraindicated in systemic fungal infections. Should be used cautiously in patients with GI ulceration or kidney disease, high blood pressure, diabetes, chicken pox, osteoporosis, Cushing's syndrome, blood-clotting disorders, seizures, myasthenia gravis (*see*), congestive heart failure, tuberculosis, herpes, and emotional instability. When taking the drug, patients may need low-sodium diets and potassium supplements. Barbiturates, phenytoin, and rifampin (*see all*) increase its effects. Indomethacin and aspirin may increase the risk of GI distress and bleeding. Prednisolone is also used in eyedrops to treat eye inflammation. Potential adverse reactions for that use include increased eye pressure, thinning of the cornea, interference with corneal wound healing, increased susceptibility to viral or fungal corneal infections, corneal ulceration; with excessive or long-term use, cataracts, worsening of glaucoma, eye-nerve damage, and systemically, such effects as suppression of adrenal hormones. Contraindicated for eye use if there are viral, fungal, or bacterial infections of the eye present.

PREDNISONE (Rx) • **Meticortin. Deltacortisone. Deltasone. Liquid Pred. Novo-Prednisone. Orasone. Panasol. Prednicen-M. Prednisone Intensol. Sterapred.** Introduced in 1955 and related chemically to cortisone (*see*), prednisone is widely used to treat severe inflammation and as an immunosuppressant; also to treat acute attacks of multiple sclerosis, arthritis, and irritable bowel syndrome (*see*). Most adverse reactions are the result of dosage or length of time between administration of doses. Should be taken with food or milk to reduce GI irritation. Potential adverse reactions include euphoria, insomnia, psychotic behavior, high blood pressure, swelling, cataracts, glaucoma, peptic ulcer, GI irritation, increased appetite, high blood sugar, growth suppression in children, delayed wound healing, acne, skin eruptions, muscle weakness, pancreatitis (*see*), hairiness, decreased immunity, irregular menstruation, male infertility, and acute adrenal gland insufficiency. When withdrawn, there may be rebound inflammation, fatigue, weakness, joint pain, fever, dizziness, lethargy, depression, fainting, a drop in blood pressure upon rising from a seated or prone position, shortness of breath, loss of appetite, and high blood sugar. Sudden withdrawal may be fatal. Contraindicated in systemic fungal infections. Should be used cautiously in patients with GI ulceration or kidney disease, high blood pressure, diabetes, chicken pox, osteoporosis, Cushing's syndrome, blood-clotting disorders, seizures, myasthenia gravis (*see*), congestive heart failure, tuberculosis, herpes, and emotional instability. When taking the drug, patients may need low-sodium diets and potassium supplements. Vitamin D supplements should be taken with long-term use, and zinc, if in need of wound repair. Barbi-

turates, phenytoin, ephedrine, rifampin (*see all*), and tobacco smoking increase its effects. Indomethacin and aspirin may increase the risk of GI distress and bleeding. Prednisone should be taken with food or with a small amount of antacid.

PREDNISONE INTENSOL • *See* Prednisone.

PREDSOL EYE DROPS • *See* Prednisolone.

PREECLAMPSIA • Development of high blood pressure with protein in the urine, or edema, or both, due to pregnancy. Usually occurs after the twentieth week of pregnancy.

PREFRIN • *See* Phenylephrine.

PREFRIN LIQUIFILM • *See* Phenylephrine.

PREGNANCY TESTS (OTC) • Home pregnancy test kits became available in 1976. Prior to that time, women had to visit doctors to have their blood or urine analyzed to determine if they were pregnant. Home tests detect the presence of the hormone human chorionic gonadotropin (HCG) in urine. Normally, this hormone is produced only by pregnant women. Home tests can now detect HCG as quickly as one day after a missed period. Some manufacturers claim their tests accurately detect pregnancy over 99 percent of the time when used by laboratory technicians. This makes home tests as accurate as those available to physicians and commercial laboratories. However, tests must be done exactly as described on the package in order to achieve these results. A study published in the *New England Journal of Medicine* indicated that the accuracy of home pregnancy tests in the hands of consumers was slightly less than 94 percent. Some medical conditions can affect the test results, such as an incomplete or recent abortion, cancer, certain problems of the ovaries, endometriosis, menopause, thyroid disease, and urinary-tract infection.

PREGNANEDIONE • *See* Progesterone.

PREGNENOLONE • A precursor—a building material—for other steroid (*see*) hormones. A great deal of research is under way to determine if this drug can enhance memory or have other benefits in older adults.

PREGNYL • *See* Gonadotropin.

PRELATE • *See* Barley.

PRELONE • *See* Prednisolone.

PRELUDIN • *See* Phenmetrazine.

PRELU-2 • *See* Phendimetrazine.

PREMARIN • *See* Estrogens, Conjugated.

PREMPHASE (Rx) • Estrogen hormone replacement with progestin in a single pack. *See* Estrogens, Conjugated, and Progestin.

PREMPRO (Rx) • Estrogen hormone replacement with progestin in a single pack. *See* Estrogens, Conjugated, and Progestin.

PRENATE (OTC) • A multivitamin and mineral preparation.

PRE-PAR • *See* Ritodrine.

PRE-PEN • *See* Benzylpenicilloyl-Polylysine.

PRESALIN (OTC) • A combination of acetaminophen, aspirin, and salicylamide (*see all*), used as a painkiller.

PRESBY- • Prefix meaning old, as in *presbyopia*, eye changes linked to aging.

PRESCRIPTION DRUG • Medicine available from a pharmacy only with a doctor's written order and instructions for use.

PREVACID • **Lansoprazole.** An ulcer treatment developed by Abbott Laboratories and a Japanese partner; approved by the FDA in 1995. It is a proton pump (acid) inhibitor and will be marketed for short-term treatment for healing and symptom relief of erosive esophagitis and active duodenal ulcers.

PREVIDENT • *See* Sodium Fluoride.

PRIAPISM • Persistent erection of the penis, accompanied by pain and tenderness. Among the substances that may cause priapism are the male hormones and the following drugs: chlorpromazine, guanethidine, haloperidol, heparin, levodopa, molindone, prazosin, prochlorperazine, trazodone, trifluoperazine, and warfarin.

PRICKLY ASH BARK (H) • *Zanthoxylum americanum.* **Toothache Tree.** A native American herb, the bark and berries have been used for more than two hundred years by herbalists to treat cholera, syphilis, rheumatism, gonorrhea, fever, dysentery, neuritis, toothaches, and ulcers. It has been found to contain coumarins, alkaloids (*see both*), and lignins. One of the lignins, asarin, has been found by modern pharmaceutical researchers to have antitubercular action. The plant is a stimulant. It was also used to produce perspiration. A popular remedy for chronic rheumatism, it was used extensively in the United States for this purpose. The bark was chewed raw or inserted into cavities as toothache remedy. Prickly ash bark was also used in the treatment of flatulence and diarrhea.

PRICKLY LETTUCE (H) • *Lactuca virosa* or *scariola.* A biennial plant with a round stem native to Europe and cultivated in many areas. Homeopathic physicians use an extract to treat asthma, cough, and urinary tract infection. It contains traces of hyoscyamine (*see*). The plant is toxic.

PRILOSEC • *See* Omeprazole.

PRIMADERM • *See* Vitamin A and Vitamin D.

PRIMAQUINE (Rx) • **Articulose. Key-Pred. Niscort.** A strong antimalarial drug introduced in 1952. Its effect is decreased if taken with antacids. Potential side effects include blood problems, headache, visual disturbances, nausea, vomiting, stomach pain, and hives. Contraindicated in lupus erythematosus (*see*) and in rheumatoid arthritis patients taking immunosuppressant drugs. Antacids containing magnesium and aluminum salts may decrease its effectiveness if taken concurrently. Should be taken with meals.

PRIMARY INFECTION • The very first infection with a particular virus. Primary infections may or may not cause symptoms such as aches or fatigue.

PRIMATENE • *See* Ephedrine.

PRIMIDONE (Rx) • **Myidone. Mysoline. Neurosyn.** An anticonvulsant introduced in 1953. Its action is unclear, but it is effective for generalized tonic-clonic and complex-partial seizures. Potential adverse reactions include a low white blood count, drowsiness, loss of balance, emotional disturbances, dizziness, irritability, fatigue, double vision, jerky movement of the eyes, loss of appetite, swelling of the eyelids, nausea, vomiting, impotence, frequent urination, rash, hair loss, decreased libido, impotence, swelling, and thirst. Carbamazepine (*see*) increases primidone levels and may cause toxicity. Because of primidone's relation to barbiturates, it may affect oral blood thinners. It makes oral contraceptives less effective. Caution should be used when taken with other central nervous system depressants, including alcohol, antidepressants, or strong painkillers, because side effects may be increased. The drug should not be discontinued abruptly. May be taken with food.

PRIMROSE (H) • *Primula vulgaris.* **Easter Rose.** A perennial native to Britain and Europe, it flourishes in meadows, hedges, and ditches. The name comes from the Latin word *primu,* meaning first, because it was the first rose of spring. Herbalists used it in a tea to treat arthritis, gout, and migraine, and as a general blood cleanser. A decoction of the root is given for catarrh, coughs, and bronchitis. It is also used to cure insomnia. *See also* Evening Primrose Oil.

PRIMULA VULGARIS • *See* Primrose.

PRINCE'S PINE • *See* Pipsissewa Leaves Extract.

PRINCIPEN • *See* Ampicillin.

PRINIVIL • *See* Lisinopril.

PRISCOLINE HYDROCHLORIDE • *See* Tolazoline Hydrochloride.

PRIVET FRUIT (H) • *Ligustrum.* A common plant used as a hedge in many yards, its fruits contain mannitol and glucose (*see both*), as well as oleanolic acid and fatty oil. It is used to treat liver, kidney, and adrenal gland problems. Herbalists also claim that it can prevent premature graying of the hair or loss of vision.

PRIVINE • *See* Naphazoline.

PROAQUA • *See* Benzthiazide.

PROBALAN • *See* Probenecid.

PRO-BANTHINE • *See* Propantheline.

PROBENECID (Rx) • **Benemid. Benn. Col-Benemid. Probalan. Proban. Robenecid.** An anti-uric-acid medicine introduced in 1951 that is used to treat gout and as an adjunct (*see*) to penicillin or cephalosporin therapy in the treatment of gonorrhea. Preferred by some doctors because it causes fewer side effects than sulfinpyrazone. Contains no analgesics or anti-inflammatory agents and is of no value during acute gout attacks. Potential adverse reactions include nausea, vomiting, headache, dizziness, anemia, low blood pressure, urinary frequency, kidney pain, rash, hair loss, flushing, sore gums, and fever. Contraindicated in blood problems, acute gout attacks, kidney dysfunction, kidney stones, radiation, and certain cancers. Should be used cautiously in peptic ulcer disease. Indomethacin and methotrexate (*see both*) may have more adverse side effects if taken with probenecid. Oral diabetes medications may have increased blood-sugar-lowering effects. Should not be used with salicylates (including aspirin) because they cause uric acid salts retention. May be taken with food to reduce stomach upset.

PROBUCOL (Rx) • **Lorelco.** A blood-fat-lowering drug introduced in 1971 that inhibits cholesterol transport from the intestine and may also decrease cholesterol manufacture. Potential adverse reactions include irregular heartbeat, diarrhea, flatulence, headache, anemia, irregular menses, impotence, itching, rash, ringing in the ears, heartburn, stomach or intestinal bleeding, easy bruising, goiter, the need to urinate at night, abdominal pain, nausea, vomiting, sweating (sometimes bad-smelling), changes in taste and smell, and swelling. Clofibrate produces additive effects. Tricyclic antidepressants, some antiarrhythmics, phenothiazines, beta-blockers, digitalis glycosides, and calcium channel blockers (*see all*) increase the risk of irregular heartbeat when used with probucol. This drug's effect is enhanced when taken with food.

PROCAINAMIDE (Rx) • **Procan SR. Procainamide BID. Promine. Pronestyl-SR. Rhythmin.** Introduced in 1950, it is an antiarrhythmic drug that controls premature contractions of the heart and irregular heartbeat. Potential adverse reactions, which reportedly occur less often than with other antiarrhythmics, include hallucinations, confusion, seizures, depression, severe low blood pressure, increased heart irregularities, nausea, vomiting, loss of appetite, diarrhea, bitter taste, rash, fever, lupus erythematosus (*see*), muscle pain, and blood problems such as anemia. When used with procainamide, blood-pressure-lowering drugs may cause blood pressure to drop too far. Procainamide reduces the effect of anticholinergic (*see*) drugs. Neuromuscular drugs increase the risk of adverse effects with procainamide. Over-the-counter stimulants, including those in cold and allergy medications, should be avoided because they counteract procainamide's effectiveness. Nicotine can cause irritability of the heart and reduce the effectiveness of this drug. Procainamide should not be discontinued suddenly. Most effective when taken on an empty stomach.

PROCAINE (Rx) • **Novocain.** A local anesthetic used for spinal anesthesia during childbirth or in operative vaginal procedures. Onset is two to five minutes and duration is sixty minutes. Potential adverse reactions include skin reactions, swelling, continuous asthma attacks, severe allergic reactions, anxiety, nervousness, and respiratory arrest. Other potential reactions include blurred vision, seizures followed by drowsiness, unconsciousness, tremors, twitches, shivering, ringing in the ears, nausea, vomiting, and cardiac arrest. Contraindicated in traumatized urethra (urine outlet) and in hypersensitivity to chloroprocaine, tetracaine, or other para-aminobenzoic acid (*see*) derivatives.

PROCAN SR • *See* Procainamide.

PROCANABID EXTENDED-RELEASE (Rx) • A long-acting drug for irregular heartbeat. *See* Procainamide.

PROCARBAZINE (Rx) • **Ibenzmethyzin. Matulane.** An alkylating (*see*) anticancer drug used to treat Hodgkin's disease, lymphomas, and brain and lung cancers. Potential adverse reactions include nausea, vomiting, bleeding, anemia, nervousness, depression, insomnia, nightmares, hallucinations, confusion, retinal hemorrhage, light hurting the eyes, rash, dry mouth, diarrhea, reversible hair loss, fluid in the lungs, and constipation. Alcohol causes a disulfiram-like reaction; central nervous depressants add to depressant effects; meperidine may cause severe low blood pressure and even death. Local anesthetics, antidepressants, and foods high in tyramine (*see*) (Chianti wine, cheese, herring) may cause tremors, heart palpitations, and increased blood pressure.

PROCARDIA • *See* Nifedipine.

PROCHLOR-ISO • *See* Prochlorperazine.

PROCHLORPERAZINE (Rx) • **Compazine. Prochlor-Iso. Pro-Iso.** An antinausea, antivomiting drug introduced in 1956 that inhibits the vomiting center in the brain. Used to treat preoperative nausea, severe nausea, and vomiting, and for symptomatic management of severe psychosis. It is not effective in motion sickness. Potential adverse reactions include a temporary drop in white blood cells, sedation, pseudoparkinsonism, dizziness, a drop in blood pressure when rising from a seated or prone position, visual changes, dry mouth, constipation, urinary retention, menstrual irregularities, enlargement of the male breast, inhibited ejaculation, jaundice, mild photosensitivity (*see*), increased appetite, and weight gain. Sudden death has occurred in patients who have taken this drug due to its effect on the cough reflex. Because it reduces vomiting, it can hide signs of toxicity due to overdose of other drugs or symptoms of disease. Contraindicated in those hypersensitive to phenothiazines, in central nervous system depression, bone marrow suppression, brain damage, and in use with certain anesthetics. Antacids inhibit its absorption if the drug is taken by mouth. Anticholinergics (*see*), including antidepressants and antiparkinsonian agents, may increase side effects. Barbiturates may decrease prochlorperazine's beneficial effects. Prochlorperazine may cause false-positive pregnancy-test results. The antipsychotic effectiveness of prochlorperazine may be counteracted by alcohol or caffeine-containing foods such as coffee, tea, cola drinks, or chocolate. Exposure to a hot environment should be avoided since this drug can affect the body's temperature-adjustment mechanism. This drug may be taken with food.

PROCRIT • *See* Erythropoietin.

PROCTITIS • Inflammation of the rectum.

PROCTO- • Prefix meaning pertaining to the anus or rectum.

PROCTOCORT • *See* Hydrocortisone.

PROCTOFOAM-HC • *See* Hydrocortisone and Pramoxine Hydrochloride.

PROCYCLE GOLD (OTC) • A product aimed at menopausal women. It includes vitamins A, B_1, B_2, B_6, B_{12}, C, E, D_3, folic acid, niacinamide, biotin, and pantothenic acids. Minerals in the product include calcium citrate, magnesium, iodine, iron, copper, zinc, manganese, potassium, selenium, and chromium.

PROCYCLIDINE (Rx) • **Kemadrin.** An antiparkinsonian drug that helps to regulate nerve-stimulation activity in the brain. It is used to treat muscle rigidity. Contraindicated in glaucoma and used with caution in persons with irregular heartbeat, low blood pressure, urine retention, and enlarged prostate. Potential adverse reactions include light-headedness, blurred vision, constipation, dry mouth, nausea, vomiting, stomach distress, rash, and muscle weakness. In severe parkinsonism, tremors may increase while spasticity is relieved. Should be taken after meals to minimize GI distress.

PRO-DEPO • *See* Hydroxyprogesterone.

PRODOX • *See* Hydroxyprogesterone.

PRODRUGS • Inactive drugs that can be converted to the active form by the body's chemistry. Scientists are working on developing soft anticancer drugs, those that fall apart to nontoxic compounds after performing their therapeutic tasks.

PROFASI HP • *See* Gonadotropin.

PROFENAL • *See* Suprofen.

PROFERDEX • *See* Iron.

PROGENS • *See* Estrogens, Conjugated.

PROGESTAJECT • *See* Progesterone.

PROGESTASERT • *See* Progesterone.

PROGESTERONE (Rx) • **Gesterol 50. Pregnanedione. Progestaject. Progestasert.** A progestin drug that suppresses ovulation, possibly by inhibiting pituitary gonadotropin secretion. It forms a thick cervical mucus. Used to treat absent menstruation or abnormal uterine bleeding. Potential adverse reactions include nausea, vomiting, dizziness, migraine, lethargy, depression, high blood pressure, blood clots, swelling, bloating, and abdominal cramps. May cause breakthrough bleeding, altered menstrual flow, painful or absent menstruation, enlargement of benign tumors of the uterus, cervical erosion, abnormal secretions, and vaginal candidiasis. There may be jaundice, high blood sugar, dark spots appearing on the skin, breast tenderness, enlargement, and secretion, and decreased libido. Contraindicated in persons with blood-clotting disorders, cancer of the breast, undiagnosed abnormal vaginal bleeding, and in pregnancy. Should be used with caution in patients with high blood pressure, seizures, migraine, and mental depression. Twice as potent as norethindrone. Rifampin (*see*) decreases progesterone's effectiveness.

PROGESTINS (Rx) • **Hydroxyprogesterone. Medroxyprogesterone. Amen. Curretab. Delalutin. Depo-Provera. Duralutin. Gesterol. Hylutin. Hyprogest. Megace. Megestrol. Micronor. Norethindrone. Norethynodrel. Norgestrel. Norlutin. Pro-Depo. Prodrox. Provera. Ovrette.** Progestins are produced by the body and are necessary during the childbearing years for the development of milk-producing glands and for the proper regulation of the menstrual cycle. They are used to adjust irregular menstrual cycles, treat certain uterine problems such as endometriosis, prevent pregnancy when used in birth-control pills, help treat certain cancers, and test the body's production of certain hormones. Potential adverse reactions include nausea, changes in appetite and weight, swelling of ankles and feet, fatigue, acne, brown, blotchy spots on exposed skin, fever, increased body and facial hair, increased breast tenderness, some loss of scalp hair, insomnia, headache, changes in vaginal bleeding, and other sudden conditions that may signal a blood clot. *See* Progesterone.

PROGLYCEM • *See* Diazoxide.

PROGNOSIS • A prediction of what might happen in a specific case of a disease.

PROGRAF • *See* Tacrolimus.

PROGYNON • *See* Estradiol.

PROHANCE • *See* Gadoteridol.

PRO-ISO • *See* Prochlorperazine.

PROKINE • *See* Sargramostim.

PROLAMINE • *See* Phenylpropanolamine.

PROLASTIN • *See* Alpha-1 Proteinase Inhibitor.

PROLEUKIN • *See* Aldesleukin.

PROLIXIN • *See* Fluphenazine Hydrochloride, Decanoate, or Enanthate.

PROLOPRIM • *See* Trimethoprim.

PROMAZINE (Rx) • **Sparine.** A phenothiazine (*see*) medication introduced in the late 1950s, it is used to treat psychosis and to prevent vomiting. Potential adverse reactions include a low white blood cell count, tardive dyskinesia (*see*), sedation, pseudoparkinsonism, dizziness, a drop in blood pressure when rising from a sitting or prone position, vision changes, dry mouth, constipation, urine retention, menstrual irregularities, enlargement of the male breast, inhibited ejaculation, mild photosensitivity, allergic skin reactions, weight gain, increased appetite, fever, irregular heartbeat, and sweating. Abrupt withdrawal of promazine may cause gastritis, nausea, vomiting, dizziness, tremors, irregular heartbeat, headache, and insomnia. Alcohol and other central nervous system depressants may cause increased central nervous system depression. Antacids inhibit absorption and should not be used within two hours of promazine. Anticholinergics (*see*) aggravate parkinsonian symptoms. Barbiturates and lithium may decrease promazine's effects. Blood pressure medications that act on the brain and oral blood thinners may be less effective. Propranolol may increase serum levels of both propranolol and promazine. Contraindicated in coma, central nervous system depression, bone-marrow suppression, brain damage, and with use of spinal or epidural anesthetic or adrenergic-blocking agents (*see*). Should be used with caution in elderly or debilitated patients, those with liver disease, cerebrovascular disease, respiratory disorders, low blood calcium, seizure disorders, intestinal obstruction, glaucoma, and enlarged prostate, and in acutely ill children. Should not be discontinued abruptly.

PROMETA • *See* Metaproterenol.

PROMETHAZINE (Rx) • **Anergan. K-Phen. Mallergan-VC. Mepergan. Pentazine. Phenameth. Phenazine. Phenergan. Phenoject-50. Pherazine-VC. Promethegan. Prometh-25. Prorex. Prothazine-25. Remsed. V-Gan-50.** A phenothiazine (*see*) derivative introduced in 1945 that differs structurally from antipsychotic phenothiazines. It has antihistamine action and antivomiting effects. Used to relieve symptoms of allergies such as stuffy nose, red eyes, rash, and allergic reactions to drugs. It is effective within twenty minutes and generally lasts four to six hours, but may persist as long as twelve hours. It is also used as a sedative for adults and children, to treat motion sickness, and for nausea after an operation. It was a candidate for OTC, but a review of data suggested a link to severe respiratory problems in infants, so the switch was not made. Potential adverse reactions include dizziness, dry mouth, drowsiness, rash, increased or decreased blood pressure, tongue protrusion, jaundice, nausea and vomiting, a low white blood cell count, sedation and confusion (especially in elderly patients), restlessness, temporary nearsightedness, stuffy nose, loss of appetite, constipation, urine retention, and photosensitivity. Should not be taken with other central nervous system depressants, including alcohol, narcotic analgesics, tranquilizers, and sleeping pills. Promethazine may lower seizure threshold. Coffee or tea may reduce drowsiness. Use with MAO inhibitors (*see*) may cause blood pressure to shoot up. Should be used cautiously in elderly patients, those with narrow angle glaucoma, overactive thyroid, heart or kidney disease, high blood pressure, bronchial asthma, enlarged prostate, bladder-neck obstruction, and peptic ulcer. Because of possible photosensitivity, sunscreen and sunglasses should be worn as a precaution. Medication should be discontinued four days before taking a skin allergy test because it can lead to inaccurate results. Should be taken with a full glass of water.

PROMETHEGAN • *See* Promethazine.

PROMETH-25 • *See* Promethazine.

PROMINE • *See* Procainamide.

PROMISE TOOTHPASTE • *See* Potassium Nitrate.

PROMIST (OTC) • A combination of pseudoephedrine and guaifenesin (*see both*).

PROMIT • *See* Dextran.

PROMOTION • An intermediate stage of cancer development during which initiated (*see*) cells, in the presence of promoters, move further along the pathway to cancer. The promotion stage may take several decades in humans.

PROMPT • *See* Psyllium.

PRONESTYL-SR • *See* Procainamide.

PRONTO LICE KILLING SHAMPOO • *See* Piperonyl Butoxide.

PROPADRINE • *See* Phenylpropanolamine.

PROPAFENONE HYDROCHLORIDE (Rx) • **Rythmol.** An antiarrhythmic drug used to treat life-threatening, irregular beating of the heart. Potential adverse reactions include loss of appetite, anxiety, dizziness, drowsiness, fatigue, headache, fainting, tremor, weakness, chest pain, worsened heart irregularities and congestive heart failure, water retention, low blood pressure, blurred vision, abdominal pain, cramps, constipation, diarrhea, heartburn, gas, nausea, vomiting, dry mouth, unusual taste, shortness of breath, rash, sweating, and joint pain. Use of propafenone with other antiarrhythmics increases the possibility of congestive heart failure. Use with cimetidine may increase propafenone's toxicity. Local anesthetics increase the risk of central nervous system toxicity. Propafenone slows the metabolism of propranolol, and metoprolol increases the possibility of side effects. Doses should be evenly spaced throughout the day to maintain blood levels of the drug.

PROPAGEST • *See* Phenylpropanolamine.

PROPANOIC ACID, CALCIUM SALT • *See* Calcium Propionate.

PROPANTHELINE (Rx) • **Norpanth. Pro-Banthine.** An anticholinergic, antispasmodic drug used to treat irritable bowel syndrome, and as an adjunctive therapy (*see* Adjunct) in peptic ulcers and other GI disorders, and urinary incontinence. Potential adverse reactions include confusion, irritability, incoherence, weakness, nervousness, drowsiness, dizziness, headache, heart palpitations, rapid heartbeat, slow heartbeat, blurred vision, sensitivity to light, increased eye pressure, difficulty in swallowing, constipation, dry mouth, nausea, vomiting, epigastric distress, urinary retention, impotence, hives, decreased sweating, and fever. Contraindicated in glaucoma, obstructions in the urinary or GI tract, myasthenia gravis (*see*), intestinal paralysis, intestinal flaccidity, unstable heart function in acute hemorrhage, and toxic enlargement of the colon. Should be used with caution in patients with nerve damage, overactive thyroid, coronary artery disease, irregular heartbeat, congestive heart failure, high blood pressure, hiatal hernia, liver or kidney disease, and ulcerative colitis. Should also be used with caution in people over forty years of age due to the possibility of glaucoma. Interaction with antihistamines, phenothiazines, corticosteroids, tranquilizers, antidepressants, and some narcotic painkillers may cause blurred vision, dry mouth, or drowsiness. Antacids affect propantheline's effectiveness and should not be taken within two hours of taking it. Should not be used with tranylcypromine sulfate, isocarboxazid, phenelzine (*see all*), or other MAO inhibitor (*see*) drugs, which may raise propantheline to toxic levels in the body. Should be taken thirty minutes to one hour before meals. Most effective when taken on an empty stomach, but may be taken with a small amount of food if stomach upset is a problem.

PROPARACAINE (Rx) • **Alcaine. Kainair. Ophthaine. Ophthetic.** A local anesthetic used in eye treatments, and for the removal of cataracts and of foreign bodies in the cornea. Potential adverse effects include redness, transient pain, and hypersensitivity reactions. Should be used cautiously in patients with heart disease or overactive thyroid gland.

PROPELLANT • A compressed gas used to expel the contents of containers in the form of aerosols. Chlorofluorocarbons were widely used because of their nonflammability. The strong possibility that they contribute to depletion of the ozone layer of the upper atmosphere has resulted in prohibition of their use for this purpose. Other propellants used are hydrocarbon gases such as butane, propane, carbon dioxide, and nitrous oxide.

PROPHENE-65 • *See* Propoxyphene.

PROPHYLACTIC • Used to prevent the occurrence of a specific condition. Also used to refer to condoms.

PROPHYLAXIS • Treatment intended to preserve health and prevent the spread of disease.

PROPINE • *See* Dipivefrin.

PROPIOMAZINE (Rx) • **Largon.** A phenothiazine compound with sedative, antivomiting, and antihistamine properties. It is given before surgery and during labor. It has a short duration of action. Potential adverse reactions include drowsiness, moderate elevation or drop in blood pressure, dry mouth, and fatal seizures.

PROPIONATE • *See* Propionic Acid.

PROPIONIC ACID (OTC) • **Propionate.** Occurs naturally in apples, strawberries, tea, and violet leaves. It can be obtained from wood pulp and by fermentation. Used as a mold inhibitor, antioxidant, and preservative in cosmetics. Its salts have been used as antifungal agents to treat skin mold. In 1992, the FDA issued a notice that propionic acid had not been shown to be safe and effective as claimed in OTC products.

PROPOFOL (Rx) • **Diprivan.** A hypnotic for use in the induction and maintenance of anesthesia. Given by injection, it works rapidly, usually within forty seconds. It may cause shortness of breath, decreased blood flow to the brain, low blood pressure, headache, dizziness, vomiting, tingling in the arms and legs, flushing of the skin, eye pain, ringing in the ear, urine retention, irregular heartbeat and other heart effects, depression, and hysteria.

PROPOLIS (H) • **Bee Bread. Hive Dross.** A resinous substance found in beehives. A greenish brown, sticky mass with a hyacinthlike odor, it contains up to 10 percent cinnamyl alcohol. Promoted by herbalists as a protectant against pollution.

PRO-POX (Rx) • *See* Propoxyphene.

PROPOXYCON (Rx) • *See* Propoxyphene.

PROPOXYPHENE (Rx) • **Dextropropoxyphene Hydrochloride. Darvon. Dolene. Doxaphene. Genagesic. Lorcet. Lorcet Plus. Prophene.** In combination with aspirin and caffeine: **Bexophene. Darvon Compound. Dolene Compound. Doxaphene Compound.** In combination with acetaminophen: **Darvocet N 100. Dolene AP-65. Doxapap N. Genagesic. Lorcet. Propacet. Prox/APAP. Wygesic.** In combination with aspirin: **Darvon N with ASA.** In combination with napsylate: **Darvocet-N. Darvon-N. Doraphen. Doxaphene. ProPox. Propoxycon.** A chemical derivative of methadone (*see*), propoxyphene was introduced in 1957 to treat mild or moderate pain. Longer lasting than many other drugs of this class, it may be more convenient for relief of chronic pain. Also less addictive than other drugs of its type, but it may cause physical dependence. Given in combination with another painkiller such as aspirin to boost its effect. Potential adverse reactions include nausea, drowsiness, headache, dizziness, euphoria, weakness, minor visual disturbances, constipation, confusion, and rash. Alcohol and sedatives may increase propoxyphene's central nervous system depression. Potential adverse effects with the combination of napsylate include sedation, dizziness, euphoria, paradoxical excitement, insomnia, nausea, vomiting, and constipation. Alcohol and central nervous system depressants are additive. If taken with MAOIs (*see*), propoxyphene may cause a dangerous rise in blood pressure. Heavy smoking may reduce the effectiveness of this drug. If you have been taking this drug for more than two weeks, you may need advice on gradually reducing your intake. Propoxyphene should be taken with food to avoid gastrointestinal upset.

PROPOXYPHENE NAPSYLATE (Rx) • **Dextropropoxyphene Napsylate. Davarocet-N. Darvon N.** Binds with opiate receptors in the brain and spinal cord, altering both perception of and emotional response to pain through an unknown mechanism. It is used for mild to moderate pain. Potential adverse reactions include dizziness, headache, sedation, euphoria, excitement, insomnia, vomiting, nausea, constipation, and dependence. Should not be used with alcohol or other central nervous system depressants.

PROPRANOLOL (Rx) • **Inderal. Intensol. Ipran.** A beta-blocker (*see*) introduced in 1968, it was the first of the beta-blockers made available in the United States. Most often used to treat hypertension, it is also an effective drug in controlling irregular heartbeat, chest pain, and reducing the heart's demand for oxygen. Also prevents vasodilation of the brain's arteries. It is used to reduce mortality following a heart attack. Also used to reduce heart palpitations, sweating, and tremor caused by the anxiety associated with stage fright, and effective in the prevention of migraine headaches. Potential adverse reactions include fatigue, lethargy, vivid dreams, hallucinations, irregular heartbeat, slow heartbeat, mental depression, tingling in the extremities, cramps, allergic reactions, low blood pressure, low blood sugar, congestive heart failure, nausea, vomiting, diarrhea, rash, joint pain, and fever. Because propranolol affects breathing, it is not prescribed to anyone suffering from asthma, decreased libido, impaired erection, impotence, male infertility, Peyronie's disease (see), chronic bronchitis, or emphysema. It also affects the body's response to low blood sugar and should be used with caution by diabetics. Aminophylline may reduce propranolol's effectiveness. Verapamil may cause increased adverse effects on the heart. Cimetidine may inhibit the metabolism of propranolol. Propranolol will interact with any psychoactive drug, including MAO inhibitors (see), which simulate the adrenal gland's effect on the nervous system. Propanolol may increase the effectiveness of medicines for diabetics, requiring dosage adjustments. Nicotine may reduce the effectiveness of this drug. Propranolol may reduce the effectiveness of digitalis. Over-the-counter stimulants in cold and allergy medications may counteract the effectiveness of propranolol. Should not be discontinued abruptly. Most effective when taken before meals.

PROPULSID • *See* Cisapride.

PROPYLENE GLYCOL (OTC) • **1,2-Propanediol. Eucerin Dry Skin Care Lotion. Keralyt. Lac-Hydrin. Preparation H Cleansing Tissues.** A clear, colorless liquid, it is the most common moisture-carrying vehicle in skin preparations, other than water itself. Its use is being reduced, and it is being replaced by safer glycols such as butylene and polyethylene glycol. In 1992, the FDA proposed a ban on propylene glycol in lice-killing products because it had not been shown to be safe and effective as claimed.

PROPYLHEXEDRINE (OTC) • **Benzedrex Inhaler.** Derived from phenol, it is used as a nasal decongestant. Should not be used continuously for more than three days.

PROPYLPARABEN • **Propyl p-Hydroxybenzoate.** Developed in Europe, the esters of hydroxybenzoic acid are widely used as preservatives, bactericides, and fungicides. Parabens are active against a variety of organisms, are neutral, low in toxicity, slightly soluble, and active in all solutions, alkaline, neutral, or acid. Used medicinally to treat fungal infections. Can cause contact dermatitis. Less toxic than benzoic or salicylic acids (*see both*). In 1992, the FDA issued a notice that propylparaben had not been shown to be safe and effective as claimed in OTC products.

PROPYL p-HYDROXYBENZOATE • *See* Propylparaben.

PROPYLTHIOURACIL (Rx) • **Propyl-Thyracil. PTU.** An anti-thyroid-hormone medication introduced in 1947 to treat overactive thyroid (*see*). Potential adverse effects include a drop in white blood cells and platelets, headache, drowsiness, dizziness, visual disturbances, diarrhea, nausea, vomiting, jaundice, liver toxicity, rash, hives, skin discoloration, itching, joint and muscle pain, swollen glands, loss of taste, drug fever, and skin hemorrhages. May be advisable to avoid foods high in iodine. Full beneficial effects may not be felt for several weeks. The drug should not be discontinued without consulting a physician.

PROPYL-THYRACIL • *See* Propylthiouracil.

PROREX • *See* Promethazine.

PROSCAR • *See* Finasteride.

PROSOBEE (OTC) • A multivitamin and mineral preparation.

PROSOM • *See* Estazolam.

PROSTAGLANDINS • **PGA. PGB. PGC. PGD.** A group of extremely potent hormonelike substances present in many tissues. There are more than sixteen known with effects such as dilating or constricting blood vessels, stimulating intestinal or bronchial smooth muscle, uterine stimulation, antagonism to hormones, and influencing metabolism of fat. Various prostaglandins in the body can cause fever, inflammation, and headache. Prostaglandins or drugs that affect prostaglandins are used medically to induce labor, prevent and treat peptic ulcers, control high blood pressure, treat bronchial asthma, and induce delayed menstruation. Aspirin and other NSAIDs (*see*) tend to inhibit prostaglandin production.

PROSTAPHLIN • *See* Oxacillin Sodium.

PROSTATE GLAND • A walnut-sized gland in the male pelvis, it produces fluid that helps to nourish and transport sperm. Enlargement of the prostate is a noncancerous condition of unknown cause that is increasingly common after fifty years of age. The prostate surrounds the urethra, the tube that carries urine from the bladder through the penis. As men age, noncancerous tumors often enlarge the prostate and block the flow of urine through the urethra, leading to more frequent urination and other symptoms such as hesitancy or difficulty in starting urination.

PROSTATISM • Refers to the difficulties associated with an enlarged prostate gland (*see*).

PROSTEP (Rx) • A nicotine patch with dosages from 11 mg to 22 mg per twenty-four hours. Recent data indicate that treatment with nicotine patches doubles or triples long-term smoking cessation rates. One double-blind, placebo-controlled trial in 220 smokers treated for eighteen weeks with a sixteen-hour nicotine patch without intensive group counseling found that 25 percent of those who received nicotine were not smoking one year later, compared to 9 percent of those who received a placebo. Manufacturers recommend wearing the patches for four to twelve weeks, but the optimal duration of patch use is unknown. This is the most expensive, as of this writing, of the nicotine patches. Use of Prostep transdermal system is contraindicated in patients with hypersensitivity or allergy to nicotine or to any of the components of the therapeutic system. Prostep should be used during pregnancy only if the likelihood of smoking cessation justifies the potential risk of use of nicotine replacement by the patient, who may continue to smoke. Smoking while using Prostep can be extremely dangerous. Prostep should be used with caution in patients with overactive thyroid, pheochromocytoma (*see*), or insulin-dependent diabetes. Nicotine delays the healing of peptic ulcer and should be used by those with active ulcers only if nicotine-replacement therapy outweighs the risks of smoking. Spontaneous abortion during nicotine-replacement therapy has been reported; as with smoking, nicotine as a contributing factor cannot be excluded. Although it has been difficult to separate out the effects of nicotine-replacement therapy from withdrawal symptoms of smoking cessation, reported probable adverse reactions include diarrhea, heartburn, dry mouth, joint and muscle aches, abnormal dreams, insomnia, nervousness, and sweating. Possible but unproven effects may be weakness, back, chest, or abdominal pain, constipation, nausea, vomiting, dizziness, headache, numbness, increased cough, sore throat, sinusitis, rash, taste perversion, and painful menstruation. Nicotine from any source can be toxic. A candidate for OTC status. *See* Nicotine.

PROSTIGMIN • *See* Neostigmine.

PROSTIN/15M • *See* Carboprost.

PROSTIN VR • *See* Alprostadil.

PROTEASE (OTC) • An enzyme that breaks down protein. In 1992, the FDA issued a notice that protease had not been shown to be safe and effective as claimed in OTC digestive-aid products.

PROTEASE INHIBITORS • Found in plants' reproductive parts, including those of soybeans and other beans, rice, and potatoes. Believed to provide these edibles with natural protection against insect predation. They are now being intensively studied because they seem to be capable of neutralizing the effect of a wide range of cancer-causing agents, from radiation and steroid hormones to potent components of diesel exhaust. Several protease inhibitors have been rushed to market to treat AIDS infections and are said to be the biggest advance in AIDS treatment. In combination with other drugs, protease inhibitors give a one-two punch to the virus to keep it knocked down. *See* Crixivan Invirase, zalcitabine, zidovudine, and lamivudine.

PROTEINS • The chief nitrogen-containing constituents of plants and animals—the essential constituents of every living cell. They are complex, but by weight contain about 50 percent carbon, 20 percent oxygen, 15 percent nitrogen, 7 percent hydrogen, and some sulfur. Some proteins also contain iron and phosphorus. Proteins are colorless, odorless, and generally tasteless. They vary in solubility, but readily undergo putrefaction, hydrolysis, and dilution with acids or alkalies. They are regarded as combinations of amino acids (*see*).

PROTEINURIA • Presence of protein in the urine.

PROTEUS • Gram-negative (*see*) bacteria found in fecal matter and putrefying materials. Some species cause urinary-tract infections, diarrhea, and gastroenteritis. May be found in abscesses.

PROTHAZINE-25 (Rx) • *See* Promethazine and Codeine.

PROTHIADEN • *See* Dothiepin.

PROTHROMBIN • A protein that is converted by enzymes to thrombin (*see*).

PROTHROMBIN TIME • The time required for blood to clot.

PROTIRELIN (Rx) • A synthetic thyrotropin-releasing hormone produced by the hypothalamus. Protirelin increases release of thyroid-stimulating hormone (TSH) from the anterior pituitary. Prolactin release is also increased from the pituitary. Administered by injection into the vein. Potential adverse reactions include blood pressure changes, breast enlargement, nausea, increased urination, skin flushing, light-headedness, bad taste in the mouth, abdominal discomfort, headache, sweating, convulsions, and dry mouth. Levodopa (*see*) may inhibit its effectiveness.

PROTOPAM • *See* Pralidoxime.

PROTOSTAT • *See* Metronidazole.

PROTRIPTYLINE (Rx) • **Vivactil.** A tricyclic antidepressant (*see*) drug, it is the least sedating of this category. Potential adverse side effects include drowsiness, dizziness, excitation, seizures, tremors, weakness, confusion, headache, nervousness, irregular heartbeat, high blood pressure, blurred vision, ringing in the ears, dry mouth, constipation, nausea, vomiting, loss of appetite, hallucinations, low body temperature, intestinal paralysis, urine retention, rash, hives, sweating, and allergy. Sudden stoppage may cause nausea, headache, and malaise. Barbiturates decrease its effectiveness; also large doses of vitamin C. Cimetidine and methylphenidate may increase its effects, as will bicarbonate of soda or acetazolamide (*see both*). Epinephrine and norepinephrine may increase protriptyline's blood-pressure-raising effects. MAO inhibitors (*see*) may cause severe excitation, high fever, or seizures. Contraindicated during recovery from a heart attack, in prostate enlargement, patients with cardiovascular disease, urine retention, glaucoma, thyroid disease, impaired liver function, or blood abnormalities, and patients who are suicidal or undergoing elective surgery. Other drugs, including over-the-counter ones, should not be used without consulting a physician. Most effective when taken on an empty stomach, but can be taken with a little food if stomach upset is a problem.

PROTROPIN • A growth hormone. *See* Somatrem.

PROVENTIL • *See* Albuterol.

PROVERA • *See* Medroxyprogesterone.

PROVIDENCIA • Gram-negative (*see*) bacteria that cause urinary-tract infections and diarrhea.

PROVIDONE-IODINE (OTC) • **Acu-dyne. Betadine. Biodine. Etodine. Iodex. Isodine. Pharmadine.** Preoperative skin preparation and scrub; germicide for surface wounds; postoperative application to incisions and used to prevent infections in patients with catheters. Ointment and solution kill bacteria, fungi, and viruses. It has the same action as iodine but is less irritating. Contraindicated in patients sensitive to iodine. Should not be used near eyes and mouth. May stain skin and mucous membranes.

PROVIR • An oral treatment for respiratory viral infections that are particularly prevalent among children. It is being developed by Shaman Pharmaceuticals, a small company that develops drugs from tropical plants. It is expected, if all goes well, to be on the market in 1996.

PROVOCHOLINE • *See* Methacholine.

PROXIGEL • *See* Carbamide Peroxide.

PROZAC • *See* Fluoxetine Hydrochloride.

PRULET • *See* Phenolphthalein.

PRUNELLA VULGARIS • *See* Self-Heal.

PRUNE POWDER and PRUNE CONCENTRATE • Banned as ingredients in laxatives by the FDA, May 1992.

PRURITUS • Severe itching.

PSEUDOEPHEDRINE (OTC) (H) • **Actifed. Afrinol. Allerest. Benadryl. Benylin. Bromfed. Comtrex. Congestac. Contac. Cenafed. Decofed. Deconsal II. Dimacol. Dorcol. Dristan. Fedahist. Fedrazil. Genac. Genaphed. Guaifed. Halofed. Histalet. Historal. Isoclor. Kronofed. Medi-Flu. NeoFed. Novahistine. Novated. Novated A. Nucofed. Ornex. PediaCare. Pseudogest. Pseudo-Hist. Robidrine. Robitussin. Ryna. Sinarest. Sine-Aid. Sine-Off. Singlet. Sinufed. Sinus Excedrin. Sinutab. Sudafed. Sudrin. Sufedrin. TheraFlu Flu and Cold Medicine. Triaminic Nite Light. Triposed. Tylenol Allergy Sinus Medication. Ursinus. Vicks Daycare. Vicks NyQuil.** More than two hundred products on the market contain this drug, which contracts blood vessels. Changed from Rx to OTC. Used for nasal and middle-ear decon-

gestion. Potential adverse reactions include anxiety, transient stimulation, tremors, dizziness, headache, insomnia, nervousness, arrhythmia (*see*), heart palpitations, rapid heartbeat, dry mouth, anorexia, nausea, vomiting, difficulty in urinating, pallor, excessive drowsiness, and fatigue. Contraindicated in severe high blood pressure or coronary artery disease, in patients receiving MAO inhibitors (*see*), and in breastfeeding women. Should be used cautiously in persons with high blood-pressure, diabetes, glaucoma, heart disease, overactive thyroid, and enlarged prostate. Elderly patients are more sensitive to the drug. Use of high blood pressure medications may increase blood-pressure-lowering effects. MAO inhibitors taken at the same time may cause severe high blood pressure. Alcoholic beverages may cause excessive drowsiness. Over-the-counter stimulants in cold medications, diet pills, and allergy medication may increase pseudoephedrine's side effects. Should be taken with food to avoid stomach upset. *See* Ephedrine.

PSEUDOEPHEDRINE SULFATE (OTC) • **Afrin. Chlor-Trimeton. Drixoral Non-Drowsy Formula. Sudafed 12 Hour Tablets.** A nasal decongestant changed from Rx to OTC. Doses should not be exceeded because at higher doses nervousness, dizziness, or sleeplessness may occur. Contraindicated in patients with heart disease, high blood pressure, thyroid disease, diabetes, or difficulty in urination due to enlargement of the prostate gland, unless directed by a physician. Should not be taken without consulting a physician by those presently taking a prescription drug for high blood pressure or depression. *See* Ephedrine.

PSEUDOGEST • *See* Pseudoephedrine.

PSEUDO-HIST • *See* Chlorpheniramine and Pseudoephedrine.

PSEUDOMONAS AERUGINOSA • Gram-negative bacteria (*see*) that occur in fresh water and salt water. One species is found in wound infections, burns, and urinary-tract infections. Another is found in soil and water and is commonly associated with food spoilage (eggs, milk, cured meats, and fish).

PSEUDOMONAS INFECTIONS • *See* Pseudomonas Aeruginosa.

PSORALEN • A chemical found in plants and used in medicines and perfumes. Exposure to psoralen and then to sunlight may increase the risk of severe burning.

PSORIASIS • A chronic disease of the skin of unknown cause, usually persisting for years with periods of remission and recurrence. Characterized by elevated lesions in various parts of the body that are covered with dry silvery scales that drop off. Psoriasis appears most often between the ages of ten and thirty and tends to run in families. In most cases, it does not affect general health if it is attended to.

PSORIGEL • *See* Coal Tar.

P & S TAR GEL • *See* Ethyl Alcohol.

PSYCH- • Prefix meaning pertaining to the mind.

PSYCHE • The mind.

PSYCHOSIS • A major mental disorder of organic or emotional origin in which the personality is seriously disorganized and contact with reality usually impaired.

PSYLLIUM (OTC) (H) • *Plantago psyllium.* **Cillium. Effer-Syllium. Fiberall. FiberCleanse. Flea Seed. Hydrocil. Konsyl. Metamucil. Modane Bulk. Naturacil. Perdiem Plain. Prompt. Reguloid. Serutan Toasted Granules. Siblin. Syllact. V-Lax.** A laxative in use since the early 1930s that absorbs water and expands to increase the bulk and moisture content of the stool to encourage bowel movement. Used to treat constipation, especially after delivery of a baby. Potential adverse reactions include nausea, vomiting, diarrhea, and narrowing of the esophagus, stomach, or intestines when the drug is taken in dry form. Contraindicated in abdominal pain, nausea, vomiting, or other symptoms of appendicitis, and intestinal obstruction or ulceration, disabling adhesions, or difficulty in swallowing. The laxative effect usually takes from twelve to twenty-four hours to three days. Not absorbed systemically. Should be taken with at least eight ounces of water. Taking a psyllium product without sufficient fluid may cause it to swell, block the throat or esophagus, and possibly cause choking. Contraindicated in those who have problems swallowing or any throat problems. If chest pain, vomiting, or difficulty in swallowing or breathing occur after taking a psyllium product, prompt medical attention should be sought. Severe allergic reactions may occur.

PTEROCARPUS MARSUPIUM • *See* Kino.

P-200 • *See* Papaverine Hydrochloride.

PTH • Abbreviation for parathyroid hormone.

PTU • *See* Propylthiouracil.

PUCCOON ROOT • *See* Goldenseal.

PUERARIA (H) • *Pueraria lobata.* **Ko Ken. Kuzu Root.** The root or vine is used by Chinese herbalists as a treatment for colds, flu, and digestive problems. It is high in starch. It grows wild in the southern states, where it is considered the scourge of the South. Its fast-growing, hardy vines that creep over everything are difficult to eradicate.

PU GONG YING • *See* Dandelion.

PULMONARY • Referring to the lungs.

PULMONARY EDEMA • Accumulation of fluids in the lungs resulting from inefficient pumping of blood from the heart, one of the signs of congestive heart failure.

PULMONARY EMBOLISM • A blood clot that obstructs the pulmonary artery, which transports blood from the heart to the lungs. More than 90 percent of pulmonary emboli originate as clots in the deep veins of the lower extremities (deep-vein thrombosis). They can result in sudden death.

PULMONARY HYPERTENSION • High blood pressure in the arteries supplying the lungs due to resistance to blood flow through the lungs.

PULMOZYME • *See* Dornase.

PULS • Homeopathic abbreviation for pulsatilla (*see*).

PULSATILLA (H) • **Puls.** Widely used in homeopathic medicine to treat a variety of ills including teething and toothache, to dry up the milk supply upon stopping nursing, painful periods, and abdominal pains. It is also used to treat asthma, cystitis, bronchitis, arthritis, and migraine. The plant is irritating and toxic. *See* Anemone and Pasqueflower.

PUMPKIN SEED (H) • *Cucurbita pepo.* Native Americans used this seed to treat problems with enlarged prostate. It has a reputation among herbalists as being a nonirritating diuretic. Among its ingredients are fatty oil, albumin, lecithin, and phytosterol, an alcohol. Used by herbalists today to get rid of worms.

PUR-, PUS-, PYO- • Prefixes meaning pertaining to pus, as in *purulent.*

PURGE CONCENTRATE • *See* Castor Oil.

PURI-CLENS • *See* Methylbenzethonium Chloride.

PURINETHOL • *See* Mercaptopurine.

PURODIGIN • *See* Digitoxin.

PURPURA • Hemorrhages into the skin.

PURSLANE (H) • *Portulaca oleracea.* Identified by Norman Salem, Jr., a lipid biochemist with the National Institute of Alcohol Abuse, Bethesda, Maryland, as the richest known omega-3 source in the world of leafy greens. Purslane is a weedy herb sometimes thrown into salads. Salem and his collaborator, Artemis P. Simopoulos of the American Association for World Health, Washington, D.C., found that range-fed chickens at one Greek farm voluntarily feast on purslane. Just one yolk from a large-sized egg produced by these chickens contains roughly 300 mg of omega-3 fatty acids, the same amount contained in a standard fish-oil capsule and ten times more than in what's found in a typical U.S. supermarket egg. The eggs from purslane hens lack the fish taste and smell of eggs from hens feeding on fish oil. The Mediterranean diet that seems so effective in preventing heart attacks contains high amounts of alpha-linolenic acid, found in purslane.

PUSTULES • Bumps filled with pus.

PUVA • The combination of a psoralen, such as methoxypsoralen, and ultraviolet light, used to treat psoriasis.

PVC • Abbreviation for premature ventricular contractions, which are fine, rapid, chaotic movements of the ventricular muscle of the heart that replace the normal contraction.

P.V. CARPINE • *See* Pilocarpine.

P.V. CARPINE LIQUIFILM • *See* Pilocarpine.

PVF K • *See* Penicillin V.

PVK • *See* Penicillin V.

P-V-TUSSIN (OTC) • A combination of chlorpheniramine, phenylephrine, guaifenesin, hydrocodone, phenindamine, and pyrilamine (*see all*), used to treat a cough.

PYLORIC STENOSIS • A stricture at the end of the stomach.

PYLORUS • The opening between the stomach and the small intestine.

PYODERMA • Pus-producing disease, such as impetigo (*see*).

PYODICIN-OTIC (Rx) • A combination of hydrocortisone and polymyxin B (*see both*).

PYOPEN • *See* Carbenicillin Disodium.

PYR-, PYRET- • Prefixes referring to fever.

PYR • Homeopathic abbreviation for pyrethrum and for pyrogen. *See* Pyrethrins and Pyrogen.

PYRANISTAN • *See* Chlorpheniramine.

PYRANTEL, EMBOLATE and PAMOATE (Rx) (OTC) • **Anthel. Antiminth. Combantrin. Early Bird. Helmex. Reese's Pinworm Medicine.** A medicine to combat roundworm and pinworm, introduced in 1972. It paralyzes the parasites and causes them to be expelled by normal movement of the patient's intestines. Adverse reactions may include headache, dizziness, drowsiness, insomnia, rash, loss of appetite, nausea, vomiting, stomach pain, diarrhea, fever, and weakness.

PYRAZINAMIDE (Rx) • **PMS Pyrazinamide. Tebrazid. Zinamide.** An adjunctive (*see* Adjunct) treatment of tuberculosis, introduced in 1955, for use when primary and secondary antitubercular drugs cannot be employed or have failed. Potential adverse reactions include anemia, loss of appetite, nausea, vomiting, pain when urinating, hepatitis, and problems with control of diabetes. Also may cause malaise, fever, and joint pain. Contraindicated in patients with severe liver disease or a history of gout. Ethionamide (*see*) may increase the risk of adverse side effects with pyrazinamide. Pyrazinamide may reduce the effectiveness of drugs used for gout.

PYRAZODINE • *See* Phenazopyridine Hydrochloride.

PYRETHRINS (OTC) • **A-200 Pediculicide. Barc. Licetrol-400. Pyrinyl. R&C. RID Lice Killing Shampoo. TISIT. Triple X.** Insecticidal ingredients of pyrethrum flowers used in combination with piperonyl butoxide to treat head, body, and pubic lice, and their eggs. Not effective against scabies (*see*). Potential adverse reactions include skin irritation with repeated use, sneezing, and wheezing. Contraindicated when skin is raw or inflamed. Must not be applied to open areas or acutely inflamed skin, to the face, eyes, or mucous membranes. These insecticides have been found to be less hazardous than other insecticides used to treat lice.

PYRETHROIDS (OTC) • **R&C Spray. Rid Lice Control Spray.** A highly active synthetic pyrethrin (*see*), it is used for the control of lice and louse eggs on garments, bedding, furniture, and other inanimate objects. Not for use on humans or animals.

PYRETHRUM • *See* Pyrethrins.

PYRETHRUM PARTHENIUM • *See* Feverfew.

PYREXIA • Fever.

PYRIDIATE • *See* Phenazopyridine Hydrochloride.

PYRIDIN • *See* Phenazopyridine Hydrochloride.

PYRIDINE-2-ALDOXIME METHOCHLORIDE • *See* Pralidoxime.

PYRIDIUM • *See* Phenazopyridine Hydrochloride.

PYRIDIUM plus PHENAZOPYRIDINE • *See* Phenazopyridine Hydrochloride, Butabarbital Sodium, and Hyoscyamine.

PYRIDOSTIGMINE (Rx) • **Mestinon. Regonol.** Introduced in 1962, it inhibits the destruction of acetylcholine (*see*) and is used as an antidote for neuromuscular-blocking agents, myasthenia gravis (*see*), and experimentally in the treatment of Alzheimer's disease. Potential adverse reactions include headache, weakness, sweating, seizures, slow heartbeat, low blood pressure, abdominal cramps, nausea, vomiting, diarrhea, excessive salivation, rash, blood clots, bronchospasm, increased bronchial secretion, muscle cramps, and muscle twitching. Atropine, anticholinergic agents, procainamide, and quinidine may make pyridostigmine less effective. Contraindicated in urinary or intestinal obstruction, slow heartbeat, low blood pressure, or in those allergic to bromides. Should be used with extreme caution in patients with asthma, and used with care in epilepsy, recent heart attack, overactive thyroid, irregular heartbeat, and peptic ulcer. Should be taken with food or milk to reduce stomach upset.

PYRIDOXINE HYDROCHLORIDE • *See* Vitamin B_6.

PYRILAMINE (OTC) • **Duo-Medihaler. Extra Strength Pamprin. Fiogesic. 4-Way Fast Acting Nasal Spray. Guaiahist. Histosal. Kronohist. Maximum Strength Midol. Premsyn PMS. Primatene Tablets-M. Robitussin Night Relief.** An antihistamine with a mild sedating action. It acts to open bronchial tubes so breathing is easier. It reduces congestion and helps to relieve asthma spasms. In 1992, the FDA proposed a ban for the use of pyrilamine to treat insect bites and stings, poison ivy, poison sumac, and poison oak. In 1992, the FDA also proposed a ban on pyrilamine maleate in internal analgesic products and in insect bite and sting drug products because it had not been shown to be safe and effective as claimed.

PYRIMETHAMINE (Rx) • **Daraprim.** A drug introduced in 1953 that kills or prevents the growth of protozoa, tiny one-celled animals. Protozoa may be involved in many infections. Pyrimethamine is used with other drugs to treat malaria and toxoplasmosis (*see*). Potential adverse reactions include severe vomiting, loss of taste, fever, sore throat, fatigue, easy bruising, stomach pain, blood problems, seizures, loss of appetite, diarrhea, and severe rash. Pyrimethamine may increase the side effects of a number of anticancer, antiviral, and antibiotic drugs. Should be taken with meals to reduce stomach irritation.

PYRIMETHAMINE WITH SULFADOXINE (Rx) • **Fansidar.** An antibacterial with an antimalarial drug. *See* Pyrimethamine.

PYRINYL • *See* Pyrethrins.

PYRITHIONE ZINC (OTC) • **Head & Shoulders Antidandruff Shampoo. X-Seb Shampoo. Zincon Dandruff Shampoo.** A zinc derivative that acts as an antibacterial and antifungal agent for the skin. Relieves the itching and flaking associated with dandruff and with seborrheic dermatitis of the scalp.

PYROGEN (H) • **Pyrexin. Pyrogenium. Sepsin.** A homeopathic remedy made from decomposed beef, used to treat fever, flu, and blood poisoning, especially from bacteria.

PYROGLUTAMIC ACID • *See* L-Pyroglutamic Acid.

PYROSIS • Heartburn (*see*).

PYRROXATE (OTC) • A combination of acetaminophen, chlorpheniramine, and phenylpropanolamine (*see all*), used to treat the symptoms of allergy and the common cold.

PYRUVIC ACID (Rx) • An important intermediate in fermentation and metabolism, it occurs naturally in coffee, and when sugar is metabolized in muscle. Is reduced to lactic acid (*see*) during exertion. Pyruvic acid is isolated from cane sugar. Has been used as a paste in the treatment of deep burns.

PYURIA • Pus in the urine.

Q

QUADRINAL (Rx) • A combination of ephedrine, phenobarbital, theophylline, and potassium iodide (*see all*), used to treat asthma.

QUADRIPLEGIA • Paralysis of all four limbs.

QUARZAN • *See* Clidinium Bromide.

QUASSIA (H) • *Pricrasma excelsa*. **Bitter Ash. Bitter Root. Bitterwood. Wahoo.** The quassia tree was taken to Stockholm in the 1700s by a Swede who had purchased it from a native healer in Suriname. A powerful, simple, bitter tonic, the medicine was widely used in Europe for gastric upset, as an appetite stimulant, and as a laxative in cases of chronic constipation in convalescents. In large doses, quassia causes vomiting.

QUATERNARIUM • A germicide derived from lauric acid, a common constituent of vegetable fats, especially coconut oil. Positively charged with a low irritation potential, it is effective against a wide range of organisms. It is a preservative present in skin preparations.

QUATERNARY AMMONIUM COMPOUNDS • A wide variety of preservatives, surfactants, germicides, sanitizers, antiseptics, and deodorants. Benzalkonium chloride (*see*) is one of the most popular. Quaternary ammonium compounds are synthetic derivatives of ammonia, a natural product that occurs in animal metabolism.

QUAZEPAM (Rx) • **Doral.** A benzodiazepine (*see*) sleeping drug that acts on the limbic system and thalamus of the brain by binding to specific benzodiazepine receptors. Potential adverse effects include fatigue, dizziness, daytime drowsiness, and headache. Use with alcohol or other central nervous system depressants, including antihistamines, opiate painkillers, and other benzodiazepines may cause increased central nervous system depression. Contraindicated in patients allergic to the drug or other benzodiazepines, in pregnancy, and in patients with suspected or established sleep apnea (*see*). Prolonged use of a benzodiazepine may lead to withdrawal symptoms when the medication is stopped.

QUEBRACHO (H) • *Aspidosperma quebracho blanco*. **Aspidosperma.** An evergreen tree with wide-spreading crown grown in South America. The bark contains alkaloids including yohimbine (*see*). It is used in homeopathic and folk remedies to treat shortness of breath, particularly in asthma, emphysema, and other bronchial constrictions. It is a bronchial relaxant. Contraindicated in persons with kidney and liver disease or low blood pressure. Quebracho is toxic when used in large amounts. It can cause severe gastrointestinal upset, a drop in blood pressure, and even respiratory arrest and death.

QUEEN-OF-THE-MEADOW (H) • *Filipendula ulmaria*. **Meadowroot.** An herb grown in North America that Indian medicine men used as a diuretic, stimulant, and astringent. Held sacred by the druids, it was a favorite wedding herb. Meadowroot is used by herbalists to treat kidney and bladder problems, especially when uric acid levels are high. It also is used to treat gout and arthritis because of its reputed ability to rid the body of uric acid. Because of its stimulating effect on glands and organs that clear the body of toxins and waste, it is used by herbalists to treat inflammation, but is used primarily as a diuretic.

QUEEN'S DELIGHT (H) • *Stillingia sylvatica*. The root of this North American herb contains volatile oil, tannin, and resin. It is used for the treatment of chronic skin conditions such as eczema and psoriasis. Also used by herbalists to treat bronchitis and laryngitis, especially when accompanied by loss of the voice. The astringent (*see*) qualities have led herbalists to use it for hemorrhoid problems. Potential adverse effects including burning of the mouth, vomiting, diarrhea, itching, and fatigue.

QUELICIN • *See* Succinylcholine.

QUELTUSS (OTC) • *See* Guaifenesin and Dextromethorphan.

QUERCETIN (H) • A bioflavonoid found in many plants, but usually obtained from the inner bark of a species of oak tree common in North America. The active ingredient, isoquercitin, has been found to block allergic and inflammatory reactions by inhibiting an antibody, IE, that is responsible for the majority of allergic reactions and inhibiting leukotrienes and prostaglandins involved in producing inflammation.

QUESTRAN • *See* Cholestyramine.

QUIBRON (Rx) • **Asbron G. Bronchial Capsules. Elixophyll-GG. Glyceryl T. Lanophyllin GG. Quibron-300. Slo-Phyllin GG. Synophylate-GG. Theoclate. Theolair-Plus.** These drugs are all a combination of theophylline and guaifenesin (*see both*) and xanthine (*see*). Used to treat asthma and other breathing problems. Potential adverse reactions include insomnia, drowsiness, muscle weakness, muscle spasm, nervousness, rapid heartbeat, chest pains, incoordination, irregular heartbeat, difficulty in urinating, and frequent urination. Charcoal-broiled meats may cause the drug to be less effective. Caffeine may add to the side effects, which means coffee, tea, cocoa, colas, and chocolate should be avoided while taking these drugs.

QUIBRON-T SR • *See* Theophylline.

QUICK PEP • *See* Caffeine.

QUIESS • *See* Hydroxyzine.

QUILLAJA EXTRACT (H) • **China Bark. Panama Bark. Quillay Bark. Soapbark.** The extract of the inner dried bark of *Quillaja saponaria,* a tree native to Chile. Used in flavorings, in folk medicine to treat bronchitis, and externally as a detergent and counterirritant (*see*). Contraindicated in patients with gastrointestinal inflammation.

QUINACRINE (Rx) • **Atabrine. Mepacrine.** Introduced in 1967, it was used to treat giardiasis, an intestinal parasite with flagella (stringlike projections), and tapeworm. Commonly causes nausea and vomiting. Also may cause headache, dizziness, nervousness, mood shifts, yellow discoloration of the skin, behavioral changes, nightmares and seizures, diarrhea, loss of appetite, abdominal cramps, and skin eruptions. Contraindicated in those with active liver or bone-marrow disease, a blood cell disorder, or who have previously had an allergic reaction to quinacrine. Alcohol use may cause a mild disulfiram-like reaction (*see*). Quinacrine may increase the toxic effects of primaquine. Should be taken with meals and a full glass of fluid.

QUINAGLUTE • *See* Quinidine.

QUINALBARBITONE • *See* Secobarbital Sodium.

QUIN-AMINO • *See* Quinine.

QUINAMINOPH • *See* Quinine.

QUINAMM • *See* Quinine.

QUINAPRIL HCL (Rx) • **Accupril.** An ACE inhibitor (*see*) indicated alone or in combination with thiazide diuretics for the treatment of high blood pressure. Introduced in 1991, it is promoted for its once-a-day dosage. It is also expected to be approved for treatment of congestive heart failure. Contraindicated in patients who are hypersensitive to the product, and to those with a history of angioedema (*see*) related to use of other ACE inhibitors. Angioedema of the face, extremities, lips, tongue, and throat has been reported in patients with ACE inhibitors. Should be used with caution in patients with impaired kidney function, undergoing major surgery, or with high potassium. ACE inhibitors have been shown to cause agranulocytosis and bone-marrow depression, and fetal and neonatal morbidity and mortality. Should not be taken by pregnant women. ACE inhibitors may cause excessive reduction of blood pressure when first taken by patients on diuretics. Quinapril can attenuate potassium loss caused by thiazide diuretics and increase blood levels of potassium when used alone. Quinapril may make tetracycline less effective and cause toxicity if used with lithium. Potential adverse reactions include headache, dizziness, fatigue, cough, nausea, vomiting, abdominal pain and—rarely—back pain, malaise, palpitation, irregular heartbeat, heart failure, heart attack, stroke, hypertensive crisis, angina, sleepiness, faintness, nervousness, depression, increased sweating, rash, itching, photosensitivity, double vision, sore throat, sinusitis, bronchitis, edema, or kidney dysfunction.

QUINATIME • *See* Quinidine.

QUINCE SEED (H) • *Cydonia oblonga.* The seed of a plant grown in central Asia and Europe for its fatty oil. Thick jelly is produced by soaking the seeds in water. Used in fruit flavorings for beverages and foods. Also used as a suspension in skin creams and lotions. It is soothing to the skin and is used by herbalists as a mouthwash, for ulcers on the gums and throat, and for inflamed and tired eyes. Also used by herbalists as an expectorant to treat dry coughs.

QUINDAN • *See* Quinine.

QUINE • *See* Quinine.

QUINESTROL (Rx) • **Estrovis.** An estrogen (*see*) used to treat atrophic vaginitis, hypogonadism, primary ovarian failure, symptoms of menopause, cancer of the prostate, and to prevent bone thinning.

QUINETHAZONE (Rx) • **Hydromox.** A thiazide-type diuretic (*see*) that increases urine excretion of sodium and water, it is used to treat edema and high blood pressure. Potential adverse reactions include nausea, vomiting, loss of appetite, pancreatitis (*see*), dehydration, a drop in blood pressure upon rising from a seated or prone position, liver dysfunction, anemia, a drop in platelets, low potassium, high blood sugar, fluid and electrolyte imbalances, rash, photosensitivity, and other allergic reactions. Cholestyramine and colestipol (*see both*) make it less effective. Diazoxide increases its blood-pressure-lowering and blood-sugar-raising effects. NSAIDs (*see*) decrease its effectiveness. Contraindicated in kidney and liver diseases, absence of urine formation, and hypersensitivity to quinethazones, thiazides, or other sulfonamide-derived drugs. Should be used cautiously in gout. Should be taken in the morning to avoid having to urinate during the night. A diet rich in potassium may be recommended. This includes dates, apricots, bananas, and tomatoes. If you are taking this drug, you should wear a sunscreen.

QUINIDEX • *See* Quinidine.

QUINIDINE (Rx); BISULFATE, GLUCONATE, SULFATE • **Cardioquin. Cin-Quin. Duraquin. Quinaglute. Quinatime. Quinidex. Quinora.** An antiarrhythmic drug introduced in the 1920s, it is used to treat heart flutter or fibrillation (*see*). When taken by mouth, the onset of action is slow. When given by injection in emergencies, it acts rapidly to control abnormal heartbeat. Potential adverse reactions include anemia, dizziness, confusion, restlessness, cold sweat, pallor, fainting, dementia, increased heartbeat irregularities, ringing in the ears, excessive salivation, blurred vision, diarrhea, nausea, vomiting, loss of appetite, abdominal pains, hepatitis, rash, hemorrhages in the mouth, itching, hives, acute asthmatic attacks, respiratory arrest, and fever. Acetazolamide (*see*), antacids, cimetidine (*see*), and sodium bicarbonate may increase quinidine blood levels. Barbiturates, phenytoin, rifampin, and nifedipine (*see all*) may make it less effective. Quinidine may increase digoxin (*see*) levels in the blood, making it more toxic. Verapamil (*see*) may result in low blood pressure if given with quinidine. Warfarin interacts to increase anticoagulation and may cause bleeding. To be avoided are over-the-counter drugs such as cold and allergy medications and diet pills, which may contain stimulants that can cause serious side effects while taking Quinidine. Most effective when taken on an empty stomach.

QUININE (Rx) (OTC) (H) • **Legatrin. M-Kya. Novoquinine. Quin-Amino. Quinamm. Quinamorph. Quinate. Quindan. Quinden. Quine-200. Quine-300. Quinoctal. Quiphile. Q-vel Muscle Relaxant. Strema.** A drug derived from cinchona (*see*) bark, from a tree that grows wild in South America. White, crystalline powder, almost insoluble in water, it was introduced as a

Western medication in 1888, to treat malaria. Used as a local anesthetic in hair tonics and sunscreen preparations, and to relieve muscle cramps. When taken internally, it reduces fever. Used in over-the-counter cold and headache remedies, as well as "bitter lemon" and tonic water, which may contain as much as 5 mg per l00 ml. Cinchonism (quinine poisoning), which may consist of nausea, vomiting, vision disturbances, ringing in the ears, and nerve deafness, may occur from an overdose of quinine. If there is a sensitivity to quinine, such symptoms can result after ingesting tonic water. Quinine more commonly causes a rash, blurred vision, headache, limb and back pain, loss of appetite, and unusual bleeding or bruising. In 1992, the FDA proposed a ban on quinine in internal analgesic products because it had not been shown to be safe and effective as claimed.

QUINOLINE • A coal tar derivative used in the manufacture of dyes. Also used as a preservative and solvent. It is permitted as a yellow dye in foods and drugs.

QUINOLONES (Rx) • **Cinoxacin. Ciprofloxacin. Nalidixic. Norfloxacin. Ofloxacin.** A class of synthetic broad-spectrum antibacterial agents derived from nalidixic acid, a coal tar derivative, they act by inhibiting bacterial DNA-associated enzymes.

QUINORA • *See* Quinidine.

QUINSANA PLUS • *See* Undecylenic Acid.

QUIPHILE • *See* Quinine.

R

RABIES • Hydrophobia. A potentially lethal disease caused by a virus that has an affinity for the brain and nervous tissue. The virus is transmitted to humans by the bite of an infected animal. Mere contact of saliva of a rabid animal on abraded or scratched skin can transmit the disease.

RABIES VACCINE, HUMAN DIPLOID CELL (HDCV) (Rx) • Imovax. Promotes active immunity to rabies after exposure to the virus. Adults and children receive five doses, the first as soon as possible after exposure. Potential adverse reactions include headache, nausea, abdominal pain, muscle ache, dizziness, fever, diarrhea, severe allergic reaction, serum sickness, and pain and redness at the site of injection.

RACEMIC AMPHETAMINE SULFATE • *See* Amphetamine.

RADIOACTIVE IODINE (Rx) • Sodium Iodine. Iodotope Therapeutic. Radioactive iodine destroys thyroid tissue. It is used to treat overactive thyroid and thyroid cancer. Potential adverse reactions include a feeling of fullness in the neck, metallic taste, swollen glands, underactive thyroid, inflamed thyroid, delayed food absorption, a possible increased risk of developing leukemia later in life, and possible increased risk of birth defects in offspring. Use of lithium carbonate after treatment may cause too much of a drop in thyroid activity. Contraindicated in pregnancy and lactation unless used to treat thyroid cancer. For seven days after treatment, the patient should not sleep in the same room with spouse or have prolonged close contact with small children due to increased risk of thyroid cancer in persons exposed to radioactive iodine.

RADIOPAQUE • Not permitting the passage of radiation. These agents, which contain iodine (*see*), are drugs used to help diagnose certain medical problems.

RADIOSTOL FORTE • *See* Vitamin D.

RADISH EXTRACT (H) • Extract of *Raphanus sativus.* The small seeds of the radish remain viable for years. Has been used as a food since ancient times. The extract is used as a counterirritant (*see*) in herbal preparations.

RAGWORT • *See* Life Root.

RAMIPRIL (Rx) • Altace. An ACE inhibitor that acts on enzymes in the blood to dilate blood vessels and lower blood pressure. Introduced in 1991, it decreases the secretion of aldosterone, an adrenal hormone, and thus reduces sodium and water retention. Potential adverse effects include headache, dizziness, fatigue, weakness, nausea, vomiting, impotence, and cough. If given within three days of taking diuretics, especially at the start of therapy, it may cause excessive low blood pressure. Use with potassium supplements or potassium salt substitutes may cause an overload of potassium in the blood. Ramipril increases the blood levels of lithium. Should be used with caution in pregnant women because it can prove fatal to the fetus. May be taken with or without food, but should be taken at the same time each day. This medication should not be stopped suddenly.

RAMSES • *See* Nonoxynol-9.

RANDOMIZED • Drugs are assigned to patients in no particular order during testing of the effects of a pharmaceutical.

RANGOPRA (H) • *Brachyglottis repanda.* A small shrub native to New Zealand. It is used in homeopathic medicines as a hypnotic. The plant is potentially carcinogenic in humans and is considered hazardous because it can cause severe liver damage.

RANITIDINE (Rx) (OTC) • Zantac. Zantac 75. Introduced in 1981, it is used for the short-term treatment of active duodenal ulcer. Most patients heal within four weeks. Also used to treat pathological hypersecretory conditions, and for short-term treatment of active, benign gastric ulcers. Also used to treat gastroesophageal reflux disease (GERD) (*see*). Contraindicated in patients known to be hypersensitive to ranitidine. Should be used with caution in patients with gastric malignancy, and those who have kidney or liver dysfunction. Headache, sometimes severe, seems to be related to ranitidine. Other potential adverse reactions include constipation, diarrhea, nausea, vomiting, abdominal discomfort and pain, impotence, decreased libido, male breast enlargement, and rarely, pancreatitis (*see*). There have been rare reports of malaise, dizziness, sleepiness, insomnia, rash, hair loss, edema, irregular or slow heartbeat, anaphylaxis, and joint pain. Rare cases of reversible mental confusion, agitation, depression, and hallucinations have been reported, predominantly in severely ill elderly patients. May cause a false-positive test for urine protein. Increased or decreased blood-clotting times have been reported during concurrent use of ranitidine and warfarin. Antacids may interfere with its absorption. Ranitidine may decrease the absorption of diazepam (*see*). Ranitidine is secreted in human milk. Dosage adjustments of antidiabetes drugs may be necessary if taken with ranitidine. May be taken with food. Approved for OTC status in 1995.

RAPHANUS SATIVUS • *See* Radish Extract.

RASPBERRY (H) • *Rubus strigosus*. **Red Raspberry.** Juice from the fresh ripe fruit grown in Europe, Asia, the United States, and Canada. Used as a flavoring. It has astringent properties. The leaf is used to treat diarrhea. A modern study showed a substance in the leaf is responsible for relaxing the smooth muscles of the uterus and intestines when they are in tone and causes contraction of the uterus when it is not in tone. The relaxation effect is believed to account for the use of raspberry leaves in folk medicine to aid childbirth. The contracting effect may explain the ability of the leaves to remedy sluggish bowel movements. Warm raspberry tea is also used by herbalists to soothe throat irritation and canker sores. Contraindicated in pregnancy because it may cause contractions of the uterus.

RATTLEROOT • *See* Black Cohosh.

RATTLESNAKE ANTIVENIN • *See* Crotaline Antivenin Polyvalent.

RAUDIXIN • *See* Rauwolfia.

RAUVERID • *See* Rauwolfia.

RAUWILOID • *See* Rauwolfia.

RAUWOLFIA (Rx) (H) • **Deserpidine. Raudixin. Rauverid. Rauwiloid. Rauzide. Reserpine. Wolfina.** A small shrub native to the Orient from India to Sumatra where it has been used for medicinal purposes for hundreds of years. The active ingredients are usually in the root. Rauwolfia contains the basics for many widely used modern drugs including reserpine, Serpasil, and yohimbine (*see all*). Rauwolfia extracts work by blocking nerve signals that trigger constriction of blood vessels. It should be given with meals. Contraindicated in mental depression and should be used cautiously in severe cardiac or cerebrovascular disease, impaired renal function, peptic ulcer, ulcerative colitis, and gallstones; in those undergoing surgery; in elderly or debilitated patients; in pregnant women and in those taking other antihypertensives or tricyclic antidepressants (*see*). Potential adverse reactions include mental confusion, depression, drowsiness, nervousness, nightmares, headache, a drop in blood pressure upon rising from a sitting or prone position, faintness, dry mouth, stuffy nose, glaucoma, hypersecretion of gastric acid, nausea, vomiting, GI bleeding, skin rash, impotence, and weight gain. Rauwolfia may predispose patients taking digitalis to irregular heart beating. When given with MAO inhibitors (*see*), may cause excitability and high blood pressure. Alcohol and other central nervous system depressants including antihistamines will add to the depressant effects of rauwolfia. Rauwolfia may be taken with food or milk.

RAUZIDE • *See* Rauwolfia.

RAYNAUD'S DISEASE (or PHENOMENON) • A disorder of the blood vessels in which exposure to the cold causes the small arteries supplying the fingers and toes to contract suddenly, cutting off blood flow to the digits, which then become pale.

R&C SHAMPOO • *See* Piperonyl Butoxide.

RDA • Abbreviation for recommended daily allowance (*see*).

RDI • Abbreviation for reference daily intakes (*see*).

REACTIVATION • Usually refers to a reawakening of latent virus in the body.

REA-LO • *See* Urea.

RECALCITRANT • Difficult to treat.

RECEPTOR • A protein molecule, which may also be composed of fat and carbohydrate. It resides on the surface or in the nucleus of the cell and recognizes and binds a specific molecule of appropriate size, shape, and charge. It acts like a lock for a key.

RECEPTOR BINDING ASSAY • A technique to determine the presence and amount of a drug, neurotransmitter, or receptor in a biological system.

RECEPTOR BLOCKADE • Similar to an impostor playing a role meant for a real person, a pharmaceutical "impostor" attaches to a receptor on a cell surface and the real chemical cannot get in. A drug such as a beta-blocker (*see*) masquerades as a hormone or neurotransmitter (*see*) and prevents the real hormone or neurotransmitter from taking effect.

RECOMBINANT DNA • Genetic instructions artificially introduced into a cell so that the genetic and physical characteristics of the cell are altered, and the new DNA is replicated along with the natural DNA. Recombinant DNA is one technique of genetic engineering.

RECOMMENDED DAILY ALLOWANCE • **RDA.** Recommended dietary allowances of the Food and Nutrition Board, National Academy of Sciences, National Research Council. The nutrient amounts are only recommended, not required.

RECTAL MEDICONE • *See* Benzocaine.

RECURRENCE • An infection caused by a microorganism that has infected the body in the past. A recurrence may be due to a reactivation or reinfection with a disease-causing organism. Also refers to the return of cancer cells and signs of cancer after remission.

RED CENTAURY • *See* Centaury.

RED CLOVER (H) • *Trifolium pratense.* This plant has been used in American folk medicine for more than one hundred years to treat and prevent cancer. Also used to treat gout, and as an expectorant. Used in an herbal tea for digestive disorders. Red clover has shown some estrogenic activity and has a reputation as an aphrodisiac. Some believe the enhancement of lovemaking is because of the estrogenic effect, which aids lubrication. Antibiotic tests on red clover have shown it to possess activity against several bacteria, including that which causes tuberculosis.

RED COCKSCOMB • *See* Amaranth.

REDISOL • *See* Vitamin B_{12}.

RED ROOT • *See* Bloodroot.

REDUX • *See* Dexfenfluramine.

REESE'S PINWORM MEDICINE • *See* Pyrantel Pamoate.

REFERENCE DAILY INTAKES • **RDIs.** A set of dietary references introduced in 1994 by the FDA based on and replacing the recommended daily allowances (RDAs) for essential vitamins and minerals and, in selected groups, protein. Vitamins and minerals are still expressed as percentages on the label, but these figures now refer to daily values. *See also* Daily Reference Values.

REFRACTORY • Not responsive to treatment.

REFRESH • *See* Artificial Tears.

REGITINE • *See* Phentolamine Mesylate.

REGLAN • *See* Metoclopramide.

REGONOL • *See* Pyridostigmine.

REGRESSION • Growing smaller or disappearing. Used to described the shrinkage or disappearance of a cancer.

REGROTON (Rx) • **Demi-Regroton.** A combination of chlorthalidone and reserpine, it is used to treat high blood pressure. The ingredients complement each other, so for certain patients their combined effect is better than that of each alone. Potential adverse reactions include nausea, vomiting, drowsiness, cramps, dizziness, diarrhea, tingling in the arms and legs, headache, restlessness, chest pains, irregular heartbeat, glaucoma, nightmares, muscle spasms, weakness, high blood sugar, blurred vision, stuffy nose, dry mouth, rash, decreased sex drive, and impotence. Must be used with caution in people with a history of mental depression, active peptic ulcer, and ulcerative colitis. Should not be taken by those sensitive to regroton's ingredients. Interaction with digitalis or quinidine may cause irregular heartbeat. Other high blood pressure medications such as guanethidine, methyldopa, chlorthalidone, and hydralazine (*see all*) may cause blood pressure to drop too low. MAO inhibitors (*see*) taken with regroton may raise the blood pressure dangerously high. Should not be used with lithium because it may lead to toxic levels of that drug. Over-the-counter medications for colds, coughs, allergy, or sleepiness may counteract the effects of regroton. A physician may recommend the patient eat a diet high in potassium or take a potassium supplement because regroton can deplete potassium in the body. May be taken with food, usually at breakfast time.

REGULOID • *See* Psyllium.

REHMANNIA (H) • *Rehmannia glutinosa.* **Sok Day–Sang Day.** The root is used by Chinese herbalists to purify and nourish the blood, strengthen the kidneys, and heal the bones and tendons. Herbalists say it is useful in building the body during recovery from an illness. It is given to women to treat menstrual irregularities and infertility, as a tonic during pregnancy, and to stop postpartum hemorrhage.

RELAFEN • *See* Nabumetone.

RELAXADON (Rx) • *See* Hyoscyamine, Atropine, Scopolamine, and Phenobarbital.

RELEASING FACTORS • Produced by the hypothalamus and then sent to the pituitary gland (*see*), where they cause the release of appropriate hormones. Among those that have been found are luteinizing hormone-releasing hormone (LHRH) (*see*), which affects the release of the sex hormones, and thyroid hormone-releasing factor (TRF), which affects the release of the thyroid hormone. Both LHRH and TRF have behavioral effects. LHRH, for example, enhances mating behavior. TRF may cause stimulation of activity.

RELEFACT TRH • *See* Protirelin.

RELIEF OPHTHALMIC SOLUTION • *See* Phenylephrine.

REMEGEL (OTC) • A combination of aluminum hydroxide and magnesium carbonate used to relieve stomach activity.

REMISSION • The disappearance of symptoms, but not of the disease itself.

REMSED • *See* Promethazine.

REN- • Prefix meaning pertaining to the kidney.

RENAL • Relating to the kidney.

RENESE • *See* Polythiazide.

RENOQUID • *See* Sulfacytine.

RENORMAX • *See* Spirapril.

RENOVA (Rx) • An antiwrinkle emollient cream that contains 0.05% of trentoin (*see*). The exact mechanism of renova is unknown but it does have an effect on skin cells. Absorption through the skin of compounds containing trentoin varies from 1 to 31 percent. In a stronger version, it is used to treat acne, and that compound has been found to cause birth defects in the babies of mothers using it. Renova is used to counteract fine wrinkles and mottled skin but does not eliminate wrinkles, repair sun damaged skin, reverse photoaging, or restore a more youthful or young skin cell pattern. Most of the improvement in the skin occurred during the first 24 weeks of use. Neither the safety nor the efficacy of using renova for more than 48 weeks has been established. Possible adverse reactions include skin irritation and changes in the elasticity of the skin. It should not be used if you are taking drugs that cause photosensitization, such as tetracyclines, phenothiazines, and sulfa drugs. The effect on the fetuses of animals has been equivocal. Should not be used by pregnant women. Should not be used if you are sunburned or have eczema or other chronic skin conditions. Should be applied once a day before bedtime and only enough to cover the problem areas. It should not be applied to the eyes, ears, nostrils, or mouth. *See* Trentoin.

REOCCLUSION • The development of a new blood clot after spontaneous or pharmacologic unblocking of a vessel that had been occluded by a clot.

REOPRO • *See* Abciximab.

REPERFUSION INJURY • The formation of highly reactive forms of oxygen (radicals) in the body, resulting from a decrease or lack of oxygen, which injures normal tissues. This may occur after procedures to open clogged blood vessels.

RESCINNAMINE (Rx) • **Moderil.** An antihypertensive drug that blocks the nerve signals that trigger constriction of blood vessels, thus reducing blood pressure. Used to treat mild to moderate high blood pressure, it may be used alone or in combination with other antihypertensives. Contraindicated in mental depression. Must be used with caution in persons with severe cardiac or cerebrovascular disease, peptic ulcer, ulcerative

colitis, gallstones, in patients undergoing surgery, pregnant women, elderly or debilitated patients, and patients taking other antihypertensives. Potential adverse reactions include mental confusion, depression, drowsiness, nervousness, nightmares, parkinsonism, a drop in blood pressure when rising from a sitting or prone position, faintness, dry mouth, nasal stuffiness, glaucoma, hypersecretion of gastric acid, nausea, vomiting, GI bleeding, rash, impotence, and weight gain. Effects of this drug may last for up to ten days after it is discontinued.

RESERPINE (Rx) • **HHR. Hydropres. Hydroprin. Hydrotensin-50. Metatensin. Naquival. Ser-AP-ES. Serpalan. Serpasil. Serpate. Tri-Hydroserpine.** An antihypertensive drug that blocks the nerve signals that trigger constriction of blood vessels, thus reducing blood pressure. Used to treat mild to moderate high blood pressure. Contraindicated in mental depression. Must be used with caution in persons with severe cardiac or cerebrovascular disease, peptic ulcer, ulcerative colitis, gallstones, in patients undergoing surgery, pregnant women, and patients taking other antihypertensives. Potential adverse reactions include mental confusion, depression, drowsiness, nervousness, nightmares, parkinsonism, a drop in blood pressure when rising from a sitting or prone position, dry mouth, nasal stuffiness, glaucoma, hypersecretion of gastric acid, nausea, vomiting, GI bleeding, rash, impotence, and weight gain. Effects of this drug may last for up to ten days after it is discontinued. Use with MAO inhibitors (*see*) may cause excitability and hypertension. Should be taken with meals. *See also* Rauwolfia.

RESINS (H) • A brittle substance, usually translucent or transparent, formed from the hardened secretions of plants. Among the natural resins are dammar, elemi, and sandarac.

RESISTANCE • Condition whereby a microorganism learns to defy a previously effective antibacterial or antiviral drug.

RESONIUM A • *See* Sodium Polystyrene Sulfonate.

RESORCINOL (Rx) (OTC) • **Acnomel Cream. BiCozene Creme. Castellani Paint. Pedinol.** A preservative, antiseptic, antifungal agent, astringent, and anti-itching agent, particularly in dandruff shampoos. It may darken light-colored hair. Also an ingredient of skin preparations for the treatment of acne, dermatitis, and fungal infections. Irritating to the skin and mucous membranes. May cause allergic reactions, dizziness, diarrhea, nausea, stomach pain, headache, nervousness, slow heartbeat, shortness of breath, sweating, and fatigue. Those using resorcinol should avoid abrasive soaps or cleansers, medicated cosmetics, alcohol-containing preparations, or any other acne preparations. In 1992, the FDA issued a notice that resorcinol had not been shown to be safe and effective as claimed in OTC products.

RESORPTION • A physiological process involving the remodeling of bone during which time the old bone is dissolved and eliminated by osteoclasts, bone-cell scavengers.

RESPBID • *See* Theophylline.

RESPINOL-G (OTC) • A combination of phenylephrine, phenylpropanolamine, and guaifenesin (*see all*), used to treat coughs and stuffy nose due to allergy or the common cold.

RESPIRATORY SYNCYTIAL VIRUS DISEASE • **RSV.** One of the most important causes of lower-respiratory-tract disease in children, accounting for over 90 percent of the cases of bronchiolitis. Symptoms include wheezing, fever, cough, and difficulty feeding.

RESTLESS LEG SYNDROME • **RLS.** Occurs at bedtime and is described as "running in bed." Relief occurs with movement and symptoms occur when stationary. Symptoms are vague with twitching and muscular discomfort.

RESTORIL • *See* Temazepam.

RETICULOGEN (OTC) • *See* Thiamin Hydrochloride and Vitamin B_{12}.

RETIN-A • *See* Tretinoin and Retinoids.

RETINA • The light-receiving structure at the back of the eye.

RETINAL DETACHMENT • Separation of the light-receiving layer of the back of the eye from its underlying layer. In most instances, the filmy structure can be reattached by laser therapy or other procedures, if medical help is sought promptly.

RETINOIC ACID • A derivative of vitamin A. *See* Tretinoin and Retinoids.

RETINOIDS (RX) (OTC) • **Retin-A.** Derivative of vitamin A, created in the laboratory by altering certain aspects of the retinol molecule. Among the retinoids in use are etretinate, 13-cRA, and trans retinoic acid. Retinoids are used to treat acne and other skin disorders. *See* Vitamin A.

RETINOL • Vitamin A as found in fish, liver, oils, butter, egg yolks, and whole milk. *See* Vitamin A.

RETINOPATHY • Any abnormal condition of the retina resulting in the loss of vision.

RETINYL PALMITATE (Rx) • The ester of vitamin A and palmitic acid, sometimes mixed with vitamin D (*see all*).

RETRO- • Prefix meaning backward or behind.

RETROVIR • *See* Zidovudine.

REVERSOL • *See* Edrophonium.

REVEX (Rx) • *See* Nalmefene.

REVIA • *See* Naltrexone.

REXOLATE • *See* Sodium Thiosalicylate.

REYE'S SYNDROME • An acute, often fatal childhood illness involving swelling of the brain and toxic degeneration of the liver. It usually develops during recovery from a flulike infection, measles, or chicken pox. Scientists believe that the syndrome may be due to the interaction in a genetically vulnerable child of the viral infection and chemical toxins, including drugs. Current recommendations are that acetaminophen, aspirin, and drugs to prevent vomiting not be used in children with viral infections.

R-GEN • *See* Iodinated Glycerol.

R-GENE 10 INJECTION • *See* Arginine.

R-GER ELIXIR • *See* Iodinated Glycerol.

RHABDOMYOLYSIS • The name is derived from the Greek words *mys,* meaning muscle, and *lysis,* meaning loosening. It is an acute, fulminating, potentially fatal disease of the skeletal muscle, which entails its destruction.

RHABDOMYOSARCOMA • A malignant tumor derived from skeletal muscle, occurring in children and less commonly in adults.

RHAG-, RHAGIA- • Prefixes meaning a bursting or sudden discharge from a vessel, such as in hemorrhage.

RHAMNUS CATHARTICA • *See* Buckthorn.

RHAMNUS PURSHIANA • *See* Cascara Sagrada.

RHATANY (H) • *Krameria triandra.* The root of a shrub native to Peru; contains up to 9 percent tannin (*see*). A powerful astringent that has long been used in conventional pharmacy. Used by herbalists to treat diarrhea, hemorrhoids, and hemorrhages, or as a styptic. Rhatany is often found in herbal toothpastes and powders to treat bleeding gums. May cause dermatitis in sensitive people. Large amounts can cause nausea and vomiting. Regular internal use may cause kidney dysfunction.

RHE • Homeopathic abbreviation for rheum (*see*).

-RHEA • Suffix indicating a discharge, as in *rhinorrhea,* a runny nose.

RHEABAN • *See* Attapulgite.

RHEUM (H) • **Rhe. Rhubarbarum. Turkey Rhubarb.** A homoepathic remedy made from rhubarb, an herbaceous plant indigenous to China and Tibet. It has been cultivated in European gardens since the mid-eighteenth century. It was used medicinally by the Arabian physicians for dropsy and jaundice. It is used in homeopathy to treat discharges, diarrhea, and teething pain. *See* Rhubarb, Chinese.

RHEUMATIC FEVER • A severe inflammatory disease that can affect the brain, heart, joints, and skin, caused by the same organism responsible for strep throat.

RHEUMATREX • *See* Methotrexate.

RHIN- RHINO- • Prefixes from the Greek word *rhis,* meaning nose.

RHINALL • *See* Phenylephrine.

RHINDECON • *See* Phenylpropanolamine.

RHINITIS • Inflammation of the mucous membranes of the nose. May be caused by a cold virus or by other infections or allergies.

RHINOCORT NASAL INHALER • *See* Budesonide.

RHINOLAR • *See* Chlorpheniramine and Phenylpropanolamine.

RHINOSYN • *See* Chlorpheniramine and Pseudoephedrine.

RHOD • Homeopathic abbreviation for rhododendron (*see*).

RHODODENDRON (H) • **Rhod. Yellow Snow Rose.** Indigenous to the mountains of Siberia and now grown worldwide, it is used in

Siberia as a remedy for arthritis, gout, and syphilis. In homeopathy, it is used to treat back-ache, fear of thunderstorms, headache, joint pain, and toothache.

RHUBARB, CHINESE (H) • **Rheum offici-nale. Da Huang.** A native of China, it has been used for thousands of years as a laxative. It was one of the plants brought out of the Far East by Marco Polo. Chinese rhubarb was twice as costly as opium. In smaller doses, it is used by herbalists to treat diarrhea, dysentery, and indigestion. When chewed, it stimulates salivation. Rhubarb also reputedly promotes blood circulation in the pelvic cavity and is therefore used by herbalists to treat painful menstruation. Banned as an ingredient in commercial laxatives by the FDA, May 1992. In August 1992, the FDA issued a notice that rhubarb fluid extract had not been shown to be safe and effective as claimed in OTC digestive-aid prod-ucts. Contraindicated in persons suffering from kidney stones and gout and in cases of peptic and stomach ulcers.

RHULICAINE • *See* Benzocaine.

RHULICREAM • *See* Camphor.

RHULIGEL • *See* Benzoyl Peroxide and Camphor.

RHULISPRAY (OTC) • Used to treat the rash of poison ivy. *See* Camphor, Benzocaine, and Calamine.

RHUS AROMATICA (OTC) (H) • **Fragrant Sumac. Hyland's Bed Wetting Tablets.** An extract of a shrub native to both temperate and warm regions. Has astringent qualities. Sumac berries contain a large amount of tannin (*see*). The root was chewed by some North American Indi-ans to treat mouth sores.

RHUS TOX • *See* Rhus Toxicodendron.

RHUS TOXICODENDRON (H) • **Rhus. Tox.** A homeopathic medicine derived from a genus of shrubs and trees native to warm regions

that includes poison ivy, poison oak, and sumac. It is used to treat painful joints, swollen glands, and skin eruptions.

RHYTHMIN • *See* Procainamide.

RIBAVIRIN (Rx) • **RTCA. Virazole.** A drug used in hospitalized infants and young children for the prevention and treatment of respiratory syncytial virus (RSV) disease. Administered by inhalation of a fine mist. It may also be used to treat lower-respiratory-tract infections in adults. Potential adverse reactions include anemia, con-junctivitis, worsening of respiratory state, rash, and swelling of the eyelids. Also may cause headaches. Contraindicated in women who may become pregnant during treatment with the drug.

RIBOFLAVIN • *See* Vitamin B_2.

RIBONUCLEIC ACID • **RNA.** Found in both the nucleus and cytoplasm of the cell, it is the material that contains directions for the genetic code of the cell, DNA.

RICELYTE (OTC) • A rice-based oral solution to maintain electrolyte (*see*) balance. *See also* Potassium Citrate.

RICE SYRUP SOLIDS (Rx) • A rice-based electrolyte (*see*) maintenance solution. Rapidly replenishes fluids and electrolytes lost in diarrhea. Contraindicated in severe, continuing diarrhea or other critical fluid losses, intractable vomiting, intestinal obstruction, perforated bowel, and when kidney function is depressed. Should be used only on a doctor's orders.

RICINUS COMMUNIS • *See* Castor Oil.

RICKETTSIAL DISEASES • A group of ills caused by bacterial infections that can be trans-mitted from mice, ticks, fleas, and lice. Among the diseases are typhus, spotted fever, and Q fever.

RID-A-PAIN (OTC) • A combination of aceta-minophen, salicylamide, and caffeine (*see all*), used to treat pain and fever.

RIDAURA • *See* Auranofin.

RID LICE KILLING SHAMPOO (OTC) • *See* Piperonyl Butoxide and Pyrethrins.

RIFABUTIN (Rx) • An AIDS drug rushed to market in 1992 for the prevention of the spread of *Mycobacterium avium* complex (MAC), a life-threatening bacterial infection that often occurs in patients with advanced HIV infection.

RIFADIN • *See* Rifampin.

RIFAMATE (Rx) • *See* Isoniazid and Rifampin.

RIFAMPICIN • *See* Rifampin.

RIFAMPIN (Rx) • **Rifadin. Rifamate. Rifampicin. Rimactane. Rofact.** A drug introduced in 1967 to treat tuberculosis, and to prevent meningitis by the elimination of *Meningococcus* from the throats of carriers. Among potential adverse reactions are anemia, a drop in blood platelets, headache, fatigue, drowsiness, lack of coordination, kidney dysfunction, dizziness, mental confusion, and generalized numbness. Also, abdominal distress, loss of appetite, nausea, vomiting, diarrhea, gas, sore mouth and tongue, high blood sugar, and serious liver damage. Use with alcohol may increase the likelihood of liver damage. Rifampin may cause irregular menstrual periods and may make oral contraceptives ineffective. Also may cause rash, hives, flulike symptoms, and discoloration of body fluids. Soft contact lenses may become permanently stained. Para-aminosalicylate sodium, an antiseptic, and keto-conazole (*see*) may decrease its effectiveness. Use with probenecid (*see*) may increase its levels in the blood. Rifampin interacts with many other drugs, including antidiabetic drugs, estrogens, and male hormones. Should be taken one hour before or two hours after a meal at the same time every day.

RILUTEK (Rx) • *See* Riluzole.

RILUZOLE (Rx) • **Rilutek.** Introduced in 1995, it is the first drug approved for the treatment of amyotrophic lateral sclerosis (*see*). Potential adverse effects: fever, dizziness, nausea. Should be taken at the same time each day. Alcohol should be avoided.

RIMACTANE INH (Rx) • A combination of isoniazid and rifampin (*see both*) used to treat tuberculosis.

RIMEXOLONE (Rx) • **Vexol.** An ophthalmic corticosteroid for the treatment of postoperative inflammation following ocular surgery and anterior uveitis (*see*).

RIMSO-50 • *See* Dimethyl Sulfoxide.

RINGER'S INJECTION and RINGER'S LACTATE (Rx) • **Hartmann's Solution.** Replaces fluids and electrolytes. A potential adverse effect is fluid overload. Contraindicated in kidney failure. Must be used cautiously in heart failure.

RINGWORM • **Tinea Corporis.** A fungal (not a worm) infection, it manifests itself on the skin in round, scaly, itchy patches. Usually affects the scalp, trunk, or feet. When ringworm affects the scalp, bald patches develop. Ringworm is infectious and can be spread from a pet, such as a dog or cat, to its owner's family.

RIO-DOPA • *See* Levodopa.

RISPERDAL • *See* Risperidone.

RISPERIDONE (Rx) • **Risperdal.** Introduced in 1994, it is a drug for the treatment of schizophrenia. It controls symptoms such as delusions and hearing voices as well as apathy and emotional withdrawal. The manufacturers claim that it is the only antischizophrenia drug that helps counteract apathy and withdrawal. It should be used with caution in those with liver impairment, heart disease, and in the elderly. A potentially fatal side effect has sometimes occurred with antipsychotic drugs, called neuroleptic malignant syndrome (NMS) (*see*). A syndrome of potentially irreversible, involuntary movements may also occur.

(*See* Tardive Dyskinesia.) Other potential adverse effects include a drop in blood pressure upon standing, seizures, cognitive and motor impairment, blood clots, disruption of body-temperature regulation, dizziness, nausea, excessive muscle activity, insomnia, stuffy nose, and suicide. Risperidone may interact with high blood pressure medications, Parkinson medications, and central nervous system depressants.

RITALIN • *See* Methylphenidate.

RITODRINE (Rx) • **Pre-Par. Yutopar.** A drug introduced in 1980 for the management of premature labor. Potential adverse reactions include nausea, vomiting, alterations in blood pressure, high blood sugar, low blood potassium, heart palpitations, fluid in the lungs, rapid heartbeat, redness, tremors, nervousness, and rash. Contraindicated before the twentieth week of pregnancy and in the following conditions: antepartum hemorrhage, eclampsia, intrauterine fetal death, infection in the amniotic fluid, maternal heart disease, pulmonary hypertension, maternal hyperthyroidism, and uncontrolled maternal diabetes. Should not be used with cortisonelike medications or beta-blockers (*see both*).

RITONAVIR (Rx) • **Norvir.** A HIV virus protease inhibitor (*see*) that has been rushed to market because of the inability to control the AIDS virus. The drug has been studied in healthy volunteers and HIV-infected patients. In combination with other AIDS drugs such as Zidovudine (*see*), it increased immune cells and reduced the HIV viral cells. The manufacturer is not claiming it is a cure and warns that its long-term effects are unknown, but it is considered a big advance in treatment. Ritonavir should not be taken with certain nonsedating antihistamines, sedative hypnotics, or heart drugs that prevent irregular rhythms. It also reacts with many other drugs and must be carefully supervised by a physician experienced in treating AIDS infections with drugs. Among its potential adverse reactions include fatigue, fever, headache, shortness of breath, stomach upset, throat irritation, and taste impairment. It also tastes pretty awful, so it is recommended that it be mixed with chocolate milk or Ensure. Should be taken with food.

RIVOTRIL • *See* Clonazepam.

RMS • *See* Morphine Sulfate or Hydrochloride.

RNA • Abbreviation for ribonucleic acid (*see*).

ROBAFEN • *See* Guaifenesin.

ROBAXIN • *See* Methocarbamol.

ROBAXISAL (Rx) • A combination of aspirin and methocarbamol (*see both*), used as a muscle relaxant.

ROBENECID • *See* Probenecid.

ROBICILLIN • *See* Penicillin V.

ROBICILLIN VK • *See* Penicillin V.

ROBIDRINE • *See* Pseudoephedrine.

ROBIMYCIN • *See* Erythromycin.

ROBINUL • *See* Glycopyrrolate.

ROBITET • *See* Tetracycline Hydrochloride.

ROBITUSSIN • *See* Guaifenesin.

ROBITUSSIN-DM (OTC) • A combination of dextromethorphan and guaifenesin (*see both*) used to treat coughs.

ROBOMOL • *See* Methocarbamol.

ROCALTROL • *See* Calcitriol.

RO-CEPH • *See* Cephradine.

ROCEPHIN • *See* Ceftriaxone.

ROCKY MOUNTAIN GRAPE • *See* Oregon Grape Root.

ROCURONIUM BROMIDE (Rx) • Zemuron. A muscle relaxant used during surgery. It has a rapid onset and was approved in 1994 after a review of 8.6 months by the FDA.

RODEX • *See* Vitamin B$_6$.

ROFERON-A (Rx) • Approved in the United Kingdom for the treatment of chronic active hepatitis B, various cancers, and Kaposi's sarcoma. The product, interferon alfa-2a, has already been approved for hepatitis C in France, Italy, and Spain. In clinical trials, it has been shown to normalize the marker of liver function, alanine aminotransferase, in approximately 40 to 80 percent of chronically infected hepatitis C patients and to produce a sustained normalization after completion of therapy in around 30 percent of patients, according to the manufacturer. *See* Interferon Alpha-2a and Alpha-2b.

ROGAINE • *See* Minoxidil.

ROLAID CALCIUM RICH • *See* Calcium Carbonate.

ROLAIDS (OTC) • *See* Dihydroxyaluminum Sodium Carbonate.

RONASE • *See* Tolazamide.

RONDEC-DM (OTC) • *See* Carbinoxamine and Pseudoephedrine, and Dextromethorphan.

RONDEC DROPS • *See* Carbinoxamine and Pseudoephedrine.

RONDEC-S (OTC) • *See* Carbinoxamine and Pseudoephedrine.

RONDOMYCIN • *See* Tetracyclines.

ROSE (H) • *Rosa gallica. Rosa officinalis* **(Apothecary's Rose). French Rose. Red Rose.** The use of rose petals dates back to very ancient times. Ancient pharmacists used them for purgatives, astringents, and tonics, to treat chronic lung diseases, diarrhea, and vaginal discharges. The medicinal properties of rose petals are generally considered mild. The buds and petals are astringent. Rosebuds are high in vitamin C, astringent tannins, and phenolic compounds.

ROSE HIPS EXTRACT (H) • *Rosa canina.* **Hipberries.** An extract of the fruit of various species of wild roses, it is rich in vitamin C and is used as a natural flavoring. Widely used by organic-food enthusiasts as a tonic, to ward off colds, and to ease constipation.

ROSEMARY (H) • *Rosmarinus officinalis.* **Mi Die Xiang.** Contains rosmaricine, the derivatives of which possess smooth-muscle stimulant activity and some analgesic properties. The herb possesses essential oils that reputedly calm and soothe irritated nerves and upset stomach. Rosemary is also high in minerals such as calcium, magnesium, phosphorus, sodium, and potassium. Used in an herbal tea for headache.

ROWASA • *See* Mesalamine.

ROXANOL • *See* Morphine Sulfate or Hydrochloride.

ROXICET (Rx) • *See* Acetaminophen and Oxycodone Hydrochloride.

ROXICODONE • *See* Oxycodone Hydrochloride.

ROXIPRIN (Rx) • *See* Aspirin and Oxycodone Hydrochloride.

ROYAL JELLY (H) • A substance secreted by honey bees. It is sold in health food storse as something that can boost energy, improve the immune system, and relieve symptoms of premenstrual tension, among other attributes. It may cause severe allergic reactions in the sensitive.

RTCA • *See* Ribavirin.

RUBEFACIENT • An agent that helps stimulate blood circulation to the skin, causing redness. Pilocarpine (*see*) is an example. Ginger and horseradish are herbs used for this purpose.

RUBELLA VIRUS VACCINE, LIVE (Rx) • **Meruvax II.** Rubella—German measles—is a serious infection that causes miscarriages, still-births, or birth defects in babies when pregnant women contract the disease. Rubella virus vaccine is an active immunizing agent used to prevent the infection. Potential adverse reactions include allergic reactions, pain or tenderness of the eyes, headache, confusion, convulsions, vomiting, stiff neck, and irritability.

RUBESOL-1000 • *See* Vitamin B_{12}.

RUBEX • *See* Doxorubicin.

RUBIA TINCTORUM • *See* Madder.

RUBIDOMYCIN • *See* Daunorubicin Hydrochloride.

RUBRAMIN (OTC) • *See* Vitamin B_{12}.

RUBUS FRUITICOSUS • *See* Blackberry.

RUE (Rx) (H) • *Ruta graveolens.* **African Rue. Garden Rue. German Rue.** An evergreen shrub, the oil is a spice agent obtained from the fresh, aromatic, blossoming plants grown in southern Europe and the Orient. Rue is mentioned in the Talmud as a valuable medicine. In the sixth century A.D., it was used to treat gout. The plant is mentioned in more than thirty-five prescriptions in a fourteenth-century manuscript for almost every known disease from itch (*see* Scabies), boils, ulcers, and snakebite to tuberculosis. It was used to ward off pestilence during the Great Plague and to combat witches. Rue was considered good for toadstool poisoning, the stings of hornets, bees, and wasps, and the bites of serpents. Still used in folk medicine in an herbal tea for high blood pressure, to treat stomach upset, reduce swelling, increase local circulation, and ease arthritis pain. Also still used to fight fly infestation. In conventional medicine, the plant is a source of harmine, which is used to treat parkinsonism (*see* Parkinson's Disease). Rue causes sensitivity to light. All parts of the plant, but especially the seeds, are toxic.

RUFEN • *See* Ibuprofen.

RU-486 • *See* Mifepristone.

RUMEX CRISPUS • *See* Rumex Extract.

RUMEX EXTRACT (H) • From genus of herbs and shrubs that are mainly native to north temperate regions and have small flowers. A homeopathic medicine (*see*) that is used to treat respiratory symptoms. *See* Sorrel Extract.

RUM-K • *See* Potassium Chloride.

RUSCOGENIN (H) • A sugar from *Ruscus aculeatus.* It is used in the treatment of hemorrhoids. *See* Butcher's-Broom.

RUSCUS ACULEATUS • *See* Butcher's-Broom.

RUTA • Homeopathic abbreviation for *Ruta graveolens* (*see*).

RUTA GRAVEOLENS (H) • A homeopathic remedy for bunions, bruises, eye strain, sprains, and tennis elbow. *See* Rue.

RUTIN (H) • Pale yellow crystals found in many plants, particularly buckwheat. Used as a dietary supplement for blood- or lymph-vessel fragility.

RU-TUSS (Rx) • A combination of chlorpheniramine and phenylephrine (*see both*) used to treat coughs.

RU-VERT M • *See* Meclizine.

RYNATAN (Rx) • A combination of chlorpheniramine, phenylephrine, and pyrilamine (*see all*), used to treat the symptoms of allergy.

RYNATUSS (Rx) • A combination of chlorpheniramine, ephedrine, phenylephrine, and carbetapentane (*see all*), used to relieve coughs.

RYTHMOL • *See* Propafenone Hydrochloride.

Rx • Symbol for a medical prescription.

Rx-TO-OVER-THE-COUNTER • Term describing the shift of a prescription drug to a category where it can be bought without a prescription (*see* Introduction, pages 5–6).

S

SABADILLA ALKALOIDS • Caustic Barley. Cevadilla. The dried ripe seeds of *Schoenocaulon officinale,* grown in the Andes. In 1992, the FDA proposed a ban on sabadilla in lice-killing products because it had not been shown to be safe and effective as claimed.

SABAL • *See* Saw Palmetto.

SAC • A pouch or bag covering an organ or tissue.

SACCHARIN • An artificial sweetener in use since 1879. It is three hundred times as sweet as natural sugar. On an FDA priority list to retest for mutagenic, subacute, and reproductive effects ever since the mid-1970s when it was reported that it may be a weak cancer-causing agent.

SACCHAROMYCES BOULARDII • A yeast that is, as of this writing, being combined with an antibiotic to treat *Colstridium difficile* (*see*). Multiple research centers in the United States are testing *Saccharomyces boulardii*'s beneficial effects. *C. difficile* occurs when antibiotics or other factors disrupt the resistance of normal colonic flora. Most antibiotics share the risk of further perturbing the protective normal flora in the colon and making the patient more susceptible to *C. difficile.* The yeast achieves a high steady-state level in the colon and is not inhibited by antibiotics, does not significantly impact the normal flora, and is cleared from the colon once therapy is discontinued.

SACRED BARK • *See* Cascara Sagrada.

SAFETY COATED • A tablet with a smooth coating that helps the user to swallow it.

SAFFLOWER (H) • *Carthamus tinctorius.* **American Saffron. Bastard Saffron.** An annual plant, a native of Egypt, it is cultivated in various parts of Europe and America. In large doses it is thought to have laxative value and, when given as a warm infusion, is said to have a fever-reducing effect. Used in an herbal tea for colds.

SAFFRON • *Crocus sativus.* Used in perfumery and as a coloring in cosmetics. It is the dried stigma of the crocus cultivated in Spain, Greece, France, and Iran. Used also in bitters, liquors, and spice flavorings. Homeopathic physicians use it to induce menstruation and as an antispasmodic. Excessive doses can cause miscarriage. Severe poisoning causes bleeding from the skin, a severe lowering of the heart rate, and collapse. Fatal cases have been reported when five to ten grams of saffron have been ingested.

SAFROLE • Found in certain natural oils such as star anise, nutmeg, and ylang-ylang, it is a stable, colorless to brown liquid with an odor of sassafras and root beer. Used in the manufacture of heliotropin (*see*) and in expensive soaps and perfumes. Used as a beverage flavoring until it was banned in 1960. The toxicity of this fragrance ingredient is being questioned by the FDA. It is an animal liver carcinogen.

SAGE (H) • *Salvia officinalis.* The flowering tops and leaves of the shrubby mints. Spices include Greek sage and Spanish sage. The genus, *Salvia,* is so named for the plant's supposed healing powers. Greek sage is used for fruit and spice flavorings. Also used by herbalists to treat sore gums, mouth ulcers, as a tonic, and to remove warts. The Arabs believed that it prevents death. In 1992, the FDA proposed a ban on sage oil in astringent drug products because it had not been shown to be safe and effective as claimed. *See also* Salvia.

SAINT BARTHOLOMEW'S TEA • *See* Maté Extract.

SAINT-JOHN'S-WORT (H) • *Hypericum perforatum.* **Amber. Blessed. Devil's Scourge. Goatweed. God's Wonder Herb. Grace of God. Hypericum. Klamath Weed.** A perennial native to Britain, Europe, and Asia, it is now throughout North America. The plant contains glycosides, volatile oil, tannin, resin, and pectin (*see all*). It was believed to have infinite healing powers derived from the saint, the red juice representing his blood. It was used as an antivenereal. It is used to treat pains and diseases of the nervous system, arthritic pains, and injuries. An infusion made from its leaves is used for stomach disorders, diarrhea, depression, and bladder problems and to remove threadworms in children. A salve has been used for colds. It reputedly also eases fibrositis, sciatica, and varicose veins. It is now being studied by researchers from the National Cancer Institute and universities as a potential treatment for cancer and AIDS. The FDA listed Saint-John's-wort as an "unsafe herb" in 1977. The FDA issued a notice in 1992 that Saint-John's-wort had not been shown to be safe and effective as claimed in OTC digestive-aid products. That does not mean, however, that it cannot be used for other purposes.

SALAC • *See* Salicylic Acid.

SAL-ACID • *See* Salicylic Acid.

SALAZOSULFAPYRIDINE • *See* Sulfasalazine.

SALBUTAMOL • *See* Albuterol.

SALCATONIN (Rx) • **Miacalcin.** A salmon-derived calcitonin nasal spray approved in 1994 for increasing bone mineral density and reducing broken-bone rates in postmenopausal osteoporosis (*see*). An injectable form has been marketed in the United States since 1986 for that purpose. The nasal spray is thought to affect primarily lumbar bone, while the injectable calcitonin increases both total body calcium and lumbar bone. *See* Calcitonin.

SALETO-200 • *See* Ibuprofen.

SALFLEX • *See* Salsalate.

SALGESIC • *See* Salsalate.

SALICARIA EXTRACT (H) • **Spiked Loose-strife.** Extract of the flowering herb *Lythrum salicaria,* which has purple or pink flowers. Used since ancient Greek times to calm nerves and soothe skin.

SALICIN • A chemical derived from the bark of several species of willow and poplar trees. Aspirin and other salicylates are derived from salicin or made synthetically.

SALICYLALDEHYDE • *See* Salicylic Acid.

SALICYLAMIDE • An analgesic fungicide and anti-inflammatory agent used to soothe skin. Gives a sensation of warmth on the tongue. In 1992, the FDA proposed a ban for the use of salicylamide to treat fever blisters and cold sores, poison ivy, poison oak, and poison sumac because it had not been shown to be safe and effective as claimed in OTC products. *See* Rid-A-Pain.

SALICYLATES (OTC) • **Aspirin. Amyl-. Benzyl-. Glyceryl-. Menthyl-. Phenyl-. Salts of Salicylic Acid. Easprin. Ecotrin. Empirin. Measurin. Sportscreme. Zorprin.** Those who are sensitive to aspirin may also be hypersensitive to FD&C Yellow No. 5, a salicylate, and to a number of foods that naturally contain salicylate, such as almonds, apples, apricots, blackberries, boysenberries, cherries, cloves, cucumbers, currants, gooseberries, grapes, nectarines, oil of wintergreen, oranges, peaches, pickles, plums, prunes, raisins, raspberries, strawberries, and tomatoes. The salts are used as sunburn preventatives and antiseptics. Aspirin is acetylsalicylic acid. Non-acetylated salicylates, such as sodium salicylate, salsalate (Disalcid and others), and choline magnesium salicylate (Trilisate and others) do not interfere with platelet function as aspirin does and may be safer than acetylated salicylates for aspirin-intolerant patients. Sodium salicylate contains 46 mg of sodium in each 325-mg tablet and 92 mg of sodium in each 650-mg tablet. Salicylates interact with many medications. The effects of antidiabetic medications may be increased. Blood thinners and valproic acid may increase the chance of bleeding. Salicylates may keep tetracyclines from being effective. Aspirin may increase the blood levels of zidovudine, which may increase the chances of serious side effects. Salicylates should be taken with food to reduce the risk of stomach irritation.

SALICYLIC ACID (Rx) (OTC) (H) • **Methyl Salicylate. Salicylaldehyde. Aveeno Cleansing Bar for Acne. Buf-Puf Medicated Acne Pads. Calicylic X-Seb Creme. Clearasil. Clear Away. Compound W. Derma-Soft Cream. Duofilm Liquid. Duoplant Gel. Fostex. Freezone. Hydrisalic. Ionil. Keralyt. Komed. Mediplast. Meted 2. MG 217 Psoriasis. Noxzema Clear-Ups. Occlusal. Off-Ezy Wart Removal. Oxipor. Oxy Clean Medicated Pads. Oxy Medicated Pads. Paplex. P & S Plus Tar Gel. SalAc. Sal-Acid. Saligel. Sal-Plant. Sastid. Sebucare. Sebulex. Sebutone Cream Shampoo. Stri-Dex Dual Textured Maximum Strength Pads. Trans-Plantar. Trans-Ver-Sal. Verrex–C&M. Viranol. Wart-Off Wart Remover.** Occurs naturally in wintergreen leaves, sweet birch, and other plants. Synthetically prepared by heating phenol with carbon dioxide. It has a sweetish taste and is used as a preservative and antimicrobial. Used externally as an antiseptic agent, fungicide, and skin-sloughing agent. It is an antipuretic (anti-itch) agent. Used as an antimicrobial at 2–20 percent concentration in lotions, ointments, powders, and plasters; also used in making aspirin (*see*). It is used as a keratolytic drug applied topically to slough the skin in the treatment of acne. It can be absorbed through the skin. Absorption of large amounts may cause vomiting, abdominal pain, increased respiration, acidosis, mental disturbances, and rash in sensitive individuals. Contact with face, genitals, and mucous membranes should be avoided. In 1992, the FDA issued a notice that salicylic acid, while useful for removing warts, is not effective as an external pain or itch reliever in insect bite and sting, poison ivy, poison sumac, and poison oak OTC drug products.

SALICYLISM • A toxic condition produced by overdosage with drugs of the aspirin family (salicylates).

SALICYLSALICYLIC ACID • *See* Salsalate.

SALIGEL • *See* Salicylic Acid.

SALINE • Containing a salt. *See* Sodium Chloride.

SALIVART • *See* Saliva Substitutes.

SALIVA SUBSTITUTES (OTC) • **Moi-Stir. Orex Salvart. Salirast. Xero-Lube.** Products used for the relief of dry mouth and throat. *See* Potassium Chloride and Sorbitol.

SALMETEROL XINAFOATE (Rx) • **Severent Inhalation Aerosol.** A long-acting (twelve-hour) inhaled bronchodilator taken twice daily for prevention of asthma bronchospasm (constriction of the airways associated with asthma) and exercise-induced bronchospasm in patients twelve years and older. Approved in 1994 after a priority review by the FDA that took 25.5 months. It has been used in the United Kingdom since 1990. The improper use of this longest-acting asthma drug has caused fatalities. The drug is effective in preventing asthma attacks but doesn't treat actual asthma attacks because it takes at least thirty minutes to begin working. During the first five months it was on the market, doctors reported twenty deaths possibly but not proven to be caused by patients inhaling the drug during an attack and waiting in vain for it to help.

SALMONELLA • A type of bacteria that causes food poisoning, gastrointestinal inflammation, and disease of the genital tract.

SALSALATE (Rx) • **Salicylsalicylic Acid. Arthra-G. Disalcid. Mono-Gesic. Salflex. Salgesic. Salsitab.** A drug similar to aspirin that produces analgesia by an ill-defined effect on the hypothalamus, and by blocking the generation of pain impulses. The peripheral action may involve inhibition of prostaglandins (*see*). Used to treat arthritic disorders. Potential adverse reactions include ringing in the ears and hearing loss, nausea, vomiting, GI distress, occult bleeding, abnormal liver function, rash, bruising, hypersensitivity manifested by asthma, and anaphylaxis. Ammonium chloride and other urine acidifiers may increase blood levels of salicylates. Antacids in high doses and other urine alkalinizers decrease levels of salicylates. Corticosteroids decrease the effectiveness of salicylates and oral anticoagulants may increase the risk of bleeding. Concomitant use with alcohol, steroids, or other NSAIDs may increase the risk of GI bleeding. In 1992, the FDA proposed a ban on salsalate in internal analgesic products because it had not been shown to be safe and effective as claimed. *See* Nonsteroidal Anti-Inflammatory Drugs.

SALSITAB • *See* Salsalate.

SALURON • *See* Hydroflumethiazide.

SALUTENSIN (Rx) • **Hydropine H.P.** A combination of hydroflumethiazide and reserpine (*see both*), used to treat high blood pressure. The first drug relaxes the muscles in veins and arteries to help reduce the volume of blood flowing, while the second drug, reserpine, works on the nervous system to reduce nerve transmission. Potential adverse reactions include nausea, vomiting, cramps, dizziness, constipation, headache, tingling in the arms and legs, restlessness, chest pains, irregular heartbeat, glaucoma, nightmares, muscle spasms, blood disorders, itching, fever, shortness of breath, high blood sugar, stuffy nose, dry mouth, weakness, impotence, and decreased sex drive. Contraindicated in persons who are allergic to any of the ingredients or who have a history of mental depression, active peptic ulcer, or ulcerative colitis. If taken with digitalis or quinidine, heart rhythms may become irregular. Caution must be taken if salutensin is given with other blood-pressure-lowering drugs because it may cause the pressure to drop too low. Should not be taken with MAO inhibitors (*see*). Salutensin may raise lithium to toxic levels if taken together. It may be necessary to eat high-potassium foods if a potassium supplement is not given. These include apricots, bananas, and tomatoes. Salutensin may be taken with food.

SALVIA (H) • *Salvia militorrhiza.* **Dang Shen.** The root is used by Chinese herbalists for blood stagnation and to regulate menses. It is also used for a variety of other conditions, including abdominal distension, boils, erysipelas, itching, and rheumatism. *See* Sage.

SAMARIUM53 EDTMP (Rx) • A radiopharmaceutical used to treat bone pain caused by cancer. It is expected on the United States market soon.

SAMMAPO • Native American word for juniper berries (*see* Juniper).

SANDALWOOD • *Santalum album.* Used in perfume. It is the pale yellow, somewhat viscous volatile oil obtained by steam distillation from the dried ground roots and wood of the plant. Has strong, warm, persistent odor and is soluble in most fixed oils. Used in floral, fruit, honey, and ginger-ale flavorings for beverages, ice cream, ices, candy, baked goods, and chewing gum. Also used for incense and as a fumigant. In homeopathic and herbal medicines, it is used to treat stomach disorders, particularly flatulence and heartburn. The isolated volatile oil has been used internally in the treatment of urinary-tract inflammations. May produce skin rash in the hypersensitive. Excessive doses may cause kidney dysfunction.

SANDIMMUNE • *See* Cyclosporine.

SANDOGLOBULIN • *See* Immune Serum Globulin.

SANDOSTATIN • *See* Octreotide.

SANGUINARIA CANADENSIS • *See* Bloodroot.

SANICLE (H) • *Sanicula europaea.* A plant grown in Europe, the mountains of Africa, and the Americas. An old folk saying is, "He who has sanicle needeth no surgeon." It has had a reputation since ancient times for healing powers. It was used for burns and wounds and was taken in the form of root tea for skin problems and St. Vitus' dance, a movement disorder. Herbalists still recommend sanicle for external use to treat skin diseases, and in mouthwashes and gargles. A strong decoction of the leaves is used for infections.

SANI-SUPP • *See* Glycerin.

SANOREX • *See* Mazindol.

SAN PEDRO (H) • *Trichocereus pachanoi.* **San Pedro Cactus.** A large cactus native to South America. It contains the hallucinogen mescaline. The plant is used in folk medicine in the treatment of gastric disorders, lung ailments, and sterility. Mescalin is a common drug of abuse.

SANSERT • *See* Methysergide.

SAPONINS (H) • Any of numerous natural glycosides—natural or synthetic compounds derived from sugars—that occur in many plants such as soapbark, soapwort, and sarsaparilla. Characterized by their ability to foam in water, saponins are used chiefly as foaming and emulsifying agents and detergents. They have the ability to liberate hemoglobin, which carries oxygen to the lungs, from red blood corpuscles at great dilutions. They have also been found to have an anti-inflammatory action similar to that of cortisone. Herbs that contain saponins, including goldenrod, chickweed, and wild yam, have long been used to soothe inflammation. Saponins are also thought to reduce blood cholesterol. They can be beneficial or deleterious. They may either be steroidal or triterpenoid in structure.

SAQUINAVIR (Rx) • *See* Invirase.

SARCOMA • A form of cancer arising mainly from connective tissue.

SARGRAMOSTIM (Rx) • **Leukine. Prokine.** A genetically engineered form of GM-CSF (*see*) produced in yeast and introduced in 1991. It is used to reconstitute bone marrow after organ transplantation, to accelerate recovery in patients with non-Hodgkin's lymphoma after bone-marrow transplant, and to accelerate bone-marrow recovery after chemotherapy. Promotes the growth, differentiation, and activation of infection-fighting white blood cells.

SARISOL No. 2 • *See* Butabarbital Sodium.

SARNA LOTION (OTC) • A combination of menthol, phenol, and camphor, used to soothe itchy skin.

SARS • Homeopathic abbreviation for sarsaparilla root (*see*).

SARSAPARILLA ROOT (H) • *Smilax officinalis.* **Sars.** A member of a large family of related *Smilax* species, sarsaparilla was independently discovered in the United States, Honduras, Mexico, and China. It has long been used by herbalists to treat arthritis and syphilis. It contains saponins (*see*). The plant is a strong diuretic and contains antibiotic agents. It lowers the urea content of the blood, promotes sweating, and has been used to treat psoriasis. Indians used it for coughs, high blood pressure, pleurisy, and as a diuretic and a tonic. Externally, it is used for wounds, sore eyes, psoriasis, and burns. Until 1950, sarsaparilla was included in the USP (*see*) for the treatment of secondary syphilis. Contraindicated in kidney dysfunction.

S.A.S.-ENTERIC • *See* Sulfasalazine.

SAS-500 • *See* Sulfasalazine and Sulfa Drugs.

SASSAFRAS BARK EXTRACT (H) • *Sassafras albidium.* **Safrole. Safrole-Free. Saxafrax.** It is the yellow to reddish yellow volatile oil obtained from the root bark of the sassafras tree. It is 80 percent safrole and has the characteristic odor and taste of sassafras. Applied to insect bites and stings to relieve symptoms; also a topical antiseptic and used medicinally to break up intestinal gas. Herbalists use it as a traditional springtime tonic. May produce dermatitis in hypersensitive individuals. The extract was banned in the United States by the FDA for use in foods and drugs because sassafras is considered a cancer-causing agent.

SASTID • *See* Salicylic Acid and Sulfur.

SATRIC 500 • *See* Metronidazole.

SATUREIA HORTENSIS • *See* Savory.

SAVORY (H) • *Satureia hortensis. Satureia montana.* Both summer and winter savories are native to France and Italy and were first cultivated in England in 1562. They were brought to the United States by English settlers. A member of the mint family, savory is used for indigestion, toothache, and to soothe insect stings. Savory is also a good insect repellent.

SAW PALMETTO (H) • *Seronoa serrulata.* **Sabal. Seronoa.** The fruit is used to treat debilitating and wasting conditions, prostatic enlargement, urinary tract infections, as an aphrodisiac, and for bodybuilding. Herbalists use it to treat "honeymoon cystitis," urinary-tract problems due to frequent sexual activity. The FDA does not recognize saw palmetto as a drug, but in Germany it is used in over-the-counter treatments for benign prostate enlargement. Saw palmetto contains anti-inflammatory agents, carotene, tannin, and estrogenic substances. It is a strong expectorant. In 1992, the FDA proposed a ban on saw palmetto in oral menstrual drug products because it had not been shown to be safe and effective as claimed.

SCABANACA • *See* Benzyl Benzoate.

SCABENE • *See* Lindane.

SCABIES • **The Itch.** A transmissible parasitic skin infection characterized by intense itching and secondary infection. It is caused by the mite *Sarcoptes scabiei.* The impregnated female mite tunnels into the skin and deposits her eggs along the burrow. The larvae hatch within a few days and congregate around the hair follicles. Lesions are thought to result from hypersensitivity to the parasites.

SCAMMONY (H) • *Convolvulus scammonia.* A climbing plant native to the Mediterranean region, it is used in homeopathic medicine as a diuretic. Contraindicated in pregnancy and in gastrointestinal inflammation and kidney disease. It is toxic in excessive amounts.

SCARLET PIMPERNEL • *See* Pimpernel, Scarlet.

SCAVENGER CELLS • Any of a diverse group of cells that have the capacity to engulf and destroy foreign material, dead tissue, or other cells.

SCHAMBERG'S LOTION (OTC) • A lotion containing zinc oxide, menthol, phenol (*see all*), cottonseed oil, olive oil, and lime water. Used to treat itching and eczema.

SCHIZANDRA (H) • *Schisandra chinesis.* An herb used by Chinese women as an aphrodisiac and youth tonic. It is a mild sedative. Also believed to increase stamina. Schizandra has been shown in modern scientific laboratories to protect against the narcotic and sedative effects of alcohol and barbiturates. It is used as a tea. Contraindicated in persons with high blood pressure, epilepsy, and increased pressure on the brain.

SCHIZOPHRENIA • A large group of severe disorders of unknown cause, typically characterized by disturbances of language and communication: thought disturbances that may involve distortion of reality, misperceptions, and sometimes, delusions and hallucinations; and mood changes, and withdrawn, regressive, or bizarre behavior. These symptoms must last longer than six months to fall into the category of schizophrenia.

SCIATICA • Pain in the back of the thigh and leg along the course of the sciatic nerve.

SCLER- • Combination form meaning hardness, as in *arteriosclerosis,* hardening of the arteries.

SCLERITIS • Inflammation of the sclera (the white of the eye).

SCLERODERMA • **Systemic Sclerosis.** An autoimmune disease that involves thickening of the skin caused by swelling and thickening of fibrous tissue in a scarlike overgrowth. It causes a person to become "hidebound." Small blood vessels are also affected. Kidney, lung, gastrointestinal, and skin diseases are particularly troublesome to scleroderma patients.

SCLEROMATE • *See* Morrhuate.

SCOPARIUS • *See* Broom.

SCOPOLAMINE (RX) (OTC) • **Hyonatal. Hyoscine. Hyosophen. Isopto Hyoscine. Kinesed. Murocoll-2. Relaxadan. Spasmolin. Spasquid. Transderm Scop. Twilight Sleep.** An anticholinergic, antispasmodic drug used to treat irritable bowel syndrome, parkinsonism, and other spastic states. It is used through a skin patch to prevent nausea and vomiting associated with motion sickness. Used preoperatively to reduce secretions. Also used in eye drops to dilate the pupil. Potential adverse reactions include disorientation, restlessness, irritability, dizziness, drowsiness, headache, heart palpitations, rapid heartbeat, slow heartbeat, dilated pupils, blurred vision, sensitivity to light, increased eye pressure, difficulty in swallowing, urinary retention, flushing, rash, skin dryness, fever, and depressed respiration. Alcohol and other central nervous system depressants may increase central nervous system depression. The eye drops may cause transient stinging on instillation, increased eye pressure, blurred vision, and sensitivity to light. Also may cause some of the systemic effects mentioned above. Centrally acting anticholinergics such as tricyclic antidepressants and phenothiazine increase adverse central nervous system reactions. Use with digoxin increases digoxin levels. Contraindicated in glaucoma, obstructive diseases of the urinary or GI tracts, asthma, chronic pulmonary disease, myasthenia gravis (*see*), paralytic ileus (*see*), flaccid intestines, unstable cardiovascular status in acute hemorrhage, and toxic megacolon. Used with caution in patients with nerve damage, overactive thyroid, coronary artery disease, irregular heartbeat, hiatal hernia, liver or kidney dysfunction, ulcerative colitis, and in patients over forty years of age due to the possibility of glaucoma. Should be used with caution in hot or humid environment; drug-induced heatstroke may occur. In therapeutic doses, scopolamine may produce amnesia,

drowsiness, and euphoria. If symptoms of urinary retention occur, check with your physician promptly. The use of scopolamine hydrobromide in OTC sleep aids was deemed ineffective by the FDA in 1990, and products using it had to be reformulated or be banned.

SCOPOLIA (H) • *Scopolia carniolica.* A toxic herb native to Europe, it is a source of hyoscyamine (*see*). It is used in homeopathic medicine to treat agitation.

SCOTOMA • An area of depressed vision in the visual field, usually surrounded by an area of normal vision.

SCOTS PINE • *See* Pine, Scots.

SCOURING RUSH (H) • *Equisetum hyemale.* **Shave Grass. Hyland's Bed Wetting Tablets.** The leaves and roots of this perennial plant are used in a homeopathic preparation for temporary relief of involuntary urination and bedwetting in children. *See also* Horsetail.

SCROPHULARIA NODOSA • *See* Figwort.

SCULLCAP • *See* Skullcap.

SCURVY GRASS EXTRACT (H) • *Cochlearia officinalis.* The extract of the leaves and flower stalks. The bright green leaves of this northerly herb were collected and eaten in large quantities by European seamen to prevent scurvy. The plant has a strong odor of horseradish, to which it is related.

SCUTELLARIA LATERIFOLIA • *See* Skullcap.

SD ALCOHOL (OTC) • **Oxy Medicated Pads. Stri-Dex Pads.** Alcohols for topical use only, which have had a chemical added to them to make them unfit for drinking.

SEA HOLLY (H) • *Eryngium maritimum.* This European plant is found on sandy shores and is used by herbalists to treat many urinary ailments.

A diuretic, it is often used to treat kidney stones and gravel, especially if there is urinary retention. Herbalists maintain it will ease colic due to urinary problems, as well as reduce hemorrhage. It can help, they say, in cystitis, urethritis, and enlarged and inflamed prostate gland.

SEBAQUIN • *See* Iodoquinol.

SEBORRHEIC DERMATITIS • Skin inflammation caused by overactivity of the oil glands in the skin.

SEBUCARE • *See* Salicylic Acid.

SEBULEX (OTC) • *See* Salicylic Acid and Sulfur.

SEBULON (OTC) • An antidandruff shampoo containing zinc pyrithione (*see*).

SEBUTONE (OTC) • A shampoo containing coal tar, salicylic acid, and sulfur (*see all*).

SECOBARBITAL SODIUM (Rx) • **Quinalbarbitone. Seconal. Tuinal.** A barbiturate sleeping drug in use since the 1930s that probably interferes with the transmission of impulses from the thalamus to the cortex of the brain. Used in preoperative sedation, insomnia, continuous seizures, and acute tetanus (*see*) seizure. Potential adverse reactions include drowsiness, lethargy, hangover, paradoxical excitement in elderly patients, nausea, vomiting, rash, hives, and exacerbation of porphyria (*see*). Alcohol or other central nervous system depressants, including narcotic analgesics, may cause excessive central nervous system and respiratory system depression. MAO inhibitors (*see*) may cause prolonged effects of barbiturates. Secobarbital may decrease the effectiveness of griseofulvin, oral blood thinners, estrogens, oral contraceptives, doxycycline, and corticosteroids (*see all*). Rifampin may decrease barbiturate levels, making them less effective. Contraindicated in uncontrolled severe pain, respiratory disease with shortness of breath or obstruction, hypersensitivity to barbiturates, previous addiction to sedatives, or porphyria.

Should be used with caution in liver or kidney impairment, and in pregnant women with toxemia or a history of bleeding. Elderly patients are more sensitive to the drug's adverse central nervous system effects. When discontinued, increased dreaming may occur. Most effective when taken on an empty stomach, but may be taken with a small amount of food if stomach upset is a problem.

SECONAL • *See* Secobarbital Sodium.

SECONDARY EFFECT • A by-product or complication of a drug use that does not occur as part of the drug's primary pharmacological activity.

SECTRAL • *See* Acebutolol.

SECUROPEN • *See* Azlocillin.

SEDABAMATE • *See* Meprobamate.

SEDAPAP-50 • A combination of acetaminophen and butalbital (*see both*) used to treat pain.

SEDATIVE • A compound that calms the nervous system and reduces stress and anxiety. Phenobarbital is an example of a prescription drug for this purpose. Diphenhydramine is an example of a nonprescription sedative, and valerian and skullcap are examples of herbs used for this purpose.

SEDGE ROOT • *See* Cyperus.

SEDIMENTATION RATE • The rate at which red blood cells settle out of a prepared specimen of blood under laboratory conditions. Used in the diagnosis of certain diseases.

SEFFIN • *See* Cephalothin.

SELDANE • *See* Terfenadine.

SELEGILINE HYDROCHLORIDE (Rx) • **Eldepryl. L-deprenyl Hydrochloride. Deprenyl.** A dopamine-boosting drug introduced in 1989 related to the monoamine oxidase inhibitors (*see*). Used as an adjunctive treatment to carbidopa-levodopa (*see*) to relieve symptoms of Parkinson's disease. It reportedly provides a more effective and uniform control of Parkinson's symptoms with a reduction of some adverse affects associated with long-term carbidopa-levodopa use. Potential adverse reactions include involuntary grimacing, awkward or slow movements, jerking, tremor, behavioral changes, stiff neck, restlessness, fatigue, headache, a drop in blood pressure upon rising from a seated or prone position, low blood pressure, irregular heartbeat, swelling, faintness, nausea, vomiting, loss of appetite, weight loss, trouble in swallowing, heartburn, dry mouth, bitter taste, urinary frequency or retention, incontinence, sexual dysfunction, sweating, and hair loss. Medications for high blood pressure may cause additive low blood pressure effects. Must be careful about taking foods with tyramine (*see*), such as wine or herring, because the combination may cause the blood pressure to shoot up. Should be taken with food or milk to reduce stomach irritation.

SELENIUM (Rx) (OTC) (H) • **Selenious Acid. Episel. Exsel. Glo-Sel. Selenitrace. Selenium Yeast. Selsun Blue.** A mineral that is a yellow solid or brownish powder. Selenium was discovered in 1807 in the earth's crust. Used as a nutrient. Works in association with vitamin E to preserve elasticity in the tissues, thus slowing down aging. It also reportedly increases endurance by improving the supply of oxygen to the heart muscle. Selenium is necessary for the formation of prostaglandins (*see*). It is available over the counter in single-ingredient tablets and in capsules in combination with vitamin E. A connection between cancer of the colon and selenium deficiencies has become apparent through epidemiological studies. Also available on prescription. Deficiency may result in loss of stamina and reduced tissue elasticity. Selenium is the most toxic of the dietary minerals. Potential adverse reactions include nausea, vomiting, baldness, loss of nails and teeth, fatigue, and bad breath. A massive overdose can be fatal. *See also* Selenium Sulfide.

SELENIUM SULFIDE • **Exsel Shampoo. Head & Shoulders Intensive Treatment Dandruff Shampoo. Selsun Blue Dandruff Shampoo-Extra Medicated.** Discovered in 1807 in the earth's crust, it is used in antidandruff shampoos and applied to the skin for the treatment of tinea versicolor (*see*). Can severely irritate the eyes if it gets into them while hair is being washed. May cause dryness or oiliness of hair or scalp and, rarely, an increase in the amount of hair normally lost.

SELF-HEAL (H) • *Prunella vulgaris.* A perennial Eurasian mint native to many countries. New England settlers used it to cure "female troubles," and as a tonic. Among self-heal's ingredients are volatile oil, bitter principle, and tannin (*see all*). Used by herbalists as an infusion, as an herbal treatment and general tonic. Externally, it is used in poultice as an antiseptic for wounds and to stop bleeding. Also used to treat diarrhea, sore throat, and hemorrhoids. It is currently being studied for its ability to significantly inhibit HIV-1 replication with relatively low toxicity to the cells.

SELSUN • *See* Selenium Sulfide.

SEMETS • *See* Benzocaine.

SEMICID (OTC) • Spermicidal suppositories containing nonoxynol-9 (*see*).

SEMPERVIVUM TECTORUM • *See* Houseleek.

SEMPREX D (Rx) • A combination antihistamine and decongestant medication for the treatment of symptoms related to seasonal allergic rhinitis. Introduced in 1994 after a 22.2-month review by the FDA. It has been used in Denmark since 1992. *See* Acrivastine and Pseudoephedrine.

SEMUSTINE • **Methyl CCNU.** An investigational anticancer drug used to treat advanced intestinal tumors, brain tumors, and Hodgkin's and non-Hodgkin's lymphomas.

SENECIO AUREUS (OTC) (H) • Golden Ragwort. Life Root. Squaw Weed. Dried plant of *Senecio aureus,* which grows in Canada and the eastern United States. It is used to increase menstrual flow. In 1992, the FDA proposed a ban on *Senecio aureus* in oral menstrual drug products because it had not been shown to be safe and effective as claimed.

SENEGA SNAKEROOT (H) • *Polygala senega.* Snake Root. The North American Indians, particularly the Seneca, used this for snakebite. It contains saponins, mucilage, salicylic acid, and resin. Used by herbalists as an expectorant in the treatment of bronchial asthma. Also used to stimulate saliva, and to treat sore throats and laryngitis. If too much is taken, it irritates the lining of the gut and causes vomiting, according to herbalists.

SENNA (OTC) (H) • *Cassia angustifolia. Cassia acutifolia.* Fletcher's Castoria. Gentle Nature Natural Vegetable Laxative Tablets. Nytilax. Perdiem Granules. Senokot. Senolax. Dried leaves and pods of the genus *Cassia,* grown in India and Egypt. Contains anthraquinones (*see*), tartaric acid, mucin, salts, and traces of tannin (*see*). Used as a laxative. In 1992, the FDA issued a notice that senna had not been shown to be safe and effective as claimed in OTC digestive-aid products. *See* Laxative.

SENOKOT • *See* Senna.

SENOLAX • *See* Senna.

SENSITIVITY • Hypersensitivity. An increased reaction to a substance that may be quite harmless to nonallergic persons. An adverse reaction, usually allergic, to a drug.

SENSITIZE • To administer or expose to an antigen provoking an immune response so that, on later exposure to that antigen, a more vigorous secondary response will occur.

SENSODYNE TOOTHPASTE • *See* Potassium Nitrate.

SENSORCAINE • *See* Bupivacaine.

SEP • Homeopathic abbreviation for sepia (*see*).

SEPIA (H) • Sep. Cuttlefish. Squid. A homeopathic medicine made from mollusks. The name *sepia* is derived from the dried brownish black ink, which is used by artists. The pure pigment is used in remedies for colds, anger, backache, cold sores, cystitis, constipation, exhaustion, eye inflammation, fever, hair loss, headache, hot flushes, insomnia, labor pains, nausea, menstrual problems, toothache, and vomiting.

SEPSIS • Blood Poisoning. Fever, chills, and other reactions of the body to bacteria or to their toxins in the bloodstream.

SEPTICEMIA • The presence of bacteria or other microorganisms in the bloodstream. A potentially fatal condition.

SEPTISOL • *See* Triclosan.

SEPTRA (Rx) • Bactrim. Bethaprim. Comoxol. Cotrim. Co-Trimoxazole. Sulfatrim. Sulmeprim. TMP-SMZ. All are combinations of sulfamethoxazole and trimethoprim (*see both*), an inexpensive antibiotic that has been found to be useful in treating *Pneumocystis carinii* pneumonia (PCP), the most common, life-threatening opportunistic infection affecting Americans with AIDS. Potential adverse reactions include nausea, vomiting, allergic reactions, blood disorders, arthritis-like pain, abdominal pain, diarrhea, headache, tingling in the arms or legs, depression, convulsions, hallucinations, ringing in the ears, dizziness, insomnia, malaise, weakness, kidney dysfunction, sensitivity to light, and nervousness. Contraindicated if a folic-acid deficiency is present or allergy exists to any of the ingredients. Septra and the other versions of this compound may prolong the effects of blood thinners such as warfarin and antidiabetic oral drugs. Each dose should be taken with a full glass of water, and fluids should be continued throughout the day to decrease the chances of kidney problems. *See* Co-Trimoxazole.

SER-AP-ES (Rx) • **Cam-Ap-Es. Cherapas. H-H-R. Ser-A-Gen. Seralazide. Tri-Hydroserpine. Unipres.** A combination of hydralazine, hydrochlorothiazide, and reserpine to treat high blood pressure. Potential adverse reactions include nausea, vomiting, headache, loss of appetite, diarrhea, irregular heartbeat, chest pains, drowsiness, cramps, tingling in the arms and legs, restlessness, depression, anxiety, nightmares, glaucoma, blood disorders, rash, itching, fever, difficulty breathing, muscle spasms, weakness, high blood sugar, blurred vision, stuffy nose, dry mouth, rash, impotence and decreased sex drive, flushing, tearing of the eyes, red eyes, confusion, and for long-term users, possible liver dysfunction. Contraindicated in persons allergic to any of its ingredients, or with a history of mental depression, active peptic ulcer, and ulcerative colitis. Long-term use in large doses may produce arthritis-like symptoms. Loss of potassium may occur, and if a potassium supplement is not prescribed, your physician may want you to increase high-potassium foods such as bananas, citrus fruit, and tomatoes. Should be taken with food.

SERAX • *See* Oxazepam.

SERENTIL • *See* Mesoridazine Besylate.

SEREVENT INHALATION AEROSOL • *See* Salmeterol Xinafoate.

SEROLOGICAL TESTS • Blood tests that detect the presence of antigens or antibodies in the blood.

SEROMYCIN • *See* Cycloserine.

SEROPHENE • *See* Clomiphene Citrate.

SEROTONIN • A natural neurotransmitter (chemical messenger between nerve cells) in the brain. Low levels are associated with depression, and some antidepressants seem to work by triggering increased production of serotonin. The substance also plays a role in temperature regulation and sleep. A class of antidepressant drugs such as Prozac and Zoloft work by raising the serotonin levels in the brain. They are reportedly effective in two-thirds of the patients taking them but, as of this writing, are more expensive than the tricyclics (*see*). Serotonin enhancers are also reportedly less potentially toxic than tricyclic antidepressants.

SERPALAN • *See* Reserpine.

SERPASIL • *See* Reserpine.

SERPATE • *See* Reserpine.

SERPENTARY • *See* Echinacea.

SERPENT'S TONGUE • *See* Adder's-Tongue.

SERRATIA • Gram-negative (*see*) bacteria found in water, soil, milk, foods, and insects. May be found in hospital-acquired infections in patients with impaired immunity.

SERTRALINE HCL (Rx) • **Zoloft.** A selective serotonin increaser introduced in 1991, it is indicated for the treatment of depression and promoted as a once-a-day medication. It reportedly has a lower incidence of tricycliclike side effects, and a low incidence of nervousness, anxiety, and agitation. The most common side effects are nausea, diarrhea, tremor, insomnia, sleepiness, and dry mouth. Other potential side effects include sweating, heart palpitations, chest pain, headache, dizziness, numbness, twitching, rash, constipation, heartburn, vomiting, gas, loss of appetite, abdominal pain, increased appetite, fatigue, hot flushes, fever, back pain, thirst, muscle pain, impotence, agitation, nervousness, anxiety, yawning, female sexual dysfunction, stuffy nose, menstrual disorder, abnormal vision, ringing in the ears, taste perversion, and urinary frequency. May cause warfarin and digitoxin to become more toxic. No contraindications, but when patients receiving other serotonin increasers also receive MAO inhibitors (*see*), sometimes fatal reactions have occurred.

SERUM • The clear portion of the blood, separated from its solid elements.

SERUM SICKNESS • Animals are injected with toxins to build up antibodies. Their serum is used to make antitoxins for humans. But such "foreign" serum can produce an allergic reaction that appears eight to twelve days after serum is injected. Other drugs, notably penicillins, given by needle or by mouth, may produce a syndrome indistinguishable from serum sickness. With the development of biotechnology and the use of laboratory-multiplied human antibodies, serum sickness will become less common.

SERUTAN • *See* Psyllium.

SERZONE • *See* Nefazodone.

SESQUITERPENES • In recent years, more than six hundred plants have been identified as containing these substances, and more than fifty are known to cause allergic contact dermatitis. Among them are arnica, chamomile, and yarrow.

SEVEN BARKS • *See* Hydrangea.

SEVERE COMBINED IMMUNODEFICIENCY DISEASE • **SCID.** Combined deficiency of white blood cells, leaving a patient virtually defenseless against all types of infection.

SEVIN • *See* Carbaryl.

SEVOFLURANE (Rx) • **Ultrane.** A rapid-acting inhalation anesthetic introduced in 1995.

SHANKA PUSPI (H) • *Confolvulus mycrophyllus.* An herb used in India to treat anxiety and mild pain.

SHAO-YAO • *See* Peony.

SHARK • **Shark Cartilage. Squalamine.** The killer of the deep is being studied as a source of antibiotics and anticancer drugs. Shark cartilage has been used in alternative medicine as an anti-cancer and anti-AIDS compound because sharks apparently do not suffer from cancer. Mainstream medical researchers are now studying squalamine, a unique compound isolated from sharks that kills a variety of bacteria, fungi, and parasites. Sharks' immune systems are different from humans', and shark derivatives are now under intensive study for treatment of AIDS and cancers.

SHARK LIVER OIL (OTC) (H) • **Preparation H Hemorrhoidal Ointment. Wyanoids Relief Factor Hemorrhoidal Suppositories.** A brown, fatty oil obtained from the liver of the large predatory fish. A rich source of vitamin A; believed to be beneficial to the skin. Used in lubricating creams and lotions, and suppositories.

SHAVE GRASS • *See* Horsetail and Scouring Rush.

SHEPHERD'S PURSE EXTRACT (H) • **Shepherd's Heart.** Extract of the herb *Capsella bursa-pastoris,* a member of the mustard family. Pungent and bitter, it was valued for its astringent properties by early American settlers. Cotton moistened with its juice was used to stop nosebleed. In an oil-in-water emulsion, it is used as a base for skin preparations. Among its constituents are saponins, choline, acetylcholine, and tyramine (*see all*). These preparations are used in modern medicine to stimulate neuromuscular function. The herb also reduces urinary tract irritation and has been shown to contract the uterus and lower blood pressure.

SHIGELLA BACILLUS • An acid-producing type of bacterium that causes acute inflammation of the intestines.

SHIGELLOSIS • **Bacillary Dysentery.** Acute diarrhea, acquired by person-to-person contact, through eating contaminated food or handling contaminated objects, or through spread of contamination by flies. The causative germs are present in the excretions of infected persons. Infection is caused by rod-shaped bacteria, *Shigella* bacilli.

SHIITAKE MUSHROOM (H) • *Lentinus edodes.* The mushrooms contain lentinan, a type of sugar that has been shown to slow the growth of cancerous tumors in animals. Used as a cancer-fighting agent in Japan and China. Shiitake also reportedly lowers cholesterol. Lentinan is now being studied as a candidate to treat AIDS.

SHINGLES • *See* Herpes Varicella-Zoster Virus.

SHOHL'S SOLUTION (Rx) • A urinary alkalinizer. *See* Sodium Citrate and Citric Acid.

SHUR-SEAL • *See* Nonoxynol-9.

SIALOGOGUE • A medication that promotes the flow of saliva. Herbs used for this purpose are cayenne and gentian. Glandosane is a prescription spray used as a substitute for saliva, and Salivart is an OTC saliva substitute.

SIBLIN • *See* Psyllium.

SICKLE-CELL ANEMIA • An inherited blood disorder in which red cells are abnormal in shape and contain an abnormal oxygen-carrying pigment, resulting in chronic, severe anemia and the characteristic sickle shape of the red cell. *See* Hydroxyurea.

SIDE EFFECT • An unintended but sometimes not unexpected effect of a medication on the body, apart from the medication's principal and intended action.

SIGAMINE • *See* Vitamin B_{12}.

SIL • Homeopathic abbreviation for silica. *See* Silicea.

SILAIN • *See* Simethicone.

SILAIN GEL • *See* Aluminum Hydroxide, Magnesium Hydroxide, and Simethicone.

SILERIS (H) • *Ledebouriella divaricata.* **Fangfeng.** The root is used by Chinese herbalists to treat spasm, flu, headache, chills, numbness, pain in the joints, and tetanus.

SILICA • *See* Silicea.

SILICEA (H) • **Sil. Silica. Silicic Acid.** A homeopathic medicine (*see*) composed of an odorless, tasteless substance that is abundant in nature. It is used as an adsorbent food additive and in toilet products because it is soothing to the skin. It is used by homeopaths to treat thick, yellow mucous discharges, swollen glands, nausea, headache, sweating, and vomiting. *See* Silicic Acid.

SILICIC ACID • **Silica Gel.** A white, gelatinous substance obtained by the action of acids on sodium silicate. Absorbs water readily. Soothing to the skin.

SILVADENE • *See* Silver Sulfadiazine.

SILVER NITRATE (Rx) (H) • A topical antibacterial and astringent used to prevent gonorrheal infections of the eyes in newborns. Potential adverse reactions include swelling around the eyes and eye irritation. In 1992, the FDA proposed a ban on silver nitrate in astringent (*see*) drug products because it had not been shown to be safe and effective as claimed. Homeopaths use it under the name argentum nitricum (*see*).

SILVER PROTEIN (OTC) • **Argyrol.** Combined with protein, it is used as an antiseptic in treating eye infections. Has no astringent (*see*) in it and so is less irritating to the eyes.

SILVER SULFADIAZINE (Rx) • **Flamazine. Silvadene. SSD. Thermazene.** An antibacterial cream used to prevent and treat wound infections, especially for second- and third-degree burns. Potential adverse reactions include a drop in white blood cells, pain, burning, rash, and itching. Should not be used by persons sensitive to sulfonamides.

SILVERWEED (H) • *Potentilla anserina.* This weed contains tannins, flavonoids, bitter principle (*see all*), and organic acids. It is an astringent used by herbalists to control the overproduction of mucus. Taken internally for hemorrhoids, or used in a compress. Also used in a mouthwash for inflamed gums and mouth ulcers, and in an infusion for sore throat.

SIMECO • *See* Simethicone.

SIMETHICONE (OTC) • **Di-Gel. Extra Strength Gas-X. Flatulex. Gelusil. Maalox. Mylanta. Mylicon Drops. Mylicon-80. Phazyme. Phazyme-95. Riopan. Silain. Tums Plus Antacid Anti-Gas Tablets.** A silicone-based substance derived from silica, which occurs abundantly in nature. It is included as an antifoaming agent in many medications for the relief of excess gas and indigestion. A potential adverse reaction is excessive expulsion of gas as belching and rectal flatus. Should not be taken indiscriminately. Tablets should be chewed before swallowing. In 1992, the FDA issued a notice that simethicone had not been shown to be safe and effective as claimed in OTC poison ivy, poison oak, and poison sumac products.

SIMILASAN • Homeopathic (*see*) eye drops containing belladonna HPUS 6X, Eurphrasia HPUS 6X, Mercurius sublimatus HPUS, SoluSept, natrium chloratum and purified water. Aimed at giving the user relief from dry, red, irritated eye, inflammation of the eyelids, hypersensitivity to light, tired, strained eyes and watery eyes.

SIMILIMUM • A homeopathic remedy that matches the symptom of the patient most closely. Based on the law *Similia similibus curantur*—like is cured by like *(see* page 9).

SIMRON • *See* Ferrous Gluconate.

SIMVASTATIN (Rx) • **Zocor.** A cholesterol-lowering drug introduced in 1991. Potential adverse reactions include headache, abdominal pain, constipation, upper-respiratory infection, diarrhea, flatulence, weakness, nausea, heartburn, and hypersensitivity reactions. Liver dysfunction may occur, thus liver-function tests are indicated before and during therapy with simvastatin. If there is muscle tenderness or weakness, you should advise your physician promptly, especially if accompanied by malaise or fever. Rare cases of potentially fatal rhabdomyolysis *(see)* with acute kidney failure have been associated with simvas-

tatin therapy. Rhabdomyolysis has also been associated with other lipid-lowering drugs. Simvastatin enhances warfarin's blood-thinning effects. *See* HMG-COA Reductase Inhibitors.

SINAREST NASAL SOLUTION • *See* Phenylephrine.

SINCALIDE (Rx) • A substance secreted by the stomach, intestines, and the pancreas, it is used as a drug to stimulate bile *(see)*.

SINE-AID (OTC) • *See* Acetaminophen and Pseudoephedrine.

SINEMET (Rx) • A combination of carbidopa and levodopa *(see both)* prescribed for Parkinson's disease. Carbidopa prevents vitamin B_6 from destroying levodopa, the active ingredient that treats the symptoms of Parkinson's. The combination is so effective that the amount of levodopa can be reduced by about 75 percent, which results in fewer side effects. Potential adverse reactions include nausea, vomiting, loss of appetite, uncontrolled muscle movements, dry mouth, difficulty in swallowing, dribbling of saliva, shaking of the hands, headache, dizziness, numbness, weakness, faintness, tooth grinding, agitation, anxiety, hallucinations, nightmares, fatigue, euphoria, heart palpitations, a drop in blood pressure when rising from a seated or prone position, lack of alertness, mental changes including paranoia, psychosis, and depression, and burning tongue, bitter taste, diarrhea, constipation, stomach gas, flushing, sweating, double or blurred vision, respiratory changes, dilation of the pupils, hot flashes, changes in body weight, stomach ulcer, high blood pressure, blood disorders, convulsions, fluid retention, hair loss, hoarseness of the voice, persistent penile erection, and bleeding of the stomach. Should not be taken if sensitivity has occurred with either component of the drug. The effectiveness of Sinemet may be increased by taking drugs with an anticholinergic *(see)* effect, such as Donnatal. Methyldopa, a blood-pressure-lowering medication, has the same effect on levodopa as does carbidopa. It can increase the amount of levodopa available to the brain. Patients taking guanethidine or a diuretic to treat high blood pressure may need less antihypertensive medication. Reserpine, benzodiazepine tranquilizers, major tranquilizers, phenytoin, and papaverine (*see all*) may interfere with the effects of Sinemet. Diabetics may need diabetes medication adjustment when taking Sinemet. MAO inhibitors (*see*) may cause a dangerous rise in blood pressure if taken within two weeks of taking Sinemet. Sinemet may increase the effects of ephedrine, amphetamines, epinephrine, and isoproterenol (*see all*) and may adversely affect the heart. This reaction may also occur with some antidepressants. This drug may be taken with food.

SINEQUAN • *See* Doxepin.

SINEX • *See* Phenylephrine.

SINEX LONG-ACTING • *See* Oxymetazoline.

SINGLET (OTC) • **Comtrex A/S. Drixoral Plus. Sine-Off Extra Strength. Sinus Nighttime Formula. Sinutab Maximum Strength. Sinutab Tablets. Teldrin MultiSymptom.** All these medications contain a combination of acetaminophen, chlorpheniramine, and phenylephrine (*see all*) to treat symptoms of the common cold, influenza, and other upper-respiratory diseases. Potential adverse reactions include nausea, vomiting, drowsiness, high blood pressure, restlessness, tension, tremor, weakness, insomnia, headache, heart palpitations, loss of appetite, dizziness, and constipation. Interaction with alcoholic beverages, sedatives, tranquilizers, antihistamines, and sleeping pills may produce excessive drowsiness and inability to concentrate. Over-the-counter drugs for the relief of cold symptoms may increase the side effects of singlet and similar drugs. None should be taken with MAO inhibitors (*see*) since severe high blood pressure may result. Singlet and the other medications may be taken with food.

SINTISONE • *See* Prednisolone.

SINUBID (OTC) • A combination of acetaminophen, phenylpropanolamine, and phenyltoloxamine (*see all*) to treat runny nose, congestion, and other symptoms of the common cold, influenza, and other upper-respiratory diseases. Potential adverse reactions include nausea, vomiting, drowsiness, high blood pressure, sweating, dizziness, constipation, insomnia, weakness, nervousness, tremor, headache, heart palpitations, and loss of appetite. Contraindicated in glaucoma and in difficulty urinating. Alcoholic beverages, sedatives, tranquilizers, other antihistamines, and sleeping pills may increase drowsiness and inability to concentrate if taken with Sinubid. Over-the-counter medications for cold symptoms taken with Sinubid may increase blood pressure and aggravate heart disease, diabetes, or thyroid disease. Sinubid should not be taken with MAO inhibitors (*see*) as severe high blood pressure may result. This medicine may be taken with food.

SINUFED • *See* Pseudoephedrine.

SINULIN (OTC) • A combination of acetaminophen, chlorpheniramine, and phenylpropanolamine (*see all*).

SINUS FORMULA (H) • **Sinuspax.** A homeopathic remedy to relieve sneezing, itching in nose or throat, watery eyes, runny nose, nasal congestion and headache due to sinusitis, hay fever, upper respiratory allergies, or the common cold. Contains kalium bichromicum 5x to relieve nasal symptoms, cough, and bronchitis; silicea 5x to relieve nasal inflammation and sore throat; and mercurius sulphuratus ruber 4x to relieve dry cough, chills, and runny nose. (*See* Kali Bichromicum, Silica, and Mercurius Corrosivus.) It also contains, among other things, belladonna 3x (*see*) and thuja 2x (*see*).

SINUSOL-B • *See* Brompheniramine.

SINUTAB (OTC) • A combination of acetaminophen, chlorpheniramine, and pseudoephedrine (*see all*). A decongestant and pain reliever for symptoms of cold or allergy.

SJOGREN'S SYNDROME • A condition in which the eyes, mouth, and vagina become excessively dry.

SKELAXIN • *See* Metaxalone.

SK-POTASSIUM CHLORIDE • *See* Potassium Chloride.

SK-PRAMINE • *See* Imipramine.

SKULLCAP (H) • *Scutellaria laterifolia.* **Mad Dog. Mad Weed. Huang Chi. Quaker Bonnet. Scullcap.** Grown throughout the world, there are about ninety known species. Skullcap was used to cure infertility. The sedative and antispasmodic properties led to its use in treating rabies, hence its popular name, "mad dog scullcap." It was also used to treat delirium tremens and infants' teething. Herbalists use it today for relief of epilepsy, convulsions, and withdrawal from drug and alcohol addiction. It is also used as a sedative. Widely used during the nineteenth century to treat nervous diseases, convulsion, neuralgia, insomnia, restlessness, and even tetanus. Modern scientists have found that it stabilizes blood pressure. Skullcap tea is used as a mild tranquilizer. Cases of liver toxicity caused by the use of this herb have been reported to the Centers for Disease Control.

SKUNK CABBAGE (H) • *Symplocarpus foetidus.* A swamp plant, a member of the arum family, it gives out a smell like a skunk. A poultice of the root was used to cover open wounds. The leaf bases were applied to reduce swellings. Herbalists still use it in a tea for coughs and catarrh. Credited with antispasmodic, emetic, diuretic, and narcotic properties, skunk cabbage has been used to treat tuberculosis, pleurisy, whooping cough, chronic coughing spells, fluid retention, twitching, hysteria, asthma, and hay fever. Contact with the skin may cause blistering of the skin.

SLEEP APNEA • A potentially fatal disorder in which breathing stops during sleep for ten seconds or more, sometimes more than three hundred times a night.

SLEEP-EZE (OTC) • Approved as a sleep aid by the FDA. *See* Diphenhydramine.

SLEEPINAL MEDICATED NIGHT TEA (OTC) • Approved by the FDA as a sleep aid. *See* Diphenhydramine.

SLEEPINOL (OTC) • Approved by the FDA as an effective sleep aid.

SLIMMING FORMULA (H) • **Fucus Complex.** A homeopathic weight loss remedy containing thryroidium 8x to balance appetite, calcarea acetica 2x to reduce hunger, and fucus vesiculosus 2x as an iodine source. *See* Calc. Carb., Bladder Wrack, and Thyroid.

SLIPPERY ELM (H) • *Ulmus fulva.* **Indian Elm. Moose Elm. Red Elm.** A widely used herbal medicine, it comes from a small tree abundant in North America, from north of the Carolinas to Quebec. Its inner bark, which contains a lot of mucilage, is used for poultices. In a solution, it is used to treat bowel and bladder problems, lung ailments, diarrhea, toothache, stomach and kidney illnesses, boils and ulcers, and infected sores. Also used in cough drops. Its mucilaginous properties supposedly ease childbirth, and it is made into pessaries and suppositories. Also used in an herbal tea for upset stomach, colitis, cough, and sore throat. Among its constituents are mucins, amino acids, and iodine (*see all*).

SLO-BID • *See* Theophylline.

SLO-MAG • *See* Magnesium Chloride and Sulfate.

SLO-NIACIN • *See* Niacin.

SLO-PHYLLIN (Rx) • *See* Theophylline and Guaifenesin.

SLO-SALT • *See* Sodium Chloride.

SLOW FE TABLETS • *See* Ferrous Sulfate.

SLOW-K • *See* Potassium Chloride.

SLYN-LL • *See* Phendimetrazine.

SMELLING SALTS • Smelling preparations, such as ammonia, used as a stimulant.

SMZ-TMP-DS • *See* Sulfamethoxazole and Trimethoprim.

SNAKEROOT • *See* Echinacea.

SNAKEWEED • *See* Bistort.

SNOWDROP (H) • *Galanthus nivalis.* **Bulbous Violet.** A small, herbaceous perennial native to Asia and Europe. It contains nivaline (galanthamine), which is used to treat polio and myasthenia gravis (*see*). It is used in folk medicine to treat spasms and as an emetic. It is toxic in overdose. Symptoms include excessive salivation, vomiting, diarrhea, and in severe cases, paralysis and convulsions.

SOAPWORT (H) • *Saponaria officinalis.* **Bouncing Bet. Bruisewort. Fuller's Herb. Sheep Weed.** The name is derived from the fact that when agitated in water, it lathers. The principal active ingredient, saponin, is a detergent. Soapwort was prescribed by medieval Arab physicians for leprosy and other skin complaints. The leaves yield an extract that has been used to promote sweating as a remedy against rheumatism, and to purify the blood. Toxic when ingested in large amounts. It can irritate the stomach and depress heart action. Contraindicated in cases of acute gastritis and internal bleeding and just after surgical operations.

SODIUM ACETATE • **Sodium Salt of Acetic Acid.** Used medicinally as an alkalizer, and as a diuretic to reduce body water.

SODIUM ACID CARBONATE • *See* Sodium Bicarbonate.

SODIUM AMINOBENZOATE • In 1992, the FDA proposed a ban on sodium aminobenzoate in internal analgesic products because it had not been shown to be safe and effective as claimed. *See* Para-Aminobenzoic Acid.

SODIUM ASCORBATE (OTC) • **Fero-Gradumet. Hyland's Vitamin C for Children. Vitamin C Sodium.** Aside from its use in vitamin C preparations, it serves as an antioxidant. *See* Ascorbic Acid and Vitamin C.

SODIUM BENZOATE • An antiseptic and preservative used in creams. Used medicinally for arthritis and tonsillitis. In 1992, the FDA proposed a ban on sodium benzoate in oral menstrual drug products because it had not been shown to be safe and effective as claimed.

SODIUM BICARBONATE (OTC) • **Baking Soda. Bell Ans. Bicarbonate of Soda. Alka-Seltzer Effervescent Antacid. Arm & Hammer Baking Soda. Citrocarbonate Antacid. Massengill Liquid Concentrate. Neut. Soda Mint.** An alkali prepared by the reaction of soda ash with carbon dioxide. It is used to neutralize excess acid in cardiac arrest, as a systemic or urinary alkalizer, and as an antacid. Potential adverse reactions include gastric distension, belching, kidney stones, and with an overdose, alkalosis, or rebound acidosis, high blood sodium, and high blood potassium. Also used in effervescent bath salts, mouthwashes, and skin-soothing powders. Its white crystals or powder are used as a gastric antacid, alkaline wash, and to treat burns. Essentially harmless to the skin, but when used on very dry skin in preparations that evaporate, it leaves an alkaline residue that may cause irritation. May alter the urinary excretion of other drugs, thus making those drugs either more toxic or less effective. May cause enteric-coated drugs to be prematurely released in the stomach. There are no contraindications for use in life-threatening emergencies. Contraindicated in high blood pressure, in patients with a tendency toward water retention, and in those who are losing chlorides by vomiting or from continuous GI suction. Should not be taken with milk because it can cause high levels of calcium in the blood. *See* Sodium Lactate.

SODIUM BIPHOSPHATE (Rx) • **Uro-Phosphate.** Used to increase urinary acidity.

SODIUM BORATE (OTC) • Collyrium for Fresh Eyes. Eye Wash. A weak antiseptic and astringent for mucous membranes, it is used in eye lotions. Has a drying effect on the skin. In 1992, the FDA issued a notice that sodium borate had not been shown to be safe and effective as claimed in OTC products including insect bite and sting drug products, and in astringent (*see*) drugs. It is, as of this writing, still used in eye products.

SODIUM CAPRYLATE (OTC) (H) • Palm Oil. Oil used in baby soaps, liniments, and ointments. Obtained from the fruit or seed of the palm tree. In 1992, the FDA issued a notice that sodium caprylate had not been shown to be safe and effective as claimed in OTC products.

SODIUM CARBONATE (OTC) • Soda Ash. Small, odorless crystals or powder that occurs in nature in ores and is found in lake brines or seawater. Absorbs water from the air. It is used to treat skin rash and as a water softener. Has been used as a mouthwash and vaginal douche. Sodium carbonate is the cause of scalp, forehead, and hand rash when those who are hypersensitive use cosmetics containing it. Ingestion of large quantities may produce corrosion of the gastrointestinal tract, vomiting, diarrhea, circulatory collapse, and death.

SODIUM CELLULOSE PHOSPHATE (Rx) • Calcibind. A phosphate and agent used for reducing calcium in the urine to prevent kidney stones. Potential adverse reactions include nausea, vomiting, drowsiness, trembling, seizures, mood changes, loss of appetite, heartburn, diarrhea, low magnesium in the blood, and acute joint pain.

SODIUM CHLORIDE (OTC) • Common Table Salt. Adsorbonac Ophthalmic Solution. Afrin Saline Mist. Ayr Saline Nasal Drops. Chlor-3 Condiment. Humist. Muro-128 Ointment. Muro Ophthalmic. NaSal Moisturizing Nasal Spray. Ocean Nasal Mist. Ricelyte Rice-Based Oral Electrolyte Maintenance Solution. Saline. Salinex Nasal Mist. Slo-Salt. Sodium Chloride Ointment. Star-Optic Eye Wash. Thermotabs. Used as an astringent and antiseptic in mouthwashes, dentifrices, and eye lotions. In eyedrops and ointments it removes excess fluid from the cornea. Odorless, with a characteristic salty taste, it absorbs water. Used topically to treat inflamed lesions. Diluted solutions are not considered irritating, but upon drying, water is drawn from the skin and may produce irritation. Salt workers have a great number of skin rashes. Also reported to irritate the roots of the teeth when used for a long time in dentifrices. Not considered toxic, but can adversely affect persons with high blood pressure and kidney disease. It is used in tablet form to replace and maintain sodium and chloride levels, and in the management of heat cramp caused by excessive perspiration. Potential adverse reactions include aggravation of congestive heart failure, edema, and fluid in the lungs if too much sodium chloride is ingested too rapidly. High salt in the blood and serious electrolyte disturbance can be side effects. In eye preparations, it may cause slight stinging upon instillation, and hypersensitivity reactions. The ointment may cause blurred vision. In 1992, the FDA issued a notice that sodium chloride had not been shown to be safe and effective as claimed in OTC digestive-aid products.

SODIUM CITRATE (Rx) • Bicitra. Citrocarbonate Antacid. Oracit. Rice-Based Oral Electrolyte Maintenance Solution. Ricelyte. Shohl's Solution. An antacid used to treat acidosis and for long-term maintenance of an alkaline urine.

SODIUM COMMON • Table salt.

SODIUM DIACETATE (OTC) • A compound of sodium acetate and acetic acid (*see*). Used as a preservative that inhibits molds and bacteria. In 1992, the FDA proposed a ban on sodium diacetate in astringent (*see*) drug products because it had not been shown to be safe and effective as claimed.

SODIUM ETIDRONATE • *See* Etidronate.

SODIUM FLUORIDE (OTC) • Fluoride. Fluor-A-Day. Fluoritab. Flura. Karidium.

Luride. Pediaflor. Phos-Flur. ACT. Check-mate. Fluorigard. Fluorinse. Flura-Drops. Gel II. Gel-Kam. Gel-Tin. Home Treatment Fluoride Gelution. Karigel. Karigel N. Listermint with Fluoride. Luride. Minute-Gel. Point-Two. PreviDent. Stop. Thera-Flur Gel. Thera-Flur-N. Fluoride tablets, drops, and rinses to aid in the prevention of dental cavities. Changed from Rx to OTC. Potential adverse reactions include stomach upset, headache, weakness, and allergic reactions such as rash, eczema, and hives. Contraindicated when fluoride intake from drinking water exceeds 0.7 parts per million. Chronic toxicity can result from prolonged use of high doses.

SODIUM HYALURONATE • The sodium salt of hyaluronic acid found in the umbilical cord and in the fluid between joints.

SODIUM HYDROGEN CARBONATE • *See* Sodium Bicarbonate.

SODIUM HYDROXIDE • **Caustic Soda. Soda Lye.** An alkali and emulsifier in soaps and creams. Readily absorbs water. If too much alkali is used, a rash of the scalp may occur. Its ingestion causes vomiting, prostration, and collapse. Inhalation causes lung damage.

SODIUM IODIDE (Rx) • **Lugol's Solution.** A form of iodine used to treat hyperthyroidism and thyroid cancer.

SODIUM IODINE • *See* Radioactive Iodine.

SODIUM LACTATE (Rx) • An injection that metabolizes to sodium bicarbonate and is used to alkalize urine. *See* Sodium Bicarbonate.

SODIUM METHICILLIN • *See* Methicillin Sodium.

SODIUM NAFCILLIN • *See* Nafcillin.

SODIUM NITRATE (OTC) • **Chile Niter. Chile Saltpeter.** Occurs as a mineral found in the mountains of Chile. In 1992, the FDA proposed a ban on sodium nitrate in oral menstrual drug products because it had not been shown to be safe and effective as claimed.

SODIUM NITROFERRICYANIDE • *See* Nitroprusside.

SODIUM OXACILLIN • *See* Oxacillin Sodium.

SODIUM PANTOTHENATE (OTC) • Vitamins D_1 and D_2. Used as a dietary supplement.

SODIUM PERBORATE (OTC) • **Professional Strength Efferdent.** White crystals, soluble in water, used as an antiseptic, deodorant bleach, in dentifrices as a tooth whitener, and in footbaths. Strong solutions that are very alkaline are irritating.

SODIUM PHOSPHATE (OTC) • **Fleet Phospho-Soda. Neutra-Phos.** Liquid or enema laxative. Potential adverse reactions include abdominal cramping and fluid and electrolyte disturbances if used daily. May lead to dependence in long-term or excessive use. Contraindicated in abdominal pain, nausea, vomiting, or other symptoms of appendicitis or acute abdomen, intestinal obstruction or perforation, edema, congestive heart failure, megacolon (*see*), impaired kidney function, and in patients on salt-restricted diets. The enema form works within five to ten minutes.

SODIUM POLYSTYRENE SULFONATE (Rx) • **Kayexalate. Resonium A. SPS.** A potassium-removing resin that exchanges sodium ions for potassium in the intestine. Used to treat high potassium in the blood. Potential adverse reactions include nausea, vomiting, diarrhea, constipation, loss of appetite, stomach irritation, low blood calcium, low potassium, low magnesium, and high sodium. Antacids and laxatives reduce its effectiveness. Should be used with caution in elderly patients and those on digitalis therapy, with severe congestive heart failure, severe high blood pressure, and marked fluid retention.

SODIUM PROPIONATE • Colorless crystals that gather water in moist air. Used as a preservative in products to prevent mold and fungi. Has been used to treat fungal infections of the skin, but can cause allergic reactions. In 1992, the FDA issued a notice that sodium propionate had not been shown to be safe and effective as claimed in OTC products.

SODIUM SALICYLATE (Rx) • **Uracel-5.** A drug similar to aspirin that produces analgesia by an ill-defined effect on the hypothalamus, and by blocking the generation of pain impulses. The peripheral action may involve inhibition of prostaglandins (*see*). Used to treat arthritic disorders. Potential adverse reactions include ringing in the ears and hearing loss, nausea, vomiting, GI distress, occult bleeding, abnormal liver function, rash, hypersensitivity manifested by asthma, and anaphylaxis. Ammonium chloride and other urine acidifiers may increase blood levels of salicylates. Antacids in high doses and other urine alkalinizers decrease levels of salicylates. Corticosteroids decrease the effectiveness of salicylates, and oral anticoagulants may increase the risk of bleeding. Contraindicated in GI ulcer, GI bleeding, and aspirin hypersensitivity. Should be used cautiously in vitamin K deficiency, bleeding disorders, and asthma with nasal polyps. Because of epidemiologic association with Reye's syndrome, the Centers for Disease Control recommends that children or teenagers with chicken pox or influenzalike illness should not be given salicylates. Feverish, dehydrated children can develop toxicity rapidly. Should be given with food, milk, antacid, or a large glass of water to reduce GI adverse reactions. Concomitant use with alcohol, steroids, or other NSAIDs (*see*) may increase risk of GI bleeding. In 1992, the FDA issued a notice that sodium salicylate had not been shown to be safe and effective as claimed in OTC digestive-aid products.

SODIUM TETRADECYL SULFATE • A compound that is used to harden or otherwise affect nerve fibers.

SODIUM THIOSALICYLATE • The sodium salt of thiosalicyclic acid. It is prepared from benzoic acid (*see*) and is related to aspirin.

SODIUM THIOSULFATE • Used as a reagent in the laboratory and as an antidote to cyanide. It is used externally for ringworm.

SODOL • *See* Carisoprodol.

SOK DAY–SANG DAY • *See* Rehmannia.

SOLATENE • *See* Beta-Carotene.

SOLFOTON • *See* Phenobarbital.

SOLGANAL • *See* Aurothioglucose.

SOLOMON'S SEAL (H) • *Polygonatum officinale.* A perennial herb, the root was formerly used for its emetic properties, and externally for bruises near the eyes, as well as for treatment of tumors, wounds, poxes, warts, and pimples. It was thought to help mend broken bones. In sixteenth-century Italy, it was used in a wash believed to maintain healthy skin. The roots contain allantoin (*see*), used today as an anti-inflammatory and healing agent.

SOLUCAP C • *See* Vitamin C.

SOLU-CORTEF • *See* Hydrocortisone.

SOLU-MEDROL • *See* Methylprednisolone.

SOMA • *See* Carisoprodol.

SOMA COMPOUND • *See* Aspirin and Carisoprodol.

SOMAT-, SOMATO- • Prefixes meaning pertaining to the body.

SOMATOMEDIN C (Rx) • **Mecasermin. Somazon.** A Japanese-developed recombinant human-growth factor for various insulin-receptor disorders, and for growth-hormone-resistant dwarfism. It is the first effective therapy for dwarfism. It was introduced in Japan and is now also being used in Sweden.

SOMATREM (Rx) • **Protropin.** Purified growth hormone made through biotechnology, used to treat children with growth failure due to lack of adequate growth-hormone secretion from the pituitary gland. Potential adverse reactions include a drop in thyroid hormone, high blood sugar, and antibodies to the growth hormone. Adrenal hormones may inhibit growth-promoting action of somatrem. Contraindicated in patients with closed epiphyses (*see*), an active, underlying intracranial lesion, and known sensitivity to benzyl alcohol.

SOMATROPIN (Rx) • **Humatrope Vials.** Introduced in 1987, it is a genetically engineered human growth hormone used to treat children with growth hormone deficiency. Contraindicated in children who have tumors. Must be administered by a physician skilled in treating this condition.

SOMINEX-2 PAIN RELIEF FORMULA (OTC) • *See* Diphenhydramine and Acetaminophen.

SOMINEX-2 TABLETS (OTC) • Approved by the FDA as a sleep aid. *See* Diphenhydramine.

SOMOPHYLLIN • *See* Aminophylline.

SOMOPHYLLIN CRT • *See* Theophylline.

SOOTHE EYE DROPS (OTC) • *See* Tetrahydrozoline Hydrochloride.

SOPAMYCETIN • *See* Chloramphenicol.

SOPORIFIC • A drug or herb that induces sleep.

SOPRODOL • *See* Carisoprodol.

SORBIC ACID • A white powder obtained from the berries of the mountain ash. It is also made from chemicals in the factory. Produces a velvetlike feel when rubbed into the skin. Practically nontoxic, but may cause skin irritation in susceptible people.

SORBITOL (OTC) • **Actidose with Sorbitol. Salivart Saliva Substitute.** First found in the ripe berries of the mountain ash, it also occurs in other berries. Consists of a white, water-absorbing powder, flakes, or granules, with a sweet taste. Used to reduce body water and for intravenous feedings. Also given as a laxative and to treat dry mouth. No known toxicity, but if ingested in excess, it can cause diarrhea and gastrointestinal disturbance; also, it may alter the absorption of other drugs, making them less effective or more toxic. *See* Salivart.

SORBITRATE • *See* Isosorbide Dinitrate.

SORIDOL • *See* Carisoprodol.

SORREL EXTRACT (H) • **Rumex Extract.** An extract of the various species of genus *Rumex*. Europeans imported this to the Americas, where the Indians adopted it. Originally, the root was used as a laxative and mild astringent. It also was used for scabs on the skin and as a dentifrice. Was widely used in twentieth-century American medical circles to treat skin diseases. Contraindicated in persons suffering from arthritis, gout, and kidney stones as well as gastric hyperacidity.

SOTALOL (Rx) • **Betapace.** A beta-blocker (*see*) long available in Europe that is effective in preventing heart-rhythm disturbances that may lead to cardiac arrest and death. An estimated 600,000 deaths a year in the United States are caused by arrhythmia, and sotalol reportedly reduces heartbeat problems by 50 percent. It was introduced to the American market in 1992 on a priority approval by the FDA. Potential adverse effects include fatigue, slow heartbeat, labored breathing, irregular heartbeat, weakness, and dizziness. May interact with drugs for diabetes and other heart drugs. May depress the contractions of the heart and precipitate heart failure. It should not be withdrawn suddenly.

SOTRADECOL • *See* Sodium Tetradecyl Sulfate.

SOUR DOCK (H) • A weed with coarse leaves that is a member of the sorrel family and contains a sour juice. Used by herbalists to treat wounds and sore throats. *See* Sorrel Extract.

SOUTHERNWOOD (H) • *Artemisia abrotanum.* Native to southern Europe and widely grown in English gardens, it belongs to the Compositae family. Pliny thought it had aphrodisiac qualities when placed under a mattress. It reputedly made hair grow on bald heads. Used in herbal teas as a sedative. Used by herbalists to bring on delayed menstruation, which gave it the nickname "lad's love." Also used to remove threadworm in children.

SOYBEANS • Soybeans contain genistein, now in clinical testing against breast cancer. They also contain other anticancer chemicals such as HEMF, which may help explain why the Japanese, who use a lot of soy products, have far less breast and prostate cancer than Americans. Japanese-style soy sauce (shoyu) is produced through a complex microbial fermentation of soybeans and wheat. During its manufacture, characteristic flavors and aromas develop due to the action of microbes and reactions between various chemical substances. Shoyu has been reported to have anticancer activity and significantly reduced stomach cancer in mice exposed to a powerful cancer-causing agent, benzopyrene. Tofu, an increasingly popular soybean-based food in the United States, contains high levels of daidzein, which is also believed to be an anticancer chemical.

SPAN CAP NO. 1 (Rx) • *See* Dextroamphetamine.

SPANISH MOSS (H) • *Tillandsia usneodes.* **Florida Moss.** It is found festooning trees and telephone poles in southeastern United States. It is used for chair stuffing and insulation. Researchers at Purdue have isolated a compound in Spanish moss that reduces blood sugar in persons suffering from most forms of diabetes.

SPANISH RADISH • *See* Radish Extract.

SPAN R/D • *See* Phentermine.

SPARINE • *See* Promazine.

SPARROWGRASS • *See* Asparagus.

SPASM • Sudden involuntary muscle contraction.

SPASMOLIN (Rx) • *See* Hyoscyamine, Atropine Sulfate, Scopolamine, and Phenobarbital.

SPASQUID (Rx) • *See* Hyoscyamine, Atropine Sulfate, Scopolamine, and Phenobarbital.

SPASTICITY • Rigidity of the muscles, causing stiffness and restriction of movement.

SPEARMINT (H) • *Mentha spicata. Mentha viridis.* **Garden Mint.** The leaves are used for many minor ailments including colds, fever, indigestion, gas, cramps, nausea, and spasms. The major active oil is carvone, used as a flavoring in food and in medications to break up intestinal gas and as a stimulant. *See* Mint.

SPECT • Abbreviation for single photon emission computed tomography. A diagnostic technique that shows a pattern of changes in blood flow and metabolism in the brain.

SPECTAM • *See* Spectinomycin.

SPECTAZOLE • *See* Econazole.

SPECTINOMYCIN (Rx) • **Spectam. Trobicin.** An antibiotic used to treat penicillin-resistant gonorrhea. Given by injection. Potential adverse reactions include dizziness, insomnia, nausea, decreased urine output, hives, fever, and chills. It may mask or delay symptoms of incubating syphilis.

SPECTROBID • *See* Bacampicillin.

SPECTROCIN • *See* Gramicidin and Neomycin.

SPEEDWELL (H) • *Veronica officinalis.* A common hairy perennial herb grown in Europe, with pale blue or lilac flowers. It has a reputation among herbalists for inducing sweating and restoring healthy body functions; also an expectorant tonic, a treatment for hemorrhage, and a medication for skin diseases.

SPERMICIDES (OTC) • **Conceptrol Gel. Delfen. Emko. Encare. Gynol II. Koromex. Nonoxynol-9. Octoxynol-9. Ortho-Creme. Pre-Fil. Semicid. Today. VCF.** Spermicides are inserted in the vagina prior to sexual intercourse. They damage and kill sperm in the vagina; thus, the sperm is unable to travel to the uterus and fallopian tubes. Used alone, vaginal spermicides prevent pregnancy only 79 percent of the time. The number of pregnancies is reduced when spermicides are used with condoms or other methods. Nonoxynol-9 has been shown to kill viruses and may be effective against a number of sexually transmitted diseases.

SPHINCTER • A purse-string muscle that surrounds and controls the opening and closing of a natural orifice such as the bladder.

SPIGELIA (H) • **Carolina Pink. Indian Pink. Maryland Pink. Pinkroot. Worm Grass.** Dried rhizome and roots of *Spigelia marilandica,* which grows from New Jersey to Florida and west to Wisconsin. Contains resin, tannin, bitter principle, and volatile oil (*see all*). It is used in homeopathic medicine (*see*) as a remedy for headaches and other pains. It is used by herbalists to rid the body of worms. *See also* Pinkroot.

SPIKENARD (H) • *Aralia racemosa.* **Nard.** American herb of the ginseng family used for skin ailments such as acne, rash, and general skin problems. Also used for coughs, colds, and other chest problems.

SPIRAEA ULMARIA • *See* Meadowsweet.

SPIRAPRIL (Rx) • **Renormax.** An ACE inhibitor (*see*) approved in 1994, after a thirty-six-month review by the FDA, for the treatment of high blood pressure. Spirapril is contraindicated in patients with known hypersensitivity to the product, and in patients with a history of angioedema (*see*) related to previous treatment with ACE inhibitors. A big drop in blood pressure may occur when the drug is first administered. If that occurs, the patient should lie down. The use of spirapril with potassium supplements or potassium-sparing diuretics may lead to a significant and potentially dangerous increase in blood potassium. Spirapril may also cause a change in kidney function in patients with kidney-associated high blood pressure. ACE inhibitors are contraindicated if a woman becomes pregnant. Ingestion of this drug with a high-fat meal has no significant effect on the body's use of the drug, but it may delay its absorption by about one hour. The most frequently reported adverse effects are headache, dizziness, upper-respiratory symptoms (including cough), and fatigue. Angioedema of the face, extremities, lips, tongue, glottis, and/or larynx has been reported in patients treated with ACE inhibitors. In the case of spirapril, the company reports that most patients experiencing this complication had been subjected to extended periods of therapy, at daily doses five to ten times the recommended dose.

SPIRONAZOLE • *See* Hydrochlorothiazide and Spironolactone.

SPIRONOLACTONE (Rx) • **Aldactone. Spironazole. Spirozide.** A potassium-sparing diuretic introduced in 1959 that combats the adrenal-gland hormone aldosterone, increasing the excretion of sodium and water, but sparing potassium. Used to treat fluid retention, high blood pressure, diuretic-induced low potassium, and in the detection of primary hyperaldosteronism (*see*). Potential adverse reactions include nausea, vomiting, diarrhea, headache, low sodium, hives, enlarged breast in men, impotence, and in women, breast soreness, decreased vaginal secretions, and menstrual disturbances. Contraindicated in the absence of urine formation, in kidney disease, and in high blood potassium. Should be used cautiously in fluid or electrolyte imbalances. Response to the drug may be delayed from two to three days when used by itself. Breast cancer has been reported in some patients taking spironolactone, but a causal relationship has not been confirmed. Because of its anti-male hormone properties, it has been used to treat hairiness in women. ACE inhibitors and potassium supplements used with this drug may cause too high a level of potassium in the blood. Aspirin may block spironolactone's effectiveness. The toxicity of digoxin (*see*) may be increased if used with this drug. Over-the-counter medications for colds or allergies that contain stimulants may counteract the effectiveness of spironolactone and have an adverse effect on the heart. Should be taken with meals to enhance absorption.

SPIROZIDE • *See* Spironolactone.

SPLEEN • A lymphoid organ in the abdominal cavity that is an important center for immune system activities.

SPO • Homeopathic abbreviation for spongia. *See* Sponge.

SPONGE (H) • *Spongia tosta.* **Hyland's Cough Syrup with Honey.** Named for the Greek word *spongos,* for fungus, sponges are elastic, porous masses of horny fibers that form the skeletons of marine animals of the lower species. *Spongia tosta* is a genus of subtropical sponges that are commercially important. They absorb water. Homeopathic medicines use sponge as a remedy for coughs and dry mucus.

SPONGIA • *See* Sponge.

SPORANOX • *See* Itraconazole.

SPORTSCREME • *See* Triethanolamine and Salicylates.

SPRX-105 • *See* Phenazopyridine Hydrochloride.

SPS • *See* Sodium Polystyrene Sulfonate.

S-P-T • *See* Thyroid.

SQUALAMINE • *See* Shark.

SQUAWROOT • *See* Blue Cohosh.

SQUAWVINE (H) • *Mitchella repens.* **Checkerberry. Partridgeberry.** An American trailing plant used for painful or absent menstruation. Also used to prepare the womb for childbirth. It acquired its name because it was popular among American Indian tribes during pregnancy.

SQUILL (H) • *Urginea maritima.* The bulb of this plant contains glycosides, mucilage, and tannin (*see all*). Used by herbalists as a powerful expectorant to treat chronic bronchitis. The mucilage content eases and relaxes the bronchioles. It was formerly used to stimulate heart action in treating heart failure and fluid retention. Contraindicated in heart disease or kidney disease. Today, it is considered highly toxic.

SSKI • *See* Potassium Iodide.

STADOL • *See* Butorphanol.

STANNOUS FLUORIDE • *See* Fluoride.

STANOZOLOL (Rx) • **Winstrol.** An anabolic steroid (*see*) that promotes tissue-building processes and reverses loss of tissue. Also stimulates the manufacture of red blood cells. Used to prevent hereditary angioedema (*see*), and in children only, to treat an attack of angioedema. Potential adverse reactions in women include acne, oily skin, weight gain, hairiness, hoarseness, clitoral enlargement, changes in libido, flushing, sweating, and vaginitis with itching. In prepubescent males, premature epiphyseal closure, priapism (*see*), growth of body and facial hair, phallic enlargement; in postpubescent males, testicular atrophy, scanty sperm, decreased ejaculatory volume, impotence, breast enlargement, and epididymitis. In both sexes, edema, gastroenteritis, nausea, vomiting, diarrhea, constipation, changes in appetite, bladder irritability, jaundice, liver toxicity, and high levels of calcium in the blood. Contraindicated in men with enlarged or cancerous prostates; carcinoma of the male breast; high levels of calcium in the blood; heart, liver, or kidney dysfunction; and in premature infants. Should be used cautiously in prepubescent males, patients with diabetes or heart disease, and those taking ACTH, corticosteroids, or anticoagulants. Should be taken with food.

STAPHCILLIN • *See* Methicillin Sodium.

STAPHYLOCOCCI • Spherical bacteria that tend to grow in clumps like bunches of grapes. They are common inhabitants of the skin and of nasal passages. Some strains cause little trouble, but some, called resistant staph, tend to proliferate and are difficult to treat. *Staphylococcus aureus* is the most virulent type and is a frequent cause of boils, sties, abscesses, bone-marrow infection, and pneumonia.

STAPHYLOCOCCUS AUREUS • A common species of staphylococci (*see*) found in the nose and in hair follicles in the skin. It causes infections of the skin, bladder, lung, bone, and heart. It also causes wound infections and food poisoning.

STAR ANISE (H) • *Illicium verum.* **Chinese Anise. Yellow-Flowered Starry Aniseed Tree.** A small tree grown in Asia and North America, the fruit has been employed in Chinese medicine for centuries, particularly to cure arthritis. The seeds and oil have stimulant, carminative, diuretic, and digestive properties. Star anise is also used to soothe inflamed mucous membranes of the nasal passages. The fruit is used today in herbal teas. In China, the seeds are used to treat toothache, and the essential oil is given to children with colic. In scientific experiments, alcoholic extracts of the fruit were effective against gram-positive and gram-negative bacteria (*see both*) and fungi. Star anise contains a high level of anethole, which can produce hives, scaling, and blisters when applied directly to the skin.

STARGRASS • *See* True Unicorn Root.

STARWEED • *See* Chickweed.

STASIS • Stagnation or slowing of the normal flow of body fluids.

STATICIN • *See* Erythromycin.

STATISTICAL SIGNIFICANCE • The likelihood that a given result did not occur by chance, usually indicated by a ρ value of 0.05 or less. For example, in a clinical trial of a drug, a ρ value 0.03 means that there is a 97 percent chance that the result occurred because of the drug and a 3 percent likelihood that the result occurred by chance.

STATOBEX • *See* Phendimetrazine.

STATOBEX-105 • *See* Phendimetrazine.

STATROL (Rx) • A combination of neomycin, benzalkonium chloride, methylparaben, and propylparaben (*see all*), used to combat eye infections.

STAVESACRE (H) • *Delphinium staphisagria.* **Lousewort. Licebane.** An annual or biennial plant native to Europe and Asia and cultivated elsewhere. It is used in homeopathic medicines to treat parasites. It should never be used internally because it is highly poisonous.

STAVUDINE (Rx) • **Zerit.** An antiretroviral for the treatment of adults with advanced HIV (*see*) infections who are intolerant of approved therapies or who have experienced significant clinical or immunologic deterioration while receiving these therapies or for whom such therapies are contraindicated. Stavudine was approved by the FDA under a priority review in 5.9 months and its first market was the United States. The drug sometimes causes peripheral neuropathy, which is characterized by pain and tingling or numbness in the hands and feet. About 15 to 21 percent of the patients in stavudine clinical trials had the problems. Stavudine was the first drug approved under the FDA's parallel-track policy, which permits the drug to be made available to patients before approval. During the two years of clinical trials, thirteen thousand patients received the drug.

STAY TRIM • *See* Phenylpropanolamine.

STD • Abbreviation for sexually transmitted disease.

STEARIC ACID • Occurs naturally in butter acids, tallow, cascarilla bark, and other animal fats and oils. It is used to make bar soap and lubricants. It is also used for suppositories. It is a possible sensitizer for allergic people.

STEARYL ALCOHOL • **Stenol.** A mixture of solid alcohols prepared from sperm whale oil. Unctuous white flakes, insoluble in water, soluble in alcohol and ether. Used in pharmaceuticals, cosmetic creams, for emulsions, and as an antifoam agent and lubricant.

STELAZINE • *See* Trifluoperazine.

STELLARIA MEDIA • *See* Chickweed.

STEMETIC • *See* Trimethobenzamide.

STEMEX • *See* Paramethasone.

STENOL • *See* Stearyl Alcohol.

STERANE • *See* Prednisolone.

STERAPRED • *See* Prednisone.

STERCULIA GUM • *See* Karaya Gum.

STEROIDS (Rx) (OTC) • A class of compounds that includes certain drugs of hormonal origin, such as cortisone, and is used to treat the inflammations caused by allergies. Glucocorticoids reduce white blood cell production; also prostaglandins and leukotrienes (*see both*). Natural and synthetic steroids have four rings of carbon atoms, but have different actions according to what is attached to the rings. Cortisone and oral contraceptives are steroids. The following toxic effects, all of which relate to the length and level of dosage, may occur: susceptibility to infection, osteoporosis, muscle weakness and wasting, diabetes, high blood pressure due to sodium and water retention, weight gain, edema, bruising, moon face (round, swollen), psychotic reactions, hairiness, menstrual disturbance, pancreatitis (*see*), cataracts, and growth retardation.

STEROL • Any class of solid complex alcohols from animals and plants. Cholesterol is a sterol and is used in hand creams. Sterols are lubricants in baby preparations, emollient creams and lotions, emulsified fragrances, hair conditioners, hand creams, and hand lotions. No known toxicity.

S-T EXPECTORANT • *See* Guaifenesin.

STICKLEWORT • *See* Agrimony.

STILBESTROL • *See* Diethylstilbestrol.

STILLINGIA ROOT (H) • *Stillingia sylvatica.* **Euphorbiaceae. Queen's Delight.** An herb from the Chinese tallow tree, widely used in the late 1800s by physicians to treat syphilis, cancer, and tuberculosis. Indians of the southern United States used this herb for venereal diseases long before that.

STILPHOSTROL • *See* Diethylstilbestrol.

STIMATE • *See* Desmopressin.

STIMULANT • An agent that increases the activity of a body part or system.

STINKWEED • *See* Jimsonweed.

ST. JOSEPH ASPIRIN-FREE FEVER REDUCER FOR CHILDREN • *See* Acetaminophen.

ST. JOSEPH MEASURED DOSE NASAL DECONGESTANT • *See* Phenylephrine.

STOM-, STOMATO- • Prefixes meaning pertaining to the mouth.

STONEROOT • *See* Collinsonia.

STOP • *See* Sodium Fluoride.

STOXIL • *See* Idoxuridine.

STRABISMUS • Deviation of eye movement that prevents the eyes from moving in a parallel fashion.

STRAWBERRY (H) • *Fragaria vesca.* A perennial, it is native to the Northern Hemisphere. Lotions and gargles were prescribed for mouth, throat, and eyes, and to fasten loose teeth. Also used to treat diarrhea, jaundice, heart conditions, and fever. Strawberry was said to stop bleeding, slow excessive menstruation, and cure gout. Externally, it was used as a lotion for eczema, and to prevent wrinkles. A concoction of the root and herb is said to be good for ulcers and liver disorders. In 1992, the FDA issued a notice that strawberry had not been shown to be safe and effective as claimed in OTC digestive-aid products.

STREPTASE • *See* Streptokinase.

STREPTOCOCCUS • A bacterium named from the Greek word *kokkus,* meaning "berry," because it looks like a bunch of berries under a microscope. Streptococci are found in the mouth and intestines of humans and animals, in dairy and other food products, and in fermenting juices. Not all cause infections.

STREPTOCOCCUS PNEUMONIAE • Bacteria that normally inhabit the respiratory system and may cause lobar pneumonia. They may also cause meningitis, sinusitis, and other infections.

STREPTOKINASE (Rx) • **Kabikinase. Streptase.** An enzyme that dissolves blood clots in acute heart attack, blood clots in the lungs, and deep-vein blood clots. In a European trial reported in *Lancet,* January 7, 1995, the drug increased both brain hemorrhage and mortality in patients with severe ischemic stroke, in which symptoms are caused by lack of blood to the brain. Potential adverse reactions include severe, spontaneous bleeding, stroke, low blood pressure, irregular heartbeat, hypersensitivity, and hives. Aspirin, dipyridamole, heparin, and coumarin (*see all*) increase the risk of bleeding. A British study of clot-busting drugs involving 41,299 patients from 924 hospitals reported in 1992 that streptokinase was equally as effective as and slightly safer than newer and more expensive drugs.

STREPTOMYCIN SULFATE (Rx) • An aminoglycoside (*see*) antibiotic, it is given by injection; active against streptococcal endocarditis, an infection of the heart. Potential adverse reactions include ear problems, muscle problems, kidney dysfunction, local pain, irritation and sterile abscesses at the site of injection, and skin disorders. Interacts with cephalothin, dimenhydrinate, general and local anesthetics, and IV loop diuretics (*see all*). Use with a wide range of drugs increases the risk of hearing loss and/or kidney failure. Such drugs include other aminoglycosides, furosemide, polymyxins, amphotericin B, cisplatin, methotrexate, lithium carbonate, and cyclosporine (*see all*).

STREPTOZOCIN (Rx) • **Zanosar.** An anticancer antibiotic that is used to treat islet-cell carcinoma of the pancreas that has spread, colon cancer, and carcinoid tumors. Potential adverse reactions include nausea, vomiting, diarrhea, a drop in white blood cells, high or low blood sugar, kidney toxicity, and severe irritation at the site of injection. Takes longer to eliminate doxorubicin (*see*) if administered with streptozocin. Other potential kidney-damaging drugs such as aminoglycoside increase the risk of toxicity. Phenytoin may make streptozocin less effective. A physician may recommend drinking extra fluids to help protect the kidneys while taking this drug.

STRIFON FORTE • *See* Chlorzoxazone.

STRONG AMMONIA SOLUTION (OTC) • Obtained by blowing steam through incandescent coke. In 1992, the FDA proposed a ban for the use of strong ammonia solution to treat fever blisters and cold sores because it had not been shown to be safe and effective as claimed in OTC products.

STRONG IODINE (Rx) • **Lugol's Solution.** Used to treat overactive thyroid, iodine deficiency, and to protect the thyroid gland from the effects of radiation from radioactive forms of iodine. May be used before and after administration of a radioactive medicine containing radioactive iodine, or after accidental exposure to radiation. Potential adverse reactions include hives, joint pain, swelling of limbs, face, lips, and throat, swollen glands, burning of mouth or throat, confusion, headache, increased watering of the mouth, irregular heartbeat, metallic taste, stomach upset, fatigue, weakness, and numbness. Should be taken with food to avoid stomach upset.

STROPHANTHUS (H) • *Strophanthus kombe. Strophanthus hispidus.* Shrubs native to Africa and Asia, originally used by natives in Tanganyika and Nyasa for arrow poison. A heart stimulant with action similar to but less predictable than that of digitalis (*see*), and with quicker effect. Used in homeopathic medicines. A reported side effect is diarrhea. Because its effect is more rapid than that of digitalis, it is a candidate for use during emergency heart failure, given intravenously.

STRYCHNINE (OTC) • *Strychnos nux vomica.* Extremely poisonous. Used as an antidote for barbiturate poisoning. Some strychnine compounds are used as a tonic. In 1992, the FDA issued a notice that strychnine had not been shown to be safe and effective as claimed in OTC digestive-aid products.

STYPTIC • An agent that reduces or stops external bleeding. Among the herbs that are used for this purpose are raspberry and yellow dock.

SUBACUTE • A zone between acute and chronic, or the process of a disease that is not readily identifiable. Subacute endocarditis, for example, is an infection of the heart that is usually due to a strep germ and may follow temporary infection after a tooth extraction.

SUBARACHNOID HEMORRHAGE • When blood from a ruptured artery spreads over the brain's surface.

SUBLIMAZE • *See* Fentanyl.

SUBSTANCE P • A neurotransmitter (*see*) believed to carry pain messages from the body to the brain and vice versa.

SUCCIMER (Rx) • **Chemet.** An orphan drug (*see*) introduced in 1991 to treat lead poisoning in children.

SUCCINIC ACID • **Butanedioic Acid. Amber Acid.** Prepared from acetic acid (*see*), succinic acid occurs naturally in fungi and moss. It is used in perfumes and in the manufacture of medicines.

SUCCINIMIDES (Rx) • Made from ammonia and succinic acid, which occurs in fungi and moss. It is prepared from acetic acid (*see*). Used to treat epileptic seizures. Potential adverse effects include gastric upsets, drowsiness, rash, and serious blood abnormalities. Must be withdrawn slowly.

SUCCINYLCHOLINE (Rx) • **Suxamethonium Chloride. Anectine. Quelicin. Sucostrin.** A muscle relaxant used as an adjunct (*see*) to anesthesia. Potential adverse reactions include slow or rapid heartbeat, increased eye pressure, irregular heartbeat, very high fever, muscle twitches, excessive salivation, allergic or unusual hypersensitivity reactions, low blood pressure, and respiratory distress. Must be used with caution in persons with personal or family histories of very high blood pressure or very high fever.

SUCCUSSION • Vigorous shaking while a homeopathic remedy is being diluted.

SUCOSTRIN • *See* Succinylcholine.

SUCRALFATE (Rx) • **Carafate.** Introduced in 1978 to treat duodenal ulcers. There are no known contraindications. Although it contains aluminum, it is not considered an antacid. When sucralfate is administered orally, small amounts of aluminum are absorbed from the gastrointestinal tract. Concomitant use of sucralfate with other products that contain aluminum such as aluminum-containing antacids may increase the total body burden of aluminum. This may be a problem with patients who have kidney dysfunction, especially those on dialysis. Sucralfate may reduce absorption of cimetidine, ciprofloxacin, digoxin, norfloxacin, phenytoin, ranitidine, tetracycline, and theophylline. Therefore, it is recommended that such drugs be taken two hours before sucralfate is ingested. Potential adverse reactions are minor and include diarrhea, nausea, vomiting, gastric discomfort, indigestion, gas, dry mouth, itching, rash, dizziness, sleepiness, and back pain. Should be taken on an empty stomach. It is a candidate for OTC status, as of this writing.

SUCRETS • *See* Dyclonine.

SUCRETS COLD DECONGESTANT FORMULA • *See* Phenylpropanolamine.

SUCRETS COUGH CONTROL FORMULA • *See* Dextromethorphan.

SUCROSE • **Sugar. Cane Sugar. Saccharose.** A sweetening agent, a preservative and antioxidant in pharmaceuticals, a demulcent, and a substitute for glycerin. In 1992, the FDA proposed a ban on sucrose in oral menstrual drug products because it had not been shown to be safe and effective as claimed.

SUDAFED • *See* Pseudoephedrine.

SUDAHIST • *See* Triprolidine and Pseudoephedrine.

SUDORIFIC • Causes profuse perspiration.

SUDRIN • *See* Pseudoephedrine.

SUFEDRIN • *See* Pseudoephedrine.

SUFENTA • *See* Sufentanil Citrate.

SUFENTANIL CITRATE (Rx) • **Sufenta.** A narcotic analgesic altering both the perception of and reaction to pain. Used as an adjunctive to anesthesia. Potential adverse effects include chills, low blood pressure, high blood pressure, slow or fast heartbeat, nausea, vomiting, itching, chest-wall rigidity, and respiratory depression. Alcohol and central nervous system depressants are additive. Must be used cautiously in head injury, lung disease, and decreased respiratory reserve.

SUL • Homoepathic abbreviation for sulfur. *See* Sulfur.

SUL-AC • Homeopathic abbreviation for sulfuric acid. *See* Sulfuric Acid.

SULAMYD • *See* Sulfacetamide.

SULAR • *See* Nisoldipine.

SULBACTAM SODIUM • *See* Ampicillin.

SULCONAZOLE NITRATE (Rx) • **Exelderm. Sulcosyn.** A topical solution that inhibits the growth of fungi and yeast. Potential adverse reactions include itching, burning, and stinging. Efficacy against athlete's foot has not been proven.

SULCOSYN • *See* Sulconazole Nitrate.

SULFA • Any of a group of fifty or more compounds containing sulfur and nitrogen that are antibacterial. Before the advent of other antibiotics, they were widely used but because of their potential serious side effects, their use is limited. *See* Sulfanilamide and Gantricin.

SULFABENZAMIDE • A sulfa drug that kills microbes and is used primarily in vaginal creams to treat infections. *See* Sulfa Drugs.

SULFACETAMIDE (Rx) • **AK-Sulf. Belph-10. Cetamide. Gyne-Sulf. Isopto-Cetamide. Ispid. I-Sulfacet. Metimyd. Sodium Sulamyd. Sulfair. Sulf 10. Sulphrin. Sultrin.** A sulfonamide antibacterial drug in use since the 1930s, it was one of the earliest sulfa drugs. Available as eyedrops or ointment, it is used to treat bacterial conjunctivitis and to prevent infection after an eye injury. Resistance to sulfacetamide develops easily, and pus contains an acid that inactivates it. Potential adverse effects include stinging or burning on application, itching, and redness. Other effects include pain on instilling eyedrops, headache or brow pain, and light hurting the eyes. Sulfacetamide is incompatible with silver eye preparations and zinc sulfate eyedrops. Local anesthetics and PABA derivatives decrease its effectiveness. *See* Sulfa Drugs.

SULFACET-R ACNE LOTION • A combination of sodium sulfacetamide and sulfur (*see both*).

SULFACYTINE (Rx) • **Renoquid.** An antifungal drug used in the treatment of urinary tract infections.

SULFADIAZINE (Rx) • **Microsulfon.** A sulfonamide drug, it is used to treat urinary tract infection, prevent rheumatic fever, and as an adjunctive treatment in toxoplasmosis. Potential adverse reactions include anemia, headache, mental depression, convulsions, hallucinations, nausea, vomiting, diarrhea, abdominal pain, loss of appetite, kidney dysfunction, jaundice, rash, local irritation, hypersensitivity, serum sickness, drug fever, and potentially fatal allergic reactions. Incompatible with ammonium chloride, vitamin C, oral blood thinners, oral contraceptives, oral diabetes drugs, and PABA-containing drugs. *See* PABA and Sulfa Drugs.

SULFA DRUGS (Rx) (OTC) • **Azulfidine. Gamazole. Gantanol. Gantrisin. Gulfasin. Gyne-Sulf. Microsulfon. Proklar. Renoquid. SAS-500. Septra. Sulfabenzamide. Sulfacytine. Sulfadiazine. Sulfamethizole. Sulfasalazine. Sulfisoxazole. Terfonyl. Thiosulfil. Triple Sulfa. Trisulfapyrimidines. Urobak.** Sulfa drugs are prescribed for infections in various parts of the body. They are particularly useful in treating urinary tract infections because they concentrate in the urine when they pass out of the body. They kill bacteria by interfering with the organisms' metabolism. Sulfasalazine (*see*) varies from the other sulfas because a good portion of it stays in the intestines; thus it has been found effective against colitis and other intestinal problems. Many people are allergic to sulfa drugs including thiazide-type diuretics and oral antidiabetes drugs. Sulfas are contraindicated in people with severe kidney or liver disease. Sulfa drugs often cause sensitivity to the sun. Potential adverse reactions include nausea, vomiting, drowsiness, headache, rash, cramps, malaise, hallucinations, dizziness, ringing in the ears, chills, blood disorders, arthritic pain, itchy eyes, diarrhea, loss of appetite, hearing loss, fever, hair loss, yellowing of eye whites and skin, and reduced sperm count. Sulfa drugs may interact with oral antidiabetes drugs, methotrexate, warfarin, phenylbutazone, and NSAIDs (*see*) to increase the level of these drugs or sulfa drugs in the blood. Drinking alcohol while on a sulfa medication may cause nausea. Sulfas may reduce the effectiveness of oral contraceptives. Women taking this combination may have breakthrough bleeding. Sulfa drugs may interfere with tests for sugar in the urine. Sulfasalazine may decrease the effectiveness of digoxin and deplete folic acid. Sulfa drugs should be taken on an empty stomach with a full glass of water for greatest effect.

SULFAIR • *See* Sulfacetamide.

SULFAMETHIZOLE (Rx) • **Thiosulfil. Urobiotic.** An antibacterial sulfonamide (*see*) used to treat urinary tract infections, primarily pyelonephritis, pyelitis, and cystitis when these infections are caused by susceptible strains of *Escherichia coli, Klebsiella, Enterobacter, Staphylococcus aureus, Proteus mirabilis,* and *Proteus vulgaris.* Because of the rapid kidney clearance of sulfamethizole, the blood levels attained are low, and accumulation of the drug in tissues outside the urinary tract is limited. Therefore, it is not used for treatment of systemic infections. Potential adverse reactions include aplastic anemia and other blood problems, drug fever, rash, hives, serum sickness, nausea, vomiting, abdominal pain, diarrhea, kidney dysfunction, headache, peripheral neuritis, swelling around the eyes, joint pain, allergic irritation of the heart muscle, photosensitivity, loss of appetite, convulsions, mental depression, ringing in the ears, and loss of balance. Deaths associated with sulfonamides have been reported from hypersensitivity reactions and blood disorders. Contraindicated in patients hypersensitive to sulfa drugs. Should be used cautiously in patients with bronchial asthma, severe allergy, and kidney or liver dysfunction. Sulfamethizole can potentiate the effects of blood thinners, drugs for diabetes control, and anticonvulsants. Para-aminobenzoic acid makes sulfamethizole less effective. Side effects of the following drugs may be increased if taken with sulfamethizole: tolbutamide, phenytoin, and warfarin (*see all*). Stones may be formed if sulfamethizole is used with methenamine mandelate (*see*). Should be taken with a full glass of water, and fluids should be drunk throughout the day. *See also* Sulfa Drugs.

SULFAMETHOXAZOLE (Rx) • **Bactrim. Bethaprim. Cotrim. Gantanol. Septra DS. SMZ-TMP-DS. Uroplus.** A sulfonamide antibacterial introduced in 1961, it is used to treat many bacterial infections, including urinary tract infections, conjunctivitis, and ear infections. Combined with trimethoprim (*see*) it is widely used for bacterial infections of the respiratory, genital, and urinary tracts, gastroenteritis, gonorrhea, typhoid fever, and pneumocystis. A long-acting drug, its side effects are less than those of most antibacterials. Potential adverse effects include anemia, nausea, vomiting, loss of appetite, diarrhea, headache, dizziness, fever, jaundice, aching joints and muscles, and rash. It is important to drink a lot of fluids to prevent crystals in urine. Should not be used with oral antidiabetic drugs, oral blood thinners, phenytoin, aspirin and other salicylates, ammonium chloride, oral contraceptives, probenecid, phenylbutazone, or PABA-containing drugs (*see all*). Should be taken with a full glass of water, and water should be drunk liberally throughout the day. *See also* Sulfa Drugs.

SULFAMYLON • *See* Mafenide.

SULFANILAMIDE (Rx) • **AVC Cream. AVC Suppository. Vagitrol.** An antibacterial primarily used in the treatment of inflammation of the vagina caused by *Candida albicans*. *See* Sulfa Drugs.

SULFAPYRIDINE • *See* Sulfonamides and Sulfa Drugs.

SULFASALAZINE (Rx) • **Salazosulfapyridine. Azulfidine. Azulfidine EN-tabs. S.A.S.-Enteric. SAS-500.** A sulfonamide introduced in 1941, it is related to the salicylates and is used to treat ulcerative colitis and Crohn's disease (*see both*). Also used to treat rheumatoid arthritis. Potential adverse effects include nausea, loss of appetite, reversible infertility, stomach irritation, allergic reaction, fever, anemia, and in rare cases, temporary sterility among men. Contraindicated in persons allergic to sulfonamide drugs, including those used to treat diabetes or fluid retention. Also should be used with caution in patients with impaired liver or kidney function. The drug may also reduce the absorption of folic acid, leading to a deficiency. It is important to drink a lot of water to prevent crystals from forming in urine. *See also* Sulfa Drugs.

SULFATES • Salts or esters of sulfuric acid (*see*). A chemical is "sulfated" to help control the acid-alkali balance.

SULFATHIAZOLE (Rx) (OTC) • A sulfonamide (*see*) antibacterial agent.

SULFIDES • Compounds containing sulfur are in garlic and cruciferous vegetables. They are believed to help prevent cancer and are under intensive study.

SULFIMYCIN • *See* Erythromycin and Sulfisoxazole.

SULFINPYRAZONE (Rx) • **Anturane.** In use since 1959, it is prescribed to prevent gout attacks but is not used to relieve the pain and inflammation of gout once the attack has begun. It reduces the amount of uric acid in the body. It has an anticoagulant effect. Potential adverse effects include nausea and vomiting, headache, flushing, blood in urine, rash, itching, wheezing, and shortness of breath. Incompatible with alcohol, thiazide diuretics, aspirin, oral diabetic drugs, insulin, indomethacin, sulfonamides, and oral anticoagulants. Contraindicated in hypersensitivity to pyrazole derivatives, active peptic ulcer, kidney problems, bone-marrow suppression, certain cancers, radiation, and blood or liver problems. It is important to drink a lot of fluids with this drug.

SULFISOXAZOLE (Rx) • Azo Gantrisin. Gantanol. Gantrisin. Sulfamethoxazole. Sulfamycin.

A sulfonamide drug introduced in 1961, used to treat urinary tract, genital tract, anorectal, and systemic infections. Potential adverse reactions include anemia, headache, mental depression, seizures, hallucinations, nausea, vomiting, diarrhea, abdominal pain, loss of appetite, kidney dysfunction, rash, jaundice, photosensitivity, serum sickness, drug fever, and hypersensitivity, including life-threatening allergic reactions. Should not be used with ammonium chloride, ascorbic acid (vitamin C), oral blood thinners, oral contraceptives, oral diabetic drugs, phenytoin (anticonvulsant), or PABA-containing drugs. It is important to drink a lot of water when taking sulfisoxazole to prevent crystals in urine. *See* Sulfa Drugs.

SULFONAMIDES (Rx) • Co-Trimoxazole. Sulfadiazine. Sulfamethoxazole. Sulfasalazine. Sulfisoxazole.

Used to treat burn, ear, vaginal, eye, and many other infections. The presence of other medical problems may affect the use of sulfonamides. These include anemia or other blood problems, glucose-6-phosphate dehydrogenase (G6PD) deficiency, kidney disease, liver disease, and porphyria (*see*). Sulfonamides may cause blood problems. These problems may result in a greater chance of certain infections, slow healing, and bleeding of the gums. Sulfonamides may cause skin to be sensitive to sunlight. Common side effects include itching and rash. Other potential adverse effects include joint and muscle pain, difficulty in swallowing, skin irritation, sore throat and fever, bleeding and bruising, malaise, blood in urine, increased thirst, and pain or burning while urinating. Also diarrhea, dizziness, headache, loss of appetite, nausea, vomiting, and fatigue. Sulfa drugs should be taken with a lot of water. *See also* Sulfa Drugs.

SULFONYLUREAS (Rx) • Antidiabetes drugs

taken by mouth stimulate the pancreas to produce insulin (*see*). They are ineffective if no insulin-secreting cells remain in the organ. They are chemically related to the sulfonamides (*see*). The administration of oral diabetes medications has been reported to be associated with increased heart and blood-vessel deaths, as compared to treatment with diet alone or diet plus insulin. This warning is based on a study conducted by the University Group Diabetes Program (UGDP), a long-term prospective clinical trial designed to evaluate the effectiveness of blood-sugar-lowering drugs in preventing or delaying vascular complications in patients with non-insulin-dependent diabetes. The study involved 823 patients who were randomly assigned to one of four treatment groups. In 1970, UGDP reported that patients treated for five to eight years with diabetic diet plus a fixed dose of tolbutamide (a sulfonylurea) had a rate of cardiovascular mortality approximately two and a half times greater than patients treated with diet alone. A significant increase in total mortality was not observed, but the use of tolbutamide was discontinued based on the increase in cardiovascular mortality, thus limiting the opportunity for the study to show an increase in overall mortality. Despite controversy regarding the interpretation of these results, the findings of the UGDP study group required that drug companies carry this warning with their sulfonylurea antidiabetes drugs: "All sulfonylureas are capable of producing severe low blood sugar." *See also* Sulfa Drugs.

SULFOXYL • *See* Benzoyl Peroxide and Sulfur.

SULF 10 • *See* Sulfacetamide.

SULFUR (OTC) (H) • Sulphur. Acnomel Cream. Aveeno Cleansing Bar. Brimstone. Buf-Bar. Clearasil Adult. Fostex. Fostex Regular Strength. Fostril. Liquimat. Lotio Alsulfa. Meted 2. Pernox. Sastid. Sebucare. Sebulex Antiseborrheic Treatment Shampoo. Sebutone Cream Shampoo. Sulfacet R. Sulpho-Lac Acne Maximum Strength Meted.

An element that occurs in the earth's crust in the free state and in combination. A mild topical antibacterial and antifungal agent used in preparations for acne and dandruff. Also a stimulant to healing when used on rash. May cause irritation of the skin. In 1992, the FDA issued a notice that sulfur had not been shown to be safe and effective as claimed in OTC products, including those for treatment of poison ivy, poison sumac, and poison oak, and sulfur (sublimed) in products to kill lice. Sulfur was also placed on the banned list for diaper rash, fever blister, and cold sore drug products because it had not been shown to be safe and effective as claimed. In homeopathic medicines, it is used to ease burning pains, eruptions, sensations, discharges, and offensive odors. It is also used for shortness of breath.

SULFURATED LIME (OTC) • Used to treat acne, scabies, and other skin disorders. Avoid using abrasive soaps or cleansers, alcohol-containing preparations, and other topical acne preparations while using sulfurated lime. May cause skin irritation.

SULFURIC ACID (H) • **Sulphuric Acid. Sul-Ac. Oil of Bitriol.** A clear, colorless, odorless, oily acid used to modify starch and to regulate acid-alkalinity in the brewing industry. It is corrosive and produces severe burns on contact with the skin and other body tissues. Inhalation of the vapors can cause serious lung damage. Dilute sulfuric acid has been used to stimulate appetite and to combat overalkaline stomach juices. It is used as a topical caustic in cosmetic products. If ingested undiluted, it can be fatal. Homeopaths used it to treat anemia, bruises, diarrhea, exhaustion, hot flushes, and thrush. The final report to the FDA of the Select Committee on GRAS Substances stated in 1980 that it should continue its GRAS status with no limitations other than good manufacturing practices. The FDA data bank has fully up-to-date toxicology information available on sulfuric acid as a food additive.

SULFURICUM (H) • A homeopathic remedy using sulfur (*see*).

SULINDAC (Rx) • **Clinoril.** Produces anti-inflammatory, analgesic, and fever-reducing effects, probably by inhibiting prostaglandins (*see*). Introduced in 1976, it is used to treat arthri-tis, bursitis, tendinitis, and gouty arthritis. Potential adverse reactions include anemia, dizziness, nervousness, headache, ringing in the ears, temporary eye problems, abdominal pain, gas, peptic ulcer, nausea, occult blood loss, vaginal bleeding, liver dysfunction, rash, and water retention. Contraindicated in GI ulcers and in people sensitive to aspirin or other NSAIDs (*see*), in patients who have GI bleeding, kidney dysfunction, heart problems, and those receiving oral blood thinners. Use with other NSAIDs or alcohol may increase the danger of GI problems. Sulindac causes sodium retention, but is reputed to have the least effect on the kidneys when compared with other NSAIDs. It may increase the effect of blood thinners. Probenecid and aspirin may increase the levels of sulindac in the blood. Sulindac may increase the effects of sulfa drugs, antidiabetes drugs, and phenytoin or other drugs for severe disorders. May be taken with food. It is a candidate for OTC status, as of this writing.

SULPH • *See* Sulfur.

SULPHASALAZINE • *See* Sulfasalazine.

SULPHRIN (Rx) • A combination of prednisolone and sulfacetamide (*see both*) used to treat eye infections.

SULPHUR • *See* Sulfur.

SULTRIN (Rx) • A combination of sulfacetamide (*see*), sulfabenzamide, sulfathiazole, and urea (*see*), used to treat vaginal infections. *See also* Sulfa Drugs.

SUMA (H) • *Pfaffia paniculata.* **Brazilian Ginseng. Para Todo.** The South American version of ginseng (*see*). Has been referred to as *para todo,* meaning "for all things," by Brazilian Indian tribes who first discovered the medicinal uses of the herb. In North America, it has been used to treat exhaustion resulting from viruses such as Epstein-Barr and chronic fatigue syndrome. Among its constituents are saponins and germanium (*see both*). A tonic to increase energy.

SUMAC (H) • *Rhus glabra*. **Sumach. Sweet Sumach.** A number of members of this genus possess poisonous properties. *Rhus* is found growing wild in all parts of the United States. The bark and fruit are astringent. Sumac berries are used as a gargle in decoction form for the chest pain angina. The decoction is also gargled for throat irritation and to help asthmatics breathe easier. The high tannin (*see*) content in the berries explains why it was used to treat diarrhea. The root was chewed by some North American Indians for mouth sores.

SUMATRIPTAN (Rx) • **Imitrex.** An injectable drug introduced in 1992 for the acute treatment of migraine and cluster headaches. In 1995, a tablet form was introduced. It does not prevent or reduce the number of attacks. Sumatriptan activates certain serotonin (*see*) receptors and has been shown to be beneficial in both conditions. In clinical trials the drug relieved pain in 80 percent of the patients within two hours of injection. Headache experts have said that other drugs are generally as effective, but that many work only when given at the beginning of a migraine episode and have side effects like drowsiness. Potential adverse effects include tingling, warm/hot sensation, pressure sensation, feeling of tightness, numbness, cold sensation, flushing, chest discomfort, weakness, neck pain, dizziness, and injection-site reaction. The FDA required Glaxo, the maker of sumatriptan, to add a warning to the drug's label in 1994. A forty-one-year-old woman who had a history of heart disease, asthma, and an allergy to codeine died shortly after receiving an injection of sumatriptan. Glaxo agreed to add a description of the incident to the label even though it felt there wasn't a positive link between the woman's death and the drug. The FDA says it wanted to make sure physicians prescribe the drug appropriately, and not for persons with heart disease. It should not be taken by pregnant women. It should also not be used within two weeks of taking an MAO inhibitor (*see*). It is now available in tablet form.

SUMOX • *See* Amoxicillin.

SUMYCIN • *See* Tetracycline Hydrochloride.

SUNDEW (H) • *Drosera rotundifolia*. The herb contains quinones, flavonoids, tannins, and citric acid (*see all*). It is used by herbalists to treat bronchitis and infections caused by the bacteria streptococcus, staphylococcus, and pneumococcus. Used to treat respiratory infections, asthma, and stomach ulcers.

SUNFLOWER (H) • *Helianthus annuus*. **Indian Sunflower. Lady Eleven O'clock. Marigold of Peru.** Introduced into the United States from Mexico and Peru, the seeds are used in medicine as a diuretic and a soothing tonic for coughs. Used today as a dietary supplement. High in vitamin E.

SUPAC (OTC) • Buffered acetaminophen, aspirin, and caffeine (*see all*), used to treat pain and fever.

SUPEN • *See* Ampicillin.

SUPERCHAR • *See* Activated Charcoal.

SUPER D PERLES • *See* Vitamin A and Vitamin D.

SUPERINFECTION • A second infection that is superimposed upon the first, which is under treatment. A superinfection is caused by germs that are not susceptible to the drug being used to treat the primary infection. Superinfections usually occur during or immediately following treatment with a broad-spectrum antibiotic.

SUPLICAL • *See* Calcium Carbonate.

SUPPAP • *See* Acetaminophen.

SUPPOSITORY • A form of medicine inserted into the vagina or rectum.

SUPPRELIN • *See* Histrelin.

SUPPRESSION • A treatment intended to keep infection under control and to prevent its progression.

SUPPRESSOR T CELLS • A subset of T cells that can turn off antibody production and other immune responses.

SUPPRETTES • *See* Belladonna.

SUPPURATE • To fester and secrete pus.

SUPRA- • Prefix meaning above or on.

SUPRANE • *See* Desflurane.

SUPRAVENTRICULAR TACHYCARDIA • An irregular rhythm of the heart that occurs when extra electrical impulses in the upper chambers or the center of the heart stimulate the lower chambers of the heart, the ventricles, to contract rapidly. *See* Arrhythmia and Antiarrhythmics.

SUPRAX • *See* Cefixime.

SURBEX (OTC) • A multivitamin preparation.

SURFAK • *See* Docusate.

SURITAL • *See* Thiamylal.

SURMONTIL • *See* Trimipramine.

SURVANTA • *See* Beractant.

SUS-PHRINE • *See* Epinephrine.

SUSTAIRE • *See* Theophylline.

SUTILAINS OINTMENT (Rx) • **Travase Ointment.** An agent applied topically to treat infected burns and skin ulcers. Promotes debridement of dead tissue.

SUXAMETHONIUM CHLORIDE • *See* Succinylcholine.

SWALLOWING DISORDERS • **Dysphagia.** Difficulty in swallowing, or the sensation that a pill or food is stuck in the neck or chest.

SWALLOWWORT (H) • *Cynanchum vincetoxicum.* Common vincetoxicum, an erect, leafy perennial native to Europe and North Africa. It is used in homeopathic medicine as a diaphoretic and diuretic. The plant may exert an adverse effect on the heart.

SWEEN CREAM • *See* Methylbenzethonium Chloride.

SWEET CICELY (H) • *Myrrhis odorata. Osmorhiza longistylis.* **Anise Root. Fern-Leaved Chervil. Sweet Anise.** A perennial herb native to Britain, it was used as a prevention against plague. In Alaska and North America, the root was used for a tonic for invalids and new mothers. It also was used in a poultice for wounds and sores and was taken for coughs, flatulence, and digestive complaints. Used in an herbal tea as a tonic.

SWEET FERN (H) • *Polypodium vulgare.* **Common Polypody. Female Fern. Rock Brake. Wood Licorice.** The root of this fern distributed throughout Europe, Africa, Siberia, Asia, and North America was used in folk medicine to treat melancholy and intestinal obstruction. The resin is considered to be useful against worms and as a purgative. It also possesses demulcent properties. Sweet fern is also reportedly useful in alleviating coughs and other lung problems, as well as being a good appetite stimulant.

SWEET FLAG • *See* Calamus.

SWEET SEDGE • *See* Calamus.

SWEET SPIRITS OF NITRE • Banned by the FDA during its review of OTC drugs.

SWEET VIOLET • *See* Violet.

SWEET WOODRUFF • *See* Woodruff.

SWIM EAR • *See* Boric Acid.

SYLLACT • *See* Psyllium.

SYMADINE • *See* Amantadine.

SYMMETREL • *See* Amantadine.

SYMPATHETIC NERVOUS SYSTEM • One of the major divisions of the autonomic nervous system (*see*); it regulates involuntary muscle action such as the beating of the heart and breathing. The sympathetic nerves that leave the brain and spinal cord pass through the nerve cell clusters (ganglia) and are distributed to the heart, lungs, intestines, blood vessels, and sweat glands. In general, sympathetic nerves dilate the pupils, constrict small blood vessels, and increase heart rate. They are the nerves that prepare us for fight or flight. The other part of the autonomic system, parasympathetic nerves, slows things down after you stop exercising or the danger has passed. The system also involves circulating substances produced by the adrenal glands.

SYMPATHOMIMETICS • Drugs that imitate the action of the sympathetic nervous system (*see*).

SYMPH • Homeopathic abbreviation for *Symphytum officinale* (*see*).

SYMPHYTUM OFFICINALE (H) • **Symph.** A homeopathic ointment used to treat rashes and sprains. *See* Comfrey.

SYMPLOCARPUS FOETIDUS • *See* Skunk Cabbage.

SYMPTOM • A specific sign of a patient's condition indicating an abnormal physical or mental state.

SYMPTOMATIC • Sick. Symptomatic patients recognize they have a disease because they are experiencing specific physical problems.

SYNACORT • *See* Hydrocortisone.

SYNACTHEN • *See* Cosyntropin.

SYNALAR • *See* Fluocinolone.

SYNALGOS-DC (Rx) • A combination of aspirin, caffeine, and dihydrocodeine (*see all*), used for mild to moderate pain relief.

SYNAPSE • A point of communication between nerve cells that come close together but do not touch. The nerve impulses are chemically transmitted.

SYNAREL • *See* Nafarelin Acetate.

SYNCOPE • Fainting.

SYNDROME • A collective set of symptoms that characterize a disease.

SYNEMOL • *See* Fluocinolone.

SYNERGISM • The interaction of two drugs to produce increased activity that is greater than the sum of the effects of the two drugs given separately.

SYNKAYVITE • *See* Menadione.

SYNOVIAL JOINT • A type of joint permitting more or less free movement, such as the joints of the limbs and the spinal column.

SYNTHETIC • Made in the laboratory and not by nature. Vanillin, for example, made in the laboratory may be identical to vanilla extracted from the vanilla bean, but vanillin cannot be called "natural."

SYNTHROID • *See* Levothyroxine.

SYNTHROX • *See* Levothyroxine.

SYNTOCINON • *See* Oxytocin.

SYPHILIS • A sexually transmitted disease caused by the bacteria *Treponema pallidum.* These bacteria easily penetrate the mucous membranes of the mouth, vagina, and penis. Syphilis may first appear as a painless skin sore, but if untreated, syphilis can appear throughout a lifetime and eventually affect the brain and cause paralysis. It may also attack the heart.

SYSTEMIC • Having a generalized effect; causing physical or chemical changes throughout the body.

SYSTEMIC LUPUS ERYTHEMATOSUS • A disease characterized by necrosis of connective tissue affecting most of the systems of the body. Caused by disturbance to the immune system. The organs affected are mostly joints. The kidney is also affected.

SYSTOLIC BLOOD PRESSURE • Blood pressure when the heart is contracting.

T

TABLET • Solid form of medication that is taken orally.

TABLOID • *See* Thioguanine.

TABRON (OTC) • A multivitamin and mineral preparation.

TACARYL • *See* Methdilazine.

TACE • *See* Chlorotrianisene.

TACHY- • Prefix indicating rapid.

TACHYCARDIA • Rapid heartbeat.

TACRINE (Rx) • **Cognex. THA.** Approved by the FDA for marketing in 1993, it is the first drug specifically aimed at treating Alzheimer's disease (*see*). It reportedly is effective in approximately 12 percent of the patients with the disease. Its use is limited by a significant incidence of liver damage and mild cognitive benefit. It does not alter the course of the disease. However, because of the devasting nature of Alzheimer's, researchers at Mt. Sinai Medical School in New York who evaluated the drug say "physicians should consider its use because it can provide some relief for patients and their families, despite its adverse event profile."

TACROLIMUS (Rx) • **Prograf.** An immunosuppressant agent introduced in 1994 for the prevention of organ rejection in patients receiving liver transplants. It was introduced to the Japanese market in 1993, and the FDA priority review took only 8.4 months. Tacrolimus reportedly does not cause excess facial hair growth—one of the adverse effects associated with cyclosporin (*see*).

TAC-3 • *See* Triamcinolone.

TAGAMET • *See* Cimetidine.

TALACEN (Rx) • An analgesic possessing fever-lowering action. *See* Acetaminophen and Pentazocine Hydrochloride or Lactate.

TALBUTAL (Rx) • **Lotusate.** A barbiturate (*see*) sleeping drug.

TALC (OTC) • **French Chalk.** A finely powdered native magnesium silicate; a mineral. Prolonged inhalation can cause lung problems because it is similar in chemical composition to asbestos, a known lung irritant and cancer-causing agent. In 1992, the FDA proposed a ban on talc in astringent (*see*) drug products because it had not been shown to be safe and effective as claimed.

TALWIN • *See* Pentazocine Hydrochloride or Lactate.

TALWIN COMPOUND (Rx) • *See* Pentazocine Hydrochloride or Lactate and Aspirin.

TALWIN NX (Rx) • *See* Naloxone and Pentazocine Hydrochloride or Lactate.

TAM • Homeopathic abbreviation for tamus (*see*).

TAMARIND EXTRACT (H) • The extract of *Tamarindus indica,* a large tropical tree grown in the East Indies and Africa. Preserved in sugar or syrup, it is used as a natural fruit flavoring. The pulp contains about 10 percent tartaric acid (*see*). Has been used as a cooling laxative drink. The medicinal properties of tamarind were employed by Arab physicians, who introduced the fruit from India into Europe. The laxative effect of the fruit is said to be due to its high concentration of sugars that are not very absorbable in the intestinal tract. Because of this, they cause water to migrate from the surrounding tissues into the intestines. This causes an expansion of the intestines, which results in a nonirritant type of bowel movement.

TAMBOCOR • *See* Flecainide Acetate.

TAMINE (OTC) • *See* Brompheniramine and Phenylpropanolamine.

TAMOXIFEN CITRATE (Rx) • **Nolvadex.** A hormonal medication introduced in 1978 for the treatment of breast cancer. It antagonizes estrogen. Used to treat advanced premenopausal and postmenopausal breast cancer. Studies have confirmed that tamoxifen, when given soon after the initial surgical or radiation treatment, can reduce the chances of cancer spreading and cure an additional twelve women per hundred treated. During the course of these studies it has been observed the chances of breast cancer occurring in the normal untreated breast are also reduced. In addition, tamoxifen has also been reported to slow osteoporosis (*see*) and lower cholesterol. Potential adverse reactions include hot flashes, nausea, depression, vaginal dryness, vaginal discharge, high blood calcium, swelling of the arms and legs, rash, vomiting, visual changes, vaginal itch, headache, loss of appetite, a transient drop in white blood cells, weight gain, drowsiness, bone pain, and a drop in platelet count. Prolonged use may be associated with an increase in uterine cancer. A study of tamoxifen for prevention of breast cancer by the National Cancer Institute has raised controversy because of an increase in the risk of uterine cancer among study participants. Although tamoxifen has fewer side effects than most anticancer medications, prolonged use may adversely affect the eyes. High doses of tamoxifen in rats have been observed to cause liver cancer. It has also been reported to cause cancer of the uterine lining in humans. Increased blood clotting has been reported very rarely in patients on tamoxifen. As of this writing, tamoxifen is being tested in healthy women who are at risk for breast cancer but who have never had it, to determine if the malignancy can be prevented. Most effective when taken on an empty stomach, but may be taken with a small amount of food if stomach distress is a problem.

TAMPER RESISTANT PACKAGING • Packaging designed to make it apparent to the user if someone has tampered with the package after it was sealed at the factory.

TAMPONADE • Fluid in the pericardium, the loose sac around the heart that keeps it from rubbing against the chest wall.

TAMUS (H) • **Tam.** A homeopathic remedy for treating chilblain, skin redness, and itching usually associated with extreme cold. *See* Black Bryony.

TANDEARIL • *See* Oxyphenbutazone.

TANGERETIN • A substance from tangerines found to be anticarcinogenic in experiments.

TANG KWEI • *See* Dong Quai.

TANG SHEN • *See* Don Sen.

TANNIC ACID (OTC) (H) • **Outgro Solution. Zilactin. Zilactin Medicated Gel. Zilactol Medicated Liquid.** Occurs in the bark and fruit of many plants, notably in the bark of the oak and sumac, and in cherry, coffee, and tea. Used medicinally as a mild astringent; when applied, it may turn the skin brown. Used in sunscreen preparations, eye lotions, and antiperspirants. Tea contains tannic acid, which explains its folk use as an eye lotion. Used in medicated gel to stop pain and speed healing of canker sores. A mild temporary stinging sensation may be experienced with this use. Excessive use in creams or lotions in hypersensitive persons may lead to irritation, blistering, and increased pigmentation. Has low toxicity when taken orally, but large doses may cause gastric distress. In 1992, the FDA issued a notice that tannic acid had not been shown to be safe and effective as claimed in OTC digestive-aid products, fever-blister treatment products, and products to treat poison ivy, poison oak, and poison sumac. Tannic acid glycerite in astringent (*see*) drugs and tannic acid in diaper-rash and cold-sore drugs were also on the list. It may still be used for other purposes.

TANNIN (H) • Any of a broad group of plant-derived phenolic compounds. Some are beneficial and some are toxic, depending upon their sources. Tannins in herbs are astringent (*see*). They are soothing to the skin and mucous membranes and can bind to the tissues of the intestines, reducing diarrhea and internal bleeding. Herbalists use them to treat burns for wound healing. *See* Tannic Acid.

TANSY (H) • *Tanacetum vulgare.* **Bitter Buttons. Parsley Fern.** A native of Greece, tansy is widespread in the United States in gardens and along highways. Its name comes from the Greek word *athanasia,* meaning "immortality," so-called because the dead flowers do not wilt. During the fifteenth century, tansy was used in a tea to treat gas, children's colic, abdominal cramps, gout, and even for the Great Plague. Was also used for centuries by young girls in a tea to alleviate slow and painful menstruation. Tansy was considered a laxative, a gentle stimulant to digestion, and even a sedative. The plant is still listed in the USP (*see*) chiefly for its use as a tea to avert colds, a cold decoction to be used during convalescence from fever and jaundice, to get rid of worms, and externally, for use on bruises and inflammation. If too much tansy is taken, it can result in vomiting, convulsions, and death.

TAO • *See* Troleandomycin.

TAPANOL • *See* Acetaminophen.

TAPAR • *See* Acetaminophen.

TAPAZOLE • *See* Methimazole.

TARACTAN • *See* Chlorprothixene.

TARAXACUM OFFICINALE • *See* Dandelion.

TARDIVE DYSKINESIA • Abnormal grimacing occurring as a side effect of some antipsychotic medications.

TARPASTE • *See* Coal Tar.

TARRAGON (H) • *Artemisia dracunculus.* A perennial herb of the wormwood family native to southern Europe, Russian, and western Asia, it is cultivated in the United States. The name is derived from *dracunculus,* meaning "little dragon." In herbal medicine, tarragon is employed as a diuretic, for digestive purposes, and to treat catarrh (*see*). It is nontoxic when used in small doses as a spice, but the oil in large doses can cause miscarriage and has been found to be carcinogenic in animals.

TARTARIC ACID • Banned by the FDA as an ingredient in saline laxatives, May 1992.

TAURINE (Rx) (H) • An amino acid found in almost every tissue of the body, and at a high level in human milk. Most infant soy protein formulas are now supplemented with taurine. Taurine is almost absent from vegetarian diets. It is believed to be necessary for healthy eyes and is an antioxidant. It is also believed to be necessary for a regular heartbeat because it affects membrane excitability by normalizing potassium flux in and out of the heart-muscle cells. Supplementation may prevent digitalis-induced irregular heartbeats.

TAVIST-D • *See* Clemastine and Phenylpropanolamine.

TAVIST-1 • *See* Clemastine.

TAXOL (Rx) • *See* Paclitaxel.

TAZICEF • *See* Ceftazidime.

TAZIDIME • *See* Ceftazidime.

T CELLS • Small white blood cells that orchestrate and/or directly participate in the immune defenses. Also known as T lymphocytes, they are processed in the thymus and secrete lymphokines.

TCN • *See* Tetracyclines.

T-DIET • *See* Phentermine.

TEA (H) • *Camellia sinensis.* The shavings of leaves, and the leaf buds and internodes of fragrant white flowers, prepared and cured to make an aromatic beverage. Cultivated principally in China, Japan, Ceylon, and other Asian countries. Tea leaves come from an evergreen of the camellia family Theaceae, and are processed in different ways to produce green, black, and oolong tea. Each emerges with different chemical properties. To produce black tea, which most Americans drink, leaves are subjected to warmth for a few hours and heated to 200° F to finish the drying process. Black tea is being studied for skin-cancer-preventing properties. Green tea is popular in Asia and is not heated, but simply steamed, rolled, and crushed. Green tea is being tested as a preventative against gastric and esophageal cancers. Oolong tea is less heated than black, but just enough to give it a character different from green. Tea in general is a mild stimulant, and its tonic properties are due to the alkaloid caffeine; tannic acid (*see*) makes it astringent. A cup of strong tea contains about 100 mg of caffeine (*see*). Used by natural cosmeticians to reduce puffiness around the eyes. No known toxicity. Green tea has recently been shown by scientists to have the most beneficial effects. It contains more polyphenols than the other teas. Polyphenols have been shown in laboratory animals to lower cholesterol and protect against cancer. Polyphenols act like antioxidants (vitamins C and E and beta-carotene, for example), which combat destructive compounds, free radicals.

TEAR-EFRIN • *See* Phenylephrine.

TEARISOL (OTC) • *See* Artificial Tears.

TEARS NATURALE (OTC) • *See* Artificial Tears.

TEARS PLUS (OTC) • *See* Artificial Tears.

TEBACIN • *See* Aminosalicylic Acid.

TEBAMIDE • *See* Trimethobenzamide.

TEBRAZID • *See* Pyrazinamide.

TECHNERIUM 99M BICISATE (Rx) • **Neurolite.** A radiopharmaceutical imaging agent for aid in localization of a stroke in patients with previously diagnosed stroke. In use in eight other countries, the FDA approved it in 1994 after a review of 32.6 months.

TEDRAL (Rx) • **Azma Aid. Phedral C.T. Primatene P. Tedrigen. Theodrine. Theofedral.** The drugs are all a combination of ephedrine, phenobarbital, and theophylline, used to treat asthma and other respiratory disorders. The combination relaxes the bronchial muscles, increases the width of breathing passages, and contains a mild tranquilizer to help relax the patient. Potential adverse reactions include dizziness, excitation, insomnia, nervousness, rapid heartbeat, chest pains, irregular heartbeat, dry nose and throat, headache, sweating, hesitation or frequency of urination, muscle weakness, drowsiness, muscle spasm, and unsteady gait. Contraindicated in severe kidney or liver disease. Taking tedral or similar medicines with MAO inhibitors (*see*) may cause severe adverse reactions. Tedral will make lithium and propranolol less effective. Erythromycin and similar antibiotics can increase the side effects of tedral. Should be taken with food.

TEGA-VERT (OTC) • *See* Dimenhydrinate.

TEGISON • *See* Etretinate.

TEGOPEN (OTC) • *See* Cloxacillin Sodium.

TEGRETOL • *See* Carbamazepine.

TEGRIN • *See* Coal Tar.

TELACHLOR • *See* Chlorpheniramine.

TELANGIECTASIS • The dilation of groups of small blood vessels, appearing as fine lines on the skin.

TELDRIN (OTC) • *See* Chlorpheniramine.

TELINE • *See* Tetracyclines.

TEMAFLOXACIN (Rx) • **Omniflox.** A broad-spectrum quinoline antibiotic introduced in 1992, indicated for the treatment of mild to moderate adult infections of the lungs, prostate, skin, and urinary tract. It was pulled from the market within three months because of severe reactions, including possibly three deaths.

TEMARIL • *See* Trimeprazine Tartrate.

TEMAZ • *See* Temazepam.

TEMAZEPAM (Rx) • **Razepam. Restoril. Temaz.** A benzodiazepine (*see*) sleeping drug introduced in 1978 that acts on the limbic system, thalamus, and hypothalamus of the central nervous system to produce hypnotic effects. Adverse reactions include drowsiness, dizziness, lethargy, incoordination, daytime sedation, confusion, loss of appetite, and diarrhea. Should be used carefully in impaired liver or kidney function, mental depression, suicidal tendencies, a history of drug abuse, and in elderly or debilitated patients. Should be used with caution in persons with narrow angle glaucoma. Alcohol and other central nervous system depressants including narcotic analgesics, tranquilizers, antihistamines, MAO inhibitors (*see*), and sleeping pills may increase the depressive effects of temazepam. Smoking may reduce the effectiveness of this drug. May take up to two and a half hours for onset of action. Should be taken at bedtime. Can be habit-forming. If you have been taking this drug for more than two weeks, check with your physician about tapering it off if you wish to stop.

TEMOVATE • *See* Clobetasol.

TEMPOROMANDIBULAR JOINT DISEASE • **TMJ.** Pain caused by misalignment of the jawbone; due to congenital and developmental anomalies, fractures, dislocations, arthritis, and tumors.

TEMPRA • *See* Acetaminophen.

TENDON • A band of tough, white, fibrous tissue that connects a muscle to a bone.

TENEX • *See* Guanfacine.

TENIDAP (Rx) • **Enablex.** A novel anti-inflammatory drug for the treatment of both osteoarthritis and rheumatoid arthritis, expected on the market as of this writing. The product is described as the first of a new class of drugs known as cytokine (*see*) modulators. It is said to ease the acute symptoms of arthritis while potentially slowing the long-term progression of the disease.

TENIPOSIDE (Rx) • **EPT. VM-26. Vumon.** An anticancer drug used in the treatment of Hodgkin's disease, non-Hodgkin's lymphomas, acute lymphocytic leukemia, bladder cancer, and neuroblastoma.

TEN-K • *See* Potassium Chloride.

TENOL • *See* Acetaminophen.

TENORETIC (Rx) • A combination of atenolol and chlorthalidone (*see both*) used to treat high blood pressure. Atenolol is a beta-blocker (*see*) and chlorthalidone is a diuretic. Potential adverse reactions include nausea, vomiting, dizziness, tingling of the scalp, taste distortion, fatigue, sweating, male impotence, urinary difficulty, diarrhea, bile-duct blockage, breathing difficulty, bronchial spasms, muscle weakness, cramps, dry eyes, blurred vision, rash, hair loss, mental depression, short-term memory loss, emotional instability, and facial swelling. Should be used cautiously in asthmatics, and in patients with severe heart failure, slow heart rate, heart block, and liver or kidney dysfunction. Beta-blockers may interact with surgical anesthetics to increase the risk of heart problems during surgery. An anesthesiologist may recommend withdrawing a beta-blocker gradually two days before surgery. Aspirin, indomethacin, estrogens, and sulfinpyrazone interfere with tenoretic's effectiveness. Other drugs used to treat blood pressure as well as antipsychotic drugs and sulfas may increase tenoretic's effects. Tenoretic may interfere with the effectiveness of asthma drugs. The combination of tenoretic and phenytoin or digitalis can result in excessive slowing of the heart and possible heart block. Tenoretic increases lithium's and quinidine's toxicity. Over-the-counter stimulants such as those in cold medications and diet pills may increase tenoretic's side effects. Should not be discontinued suddenly. Should be taken before 10 A.M. to avoid having to urinate during the night.

TENORMIN • *See* Atenolol.

TENSILON • *See* Edrophonium.

TENUATE • *See* Diethylpropion.

TERAMIN • *See* Phentermine.

TERATOGENIC • From the Greek word *terat,* meaning monster, and Latin word *genesis,* meaning origin: the origin or cause of a monster, or a defective fetus.

TERAZOL 7 • *See* Terconazole.

TERAZOSIN HYDROCHLORIDE (Rx) • **Hytrin.** A drug introduced in 1987 that blocks the nerve signals that trigger constriction of blood vessels, thus lowering blood pressure. Potential adverse effects include weakness, dizziness, headache, nervousness, numbness, sleepiness, decreased libido, impotence, heart palpitations, a drop in blood pressure upon rising from a sitting or prone position, irregular heartbeat, swelling, stuffy nose, sinusitis, blurred vision, nausea, shortness of breath, back pain, muscle pain, weight gain, and impotence. Terazosin may interact with nitroglycerin or calcium channel blockers (*see both*) to increase side effects. The blood-pressure-lowering effect of terazosin may be reduced by indomethacin. Other blood-pressure-lowering drugs increase the blood-pressure-lowering effect of terazosin, possibly causing very low blood pressure. Alcohol may exaggerate the blood-pressure-lowering actions of this drug, causing excessive reduction. May be taken with or without food.

TERBINAFINE (Rx) • **Lamisil.** An antifungal medication introduced in the United States in 1992 for the treatment of athlete's foot, jock itch, and ringworm. It is being used in twenty-three other countries.

TERBUTALINE SULFATE (Rx) • **Brethaire. Brethine. Bricanyl.** A bronchodilator introduced in 1974 to relieve bronchospasm in patients with reversible obstructive airway disease, and to counteract premature labor. Reportedly very effective in the relief of bronchospasm. Potential adverse reactions include tremors, headache, drowsiness, sweating, increased heart rate, drying and irritation of the nose and throat (inhaler form), vomiting, and nausea. MAO inhibitors (*see*) may cause severe high blood pressure. Propranolol and other beta-blockers (*see*) make it less effective. Antidepressants, some antihistamines, and levothyroxine also may make terbutaline less effective. Should be used cautiously in patients with diabetes, high blood pressure, overactive thyroid, severe heart disease, and irregular heartbeat. Terbutaline may lose its effectiveness if overused. May be taken with food.

TERCONAZOLE (OTC) • **Terazol 7 Vaginal Cream. Terazol 3 Vaginal Suppositories.** An antifungal agent used to treat vaginal candidiasis. Potential adverse reactions include headache, burning and irritation of the vaginal lining, fever, chills, and body ache. The effectiveness of this drug is not affected by menstruation. Partner should use a condom to prevent reinfection.

TEREBINTH • *See* Turpentine Tree.

TERFENADINE (Rx) • **Seldane. Seldane-D (with pseudoephedrine).** Introduced in 1977, it is used to relieve symptoms associated with seasonal allergic rhinitis such as sneezing, runny nose, itching, and tearing. Promoted as a non-sedating antihistamine. Relief begins in one hour. Contraindicated in patients with known hypersensitivity to terfenadine or any of its ingredients. Should be used cautiously in patients with liver dysfunction, low potassium, or irregular heartbeat. In July 1992, the FDA instructed the makers of terfenadine to strengthen the warning about the risk of patients developing life-threatening, abnormal heart rhythms if they have liver dysfunction or if they take one of three antibiotics—erythromycin, ketoconazole, or troleandomycin—concurrently with terfenadine. Reports received by the company of severe adverse cardiovascular effects include, in addition to irregular heartbeat, low blood pressure, heart palpitations, and fainting. Nine cases of serious side effects including one death have been reported in Japan in association with terfenadine. The adverse drug reactions were related to heart problems in patients receiving certain antibiotics, or in those with liver problems. Other potential adverse terfenadine effects include drowsiness, headache, fatigue, dizziness, nervousness, weakness, appetite increase, abdominal distress, nausea, vomiting, a change in bowel habits, dry mouth, nose, and throat, cough, sore throat, nosebleed, hair loss, menstrual irregularity, female breast enlargement with milk production, sweating, muscle ache, tingling of hands and feet, visual disturbances, liver dysfunction, itching, and rash. Unlike other antihistamines, terfenadine reportedly does not interact with alcohol and other central nervous system depressants. Medication should be discontinued four days before taking a skin allergy test because it can lead to inaccurate results. Terfenadine may be taken on an empty stomach. A candidate for OTC status, as of this writing. Also a candidate for production as a less costly generic drug.

TERFONYL • *See* Trisulfapyrimidines.

TERIPARATIDE (Rx) • Synthetic substance that has a biological activity similar to the parathyroid hormone, which helps control the level of calcium in the blood. It is used to treat osteoporosis (*see*), and as a diagnostic aid in cases of low calcium.

TERPENES (Rx) (OTC) (H) • A class of unsaturated hydrocarbons occurring in most essential oils and plant resins. Among terpene derivatives are camphor and menthol (*see both*). Some terpenes are used as antiseptics.

TERPIN HYDRATE (OTC) • An expectorant that increases the production of respiratory-tract fluids to help liquefy and reduce the viscosity of thick secretions. Used to treat excessive bronchial secretions. Potential adverse reactions include nausea, vomiting, drowsiness, and stomach pain. Contraindicated in peptic ulcer or severe diabetes. When formulated with codeine, it has a depressant effect and a potential effect on breathing and should not be taken with alcohol, sedatives, tranquilizers, antihistamines, or other depressant drugs unless prescribed by a physician. The alcohol in this medication will add to the effects of other alcohol-containing preparations and central nervous system depressants. A full glass of water should be taken with each dose to loosen mucus in the lungs.

TERRA-CORTRIL OPHTHALMIC • *See* Hydrocortisone and Oxytetracycline.

TERRAMYCIN • *See* Oxytetracycline.

TERRAMYCIN OPHTHALMIC OINTMENT • *See* Oxytetracycline and Polymyxin B.

TERSA-TAR • *See* Coal Tar.

TESLAC • *See* Testolactone.

TESPA • *See* Thiotepa.

TESSALON PERLES • *See* Benzonatate.

TESTICULAR CANCER • Tumors in the testicles, which account for the majority of solid malignancies in males under thirty years of age.

TESTODERM • A scrotal patch for testosterone (*see*) replacement therapy for conditions associated with a deficiency or absence of body testosterone. It was approved by the FDA in 1994.

TESTOLACTONE (Rx) • **Teslac.** A hormonal anticancer drug used to treat advanced postmenopausal breast cancer. Potential adverse reactions include nausea, vomiting, diarrhea, a sensation of pins and needles, increased blood pressure, fluid retention, high blood calcium, and hair loss. Oral blood thinners increase testolactone's effects. Contraindicated in male breast cancer and not recommended for premenopausal women.

TESTOSTERONE (Rx) • **Andro. Andro-cyp. Android-T. Andro-LA. Andronaq-LA. Andronate. Andryl. Delatest. Delatestryl. depAndro. Depotest. DEPO-Testosterone. Duratest T-Cypionate. Durathate-200. Everone. His-**

terone. **Malogen. Tesionate. Testa-C. Testaqua. Testex. Testoderm Scrotal Patch. Testoject. Testoject-LA. Testone LA. Testred Cypionate. Testrin PA. Virilon IM.** The male hormone, a steroid (*see*) produced by cells of the testicles. The testosterone market is expected to exceed $400 million in 1997. Given by injection or tablet, it stimulates target tissues to develop normally in androgen-deficient men. It is used to treat eunuchs and male hormonal change symptoms. Also used for breast engorgement in nonnursing mothers, and to treat breast cancer in women who are one to five years postmenopausal. Potential adverse reactions in women include acne, oily skin, weight gain, hairiness, hoarseness, clitoral enlargement, changes in libido, flushing, sweating, and vaginitis with itching. In prepubescent males, premature epiphyseal closure, priapism (*see*), growth of body and facial hair, phallic enlargement; in postpubescent males, testicular atrophy, scanty sperm, decreased ejaculatory volume, impotence, breast enlargement, and epididymitis. In both sexes, edema, gastroenteritis, nausea, vomiting, diarrhea, constipation, changes in appetite, bladder irritability, jaundice, liver toxicity, and high levels of calcium in the blood. Contraindicated in men with enlarged or cancerous prostates; carcinoma of the male breast; high levels of calcium in the blood; heart, liver, or kidney dysfunction; and in premature infants. Should be used cautiously in prepubescent males, patients with diabetes or heart disease, and in those taking ACTH, corticosteroids, or anticoagulants. Should be taken with food.

TESTRED • *See* Methyltestosterone.

TESTRIN PA • *See* Testosterone.

TETANUS • **Lockjaw.** A potentially fatal infection caused by toxins of tetanus organisms, which get into the body through perforating or penetrating or deep wounds and thrive in the absence of oxygen.

TETANUS ANTITOXIN (Rx) • **TAT.** An injection that neutralizes and binds tetanus (*see*) toxin. The injection is into the wound. Potential adverse reactions include joint pain, severe aller-gic reactions, serum sickness, and pain, numbness, and rash at the site of injection.

TETANUS TOXOID (Rx) • Tetanus causes death in 30–40 percent of all cases. This injection promotes immunity to tetanus by inducing production of antitoxin. Potential adverse reactions include slight fever, chills, malaise, aches and pains, flushing, hives, itching, rapid heartbeat, low blood pressure, and severe allergic reaction.

TETANY • Muscle twitchings and cramps due to lack of calcium in the blood.

TETRABENAZINE (Rx) • A dopamine-depleting agent used to treat psychosis and uncontrolled movements. Dopamine is a natural neurotransmitter involved in movement and mood. It is a precursor of norepinephrine and epinephrine (*see*).

TETRACAINE (Rx) • **Pontocaine. Pontocaine with Dextrose. Y-itch.** A local anesthetic introduced in 1932 for muscle sprain or saddle block in delivery of a baby. It is ten times as strong as procaine. Onset is in fifteen minutes and the duration of effect is up to three hours. Potential adverse reactions include skin reactions, swelling, continuous asthma attacks, severe allergic reactions, anxiety, nervousness, and seizures followed by drowsiness, unconsciousness, tremors, twitches, shivering, and respiratory arrest. Other potential reactions include blurred vision, ringing in the ears, nausea, and vomiting. It is also used in an eye ointment or solution used to anesthetize the eye during examination, the removal of corneal foreign bodies, and other minor surgical procedures. Potential adverse reactions include temporary stinging in the eye after instillation, and sensitization after repeated use. Cholinesterase inhibitors (*see*) may prolong eye anesthesia and increase the risk of toxicity. Tetracaine may make sulfonamides less effective.

TETRACLEAR (OTC) • *See* Tetrahydrozoline Hydrochloride.

TETRACOSACTIDE • *See* Cosyntropin.

TETRACYCLINE HYDROCHLORIDE (Rx)
• **Achromycin. Achromycin IV. Apo-Tetra. Cyclopar. KessoTetra. Robitet. Sumycin. Tetracap. Tetracyn. Tetralan.** A tetracycline antibiotic used to treat infections caused by gram-negative and gram-positive (*see both*) organisms, syphilis, gonorrhea, chlamydia, trachoma, brucellosis, shigellosis, rickettsiae, and *Mycoplasma* (*see all*). Potential side effects include nausea, vomiting, a drop in white blood cells, dizziness, headache, pressure on the brain, sore throat, sore tongue, trouble in swallowing, loss of appetite, colitis, inflammation around the anus, liver or kidney problems, and diarrhea. Tetracyclines may cause sensitivity to sunlight and result in a rash and discoloration of the skin. If tetracycline was taken during pregnancy, a child may have discolored teeth. Must be used with extreme caution in those with kidney or liver problems. Antacids, calcium supplements, milk, magnesium-containing laxatives, and baking soda should not be used with tetracyclines because they will make the drug less effective. If taken with tetracyclines, methoxyflurane (*see*) may cause severe kidney damage; oral contraceptives containing estrogen may not work properly. Iron supplements may reduce the effectiveness of tetracyclines, and they may reduce the effectiveness of penicillins. Also should not be taken with anticoagulants because tetracyclines may increase the action of these drugs; nor should they be taken with lithium, since such use may increase the levels of lithium in the blood.

TETRACYCLINES (Rx) (OTC)
• **Achromycin. Achromycin Ophthalmic. Aureomycin. Demeclocycline Hydrochloride. Doxycycline. Doxycycline Hyclate. Doxycycline Hydrochloride. Meclan. Methacycline. Minocycline Hydrochloride. Mysteclin F. Nor-Tet. Oxytetracycline Hydrochloride. Panmycin. TCN. Teline. Tetracap. Tetracycline Hydrochloride. Tetracyn. Tetralan. Tetram. Tetrex. Topicycline.** Introduced in 1953, they are among the most widely prescribed antibiotics. Used to treat acne, pneumonia, syphilis, gonorrhea, bronchitis, inflammation of the tube that carries urine, and to prevent chest infections. Also used to treat Rocky Mountain spotted fever, brucellosis, relapsing fever, cholera, trachoma, and arthritis due to infection. In skin preparations, it is used to treat acne. Potential adverse effects of skin products include pain, redness, swelling, and other signs of irritation not present before using the medication. Potential adverse effects of oral tetracyclines include nausea, vomiting, and diarrhea. Tetracyclines may cause sensitivity to sunlight and result in a rash and discoloration of the skin. Also used to prevent and treat eye infections. Eye preparations may cause eye itching and rash, allergic reactions, and overgrowth of resistant organisms with long-term use. If tetracycline is taken during pregnancy, a child may have discolored teeth. Antacids, calcium supplements, magnesium-containing laxatives, and baking soda should not be used with tetracyclines because they will make tetracyclines less effective. Oral contraceptives containing estrogen may not work properly if taken with tetracyclines. Iron supplements may reduce the effectiveness of tetracyclines, and tetracyclines may reduce the effectiveness of penicillins. Also should not be taken with anticoagulants because tetracyclines may increase the action of these drugs, nor should they be taken with lithium since such use may increase levels of lithium in the blood. Should be taken on an empty stomach one or two hours after meals, with eight ounces of water. The antibacterial effect of tetracycline may be neutralized when taken with food, some dairy products, iron-rich foods such as liver and lima beans, and antacids. Topical forms of tetracyclines are available without a prescription.

TETRACYN
• *See* Tetracyclines and Tetracycline Hydrochloride.

TETRAHYDROCANNABINOL
• *See* Dronabinol.

TETRAHYDROZOLINE HYDROCHLORIDE (OTC)
• **Colliyrium Fresh. Murine Plus. Ocu-Drop. Optigene-3. Soothe Eye Drops. Tetraclear. Tetra-Ide. Tetrasine. Tetryzoline. Tyzine Drops. Visine.** Eyedrops introduced in 1954 to produce constriction of the blood vessels in the eyes; used to "take the redness out"

and soothe irritation. Tetrahydrozoline constricts blood vessels and thus makes the eye whiter. The problem is that when the drops are used as often as several times a day, the blood vessels can become accustomed to the vasoconstriction. Consequently, redness recurs when the drops are not used. A second problem lies in the potential for the drops to wash away a protective layer on the tear film of the cornea, resulting in "paradoxical tearing"—the tear ducts begin to overwater the eye to compensate for the loss of this layer caused by the drops. Both conditions are temporary and clear once the overuse of drops has been stopped. In nose drops, tetrahydrozoline is used to counteract nasal congestion. Potential adverse reactions include transient stinging, dilation of the pupil, increased eye pressure, irritation, iris floaters in the elderly, drowsiness, central nervous system depression, heart irregularities, headache, dizziness, tremors, and insomnia. Tricyclics, guanethidine, and MAO inhibitors (*see*) may cause severe high blood pressure if tetrahydrozoline is systemically absorbed. Contraindicated in patients receiving MAO inhibitors, in those with hypersensitivity to any of the ingredients, and in those with glaucoma. Should be used cautiously in patients with overactive thyroid, diabetes, high blood pressure, or heart disease, and in the elderly.

TETRA-IDE • *See* Tetrahydrozoline Hydrochloride.

TETRALAN • *See* Tetracyclines and Tetracycline Hydrochloride.

TETRAMUNE (Rx) • A combination vaccine approved in 1993 that protects against diphtheria, tetanus, pertussis, and haemophilus b (the leading cause of meningitis). It reduces the number of vaccinations, from eight to four, that a child is required to have.

TETREX • *See* Tetracyclines.

TETRYZOLINE • *See* Tetrahydrozoline Hydrochloride.

TETTERWORT • *See* Bloodroot.

TEXACORT • *See* Hydrocortisone.

TG • *See* Thioguanine.

THA • *See* Tacrine.

THALITONE • *See* Chlorthalidone.

THAM • *See* Tromethamine.

THAM-E • *See* Tromethamine.

THC • *See* Dronabinol.

THEOBID • *See* Theophylline.

THEOBROMA OIL (OTC) (H) • **Cacao Butter. Cocoa Butter.** A yellowish white solid with a chocolatelike taste and odor. Derived from the cacao bean. Widely used in confections, suppositories, pharmaceuticals, soaps, and cosmetics. No known toxicity, but may cause allergic reactions in those who are sensitive to it.

THEOBROMINE (OTC) (Rx) • The alkaloid found in cocoa, cola nuts, tea, and chocolate products, closely related to caffeine. It is used as a diuretic, smooth-muscle relaxant, heart stimulant, and blood-vessel dilator. In 1992, the FDA proposed a ban on theobromine sodium salicylate in oral menstrual drug products because it had not been shown to be safe and effective as claimed.

THEOCHRON • *See* Theophylline.

THEOCLEAR • *See* Theophylline.

THEO-DUR • *See* Theophylline.

THEOLAIR (Rx) • *See* Theophylline and Guaifenesin.

THEON • *See* Theophylline.

THEO-ORGANIDIN • *See* Theophylline.

THEOPHYL • *See* Theophylline.

THEOPHYLLINE (Rx) (OTC) • Accurbron. Aerolate. Aquaphyllin. Asmalix. Bronkodyl S-R. Duraphyl. Elixomin. Elixophyllin. Gyrocaps. Labid. Lanophyllin. Lixolin. Lodrane. Primatene Tablets. Quibron-T/SR. Sastavie. Slo-Bid. SloPhyllin. Somophyllin CRT. Synophylate. Theobid. Theo-Dur. Theochron. Theoclear. Theolair. Theon. Theo-Organidin. Theophyl. Theophyl-SR. Theospan-SR. Theostat. Theo-Time. Theo-24. Theovent. Uniphyl. An alkaloid with caffeine found in tea leaves, it is prepared synthetically for pharmaceutical use. A smooth-muscle relaxant, diuretic, heart stimulant, and vasodilator introduced in 1929, it is used to treat bronchial asthma, angina, and peripheral vascular disease. Potential adverse reactions include nausea, vomiting, restlessness, dizziness, headache, insomnia, seizures, muscle twitching, heart palpitations, rapid heartbeat, flushing, low blood pressure, an increase in breathing rate, loss of appetite, bitter aftertaste, heartburn, diarrhea, and hives. It is often combined with other medications such as ephedrine, guaifenesin, hydroxyzine, and barbiturates (*see all*). Barbiturates, phenytoin, and rifampin make it less effective. Beta-blockers (*see*) may cause bronchospasms. Erythromycin, troleandomycin, cimetidine, flu vaccine, and oral contraceptives may make it toxic. Smoking cigarettes or marijuana makes theophylline less effective. Contraindicated in those hypersensitive to xanthine compounds such as caffeine and theobromine, and those with irregular heartbeat. Must be used cautiously in young children, and in elderly patients with congestive heart failure or other circulatory problems. Also those with kidney or liver disease, peptic ulcer, overactive thyroid, and diabetes. Those taking theophylline must be careful about over-the-counter remedies that contain ephedrine. A smoker or recent former smoker must have the medication adjusted because its effectiveness is affected by the condition of the lungs due to smoking. In 1992, the FDA proposed a ban on theophylline in oral menstrual drug products because it had not been shown to be safe and effective as claimed. Should be taken on an empty stomach, but if it causes too much of a stomach problem, it can be ingested with a small amount of food. Avoid caffeine drinks and chocolate as they may increase the drug's effects.

THEOPHYL-SR • *See* Theophylline.

THEOSPAN • *See* Theophylline.

THEOSTAT • *See* Theophylline.

THEO-TIME • *See* Theophylline.

THEOVENT • *See* Theophylline.

THEOZINE • *See* Hydroxyzine.

THERACYS • *See* Bacillus Calmette-Guerin.

THERAFECTIN • *See* Amiprilose.

THERAFLU (OTC) • *See* Chlorpheniramine, Pseudoephedrine, and Acetaminophen.

THERA-FLUR GEL (Rx) • *See* Sodium Fluoride.

THERAGESIC • *See* Methyl Salicylate and Menthol.

THERAGOLD ANALGESIC LOTION • *See* Camphor.

THERAGRAN (OTC) • A multivitamin preparation with iron.

THERALAX (OTC) • *See* Bisacodyl.

THERMAZENE • *See* Silver Sulfadiazine.

THERMOGENESIS • The production of heat. A substance that raises body or skin temperature, such as menthol.

THERMOTABS (OTC) • Used to relieve muscle cramps and heat prostration due to excessive perspiration. *See* Potassium Chloride and Sodium Chloride.

THIABENDAZOLE (Rx) • Foldan. Mintezol. Tiabendazole. Introduced in 1967, it is used to treat systemic infections of pinworm, roundworm, threadworm, whipworm, cutaneous larva migrans, and trichinosis. May cause impaired mental alertness, impaired physical coordination, headache, and dizziness. May also cause fever, flushing, chills, swollen glands, loss of appetite, nausea, vomiting, diarrhea, and heartburn. It is best taken after meals, which helps to prevent nausea, vomiting, dizziness, and loss of appetite. The topical form is used to treat creeping eruption from the larvae found on a dog or cat. These larvae cause slowly moving burrows in the skin, itching, and inflammation. There have been no significant reports of adverse skin reactions.

THIAMAZOLE • *See* Methimazole.

THIAMIN • *See* Thiamin Hydrochloride.

THIAMIN HYDROCHLORIDE (OTC) • Betalin S. Biamine. Thiamin. Thiamin Mononitrate. Vitamin B$_1$. A white, crystalline powder used as a dietary supplement. Practically all vitamin B$_1$ sold is synthetic. Makes the energy in food available to the body; helps normal functioning of the nervous system. Also acts as a helper in important energy-yielding reactions in the body, and is vital for a healthy nervous system, strong muscles, and normal heart function. The recommended daily dietary allowance (RDA) of thiamin is 0.3 mg from birth to six months; 0.5 mg for six months to one year; 0.7 mg for one to three years; 0.9 mg for four to six years; 1.2 mg for seven to ten years; 1.4 mg for males aged eleven to eighteen years; 1.5 mg for males aged nineteen to fifty; 1.2 mg for males over fifty; 1.1 mg for females aged eleven to twenty-two; 1.0 mg for females over twenty-three years of age. Beriberi, which includes tingling or burning sensation in the legs, cramps, incoordination, heartbeat irregularities, and heart failure, is caused by severe deficiency of vitamin B$_1$. Milder deficiency may cause symptoms such as fatigue, irritability, loss of appetite, and disturbed sleep. More severe deficiency may cause confusion, loss of memory, depression, abdominal pain, and constipation. Prolonged use of thiamin may deplete other vitamins; thus, it should be taken in a vitamin B complex product. Other adverse reactions include restlessness, low blood pressure after rapid IV injection, nausea, hemorrhage, diarrhea, a feeling of warmth, itching, hives, sweating, fluid in the lungs, weakness, and severe allergic reactions. Thiamin is destroyed by alkalies and alkaline drugs such as phenobarbital. In 1992, the FDA proposed a ban on thiamin hydrochloride in oral menstrual drug products because it had not been shown to be safe and effective as claimed.

THIAMYLAL (Rx) • Surital. A barbiturate solution that is used to induce and maintain general anesthesia. It is given by vein.

THIAZIDE DIURETICS (Rx) • These sulfa-derived drugs are used to rid the body of excess fluid. They may lead to potassium deficiency and are therefore often given together with a potassium supplement or combined with a potassium-sparing diuretic. They are rapidly absorbed following oral administration and demonstrate their peak effects within two to three hours. Should not be taken with calcium supplements, calcium-containing foods, or vitamin D supplements; may cause a calcium overload. Symptoms include kidney stones, loss of appetite, nausea or vomiting, constipation, and frequent urination. Examples of thiazides are cyclothiazide, maxzide, minizide, and dyazide. *See* Sulfa Drugs.

THIETHYLPERAZINE (Rx) • Norzine. Torecan. A drug that inhibits nausea and vomiting, often used to counteract those effects of anticancer drugs. Potential adverse reactions include a transient drop in white blood cells, a high incidence of movement and balance problems, a sudden drop in blood pressure when rising from a seated or prone position, rapid heartbeat, blurred vision, dry mouth, constipation, urinary retention, menstrual irregularities, enlargement of the male breast, inhibited ejaculation, jaundice, mild photosensitivity (*see*), allergic skin reactions, increased appetite, and weight gain. Contraindicated in severe central nervous system depression, liver disease, coma, and in those sensitive to phenothiazine (see). Antacids inhibit the absorption of the oral form of thiethylperazine. Drugs that act on the central nervous system increase its adverse effects. Barbiturates decrease its effectiveness.

THIMEROSAL (OTC) • Merthiolate. A mercury compound with antimicrobial and antiseptic properties.

THIOCYANOACETATE (OTC) • A colorless gas or white solid that is very acidic. In 1992, the FDA proposed a ban on thiocyanoacetate in lice-killing products because it had not been shown to be safe and effective as claimed.

THIOGUANINE (Rx) • TG. Lanvis. 6-TG. 6-Thioguanine. Tabloid. Tioguanine. An anticancer drug used to treat acute and chronic leukemias. Potential adverse reactions include nausea, vomiting, diarrhea, sore mouth, anemia, high uric acid, loss of appetite, and liver damage. This medication should be taken on an empty stomach.

THIOPENTAL (Rx) • Pentothal. Sodium Pentothal. A fast-acting barbiturate used to induce general anesthesia for short-term procedures and to treat psychiatric disorders. Potential adverse reactions include prolonged sleepiness, amnesia of recent events, irregular heartbeat, respiratory depression, and lung and throat spasms, sneezing, coughing, and shivering.

THIORIDAZINE (Rx) • Mellaril. A phenothiazine (see) introduced in 1959, it is widely used to treat psychosis, depressive neurosis, alcohol withdrawal, dementia in geriatric patients, and behavioral problems in children. Potential adverse reactions include a low white blood count, tardive dyskinesia (see), sedation, a drop in blood pressure when rising from a seated or prone position, vision changes, dry mouth, constipation, urine retention, menstrual irregularities, inhibited ejaculation, liver dysfunction, mild photosensitivity, allergic skin reactions, decreased libido, impaired female orgasm, priapism (see), male breast enlargement, female breast enlargement with milk production, weight gain, increased appetite, fever, irregular heartbeat, and profuse sweating. Sudden discontinuation of long-term drug therapy may cause gastritis, nausea, vomiting, dizziness, tremors, sweating, irregular heartbeat, headache, and insomnia. Contraindicated in coma, central nervous system depression, bone marrow suppression, high or low blood pressure, brain damage, and with use of spinal or epidural anesthetic or adrenergic-blocking agents (see). Should be used cautiously in elderly or debilitated patients, in those with liver disease, cerebrovascular disease, respiratory disorders, low blood calcium, seizure disorders, intestinal obstruction, glaucoma, enlarged prostate, and in acutely ill or dehydrated children. Use with alcohol and other central nervous depressants may increase central nervous system depression. Antacids inhibit absorption and should not be used within two hours of taking thioridazine. Barbiturates and lithium may decrease thioridazine's effects. High blood pressure medications may be less effective. Caffeine-containing foods such as coffee, tea, cola drinks, or chocolate may counteract the effects of thioridazine. The drug may cause a false-positive pregnancy-test result. May be taken with or following meals to reduce stomach irritation.

THIOS • Homeopathic abbreviation for thiosinamine (see).

THIOSINAMINE (H) • Thios. Made from mustard oil, alcohol, and ammonia, it is used by homeopaths to treat scars.

THIOSULFIL • See Sulfa Drugs.

THIOTEPA (Rx) • TESPA. An alkylating (see), anticancer agent used to treat breast and ovarian cancer, lymphomas, and lung cancer. Potential adverse reactions include nausea, vomiting, discontinuation of menses, decreased sperm, high uric acid, hives, rash, a drop in white blood cells, headache, fever, tightness of throat, dizziness, and intense pain at administration site.

THIOTHIXENE (Rx) • Navane. Tiotixene. An antipsychotic drug introduced in 1967, used to treat acute agitation and mild to severe psychosis. Potential adverse reactions include a low white blood count, tardive dyskinesia (*see*), sedation, a drop in blood pressure when rising from a seated or prone position, vision changes, dry mouth, constipation, urine retention, menstrual irregularities, enlargement of male breast, inhibited ejaculation, liver dysfunction, mild photosensitivity, allergic skin reactions, weight gain, increased appetite, fever, irregular heartbeat, and profuse sweating. Sudden discontinuation of long-term drug therapy may cause gastritis, nausea, vomiting, dizziness, tremors, sweating, irregular heartbeat, headache, and insomnia. Use with alcohol and other central nervous system depressants may increase central nervous system depression. Antacids inhibit absorption and should not be used within two hours of taking thiothixene. Barbiturates, sleeping pills, narcotics, lithium, alcohol, and other central nervous system depressants may decrease thiothixene's effects. High blood pressure medications may be less effective. Contraindicated in coma, central nervous system depression, bone marrow suppression, high or low blood pressure, brain damage, and with the use of spinal or epidural anesthetic, or ACE inhibitors (*see*). Should be used cautiously in elderly or debilitated patients, in those with liver disease, cerebrovascular disease, respiratory disorders, low blood calcium, seizure disorders, intestinal obstruction, glaucoma, enlarged prostate, and in acutely ill or dehydrated children. Care should be taken in warm weather because this drug makes patients more susceptible to heatstroke. May be taken with or without food.

THISTLE (H) • *Cnicus benedictus. Sonchus oleraceus.* Holy Thistle. Milk Thistle. Sow Thistle. Several thistles were used as medicinal herbs. Holy thistle (*see*), a native of Greece and Italy, is an annual. Sow thistle, a vile-smelling weed, appeared in English medicine in 1387 and has been mentioned frequently from that time as a tonic. *See also* Milk Thistle.

THIURETIC • *See* Hydrochlorothiazide.

THORAZINE • *See* Chlorpromazine.

THORNAPPLE • *See* Jimsonweed.

THOR-PRAM • *See* Chlorpromazine.

THROMB- • Prefix that refers to a blood clot.

THROMBIN • Thrombinar. Thrombogen. An enzyme in blood that helps it to clot.

THROMBINAR • *See* Thrombin.

THROMBOCYTHEMIA • Spontaneous bleeding, irregularly shaped platelets and aggregates of platelets. Can lead to or accompany other conditions such as leukemia and polycythemia.

THROMBOCYTOPENIA • A reduction in the number of platelet cells in the blood, which causes a tendency to bleed.

THROMBOGEN • *See* Thrombin.

THROMBOLYSIS • Dissolution of a blood clot.

THROMBOLYTIC AGENT • Agents such as streptokinase and urokinase (*see both*) that dissolve blood clots.

THROMBOLYTIC THERAPY • Treatment with a class of drugs that dissolve blood clots.

THROMBOSIS • Formation of a blood clot on the lining of a blood vessel. A thrombus (*see*) that breaks away and is carried along in the bloodstream is one type of embolus (*see*). The process can be life-saving during hemorrhage, or life-threatening when the clot obstructs blood flow to an organ or body part.

THROMBOSTAT • *See* Thrombin.

THROMBUS • A blood clot that forms within the heart or blood vessel and remains attached to its point of origin.

THRUSH • A fungal infection of the mouth.

THU • Homeopathic abbreviation for thuja (*see*).

THUJA (H) • *Thuja occidentalis*. **Thu. Northern White Cedar. Cedar Leaf Oil.** The twigs of this evergreen contain volatile oils, glycosides, flavonoids, mucilage, and tannin (*see all*). Thuja's main action is due to its stimulating volatile oil. It is used by herbalists as an expectorant, stimulant to smooth muscles, diuretic, and astringent. Has a marked antifungal effect and is used externally for ringworm. Also used to treat psoriasis and urinary incontinence due to loss of muscle tone. Thuja preparations are toxic when ingested in large amounts. They can cause miscarriage, a drop in blood pressure, spasms, coma, and even death. The oil is contraindicated in pregnancy or in persons with gastrointestinal inflammation or liver or kidney dysfunction.

THUNDER GOD VINE (H) • *Tripteryqium wilfordii*. **Lei Gong Tang. Hook F.** The Chinese have been using the root medicinally for centuries to treat arthritis, systemic lupus erythematosus (*see*), chronic hepatitis, and a variety of skin disorders. Researchers at the University of Texas have applied to the FDA for permission to administer an extract of the vine root to treat rheumatoid arthritis.

THYME (H) • *Thymus vulgaris*. Native to Europe, the name comes from the Greek word *thymon*, meaning to fumigate, make a burnt offering. In medieval medicine, thyme was used to combat nightmares, nervous disorders, and headaches. It contains essential oils including thymol, which has been used by herbalists since ancient times to treat throat and digestive illnesses, laryngitis, bronchitis, earache, toothache, whooping cough, ringworm, and as a skin antiseptic. Used in an herbal tea for fatigue. Thyme preparations are harmless when used in low doses. The oil, however, is toxic when ingested. Toxicity includes nausea, stomach upset, kidney damage, irregular heart rate, and blood in the urine. Thyme as a remedy should not be used internally by the elderly or small children nor by people with kidney or liver dysfunction. *See* Thymol.

THYMIC HUMORAL FACTOR (THF) • A natural hormone isolated from calf thymus, it reportedly increases the number of T lymphocytes and increases immunity in those with weakened or absent defenses.

THYMOL (OTC) • **Listerine Antiseptic.** Obtained from the essential oils of lavender, origanum, thyme, and other volatile oils. A topical antifungal agent with a pleasant aromatic odor, it destroys mold and preserves anatomical specimens. Used in mouthwashes to help prevent and reduce plaque and gum problems. Thymol is omitted from hypoallergenic cosmetics because it can cause allergic reactions. Also can cause vomiting, diarrhea, dizziness, and cardiac depression when taken in sufficient amounts. In 1992, the FDA issued a notice that thymol alum had not been shown to be safe and effective as claimed in OTC products, including those to treat fever blisters and cold sores, poison ivy, poison oak, and poison sumac, and astringent (*see*) drug products.

THYMOPENTIN • **Timunox.** A biologically active substance similar to the thymus (*see*) hormone thymopoietin. It is being developed for the treatment of HIV infections in people who have not yet shown the symptoms of AIDS.

THYMOSIN A-1 • A substance from the thymus gland (*see*) that is being tested against chronic active hepatitis B and C and viral infections that affect the liver.

THYMOSTIMULIN (TP2) • A substance from the thymus that has shown some slight promise against head and neck squamous cell carcinoma by Dutch researchers, however, the work is too early yet to draw definitive answers.

THYMUS GLAND • An organ in the chest that helps to activate the body's defenses against infection.

THYRAR • *See* Thyroid and Thyroid Desiccated.

THYRO-BLOCK • *See* Potassium Iodide.

THYROGLOCULIN • Proloid. *See* Thyroid and Levothyroxine.

THYROID (Rx) • Euthroid. Levothroid. Levothyroxine. Levoxine. L-Thyroxine. S-P-T. Synthroid. T4. Thyrar. Thyroglobulin. Thyrolar. Thyroxine. The thyroid is a butterfly-shaped gland located in the neck with a "wing" on either side of the windpipe. The gland produces thyroxine, which controls the rates of chemical reactions in the body. Generally, the more thyroxine, the faster the body works. Thyroxine needs iodine to function. The normal thyroid gland contains approximately 200 mcg of levothyroxine (T_4) per gram of gland and 15 mcg of triiodothyronine (T_3) per gram. The ratio of these two hormones in the circulation does not represent the ratio in the thyroid gland. Levothyroxine, introduced in 1953, is the treatment of choice for hypothyroid patients and is not combined with triiodothyronine because the latter may raise the thyroid hormone to toxic levels. Taken with excessive amounts of cabbage, carrots, cauliflower, spinach, pears, peaches, brussels sprouts, and turnips, may reduce natural thyroid hormone activity and make thyroid medications less effective. Thyroid medication may increase the effects of warfarin, increasing the risk of bleeding. Thyroid hormone may decrease the effects of digoxin. Cholestyramine may decrease the effects of thyroid hormone.

THYROID DESICCATED (Rx) • Armor Thyroid. S-P-T. Thyrar. Thyroid Strong. Thyroid USP Enseals. Thyro-Teric. A strong form of thyroid hormone that stimulates the metabolism of all body tissues by accelerating the rate of cellular oxidation. Its use includes treatment for the following: cretinism, adult myxedema (*see*), ordinary adult and juvenile hypothyroidism in patients of any age or state (including pregnancy), primary hypothyroidism resulting from functional deficiency, primary atrophy, partial or total absence of the thyroid gland, or the effects of surgery, radiation, or drugs, with or without the presence of goiter, and problems with the pituitary gland or the hypothalamus. The use of thyroid hormones in the therapy of obesity, alone or combined with other drugs, is unjustified and has been shown to be ineffective. Thyroid hormones should be used with great caution in patients with cardiovascular disease, diabetes, or adrenal cortical insufficiency. Replacement therapy is usually taken for life. Potential adverse reactions include chest pain, increased pulse rate, heart palpitations, hyperirritability, twitching, headache, excessive sweating, heat intolerance, insomnia, leg cramps, change in appetite, high blood pressure, fever, menstrual irregularities, and nervousness. May increase the effects of anticoagulants and decrease the effects of insulin or oral hypoglycemics. Cholestyramine impairs absorption of thyroid hormones and therefore should be taken at least four hours before levothyroxine (*see* Thyroid). Estrogens tend to increase the need for levothyroxine. Over-the-counter products containing stimulants such as many drugs used to treat coughs, colds, or allergies may increase the side effects of thyroid medication. Thyroid replacement may increase the effect of blood-thinning drugs. Diabetics may have to increase their dosages of insulin or oral medication. This drug is most effective on an empty stomach, but may be taken with food.

THYROID-STIMULATING HORMONE • *See* Thyrotropin.

THYROID STRONG • *See* Thyroid Desiccated.

THYROLAR • *See* Liotrix.

THYROTROPIN (Rx) • Thyroid-Stimulating Hormone. TSH. Thytropar. Stimulates the uptake of radioactive iodine in patients with thyroid cancer. Also promotes thyroid hormone production by the pituitary. Used to diagnosis thyroid cancer and other thyroid problems. Also used as therapy for thyroid cancer. Potential adverse reactions include nausea, vomiting, headache, rapid heartbeat, irregular heartbeat, low blood pressure, enlarged thyroid, fever, menstrual irregularities, allergic reactions, hives, and anaphylaxis. Contraindicated in heart attack patients and untreated Addison's disease (*see*), hypopituitarism, and insufficient output by the adrenal gland.

THYROTROPIN-RELEASING HORMONE • TRH. A naturally occurring brain hormone that regulates the activity of the thyroid gland and may also influence the cholinergic (*see*) system of the brain.

THYROXINE • *See* Thyroid.

THYTROPAR • *See* Thyrotropin.

TIABENDAZOLE • *See* Thiabendazole.

TIAZAC (Rx) • *See* Diltiazem.

TICAR • *See* Ticarcillin Disodium.

TICARCILLIN DISODIUM (Rx) • Ticar. A penicillin antibiotic used for septicemia (*see*), and skin, genital, urinary, and respiratory infections caused by susceptible strains of gram-positive and especially gram-negative (*see both*) organisms, including *Pseudomonas* and *Proteus* (*see*). Potential adverse reactions include anemia, seizures, neuromuscular excitement, nausea, diarrhea, low blood potassium, local pain at injection site, and hypersensitivity reactions, including potential fatal allergic anaphylaxis and overgrowth of non-susceptible organisms.

TICARCILLIN DISODIUM/CLAVULAN-ATE POTASSIUM (Rx) • Timentin. Ticarcillin is used to treat infections of the lower-respiratory tract, urinary tract, bones and joints, and skin, and blood poisoning when caused by beta-lactamase-producing strains of bacteria or by ticarcillin-susceptible organisms. Clavulanic acid increases ticarcillin's effectiveness by inactivating beta-lactamases, which destroy ticarcillin. Potential adverse reactions include anemia, seizures, neuromuscular excitement, nausea, diarrhea, low blood potassium, local pain at injection site, and hypersensitivity reactions, including potential fatal allergic anaphylaxis and overgrowth of nonsusceptible organisms. Is incompatible with aminoglycoside (*see*) antibiotics. *See also* Beta-Lactams.

TIC DOULOUREUX • Trigeminal Neuralgia. Stabbing, excruciating pain in the face along pathways of a cranial nerve.

TICE-BCG • *See* Bacillus Calmette-Guerin.

TICLID • *See* Ticlopidine.

TICLOPIDINE (Rx) • Ticlid. An antiplatelet drug introduced in 1991 that reduces the risk of stroke caused by blood clots to the brain in patients who have had stroke or stroke precursors.

TICON • *See* Trimethobenzamide.

TICS • Habit Spasms. Twitches of certain muscles, always in the same way.

TIENCHI (H) • *Panax notoginseng*. Yunan Baiyao. The root is used by Chinese herbalists to treat hemorrhage. May be applied directly to wounds or taken internally to stop bleeding. Also used as a tonic for the heart, and to maintain normal body weight, to prevent fatigue, and ease stress.

TIGAN • *See* Trimethobenzamide.

TILADE • *See* Nedocromil.

TIMENTIN (Rx) • *See* Ticarcillin Disodium/ Clavulanate Potassium.

TIMOLIDE (Rx) • *See* Hydrochlorothiazide and Timolol Maleate.

TIMOLOL MALEATE (Rx) • Blocadren. Timolide. Timoptic. An antihypertensive beta-blocker (*see*) introduced in 1972 that blocks the nerve signals that trigger constriction of blood vessels, thus lowering blood pressure. Also used as a prophylaxis (*see*) in patients who have survived a heart attack, and to treat glaucoma (*see*) and migraine headache. In eye preparations, it may cause headache, depression, memory impairment, fatigue, minor eye irritation, loss of appetite, and in infants, breathing problems.

Potential adverse reactions when taken systemically include fatigue, vivid dreams, low blood pressure, decreased libido, impaired erection, impotence, congestive heart failure, peripheral vascular disease, abnormal heartbeat, low blood sugar, breathing difficulty, rash, and fever. Contraindicated in diabetics, asthmatics, those with allergic rhinitis, and during ethyl ether anesthesia; also in patients with heart block or other serious heart or lung problems. Must be used with caution in patients with kidney, liver, or respiratory dysfunction, and in those taking other antihypertensives. Timolol interacts with cardiac glycosides to cause excessive slowing of the heartbeat. Indomethacin decreases the effectiveness of timolol. Timolol may alter requirements for diabetes drugs. General anesthetics may cause excessive low blood pressure. Timolol will interact with any drug used to treat mental illness, including MAO inhibitors (*see*), which stimulate the central nervous system. Over-the-counter medications containing stimulants such as cold or allergy medications may make timolol less effective. The oral medication is most effective when taken on an empty stomach. Timolol should not be discontinued suddenly.

TIMOPTIC • *See* Timolol Maleate.

TIMUNOX • *See* Thymopentin.

TINACTIN and TINACTIN CREAM • *See* Tolnaftate.

TINCTURE • A diluted alcoholic solution of herbs.

TINDAL • *See* Acetophenazine Maleate.

TINEA CORPORIS • *See* Ringworm.

TINEA CRURIS • *See* Jock Itch.

TINEA PEDIS • *See* Athlete's Foot.

TINEA VERSICOLOR • An eruption of tan or brown patches on the skin of the trunk, often appearing white in contrast with tan skin, after exposure to the summer sun.

TING SPRAY • *See* Undecylenic Acid.

TINNITUS • Derived from the Latin word meaning to tinkle or ring like a bell. A subjective experience in which one hears a sound when no external physical sound is present. Sometimes called "head noises" or "ear ringing." Problems ranging in severity from wax pressing on the eardrum to tumors can cause tinnitus.

TIOCONAZOLE (OTC) • **Vagistat.** A fungicidal ointment used in the treatment of candidiasis changed from Rx to OTC. May cause burning, itching, discharge, swelling of the vulva, and irritation. Patient should use sanitary napkins to prevent staining of clothing. Sexual intercourse should be avoided during therapy or the partner should use a condom to prevent reinfection.

TIOGUANINE • *See* Thioguanine.

TIOPRONIN (Rx) • **Thiola.** A drug for the treatment of stones in the urinary tract. Potential adverse reactions include nausea, vomiting, loss of taste, rash, itching, drug fever, and lupus-erythematosus-like reaction. Contraindicated in patients with blood problems. Whenever possible, the drug should be taken at least one hour before or two hours after meals. *See* Lupus Erythematosus.

TIOTIXENE • *See* Thiothixene.

TIREND • *See* Caffeine.

TISANE • Herbal tea.

TISIT • *See* Pyrethrins.

TISSUE CULTURE • A technique in which portions of a plant or animal are grown on an artificial culture medium. In many instances, entire plants can be grown from one tissue-culture sample. Organs and entire animals cannot be grown from tissue-culture cells, even in the case of lower forms of animals such as a starfish, which can naturally regrow parts of itself.

TISSUE PLASMINOGEN ACTIVATOR • *See* T-PA.

TISSUE SALTS • Biochemic Cell Salts. Inorganic substances in body tissues used in homeopathic medicine. Tissue salts are used in homeopathy with a "trituration" of natural minerals and milk sugar to a dilution of 1 to 1 million for 6X, the most used potency. The third-trituration 3X tablets are less potent. The tiny tissue-salt tablets sold in health-food stores are dissolved under the tongue or in a little water. Twelve such salts have been used as remedies for more than a hundred years. They are calc. fluor.; calc. phos.; calc. sulph; ferr. phos; kali. mur.; kali. phos.; kali. sulph.; mag. phos.; nat. mur.; nat. phos.; nat. sulp.; and silicea (*see all*).

TITRALAC • *See* Calcium Carbonate.

TMP • *See* Trimethoprim.

TMP-SMZ • *See* Co-Trimoxazole.

TOADFLAX (H) • *Linaria vulgaris.* **Butter and Eggs. Ramsted. Snap Dragon. Yellow Toadflax.** A woody herb native to Europe and introduced into North America and Great Britain, it is valued for both external and internal use. Employed to treat hemorrhoid and skin diseases. The flowers are sometimes mixed with vegetable oils to make a liniment. Taken internally, an infusion of the leaves has been used by herbalists to eliminate kidney stones. Toadflax is reportedly both a diuretic and a cathartic.

TOBRAMYCIN (Rx) • Tobramycin Sulphate. Nebcin. Tobrex Ophthalmic. An aminoglycoside (*see*) antibiotic introduced in 1975 for treatment of serious infections caused by *Escherichia coli, Proteus, Klebsiella, Enterobacter, Serratia, Staphylococcus aureus, Pseudomonas, Citrobacter,* and *Providencia* (*see all*). In eye ointments, it is used to treat eye infections caused

by gram-negative (*see*) bacteria. Potential adverse reactions include headache, lethargy, muscle problems, ear problems, kidney dysfunction, and hypersensitivity reactions. Eye ointments may cause burning or stinging upon instillation, lid itching, lid swelling, and blurred vision. May interact with cephalothin causing increased kidney dysfunction, dimenhydrinate, general and local anesthetics, loop diuretics, cisplatin, and parental penicillins (*see all*).

TOBREX OPHTHALMIC • *See* Tobramycin.

TOCAINIDE HYDROCHLORIDE (Rx) • Tonocard. An antiarrhythmic drug introduced in 1976, used to treat irregular heartbeat. Potential adverse reactions include anemia, light-headedness, tremors, restlessness, numbness, confusion, dizziness, low blood pressure, increased heart irregularities including congestive heart failure, blurred vision, nausea, vomiting, constipation, diarrhea, loss of appetite, hepatitis, respiratory arrest, lung problems, and rash. Beta-blockers (*see*) may increase central nervous system toxicity. Unlike other oral antiarrhythmic drugs, tocainide does not interact with digoxin. May be taken with food.

TOCOPHER • *See* Vitamin E.

TOCOPHEROLS • Vitamin E. Obtained by the vacuum distillation of edible vegetable oils. *See* Vitamin E.

TOCOPHERSOLAN • Liqui-E. *See* Vitamin E.

TOCOPHERYL ACETATE • *See* Vitamin E.

TOFRANIL • *See* Imipramine.

TOLAZAMIDE (Rx) • Ronase. Tolamide. Tolinase. A member of the sulfonylurea family, introduced in 1966, it is prescribed to reduce blood glucose levels by stimulating the pancreas to produce insulin. An adjunct (*see*) to diet to lower the blood sugar in patients with non-insulin-dependent diabetes. Potential adverse reactions include nausea, vomiting, heartburn, sodium loss, low blood sugar, rash, itching, facial flushing, and hypersensitivity reactions. Anabolic steroids (*see*), chloramphenicol, clofibrate, guanethidine, MAO inhibitors, oral blood thinners, phenylbutazone, salicylates, and sulfonamides increase blood-sugar-lowering activity. Beta-blockers (*see*) and clonidine prolong the low blood sugar effect and may also mask symptoms of low blood sugar. Corticosteroids, glucagon, rifampin, and thiazide diuretics decrease the blood-sugar-lowering effect. Contraindicated in treating insulin-dependent diabetes, in diabetes adequately controlled by diet, and in Type II diabetes complicated by ketosis, acidosis, diabetic coma, Raynaud's disease, gangrene, liver or kidney dysfunction, and thyroid or other endocrine dysfunction. The possibility of increased heart deaths is associated with the use of sulfonylureas. This medication is most effective when taken on an empty stomach, but may be taken with a small amount of food.

**TOLAZOLINE HYDROCHLORIDE (Rx) •
Priscoline Hydrochloride.** A vasodilator given to treat pulmonary hypertension in newborn infants and for arterial spasms in adults. Potential adverse effects include irregular heartbeat, anginal pain, high blood pressure, flushing, dizziness, a drop in blood pressure when rising from a seated or prone position, nausea, vomiting, diarrhea, irritated stomach, and exacerbation of peptic ulcer. Also may cause burning at the injection site, weakness, apprehension, pulmonary hemorrhage, and a paradoxical response in seriously damaged limbs due to arterial spasms. May interact with alcohol, like disulfiram (*see*). Contraindicated in coronary artery disease, active peptic ulcer, and following a stroke.

**TOLBUTAMIDE (Rx) • Apo-Tolbutamide.
Oramide. Orinase.** A member of the sulfonylurea family, introduced in 1956, it is prescribed to reduce blood glucose levels by stimulating the pancreas to produce insulin. An adjunct (*see*) to diet to lower the blood sugar in patients with non-insulin-dependent diabetes. Potential adverse reactions include nausea, vomiting, heartburn,

sodium loss, low blood sugar, rash, itching, facial flushing, and hypersensitivity reactions. Anabolic steroids (*see*), chloramphenicol, clofibrate, guanethidine, MAO inhibitors, oral blood thinners, phenylbutazone, salicylates, and sulfonamides increase blood-sugar-lowering activity. Beta-blockers (*see*) and clonidine prolong the low blood sugar effect and may also mask symptoms of low blood sugar. Corticosteroids, glucagon, rifampin, and thiazide diuretics decrease the blood-sugar-lowering effect. Thiazide diuretics may increase the need for a high dose of tolbutamide, while phenylbutazone, aspirin and other salicylates, probenecid, dicoumarol, bishydroxycoumarin, warfarin, phenyramidol, and MAO inhibitors may increase the action of tolbutamide. Interaction with alcoholic beverages will cause flushing, throbbing head pain, difficulty breathing, nausea, vomiting, sweating, thirst, dizziness, and confusion. Because of the stimulant ingredients in many over-the-counter products for the relief of colds and allergies, these should be avoided while taking tolbutamide, unless prescribed by a physician. Tolbutamide is contraindicated in treating insulin-dependent diabetes, in diabetes adequately controlled by diet, and in Type II diabetes complicated by ketosis, acidosis, diabetic coma, Raynaud's disease, gangrene, liver or kidney dysfunction, and thyroid or other endocrine dysfunction. The possibility of increased heart deaths is associated with the use of sulfonylureas. This medicine is best taken on an empty stomach, but may be taken with a small amount of food if stomach upset is a problem.

TOLECTIN • *See* Tolmetin Sodium.

TOLERANCE • The ability to live with an allergen. The term is also used to refer to an adaptation of the body that lessens responsiveness to a drug on continuous or repeated administration.

TOLINASE • *See* Tolazamide.

TOLINDATE (OTC) • An antifungal related to chloroform. In 1992, the FDA issued a notice that tolindate had not been shown to be safe and effective as claimed in OTC products.

TOLMETIN SODIUM (Rx) • Tolectin. Introduced in 1976, it is a nonsteroidal anti-inflammatory (*see*) drug that produces anti-inflammatory, analgesic, and fever-reducing effects, probably by inhibiting prostaglandins (*see*). Used to treat arthritis, gout, and painful menstruation. Potential adverse reactions include dizziness, drowsiness, headache, water retention, abdominal pain, gas, peptic ulcer, nausea, occult blood loss, kidney toxicity, rash, itching, hives, and sodium retention. Oral blood thinners may increase blood-thinning effects of tolmetin. Contraindicated in asthmatics. Must be used cautiously in patients with GI ulcers or bleeding. Serious GI toxicity can occur at any time in patients taking NSAIDs (*see*) on a long-term basis. Use with other NSAIDs, aspirin, or alcohol may increase the danger of GI problems. Should be taken with meals.

TOLNAFTATE (OTC) • Aftate for Athlete's Foot. Aftate for Jock Itch. Footwork. Fungatin. Genaspor. NP-27. Tinactin. Tinactin Cream. Ting. Zeasorb-AF. An antifungal medication introduced in 1965 that is prepared as a liquid, powder, cream, gel, or solution to treat superficial fungal infections of the skin, athlete's foot, and jock itch. No significant adverse reactions have been reported. If your skin problem does not improve in a month, seek professional advice. Adverse reactions are rare; tolnaftate reputedly does not cause skin irritation or rash as do many other antifungal drugs.

TOLRESTAT (Rx) • Alredase. A hydantoin-derived aldose reductase (*see*) inhibitor that represents a new approach to the prevention or arrest of diabetes complications. Aldose reductase is an enzyme that converts to sorbitol the blood sugar glucose. The inhibitor of aldose reductase should prevent polyol (a type of sugar) accumulation, which has been implicated in degenerative changes in the lens of the eye and nerve tissue in diabetics. *See also* Hydantoin.

TOLU-SED • See Guaifenesin and Codeine Phosphate and Sulfate.

TONKA BEAN (H) • *Dipteryx odorata*. A large tree native to Brazil and Guyana, its seeds contain from 3 to 10 percent coumarin (*see*). Tonka bean has been used in combination with other herbs as a general tonic, usually in the form of a tea. It is also used in homeopathic medicine. Tonka bean is toxic when used in large amounts and can exert an adverse effect on the heart and cause hemorrhaging. Contraindicated in peptic ulcer and during menstruation. It increases the effects of other anticoagulants. Your doctor should be informed if you are taking a tonka bean remedy.

TONOCARD • See Tocainide Hydrochloride.

TOOTHACHE TREE • See Zanthoxylum.

TOPEX • See Benzoyl Peroxide.

TOPICAL • Used to describe the application of a drug directly to the external site on the body where it is intended to have its effect.

TOPICAL STARCH • Stored by plants, it is taken from grains of wheat, potatoes, rice, and many other vegetables. In 1992, the FDA proposed a ban on topical starch in astringent (*see*) drug products and in fever blister and cold sore products because it had not been shown to be safe and effective as claimed.

TOPICORT • See Desoximetasone.

TOPICYCLINE • See Tetracyclines.

TOPISPORIN (Rx) • A combination of bacitracin, neomycin, and polymyxin B (*see all*).

TOPOTECAN (Rx) • Hycamtin. The first of a new class of drugs that inhibit an enzyme that is essential for growth of tumors. It is expected to be approved by the FDA in the near future. It does have severe side effects but they can be treated. It is supposed to be equal or better than taxol (*see*) for the treatment of ovarian cancer. It is expected to be useful for ovarian cancer patients who have not responded to taxol.

TOPSYN • *See* Fluocinonide.

TORADOL • *See* Ketorolac Tromethamine.

TORECAN • *See* Thiethylperazine.

TORMENTIL (H) • *Potentilla procumbens. Potentilla tormentilla.* **Septfoil.** Tormentil is a powerful astringent. Hippocrates used it for skin problems. The earliest citation of this Eurasian herb in England appeared in 1387 recommending it for treatment of toothache. Through the years it came to be used for piles, fevers, canker sores, and to relieve pain. The root stalk is used by herbalists as a gargle for sore mouth and throat. Supposedly, a piece of cloth soaked in a decoction of tormentil and then covering a wart will cause the growth to turn black and fall off. The same decoction is recommended for sores and ulcers. A fluid extract of the root is used by herbalists to stop the bleeding of gums and cuts. The root contains more tannin (*see*) than oak bark. May cause constipation.

TORNALATE • *See* Bitolterol.

TOROFOR • *See* Iodochlorhydroxyquin.

TOTACILLIN • *See* Ampicillin.

TOURETTE'S SYNDROME • **Gilles de la Tourette's Syndrome.** A hereditary multiple-tic disorder that begins in childhood. The tics may progress to multiple complex movements, include grunting or barking noises, and evolve into compulsive utterances.

TOXICITY • The capacity of a drug to dangerously impair body functions or to damage body tissue.

TOXIC MEGACOLON • Acute nonobstructive dilation of the colon, seen in severe ulcerative colitis (*see*).

TOXIC REACTION • Symptoms, sometimes harmful and poisonous, caused by a drug as the result of an overdose or adverse reaction.

TOXOPLASMOSIS • A disease due to infection with the protozoa *Toxoplasma gondii,* frequently causing inflammation of the brain. It may also involve the heart, lungs, adrenal glands, pancreas, and testes.

T-PA (Rx) • **Activase. Alteplase.** Abbreviation for tissue-plasminogen activator. Introduced in 1987, T-PA is an enzyme that dissolves blood clots in cases of acute heart attack. Manufactured or genetically engineered from human cells, it is used as soon as possible after a heart attack to break up the clot that is cutting off blood to the heart muscle. It was approved for the treatment of strokes in 1996. Given by infusion into a vein or directly into a coronary artery, T-PA may, if given in time, prevent the heart muscle from being damaged by the heart attack or the brain being damaged by a blood clot. Potential adverse reactions include severe, spontaneous bleeding, stroke, low blood pressure, irregular heartbeat, hypersensitivity, and hives. Aspirin, dipyridamole, heparin, and coumarin (*see all*) increase the risk of bleeding. Potential adverse reactions include hemorrhaging and stroke. On the other hand, a five-year study published in the December 14, 1995, issue of *The New England Journal* reported that T-PA is an effective treatment for acute ischemic stroke (lack of blood supply to the brain tissue). As a natural substance, it is less likely to produce allergic reactions. T-PA is expensive and there is a great deal of controversy over its use when compared to older clot-dissolving medications. According to a British study of 41,299 patients reported in the British medical journal *Lancet,* T-PA slightly increases the risk of stroke by about 0.4 percent. The study determined that an older, less expensive clot-buster, streptokinase, which costs about $300 a dose, is just as effective and slightly less risky. T-PA cost $2,200 a dose at the time of this writing. Contraindicated in recent trauma (within ten days); pregnancy; diabetic hemorrhagic retinopathy; and recent major surgery (ten days) such as coronary bypass, organ biopsy, and obstetrical delivery.

TRACE METALS • *See* Chromium, Copper, Iodine, Manganese, Selenium, and Zinc.

TRACHEA • Windpipe. Air passageway to the lungs.

TRACHOMA • A contagious eye infection.

TRAL • *See* Hexocyclium.

TRAMADOL (Rx) • **Ultram.** A painkiller designed to act like morphine and codeine but claimed to be without the side effects or potential for addiction. Introduced in 1995 in the United States, it has been used in seventy countries since 1977, when it was introduced in Germany. The first non-NSAID (*see* NSAIDs) in ten years, it is indicated for moderate to moderately severe pain associated with both acute and chronic conditions. The most frequently reported adverse reactions have been dizziness, nausea, constipation, headache, rash, and sleepiness.

TRANCOPAL • *See* Chlormezanone.

TRANEXAMIC ACID • An inhibitor of natural substances in the blood, plasminogen and plasmin, that prevent clotting. It is used to reduce or prevent hemorrhage in hemophiliacs.

TRANMEP • *See* Meprobamate.

TRANQUILIZERS • A group of medications used to relieve anxiety and agitation in the case of emotional disturbance.

TRANSAMINE SULFATE • *See* Tranylcypromine Sulfate.

TRANSDERMAL • A drug delivery system consisting of an adhesive patch containing a medication that diffuses through the skin and acts systemically in the body. Examples include nicotine-containing patches to help people stop smoking, and nitroglycerin-containing patches to treat and prevent angina (*see*) attacks.

TRANSDERM-NITRO (Rx) • A patch that is put on the skin as a way of administering systemic medication. *See* Nitroglycerin.

TRANSDERM SCŌP (Rx) • A patch that is put on the skin as a way of administering systemic medication. *See* Scopolamine.

TRANSGENIC ANIMAL, PLANT, or CROP • An animal, plant, or crop in which the hereditary DNA (*see*) has been altered through genetic engineering by adding DNA from a source other than its parent.

TRANSIENT ISCHEMIC ATTACKS • **TIS.** Temporary interruption in blood supply to a portion of the brain. May be the forerunner of a stroke. Symptoms may include loss of speech, paralysis of the arm or leg, dizziness, temporary visual changes.

TRANS-VER-SAL • *See* Salicylic Acid.

TRANXENE • *See* Clorazepate.

TRANYLCYPROMINE SULFATE (Rx) • **Parnate. Transamine Sulfate.** A monoamine oxidase inhibitor (MAOI) (*see*) used to treat depression that is refractory or intolerant to tricyclic antidepressants (*see*) or electroconvulsive therapy. Potential adverse reactions include dizziness, vertigo, headache, excitement, tremors, muscle twitching, mania, jitters, confusion, memory impairment, fatigue, a drop in blood pressure when rising from a seated or prone position, constipation, diarrhea, dry mouth, loss of appetite, irregular heartbeat, high blood pressure, blurred vision, impotence, rash, swelling, sweating, weight changes, chills, and altered libido. Use with alcohol, barbiturates, narcotics, dextromethorphan (in many over-the-counter cold and allergy medications), and tricyclic antidepressants may depress the central nervous system. Amphetamines, antihistamines, ephedrine, levodopa, meperidine, metaraminol, methotrimeprazine, methylphenidate, phenylephrine, and phenylpropanolamine may cause blood pressure to shoot up. Must be used cautiously with antiparkinsonian drugs and spinal anesthetics. Dosages of insulin and oral diabetes medicines may have to be adjusted. Contraindicated in severe liver or kidney dysfunction, congestive heart failure, high blood pressure, cerebrovascular disease, severe or frequent headaches, in people taking diuretics, and the elderly, debilitated, or suicidal. Also contraindicated during therapy with foods containing tyramine or tryptophan (*see both*). Should not be taken within seven days of elective surgery requiring general or local anesthetics.

TRASICOR • *See* Oxprenolol.

TRAVASE OINTMENT • *See* Sutilains Ointment.

TRAVELER'S JOY (H) • *Clematis vitalba.* **Old-Man's Beard.** A woody vine native to Europe and imported to North America, it is used in homeopathic medicine to treat genitourinary-tract ailments and skin diseases. Herbalists use it to relieve migraine attack. The plant is toxic and may cause skin irritation.

TRAVIST • *See* Clemastine.

TRAZODONE HYDROCHLORIDE (Rx) • **Desyrel. Trazodone HCl. Trialodine.** An antidepressant introduced in 1967 that inhibits the uptake of the neurotransmitter serotonin and is not related to tricyclic antidepressants or to MAO inhibitors (*see both*). Potential adverse reactions include drowsiness, dizziness, nervousness, fatigue, confusion, tremors, weakness, a drop in blood-pressure when rising from a sitting or prone position, blurred vision, ringing in the ears, dry mouth, constipation, nausea, vomiting, loss of appetite, urine retention, priapism (*see*), decreased male libido, increased female libido, impotence, irregular menstruation, rash, hives, and sweating. Use with alcohol and central nervous system depressants increases its central nervous system depression effects. Blood pressure medication may add to trazodone's blood-pressure-lowering effects. Trazodone may increase the effects of digoxin and phenytoin to levels of toxicity. Should not be used during the initial recovery phase of a heart attack, nor in persons receiving electroshock therapy. Should be taken after meals. Takes at least two weeks before effects are manifested.

TRECATOR-SC • *See* Ethionamide.

TREMIN • *See* Trihexyphenidyl.

TREMOR • An involuntary movement or quivering, most often in stretched-out hands.

TRENTAL • *See* Pentoxifylline.

TRETINOIN (Rx) • **Vitamin A. Retinoic Acid. Retin-A. Renova.** A cream, gel, or solution introduced in 1973 to treat severe acne and fine wrinkles from sun-damaged skin. In 1995, a former vice president of the company making Retin-A was indicted for ordering employees to shred documents subpoenaed for a U.S. government investigation into whether the company illegally promoted the drug for photoaging (wrinkles), an unapproved use. There are many reports by physicians and patients that the medication is effective for that purpose. Potential adverse effects from tretinoin include a feeling of warmth, slight stinging, local redness, peeling, chapping, swelling, blistering, crusting, temporary increase or decrease in pigmentation, and acne. Increased sensitivity to wind and cold may occur. Contact with eyes and mouth should be avoided. Topical preparations containing sulfur, resorcinol, or salicylic acid increase the risk of skin irritation and should not be used with tretinoin. Contraindicated in hypersensitivity to any tretinoin components. Should be used with caution in eczema. No medicated cosmetics should be used.

TREXAN • *See* Naltrexone.

TRIACETIN (OTC) • **Fungoid. Glyceryl Triacetate.** An antifungal agent used to treat athlete's foot. In 1992, the FDA issued a notice that triacetin had not been shown to be safe and effective as claimed in OTC products.

TRIAD (Rx) • A combination of acetaminophen, butalbital, and caffeine (*see all*), used to treat mild to moderate pain.

TRIAFED (OTC) • *See* Triprolidine and Pseudoephedrine.

TRIAM-A • *See* Triamcinolone.

TRIAMCINOLONE (Rx) • **Amcort. Aristocort. Aristospan. Articulose-LA. Atolone. Azmacort. Cenocort A. Cinonide. Flutex. Kenacort. Kenaject-40. Kenalog. Kenalone. Mycolog. Mycolog II. Myco-Triacet. Mytrex. Nasacort. N.G.T. TAC-3. Tramacort. Triam-A. Triamcin. Triamolone. Triamonide. Triderm. Tri-Kort. Trilog. Trilone. Tristoject. Trymex.** A steroid hormone introduced in 1958 with actions and uses similar to those of prednisolone (*see*). Administered in tablets, in syrup, by injection, by inhalation, and topically, it is used to treat severe inflammation, steroid-dependent asthma, and as an immunosuppressant. Most adverse reactions are the result of dosage or length of time between administration of dosages. Should be taken with food or milk to reduce GI irritation. Potential adverse reactions include euphoria, insomnia, psychotic behavior, high blood pressure, swelling, cataracts, glaucoma, peptic ulcer, GI irritation, increased appetite, high blood sugar, growth suppression in children, delayed wound healing, acne, skin eruptions, muscle weakness, pancreatitis (*see*), hairiness, decreased immunity, and acute adrenal gland insufficiency. When withdrawn, there may be rebound inflammation, fatigue, weakness, joint pain, fever, dizziness, lethargy, depression, fainting, a drop in blood pressure upon rising from a seated or prone position, shortness of breath, loss of appetite, and high blood sugar. Sudden withdrawal may be fatal. Contraindicated in systemic fungal infections. Should be used cautiously in patients with GI ulceration or kidney disease, high blood pressure, diabetes, chicken pox, osteoporosis, Cushing's syndrome, blood-clotting disorders, seizures, myasthenia gravis (*see*), congestive heart failure, tuberculosis, herpes, and emotional instability. When taking the drug, patients may need low-sodium diets and potassium supplements. Use with barbiturates, phenytoin, and rifampin (*see all*) increases its effects. Indomethacin and aspirin may increase the risk of GI distress and bleeding. In skin preparations, potential adverse reactions include burning, itching, irritation, dryness, inflammation of the hair follicles, acne, rash around the mouth, spots of pigment loss, hairiness, allergic contact dermatitis, and if covered with a dressing, secondary infection, atrophy, streaks, and blisters. Should be used cautiously in skin problems caused by viruses such as herpes, and in fungal or bacterial skin infections. Should not be used for more than two weeks due to potential absorption into the system that may cause an effect on the hypothalamus, and pituitary and adrenal glands. Should not be applied near the eyes or mucous membranes, under the arms, on the face, groin, or under the breast unless medically specified. Because of its immunosuppressant effects, care should be taken to avoid exposure to chicken pox or measles.

TRIAMCINOLONE INHALER (Rx) • **Azmacort.** The ingredient in this product is the same drug applied to the skin. In an inhaler, it relieves the inflammation of the lining of the bronchi, making it easier to breathe. It will not treat asthma attacks but is used to help prevent them. *See* Triamcinolone.

TRIAMINIC COLD SYRUP (OTC) • *See* Chlorpheniramine and Phenylpropanolamine.

TRIAMINIC EXPECTORANT (OTC) • *See* Guaifenesin and Phenylpropanolamine.

TRIAMINICOL MULTI-SYMPTOM COLD SYRUP (OTC) • *See* Chlorpheniramine, Phenylpropanolamine, and Dextromethorphan.

TRIAMOLONE • *See* Triamcinolone.

TRIAMTERENE (Rx) • **Dyazide. Dyrenium. Maxzide.** A potassium-sparing diuretic introduced in 1964 that is used to treat water retention. Potential adverse reactions include nausea, vomiting, dry mouth, sore throat, low blood pressure, anemia, dizziness, high potassium, low sodium, dehydration, photosensitivity, rash, muscle cramps, and serious allergic reactions. ACE inhibitors (*see*) and potassium supplements increase the risk of high blood potassium. Indomethacin and NSAIDs (*see both*) may increase the risk of kidney dysfunction. Contraindicated in absence of urine formation, severe or progressive kidney disease, severe liver disease, and high blood potassium. Should also be used with caution in diabetics, pregnancy, and breast-feeding mothers. Should be taken after meals to prevent nausea. Those taking this drug should be cautious about eating a diet that is too high in potassium.

TRIAPRIN • *See* Acetaminophen and Butalbital Compounds.

TRIAVIL (Rx) • **Etrafon.** A combination of amitriptyline and perphenazine, used to treat depression and anxiety. It takes at least two weeks to one month to become effective. Potential adverse reactions include nausea, dry mouth, difficulty in urinating, constipation, blurred vision, rapid heartbeat, numbness and tingling in the arms and legs, yellowing of the skin and eyes, low blood pressure, drowsiness, dizziness, excitement, fainting, twitching of the muscles, weakness, headache, heartburn, loss of appetite, stomach cramps, increased perspiration, loss of coordination, rash, sensitivity to bright light, itching, redness, peeling away of large sections of skin, breathing difficulties, fluid retention, swelling of the face and tongue, and changes in sex drive and sexual performance. Quinidine or procainamide, drugs used to control heart rhythm, will strongly increase the effects of triavil. Drugs that depress the central nervous system such as tranquilizers, sleeping pills, antihistamines, and alcohol will greatly affect alertness and the ability to concentrate. Some patients may experience changes in heart rhythm when taking this drug with thyroid medication. Over-the-counter stimulants in cold and allergy medications may increase nervousness and insomnia. Large amounts of vitamin C may make triavil less effective. Triavil may neutralize the effects of drugs to treat high blood pressure. Use with MAO inhibitors (*see*) can elevate blood pressure to dangerous levels. Most effective when taken on an empty stomach, but may be taken with a small amount of food if stomach distress is a problem.

TRIAZOLAM (Rx) • **Halcion.** A benzodiazepine sleeping drug introduced in 1974 that acts on the limbic system, thalamus, and hypothalamus of the central nervous system to produce hypnotic effects. The use of this drug has become controversial. Stories in the media in 1991 about people who experienced adverse side effects—particularly amnesia, anxiety, confusion, delusions, hallucinations, and hostility—while taking this drug led to demands that it be reevaluated by the FDA and physicians who prescribed it. In May 1992, an FDA panel recommended that the sleeping pill was safe and effective and should remain on the market, but it asked that the drug's warning label be strengthened. Adverse reactions listed for the drug include drowsiness, dizziness, headache, rebound insomnia, amnesia, lightheadedness, lack of coordination, mental confusion, nausea, and vomiting. Should be used carefully in impaired liver or kidney function, mental depression, suicidal tendencies, and a history of drug abuse, and in elderly or debilitated patients. Dependence is possible with long-term use. Use with alcohol or central nervous system depressants, including narcotic analgesics, may increase central nervous system depression. Cimetidine and erythromycin may prolong triazolam's sedative effects. Caffeine-containing beverages should not be taken within four hours of triazolam. The drug should not be discontinued suddenly. May be taken with food if stomach distress is a problem.

TRICHLORMETHIAZIDE (Rx) • **Aquazide. Diurese. Metahydrin. Metatensin. Naqua. Naquival.** A thiazide diuretic that increases urine excretion of sodium and water, it is used to treat edema and high blood pressure. Potential adverse reactions include nausea, vomiting, loss of appetite, pancreatitis (*see*), dehydration, a drop in blood pressure upon rising from a seated or prone position, liver dysfunction, anemia, a drop in platelets, low potassium, high blood sugar, fluid and electrolyte imbalances, rash, photosensitivity, and other allergic reactions. Cholestyramine, colestipol, and NSAIDs (*see all*) decrease its effectiveness. Diazoxide increases its blood-pressure-lowering and blood-sugar-raising effects. Contraindicated in kidney or liver disease, absence of urine formation, and hypersensitivity to other thiazides or sulfonamide-derived drugs.

Should be used cautiously in gout. Should be taken in the morning to avoid having to urinate during the night. A diet rich in potassium may be recommended. This includes dates, apricots, bananas, and tomatoes. If you are taking this drug, you should wear a sunscreen.

TRICHLOROACETALDEHYDE MONO-HYDRATE • *See* Chloral Hydrate.

TRICHLOROACETIC ACID (OTC) • A topical preparation containing salicylic acid; used to treat warts.

TRICHOMONAS • A type of parasite that causes infections in the urinary or genital tracts.

TRICHOSANTHES (H) • **TAP 29.** An agent from the root of *Trichosanthes kirilowii,* a Chinese herb. In 1991, researchers at New York University reported it to be effective against the AIDS virus. It is reportedly nontoxic to normal cells and may eventually be used in condoms, vaginal jellies, and toothpastes to minimize the risk of HIV transmission.

TRICLOSAN (OTC) • **Oxy Medicated Soap.** A broad-spectrum antibacterial agent that is active against bacteria. It is used in deodorant soaps, acne products, vaginal deodorant sprays, bar soaps, and in wound-cleansing products. Its deodorant properties are due to the inhibition of bacterial growth. Can cause allergic contact dermatitis, particularly when used in products for the feet.

TRICODENE (OTC) • A combination of chlorpheniramine, dextromethorphan, and phenylpropanolamine (*see all*), used to treat the symptoms of colds and allergies.

TRICYCLIC • An organic compound composed of only three-ring molecular structures, which may be identical or different. *See* Tricyclic Antidepressants.

TRICYCLIC ANTIDEPRESSANTS (Rx) • The most widely used class of antidepressant medications. Tricyclics are usually the first to be prescribed for patients with what is known as "major depression." Some tricyclics, such as amitriptyline (*see*), are given to people who have trouble sleeping, because they have a sedative effect. Others, such as imipramine or amoxapine (*see both*), have a stimulant effect and are given to people who are lethargic. Tricyclics should not be taken with breads, crackers, cookies, cheeses, peanut butter, corn, lentils, cranberries, plums, prunes, peanuts, bacon, eggs, fish, or fowl. These may make tricyclics less effective. Tricyclics, reportedly, work in only two-thirds of patients to whom they are given.

TRIDESILON • *See* Acetic Acid and Desonide.

TRIDIHEXETHYL CHLORIDE (Rx) • **Milpath. Panthilon.** An anticholinergic, antispasmodic drug used in the treatment of irritable bowel syndrome and peptic ulcer.

TRIDIL • *See* Nitroglycerin.

TRIDIONE • *See* Trimethadione.

TRIENTINE (Rx) • **Cuprid. Syprine.** A chelating agent used to remove excess copper in Wilson's disease in patients who cannot tolerate penicillamine (*see*). Potential adverse reactions include iron deficiency anemia, fever, and hypersensitivity reactions. Mineral supplements may block the drug's absorption. *See also* Chelation.

TRIETHANOLAMINE (OTC) • **Sportscreme.** Made from ethylene, a petroleum derivative that also occurs in ripe fruit. It is used in the manufacture of detergents, waxes, polishes, and toilet goods. It is a coating agent for fresh fruits and vegetables and is widely employed in cosmetic creams and body lotions. It can be an irritant.

TRIETHANOLAMINE POLYPEPTIDE OLEATE-CONDENSATE (OTC) • **Cerumenex Drops.** An ear drop that breaks up accumulated earwax. Potential adverse reactions include redness, itching, and eczema. Contraindicated in perforated eardrum, ear infection, and allergies.

TRIFLUOPERAZINE (Rx) • Stelazine. Suprazine. A phenothiazine (see) antipsychotic drug introduced in 1958 to treat anxiety states, schizophrenia, and other psychotic disorders. Potential adverse reactions include a low white blood count, tardive dyskinesia (see), sedation, a drop in blood pressure when rising from a seated or prone position, vision changes, dry mouth, constipation, urine retention, menstrual irregularities, enlargement of the male breast, inhibited ejaculation, liver dysfunction, mild photosensitivity, allergic skin reactions, weight gain, increased appetite, fever, and profuse sweating. Sudden withdrawal of long-term drug therapy may cause gastritis, nausea, vomiting, dizziness, tremors, sweating, irregular heartbeat, headache, and insomnia. Use with alcohol and other central nervous system depressants may increase central nervous system depression. Antacids inhibit absorption and should not be used within two hours of trifluoperazine. Barbiturates and lithium may decrease trifluoperazine's effects. High blood pressure medications may be less effective. Contraindicated in coma, central nervous system depression, bone marrow suppression, high or low blood pressure, brain damage, and with use of spinal or epidural anesthetics or adrenergic-blocking agents (see). Should be used cautiously in elderly or debilitated patients, in those with liver disease, cerebrovascular disease, respiratory disorders, low blood calcium, seizure disorders, intestinal obstruction, glaucoma, enlarged prostate, and in acutely ill or dehydrated children. Care should be taken in hot weather because this drug increases susceptibility to heatstroke. Vitamin B_2 supplementation may be needed. The drug may be taken with meals to reduce stomach upset.

TRIFLUPROMAZINE (Rx) • Vesprin. Used to treat psychotic disorders other than depression, to get rid of worm infections, to stop vomiting, and to halt intractable hiccups. See Phenothiazine and Promazine.

TRIFLURIDINE (Rx) • Viroptic. An eye solution used to treat herpes simplex keratitis (see) of the eye. Potential adverse reactions include stinging upon instillation, swelling of the eyelids, increased pressure within the eye, and allergic reactions. Treatment is usually not continued for more than three weeks.

TRIFOLIUM PRATENSE • See Clover, Red.

TRIGEMINAL NEURALGIA • See Tic Douloureux.

TRIGESIC • See Acetaminophen, Aspirin, and Caffeine.

TRIHEXANE • See Trihexyphenidyl.

TRIHEXY • See Trihexyphenidyl.

TRIHEXYPHENIDYL (Rx) • Artane. Tremin. Trihexane. Trihexidyl. Trihexy. A drug that regulates the transmission of nerve-stimulation chemicals in the brain. Introduced in the 1940s, it is used to treat drug-induced parkinsonism; widely used in the early stages of the disease to reduce rigidity and tremor. Potential adverse reactions include nervousness, dizziness, headache, restlessness, agitation, hallucinations, euphoria, delusions, amnesia, irregular heartbeat, blurred vision, pressure inside the eye, constipation, dry mouth, nausea, and urinary retention. Must be used cautiously in patients with glaucoma, heart, liver, or kidney disorders, high blood pressure, obstructive disease of the GI and genitourinary tracts, in patients with enlarged prostate, and those with hardening of the arteries or a history of drug hypersensitivity. Amantadine may cause confusion or hallucinations when given with trihexyphenidyl. Interaction with other anticholinergic (see) drugs, including tricyclic antidepressants, may cause severe stomach upset. Over-the-counter medications containing atropine or similar drugs should also be avoided. This drug should not be taken with alcohol. Should be taken with food.

TRI-HYDROSERPINE (Rx) • A combination of hydralazine, hydrochlorothiazide, and reserpine (see all), used to treat high blood pressure.

TRIIODOTHYRONINE • See Liothyronine.

TRI-KORT • *See* Triamcinolone.

TRILAFON • *See* Perphenazine.

TRI-LEVLEN (Rx) • *See* Estradiol and Levonorgestrel.

TRILISATE • *See* Choline Magnesium Trisalicylate.

TRILLIUM (H) • **Beth Root. Ground Lily. Indian Balm.** The dried rhizome of *Trillium liliaceae,* which contains tannin (*see*). Used by herbalists to treat painful menstrual symptoms, various types of hemorrhage, and diarrhea. In 1992, the FDA issued a notice that trillium had not been shown to be safe and effective as claimed in OTC digestive-aid products.

TRILOG • *See* Triamcinolone.

TRILONE • *See* Triamcinolone.

TRILOSTANE (Rx) • **Modrastane.** A synthetic corticosteroid drug given to treat an overactive adrenal gland in Cushing's syndrome. Potential adverse reactions include nausea, diarrhea, upset stomach, gas, bloating, flushing, rash, fever, fatigue, burning of oral and nasal membranes, headache, and a drop in blood pressure when rising from a seated or prone position. Use with aminoglutethimide and mitotane may cause a severe drop in aldosterone production. Contraindicated in patients with severe kidney or liver disease.

TRIMEPRAZINE TARTRATE (Rx) • **Alimemazine. Tartrate. Temaril.** An antihistamine introduced in 1958, used to treat itching. Potential adverse reactions include a drop in white blood cells, drowsiness and confusion (especially in the elderly), dizziness, low blood pressure, heart palpitations, restlessness, irritability, insomnia (especially in children), excitation, rapid heartbeat, loss of appetite, nausea, vomiting, dry mouth and throat, urinary frequency, urinary retention, hives, rash, and photosensitivity. Use with central nervous system depressants, including alcohol, increases sedation. Use with MAO inhibitors (*see*) may cause blood pressure to shoot up. Contraindicated in acute asthma. Should be used cautiously in elderly patients, those with glaucoma, overactive thyroid, heart or kidney disease, high blood pressure, bronchial asthma, enlarged prostate, bladder-neck obstruction, and peptic ulcer. Coffee or tea may reduce drowsiness. May cause photosensitivity, so sunscreen and sunglasses should be worn as a precaution. Medication should be discontinued four days before taking a skin allergy test because it can lead to inaccurate results. Should be taken with food or milk to reduce GI distress.

TRIMETHADIONE (Rx) • **Tridione. Troxidone.** A drug that raises the threshold for seizures but does not modify seizure pattern. Used to treat absence seizures (*see*) that are unresponsive to other medications. Potential adverse effects include anemia, drowsiness, fatigue, malaise, insomnia, dizziness, headache, numbness, irritability, high or low blood pressure, double vision, sensitivity to light, nosebleed, retinal hemorrhage, kidney dysfunction, vaginal bleeding, liver dysfunction, acne, rash, swollen glands, lupus-erythematosus-like syndrome, and myasthenia-gravis-like syndrome (*see both*). Contraindicated in paramethadione and trimethadione hypersensitivity, and severe blood or liver problems. Should be used with extreme care in retinal and optic-nerve diseases. Should not be withdrawn suddenly. May cause photosensitivy, so sunglasses should be worn.

TRIMETHAPHAN CAMSYLATE (Rx) • **Arfonad.** A drug given in an emergency to reduce blood pressure. Contraindicated in anemia and respiratory insufficiency. Must be used with caution in those with heart and blood-vessel disease, liver or renal dysfunction, Addison's disease, and diabetes. Potential adverse reactions include dilated pupils, extreme weakness, a severe drop in blood pressure upon rising from a sitting or prone position, irregular heartbeat, loss of appetite, nausea, vomiting, dry mouth, urine retention, and respiratory distress. Patients are given oxygen during administration of this drug. Interacts with anesthetics, diuretics, and procainamide (*see*) to cause a big drop in blood pressure.

TRIMETHOBENZAMIDE (Rx) • **Arrestin. Bio-Gan. Stemetic. Tebamide. T-Gen. Ticon. Tigan. Tiject-20.** A drug that inhibits the centers in the brain involved in nausea and vomiting. It is used to prevent and treat postoperative nausea and vomiting. Has little or no effect in preventing motion sickness. Potential adverse reactions include drowsiness, dizziness, low blood pressure, diarrhea, headache, convulsions, tremors, worsening of preexisting nausea, liver toxicity, and allergic skin reactions. Its antivomiting effects may mask more serious problems such as an overdose of a toxic substance or an intestinal obstruction. Contraindicated in children with viral illness because it may contribute to the development of Reye's syndrome (*see*). Trimethobenzamide suppositories are contraindicated in those hypersensitive to benzocaine or similar local anesthetics. The oral medication is best taken on an empty stomach but may be taken with a small amount of food.

TRIMETHOPRIM (Rx) • **TMP. BactrimDS. Bethaprim. Cotrim. Proloprim. SeptraDS. SMZ-TMP-DS. Trimpex. Uroplus.** An antibacterial introduced in 1967, it is used to treat and prevent urinary tract infections and sometimes gonorrheal and pneumocystic infections. Currently used in AIDS patients to prevent pneumonia due to *Pneumocystis carinii*. Potential adverse reactions include anemia, epigastric distress, nausea, vomiting, sore tongue, rash, and fever. Trimethoprim may increase blood levels of phenytoin (*see*). Most effective when taken on an empty stomach, but may be taken with food if it causes gastric distress.

TRIMETHYLPSORALEN • *See* Trioxsalen.

TRIMETREXATE GLUCONATE (Rx) • **Neu-Trexin.** A drug introduced in 1994 for the treatment of *Pneumocystis carinii* (*see*) pneumonia.

TRIMIPRAMINE (Rx) • **Surmontil.** A tricyclic antidepressant (*see*) drug that increases the amount of the neurotransmitters serotonin and norepinephrine in the brain. Potential side effects include dizziness, excitation, headache, confusion, tremors, weakness, nervousness, blurred vision, ringing in the ears, dry mouth, constipation, nausea, vomiting, loss of appetite, intestinal paralysis, urine retention, rash, hives, sweating, and allergy. If there is abrupt withdrawal, nausea, malaise, and headache can result. Barbiturates decrease trimipramine's levels in the blood. Cimetidine and methylphenidate increase it. Epinephrine and norepinephrine increase trimipramine's blood-pressure-raising effects. MAO inhibitors (*see*) may cause severe excitation, high fever, or seizures. Contraindicated during recovery from the acute phase of a heart attack, in enlargement of the prostate, in patients with seizures, and those receiving electroshock therapy. Should not be used in those receiving thyroid drugs or undergoing elective surgery, or in patients who are suicidal. Should be used with caution in patients with cardiovascular disease, urine retention, glaucoma, thyroid disease, blood problems, and impaired liver function. The drug should not be withdrawn abruptly. A full dose should be taken at bedtime to avoid daytime sleepiness. Effects will not be manifested for at least two weeks. Most effective when taken on an empty stomach, but may be taken with a small amount of food if it causes stomach upset.

TRIMOX • *See* Amoxicillin.

TRIMPEX • *See* Trimethoprim.

TRIMSTAT • *See* Phendimetrazine.

TRIMTABS • *See* Phendimetrazine.

TRINALIN • *See* Azatadine Maleate and Pseudoephedrine.

TRIND (OTC) • A combination of chlorpheniramine, dextromethorphan, and phenylpropanolamine (*see all*), used to treat symptoms of colds and allergies.

TRI-NORINYL • *See* Estradiol and Norethindrone.

TRINSICON (OTC) • A multivitamin and mineral preparation.

TRIOFED (OTC) • *See* Triprolidine and Pseudoephedrine.

TRIOXSALEN (Rx) • **Trimethylpsoralen. Trisoralen.** Used in conjunction with controlled exposure to ultraviolet light or sunlight for repigmentation of vitiligo (*see*), and to treat psoriasis. It helps to increase tolerance to sunlight for albinos. Potential adverse reactions include nausea, itching, and dizziness. There is an increased risk of developing skin cancer after use of trioxsalen.

TRIPELENNAMINE (Rx) • **PBZ. Pelamine. Pyribenzamine.** An antihistamine used to treat stuffy nose and allergy symptoms. Potential adverse reactions include drowsiness and confusion (especially in the elderly), anemia, dizziness, tremors, heart palpitations, restlessness, irritability, insomnia, loss of appetite, nausea, vomiting, dry mouth and throat, urinary frequency, urinary retention, hives, rash, and thick bronchial secretions. Use with central nervous system depressants, including alcohol, increases sedation. MAO inhibitors (*see*) may cause blood pressure to shoot up. Contraindicated in acute asthma attacks. Should be used cautiously in elderly patients, those with glaucoma, overactive thyroid, heart or kidney disease, high blood pressure, bronchial asthma, enlarged prostate, bladder-neck obstruction, and peptic ulcer. Should be taken with food or milk to reduce GI distress. Coffee or tea may reduce drowsiness. Medication should be discontinued four days before taking a skin allergy test because it can lead to inaccurate results.

TRIPHASIL • *See* Estradiol and Levonorgestrel.

TRIPHED • *See* Triprolidine.

TRI-PHEN-CHLOR (OTC) • A combination of chlorpheniramine, phenylephrine, phenylpropanolamine, and phenyltoloxamine (*see all*), used to treat symptoms of a cold or allergy.

TRIPLE ANTIBIOTIC (Rx) • A combination of bacitracin, neomycin, and polymyxin B (*see all*) to treat skin and eye infections.

TRIPLE SULFA (Rx) • A combination of sulfacetamide, sulfabenzamide, and sulfathiazole (*see all*) to treat vaginal infections.

TRIPLE X • *See* Pyrethrins.

TRIPOSED (OTC) • *See* Triprolidine and Pseudoephedrine.

TRIPROLIDINE (OTC) • **Actagen. Actidil. Actifed Plus. Allerfrin. Allerphed. Aprodrine. Cenafed. Genac. Myidil. Sudahist. Triafed. Triofed. Triphed. Triposed.** An antihistamine introduced in 1958 to treat cold and allergy symptoms. Changed from Rx to OTC. Potential adverse reactions include a drop in white blood cells, drowsiness and confusion (especially in the elderly), dizziness, low blood pressure, heart palpitations, restlessness, irritability, insomnia (especially in children), excitation, rapid heartbeat, loss of appetite, nausea, vomiting, dry mouth and throat, urinary frequency, urinary retention, hives, rash, and photosensitivity. Use with central nervous system depressants, including alcohol, increases sedation. MAO inhibitors (*see*) may cause blood pressure to shoot up. Contraindicated in acute asthma. Should be used cautiously in elderly patients, those with glaucoma, overactive thyroid, heart or kidney disease, high blood pressure, bronchial asthma, enlarged prostate, bladder-neck obstruction, and peptic ulcer. Should be taken with food or milk to reduce GI distress. Coffee or tea may reduce drowsiness. Medication should be discontinued four days before taking a skin allergy test because it can lead to inaccurate results.

TRIPTERYQIUM WILFORDII • *See* Thunder God Vine.

TRISORALEN • *See* Trioxsalen.

TRISULFAM • *See* Co-Trimoxazole.

TRISULFAPYRIMIDINES (Rx) • Terfonyl. A combination of sulfadiazine, sulfamerazine, and sulfamethazine, used to treat mild to moderate infections.

TRI-THALMIC (Rx) • A combination of bacitracin, neomycin, polymyxin B, and hydrocortisone (*see all*).

TRI-THALMIC HC (Rx) • A combination of bacitracin, neomycin, polymyxin B, and hydrocortisone (*see all*), used to treat eye inflammations and infections.

TRITICUM • *See* Dog Grass.

TRITRACID • *See* Calcium Carbonate.

TRI-VI-FLOR (OTC) • A multivitamin preparation with fluoride (*see*).

TRI-VI-SOL (OTC) • A multivitamin preparation.

TROBICIN • *See* Spectinomycin.

TROFAN • *See* Tryptophan.

TROLAMINE SALICYLATE (OTC) • Triethanolamine. Aspercreme Creme, Lotion, Analgesic Rub. Mobisyl Analgesic Creme. Myoflex Analgesic Cream. Derived from ethylene oxide and ammonia, it is used in products to treat the temporary pain of minor backache, sore muscles, and aching joints caused by arthritis. In 1992, the FDA proposed a ban for the use of trolamine salicylate in drug products to treat fever blisters and cold sores, in insect bite and sting drug products, and in those to treat poison ivy, poison oak, and poison sumac because it had not been shown to be safe and effective as claimed in OTC products. *See* Salicylates.

TROLEANDOMYCIN (Rx) • Tao. Triacetyloleandomycin. An antibiotic derived from *Streptomyces antibioticus,* it is active against certain streptococcal infections and pneumonias. Potential adverse reactions include hepatitis, nausea, vomiting, abdominal cramps, and diarrhea. During prolonged or repeated therapy, overgrowth of nonsusceptible organisms may occur. Mild allergic reactions, such as hives and other rashes, and more serious allergic reactions have been reported. Troleandomycin is principally excreted by the liver and should be used with caution in patients with liver dysfunction.

TROMETHAMINE (Rx) • Tham. Than-E. A drug used to dissolve certain types of stones in the urinary tract, and to treat acidosis associated with cardiac bypass surgery or cardiac arrest. Potential adverse reactions include respiratory depression, low blood sugar, and high potassium. Contraindicated in serious kidney dysfunction, chronic respiratory acidosis, and pregnancy, except in life-threatening situations.

TRONOLANE • *See* Pramoxine Hydrochloride.

TRONOTHANE • *See* Pramoxine Hydrochloride.

TROPAEOLIN MAJUS • *See* Nasturtium.

TROPHOBLASTIC TUMORS • Tumors of cells that form the placenta, which nourishes the fetus. The tumors may occur inside or outside the womb after pregnancy.

TROPICACYL • *See* Tropicamide.

TROPICAMIDE (Rx) • I-Picamide. Mydriacyl. Mydriafair. Ocu-Tropic. Tropicacyl. A drug that enlarges the pupil; used in eye examinations and for treatment of some cases of acute eye inflammation. Symptoms of too much drug being absorbed into the body include confusion, unsteadiness, rapid heartbeat, and flushing.

TROXIDONE • *See* Trimethadione.

TRUE UNICORN ROOT (H) • *Aletris farinosa.* Colic Root. The rhizome and root of this herb, which is often confused with false unicorn root (*see*), is used by herbalists for sluggish digestion. Its bitter principle (*see*) stimulates the digestion and increases appetite, while decreasing intestinal gas and heartburn. Also called colic root because it relieves stomach pain.

TRUPHYLLINE • *See* Aminophylline.

TRUSPOT • *See* Dorzolamide.

TRYMEGEN • *See* Chlorpheniramine.

TRYMEX • *See* Triamcinolone.

TRYPSIN (OTC) • An enzyme formed in the intestine that is administered as a drug in the treatment of indigestion.

TRYPTACIN • *See* Tryptophan.

TRYPTOPHAN (H) • **Trofan. Tryptacin.** A tremendous amount of research is now in progress with this amino acid (*see*). First isolated in milk in 1901, it is now being studied as a means to calm hyperactive children, induce sleep, and fight depression and pain. Although it is sold over the counter, tryptophan is not believed to be completely harmless and has been suspected of being a cocarcinogen (abets a cancer-causing agent) and to affect the liver when taken in high doses. As with niacin, it is capable of preventing and curing pellagra. It is used by the body to make the brain hormone serotonin and is indispensable for the manufacture of certain cell proteins.

TSH • Abbreviation for thyroid-stimulating hormone (*see*).

T-STAT • *See* Erythromycin.

TUCKS • *See* Witch Hazel.

TUINAL (Rx) • A combination of secobarbital and amobarbital, it is used as a sedative during the day and to induce sleep at night. The drug is a combination of a short- and an intermediate-acting barbiturate. Potential adverse reactions include nausea, vomiting, drowsiness, diarrhea, rash, dizziness, hangover, breathing difficulty, allergic reactions, anemia, and yellowing of the eyes. Other central nervous system depressants such as sleeping pills, tranquilizers, or sedatives increase its effects. The drug can reduce the effects of blood thinners, muscle relaxants, painkillers, anticonvulsants, quinidine, theophylline, metronidazole, phenmetrazine, birth control pills, and acetaminophen. Contraindicated in people who are sensitive to barbiturates, have liver or kidney dysfunction, or have a tendency to become addicted. Most effective when taken on an empty stomach, but may be taken with a small amount of food if stomach upset is a problem.

TUMS (OTC) • *See* Calcium Carbonate.

TURMERIC (H) • *Curcuma longa.* A perennial plant belonging to the ginger family, turmeric is native to East India and most of the Pacific islands. The hard roots are powdered by herbalists and applied to ulcers. The roots also are used for liver and bowel complaints, and for the treatment of jaundice and menstrual problems. More than three thousand years ago, Indian healers used turmeric to treat obesity. In Germany, it was used to treat gallbladder disease. Turmeric has been found to have strong anti-inflammatory and antibacterial properties. It reputedly relieves the symptoms of arthritis. Modern studies have shown that it may prevent blood clots. The active principle of turmeric, curcumin, is a potent antimutagenic agent and is being studied for its activity against cancer and inflammation. In large doses or long-term use, turmeric may cause increased gastric acidity and liver dysfunction.

TURPENTINE TREE (OTC) (H) • *Pinus taeda. Pistacia terebinthus.* **Spirits of Turpentine. Terebinth. White Turpentine.** The term *turpentine* refers to vegetable juices, liquids, or gums containing the essential oil generally procured from various species of pine; other trees, such as the European larch, also yield turpentine. *Pistacia terebinthus* is a small tree native to Greece. The common American, or white, turpentine, which is listed as terebintha in the USP (*see*), is from *Pinus taeda*. The oil or "spirit" is a local irritant and somewhat antiseptic. It was used in folk medicine as an expectorant. It was a stimulant to kidney function and was sometimes used in diluted solutions as a diuretic. In large doses, it damages the kidney. It was also used to treat intestinal gas and colic, chronic diarrhea and dysentery, typhoid fever, internal hemorrhages, bleeding, worms, vaginal discharge, and absence of menses. Turpentine baths, arranged so that vapors were not inhaled, were given to patients with chronic arthritis. Terebinth was also used in enema form to treat constipation. Applied topically as a liniment or ointment, it is used by herbalists to treat arthritis and nerve pain. It was also used topically to treat and promote the healing of burns and to heal parasitic skin diseases. Terebene, which is derived from oil of turpentine, is used orally or by inhalation as an antiseptic and expectorant. In 1992, the FDA proposed a ban for the use of turpentine oil to treat fever blisters and cold sores, in insect bite and sting drug products, and in those to treat poison ivy, poison sumac, and poison oak because it had not been shown to be safe and effective as claimed in these OTC products. The FDA also put sulfurated oils of turpentine on the ban list for oral menstrual drugs.

TUSAL • *See* Sodium Thiosalicylate.

TUSSAGESIC (OTC) • A combination of acetaminophen, dextromethorphan, phenylpropanolamine, pheniramine, and pyrilamine (*see all*), used to treat the symptoms of a cold or allergy, particularly a cough.

TUSSAR (Rx) • A combination of chlorpheniramine, codeine phosphate and sulfate, dextromethorphan, and guaifenesin (*see all*), used to treat symptoms of a cold or allergy.

TUSSAR SF (Rx) • A combination of chlorpheniramine, codeine phosphate and sulfate, and guaifenesin (*see all*), used to treat a cough.

TUSSEND • *See* Pseudoephedrine and Hydrocodone.

TUSSILAGO FARFARA • *See* Coltsfoot.

TUSSIONEX (Rx) • A combination of hydrocodone and phenyltoloxamine, it is a cough suppressant and antihistamine combination used to treat colds and other respiratory symptoms. The cough suppressant, hydrocodone, is more powerful than codeine. Potential adverse reactions include nausea, vomiting, light-headedness, drowsiness, sweating, itching, rash, sensitivity to light, chills, dry mouth, nose, and throat, euphoria, weakness, agitation, incoordination, minor hallucinations, confusion, visual disturbances, loss of appetite, constipation, flushing, rapid heartbeat, heart palpitations, difficulty in urinating, reduced sexual potency, low blood sugar, anemia, yellowing of the skin or eye whites, blurred or double vision, ringing in the ears, wheezing, and stuffy nose. Contraindicated in those allergic to codeine or ingredients found in Tussionex. Should be used with caution in those who have a history of seizures, glaucoma, stomach ulcers, thyroid disease, heart disease, or diabetes. Alcohol or other central nervous system depressant drugs may increase the depressant effects of Tussionex. This drug should not be taken with MAO inhibitors (*see*) because the combination can be dangerous. Tussionex is most effective if taken on an empty stomach, but may be taken with a small amount of food if stomach upset is a problem.

TUSSI-ORGANIDIN NR (Rx) • *See* Guaifenesin and Codeine Phosphate and Sulfate.

TUSSI-ORGANIDIN-S NR (Rx) • Liquid form. *See* Guaifenesin and Codeine Phosphate.

TUSSIREX (Rx) • A combination of codeine phosphate and sulfate, phenylephrine, caffeine, pheniramine, sodium citrate, and sodium salicylate (*see all*), used as a cough medicine.

TUSSIS • Latin for cough.

TUSSTAT • *See* Diphenhydramine.

25-HCC • *See* Calcifediol.

TWICE-A-DAY NASAL • *See* Oxymetazoline.

TWILITE • *See* Diphenhydramine.

TWIN-K • *See* Guaifenesin.

2-PAM • *See* Pralidoxime.

TYLENOL (OTC) • *See* Acetaminophen.

TYLENOL WITH CODEINE • *See* Acetaminophen and Codeine Phosphate and Sulfate.

TYLOX • *See* Acetaminophen and Oxycodone Hydrochloride.

TYMPAGESIC SOLUTION (Rx) • A combination of benzocaine, phenylephrine, and antipyrine (*see all*) to treat ear pain.

TY-PAP • *See* Acetaminophen.

TYPHOID FEVER • An acute feverish illness caused by germs of the salmonella family, contained in the feces of infected patients and unknowing carriers. Usually transmitted by contaminated water or food, or poor personal hygiene.

TYPHOID VACCINE (Rx) • Provides active immunity to typhoid fever. Potential adverse reactions include fever, malaise, headache, nausea, and severe allergic reaction.

TYRAMINE • A derivative of tyrosine (*see*), it is a chemical present in mistletoe (*see*) and many common foods and beverages. It raises blood pressure, but usually causes no problem because enzymes in the body hold it in check. When drugs are used that inhibit the major enzyme restraining its action, monoamine oxidase (MAO), blood pressure can shoot up to dangerous levels, particularly when foods and beverages containing significant levels of tyramine (*see*) are ingested. Among these foods are cheese, beer, wines, pickled herring, chicken livers, yeast extract, canned figs, raisins, bananas, avocados, chocolate, soy sauce, fava beans, meat tenderizers, eggplant, tea, cola, liver, and yogurt. Among the drugs that inhibit the enzyme and may lead to a serious rise in blood pressure are the MAO inhibitors (*see*), anti-TB drugs such as isoniazid (*see*), and anticancer drugs such as procarbazine.

TYROSINE (OTC) • **L-Form (L-Tyrosine).** A widely distributed amino acid (*see*), termed nonessential because it does not seem to be necessary for growth. Used as a dietary supplement, it is a building block of protein.

TY-TABS • *See* Acetaminophen.

TYZINE DROPS • *See* Tetrahydrozoline Hydrochloride.

U

UBIQUINONE • *See* Coenzyme Q$_{10}$.

U-CORT • *See* Hydrocortisone.

ULCER • An open sore with an inflamed base. The tissues disintegrate and there may be pus oozing from the sore.

ULCERATION • The formation of an ulcer (*see*).

ULCERATIVE COLITIS • A condition that affects the entire colon, causing sores or ulcers inside the tube and characterized most often by bloody diarrhea.

ULTANE (Rx) • *See* Sevoflurane.

ULTIMATE XPHORIA (H) • A so-called "natural high" drug promoted to young people.

ULTRACEF • *See* Cefadroxil Monohydrate.

ULTRALENTE • *See* Insulin.

ULTRAM • *See* Tramadol.

ULTRA-MIDE • *See* Urea.

ULTRA TEARS (OTC) • *See* Artificial Tears.

ULTRAVATE • *See* Halobetasol Propionate.

ULTRAVIST (Rx) • *See* Topromide.

UMBELLIFERAE • *See* Aniseed.

UNASYN (Rx) • *See* Ampicillin and Sulbactam.

UNDECYLENIC ACID (OTC) • **Breeze Mist. Cruex. Desenex. Kool Foot. Merlenate. Pedi-Dri. Quinsana Plus. Ting Spray. Undoguent.** An antifungal and antibacterial agent used to treat athlete's foot, jock itch, and ringworm of the body except nails and hairy areas. Potential adverse reactions include skin irritation in hypersensitive persons. Ointments, creams, and liquids are used as primary therapy in very mild conditions, or as prophylactic (*see*) agents, especially in moist areas. Powders with a cornstarch base may be preferred over those with a talc base. Inhaling the powders and any contact with undecylenic acid products around the eyes or other mucous membranes should be avoided. Should not be applied on blistered, raw, or oozing skin, or over deep wounds or punctures. Patients with impaired circulation, including diabetics, should consult a physician before using undecylenic acid. If a skin problem does not clear up in a month or gets worse, consult your physician.

UNDOGUENT (OTC) • *See* Undecylenic Acid.

UNGUENTINE (OTC) • Ointment used for minor burns. *See* Petrolatum and Alum.

UNGUENTINE PLUS FIRST AID & BURN (OTC) • For minor burns. *See* Lidocaine and Parachlorometaxylenol.

UNIBASE • A base for medicated creams and ointments containing lanolin and petrolatum (*see both*).

UNIFAST • *See* Phentermine.

UNILAX (OTC) • *See* Danthron and Docusate.

UNIPEN • *See* Nafcillin.

UNIPHYL • *See* Theophylline.

UNIPRES (Rx) • A combination of hydralazine, hydrochlorothiazide, and reserpine (*see all*), used to lower blood pressure.

UNI-PRO (OTC) • *See* Ibuprofen.

UNISOM (OTC) • Approved by the FDA as a sleep aid. *See* Doxylamine.

UNITED STATES PHARMACOPEIA (USP) • A compilation of the monographs covering standards for the strength and purity of drug ingredients, and directions for making medicinal preparations. *USP* is often used on nonprescription labels after the name of an ingredient to show that the substance meets specifications set forth in the USP.

UNIVASE (Rx) • *See* Moexipril.

UNNA'S BOOT • *See* Zinc Gelatin.

UNNA'S PATE • *See* Zinc.

UNPROCO (OTC) • *See* Dextromethorphan and Guaifenesin.

-UR, URE-, UREO- • Suffix and prefixes meaning pertaining to urine.

URABETH • *See* Bethanechol.

URACEL-5 • *See* Sodium Salicylate.

URACIL MUSTARD (Rx) • An anticancer agent used to treat chronic leukemia, Hodgkin's disease, non-Hodgkin's lymphomas, sarcomas, mycosis fungoides, polycythemia vera, and cancers of the ovaries, cervix, and lungs. Uracil interferes with the growth of cancer cells, which are eventually destroyed. Since the growth of normal body cells may also be affected, the drug must be supervised with great care. Potential adverse reactions include anemia, bone-marrow suppression, nausea, vomiting, diarrhea, abdominal pain, loss of appetite, loss of hair, itching, rash, dark spots on skin, irritability, nervousness, mental cloudiness, and depression. Blood thinners, including aspirin, must be used cautiously. Uracil is usually taken at bedtime to reduce nausea, but the patient should drink fluids liberally throughout the day. The taking of this drug must be carefully supervised by a physician.

UREA (Rx) (OTC) • Amino-Cerv Vaginal Cream. Aqua Care Cream. Carbamide. Carmol 20 Cream. Kera Creme. Nutraplus. Pen. Rea-Lo. Sultrin. Ultra-Mide 25. Ureacin-20. Ureaphil. A product of protein metabolism; excreted from human urine. It is included in skin preparations for the treatment of dry, scaling skin conditions and mild inflammation of the uterine cervix. It is an osmotic diuretic that enhances the flow of water into fluid outside the cells. Used to reduce pressure on the brain or within the eyes. Potential adverse reactions include nausea, vomiting, drowsiness, headache, rapid heartbeat, congestive heart failure, fluid in the lungs, and sodium and potassium depletion. Contraindicated in severely impaired kidney or liver function, and active bleeding within the head. Should be used cautiously in pregnancy, breast-feeding women, and patients with heart disease or sickle-cell anemia (*see*). In 1992, the FDA proposed a ban on urea in oral menstrual drug products because it had not been shown to be safe and effective as claimed.

UREACIN-20 (OTC) • *See* Urea.

UREA DERM (OTC) • A skin cream containing urea (*see*).

UREA PEROXIDE • *See* Carbamide Peroxide.

UREAPHIL • *See* Urea.

UREASE • An enzyme that hydrolyzes urea (*see*) to ammonium carbonate (*see*).

URECHOLINE • *See* Bethanechol.

URETHR- URETHRO- • Prefixes meaning relating to the urethra (*see*), the tube that carries urine from the bladder.

URETHRA • The canal from the neck of the bladder to the outside through which urine passes.

URETHRITIS • Inflammation of the urethra (*see*).

UREX • *See* Methenamine.

URICEMIA • Excessive amounts of uric acid in the blood.

URIDON • *See* Chlorthalidone.

URINARY TRACT INFECTION TEST KITS FOR HOME USE (OTC) • **Biotel/UTI.** A kit to be used by a nonphysician to detect bladder or kidney infections. Those likely to get frequent infections, such as women, diabetics, and patients with catheters, or those who have had urinary tract infections in the past, may find the kit helpful.

URISED (Rx) • A combination of atropine, benzoic acid, hyoscyamine, methenamine, methylene blue, and phenyl salicylate (*see all*), used to treat urinary-tract infections.

URISPAS (Rx) • *See* Flavoxate.

URITAB (Rx) • A combination of atropine, benzoic acid, hyoscyamine, methenamine, methylene blue, and phenyl salicylate (*see all*), used to treat urinary tract infections.

URI-TET • *See* Oxytetracycline.

UROBIOTIC (Rx) • *See* Oxytetracycline and Phenazopyridine Hydrochloride.

UROBLUE (Rx) • A combination of atropine, hyoscyamine, methenamine, methylene blue, and phenyl salicylate (*see all*), used to treat urinary-tract infections.

URODINE • *See* Phenazopyridine Hydrochloride.

UROFOLLITROPIN (Rx) • **Metrodin.** Used to induce ovulation in patients with polycystic ovarian disease, and to stimulate the development of multiple eggs. Potential adverse reactions include nausea, vomiting, bloating, stomach or pelvic pain, decreased amount of urine, fever and chills, rapid weight gain, shortness of breath, rash, hives, and breast tenderness.

UROGESIC (Rx) • A combination of phenazopyridine, atropine, hyoscyamine, and scopolamine to treat urinary tract infections.

UROKIN (OTC) • A combination of pumpkin-seed powder and bee pollen (*see both*).

UROKINASE (Rx) • **Abbokinase. Breokinase.** A substance that dissolves blood clots to the lungs and coronary arteries. Potential adverse reactions include severe, spontaneous bleeding, hypersensitivity, muscle and bone pain, and bronchospasm. Aspirin, dipyridamole, heparin, and coumarin (*see all*) increase the risk of bleeding if taken with urokinase.

URO-KP-NEUTRAL • *See* Potassium Phosphate and Sodium Phosphate.

UROLENE BLUE • *See* Methylene Blue.

URO-PHOSPHATE (Rx) • *See* Methenamine and Sodium Biphosphate.

UROPLUS • *See* Co-Trimoxazole.

URSODEOXYCHOLIC ACID • *See* Ursodiol.

URSODIOL (Rx) • **Actigall. Ursodeoxycholic Acid.** A naturally occurring bile acid that suppresses liver synthesis and secretion of cholesterol, as well as intestinal absorption. After long-term administration, it can dissolve cholesterol from gallstones. Potential adverse reactions include nausea, vomiting, abdominal pain, anxiety, depression, sleep disorders, cough, runny nose, gas, diarrhea, constipation, sore mouth, itching, rash, dry skin, hives, hair thinning, joint and muscle pain, and back pain. Aluminum-containing antacids, cholestyramine, and colestipol make it less effective. Estrogen, oral contraceptives, and clofibrate counteract its effects. Contraindicated in patients allergic to ursodiol or other bile acids. Also contraindicated in chronic liver disease, acute gallbladder trouble, and gallstone pancreatitis. Ursodiol will not dissolve calcified cholesterol stones. Long-term therapy with ursodiol is needed before it produces effects. Patients with unremitting acute inflammation or obstruction of the gallbladder, gallstone pancreatitis, or biliary gastrointestinal fistulas are not candidates for Actigall therapy.

URSOLIC ACID • **Bearberry. Privet Fruit.** Found in leaves and berries of *Arctostaphylos* *uva-ursi.* Used as an emulsifying agent in pharmaceuticals and foods.

URTICA DIOICA • *See* Nettle.

URTICARIA • **Hives. Nettlerash.** Whitish, raised bumps that itch; usually an allergic reaction.

URTICA URENS (H) • **Urt-u.** A homeopathic remedy for bee stings, minor burns, eczema, and sunburn. *See* Nettle.

URT-U • Homeopathic abbreviation for *Urtica urens (see).*

USNEA (H) • *Usnea barbata.* **Beard Lichen.** A lichen growing on tree branches, it is used internally and externally for fungal, viral, and bacterial infections. When combined with echinacea (*see*), it is used as a general antibiotic and antifungal medication.

USNIC ACID (H) • An antibacterial compound found in lichens. Pale yellow, slightly soluble in water. *See* Usnea.

USP • Abbreviation for United States Pharmacopeia (*see*), the official publication for drug product standards.

UTERINE TUMORS • Cancers of the uterus, the womb. They include cancer of the cervix, the opening of the womb, and of the corpus body of the womb, and of the endometrium, lining of the womb.

UTICORT • *See* Betamethasone.

UTIMOX • *See* Amoxicillin.

UVA-URSI (H) • *Arctostaphylos uva-ursi.* **Bearberry.** An astringent used to treat bladder problems, its action is believed due to the high concentration of the antiseptic arbutin. Arbutin, in passing through the system, yields hydroquinone (*see*), a urinary disinfectant. Uva-ursi leaves contain anesthetic principles that numb pain in the urinary system, and the herb has been shown to have antibiotic activity. Crude extracts of uva-ursi reportedly possess some anticancer property. In 1992, the FDA proposed a ban on uva-ursi extract in oral menstrual drug products because it had not been shown to be safe and effective as claimed. Regular use of the plant may lead to constipation.

UVEITIS • Inflammation of the eye that may cause hazy or diminished vision and floating spots.

V

VACCINE • A solution containing a killed or altered strain of a disease-producing organism. Vaccines create resistance to the diseases the organisms cause.

VACHA (H) • *Acorus calamus.* An herb used in India as a tranquilizer and aphrodisiac.

VAGILLA (Rx) • A combination of sulfabenzamide, sulfacetamide, and sulfathiazole, used to treat vaginal infections.

VAGISTAT • *See* Tioconazole.

VAGITROL • *See* Sulfanilamides.

VALACYCLOVIR (Rx) • **Valtrex.** Indicated for the treatment of herpes zoster (shingles) (*see*) in adults with a normal immune system. It is contraindicated in patients with a known hypersensitivity or inteolerance to valacyclovir, acyclovir (*see*), or any component of the formulation. Deaths have been reported in patients with advanced HIV disease and also in transplant patients. Safety and effectiveness in children and nursing mothers have not been established. The most common potential side effects include nausea, headache, vomiting, diarrhea, and constipation.

VALADOL • *See* Acetaminophen.

VALDRENE • *See* Diphenhydrazine.

VALERGEN • *See* Estradiol.

VALERIAN (OTC) (H) • *Valeriana officinalis.* **Garden Heliotrope.** A perennial native to Europe and the United States, it was reputed to be a love potion. Its vapor was found to kill the bacillus of typhoid fever after forty-five minutes. The herb has been widely studied in Europe and Russia, and the major constituents, the valepotriates, have been reported to have marked sedative, anticonvulsive, blood-pressure-lowering, and tranquilizing effects. It has been used for centuries to treat panic attacks. It is on the market as a sleep aid. In Germany, valerian preparations have been used for more than a decade to treat childhood behavioral disorders, supposedly without the side effects experienced with pharmaceuticals for that purpose. Valerian has also been reported to help concentration and energy. Prolonged use of valerian may result in side effects such as irregular heartbeat, headaches, uneasiness, nervousness, and insomnia. Large doses may cause paralysis.

VALERIANA OFFICINALIS • *See* Valerian.

VALERIC ACID • Occurs naturally in apples, cocoa, coffee, oil of lavender, peaches, and strawberries. A synthetic flavoring agent usually distilled from the root of valerian (*see*). Some of its salts are used in medicine.

VALINE • **L-Form.** An essential amino acid (*see*). Occurs in the largest quantities in fibrous protein. It is indispensable for growth and nitrogen balance.

VALISONE • *See* Betamethasone.

VALIUM • *See* Diazepam.

VALORIN • *See* Acetaminophen.

VALPIN 50 • *See* Anisotropine.

VALPROIC ACID (Rx) • **Dalpro. Depakene Syrup. Depakote. Myproic Acid. Myproic Acid Syrup.** An epilepsy drug introduced in 1967 that increases the level of the neurotransmitter gamma-aminobutyric acid (*see*), which transmits inhibitor nerve impulses to the central nervous system. It is used to treat simple and complex absence seizures (*see*), mixed seizures, and generalized, tonic-clonic seizures. This drug is also being tested and shows effectiveness against manic-depressive disorder (*see*). Potential adverse reactions are hard to identify because valproic acid is usually mixed with other anticonvulsants. It has been reported to inhibit clotting and cause sedation, emotional upset, depression, psychosis, aggression, hyperactivity, behavioral deterioration, double vision, sore mouth, muscle weakness, tremor, nausea, vomiting, indigestion, diarrhea, abdominal cramps, constipation, increased or decreased appetite, decreased libido, female breast enlargement with milk production, irregular menstruation, weight gain, pancreatitis (see), liver dysfunction, and hair loss. Serious or fatal liver toxicity may follow nonspecific symptoms such as malaise, fever, and lethargy. Contraindicated in liver dysfunction. Should be used cautiously in children under two years of age and in mentally retarded children. Aspirin may cause valproic acid toxicity. The drug may increase sodium levels in the blood. Valproic acid may increase levels of phenobarbital, causing toxicity, and may increase or decrease phenytoin levels. MAO inhibitors (see) may depress the central nervous system when taken with valproic acid. Valproic acid may increase the effects of central nervous system depressants such as sleeping pills, tranquilizers, and alcohol. It may make oral contraceptives ineffective. Depakote is enteric coated (see). Most effective when taken on an empty stomach, but may be taken with a small amount of food if stomach distress is a problem.

VALRELEASE • See Diazepam.

VALTREX • See Valacyclovir.

VANCENASE • See Beclomethasone.

VANCERIL • See Beclomethasone.

VANCOCIN • See Vancomycin Hydrochloride.

VANCOLED • See Vancomycin Hydrochloride.

VANCOMYCIN HYDROCHLORIDE (Rx) • Lyphocin. Vancocin. Vancoled. Vancor. An antibiotic used to treat severe staphylococcal infections when other antibiotics are ineffective or contraindicated. Also used to prevent heart infection in susceptible people undergoing dental work, and to prevent inflammation of the lining of the heart in patients with heart-valve disease or artificial heart valves who are allergic to penicillin. Potential adverse reactions include a low white blood count, ringing in the ears, nausea, rash, local pain at site of injection, bad taste in the mouth, drowsiness, increased thirst, chills, fever, and severe allergic reactions. Several of the side effects may occur a number of weeks after the medication has been discontinued. If vancomycin is used with aminoglycosides, amphotericin B, cisplatin, or pentamidine, the risk of kidney damage may be increased. If your doctor prescribes cholestyramine or colestipol (see both), do not take vancomycin orally within three to four hours of the time you take either of these medicines or the vancomycin may be ineffective. New Jersey State Health Department researchers reported in 1995 that this antibiotic puts people at risk of developing vancomycin-resistant enterococci (VRE), in which harmless bacteria found in everyone's intestines turns potentially deadly. The New Jersey researchers say that no conventional antibiotic works against VRE and even multidrug efforts often fail.

VANCOR • See Vancomycin Hydrochloride.

VANILLA • Extracted from the full-grown unripe fruit of the vanilla plant of Mexico and the West Indies, it is used as a flavoring in foods and medicines. It reputedly works as an aphrodisiac, possibly because it has a mildly sensitizing effect on motor nerves and has been found to stimulate the male reproductive tract. Whether or not this is proven, vanilla perfumes became popular in the midnineties.

VANILLIN • Occurs naturally in vanilla and potato parings and is used as an artificial flavoring.

VANOXIDE-HC (OTC) • See Benzoyl Peroxide.

VANQUISH (OTC) • A combination of aspirin, acetaminophen, aluminum hydroxide, magnesium hydroxide, and caffeine (see all), used to treat pain. Contains 33 mg of caffeine.

VANSIL • See Oxamniquine.

VANTIN • See Cefpodoxime Proxetil.

VAPO-ISO • See Isoproterenol.

VAPONEFRIN • *See* Epinephrine.

VARICELLA VIRUS VACCINE, LIVE (Rx) • **Varivax.** The first vaccine against chicken pox in the United States, introduced in 1995. Saying the vaccine was 70 to 90 percent effective in preventing the viral infection, the FDA approved its use for children one year or older. The FDA says that of the 30 percent who failed to be protected by the vaccine in clinical trials, almost all had much milder manifestations of the disease. The American Academy of Pediatrics recommends the vaccine for all children and for adolescents and adults who have not had chicken pox. Children twelve months to twelve years receive a single dose administered under the skin. Adolescents and adults receive two doses administered four to eight weeks apart. The duration of protection of the vaccine is unknown at this writing.

VARICELLA-ZOSTER • A virus that can infect humans, most commonly causing chicken pox, and associated with shingles in adults.

VARICOSE VEINS • Dilated superficial leg veins with incompetent valves. The condition affects 20 percent of the population, with a high incidence of family weakness in the vein wall.

VARIVAX • *See* Varicella Virus Vaccine, Live.

VASCOR • *See* Bepridil Hydrochloride.

VASCULITIS • **Angiitis.** A widespread allergic reaction of the skin or other organs characterized by inflammation of the blood vessels.

VASELINE • *See* Petrolatum.

VASERETIC (Rx) • **Enalapril Maleate–Hydrochlorothiazide.** A combination of enalapril and hydrochlorothiazide (*see both*) used to treat high blood pressure. The blood-pressure-lowering effect of the two drugs is greater than either alone. Potential adverse reactions include nausea, vomiting, diarrhea, headache, rash, cough, itching, fever, temporary loss of taste, stomach irritation, chest pain, low blood pressure, heart palpitations, tingling in the hands or feet, flushing, swelling of the limbs, and closing of the throat. The hydrochlorothiazide ingredient can cause a loss of body potassium and increase the toxicity of lithium. The blood-pressure-lowering effect of Vaseretic is additive with diuretic drugs and beta-blockers (*see*). Enalapril may increase potassium levels in the blood. Vaseretic should be used cautiously in persons with kidney dysfunction, asthma, immune/collagen diseases such as lupus erythematosus (*see*), and those who have taken other drugs that affect the white blood cell count. Vaseretic should be taken on an empty stomach.

VASOACTIVE INTESTINAL PEPTIDE • **VIP.** A neurotransmitter (*see*) present in both the gut and the brain. Its peripheral effects include lowering blood pressure by causing vasodilation, suppressing the secretion of stomach acid, and stimulating secretion in the small intestine and colon. VIP stimulates the release of a number of pituitary hormones, including growth hormone and prolactin, and may thus help to regulate the hormone glands. It may also play a part in arousal.

VASOCIDIN • *See* Sulfacetamide and Prednisolone.

VASOCLEAR (OTC) • *See* Naphazoline.

VASOCON-A • *See* Naphazoline and Antazoline.

VASOCONSTRICTION • A decrease in the diameter of a blood vessel.

VASOCONSTRICTOR • A substance that causes a narrowing of the blood vessels. Cold, stress, nicotine, and certain drugs such as ergotamine are vasoconstrictors.

VASODERM • *See* Fluocinonide.

VASODILAN • *See* Isoxsuprine.

VASODILATION • Relaxation of arterial walls, which increases the diameter of the arterioles.

VASODILATOR • An agent that relaxes smooth muscle of blood vessels, thereby increasing their diameter.

VASOMOTOR • Refers to the control of dilation or constriction of blood-vessel walls, and thus the volume of blood flowing through them. Impulses from the brain go to the muscle fibers in the walls of blood vessels, over nerves of opposite action: constriction or dilation. Feedback mechanisms of the vasomotor system are complicated. When you feel threatened, the vasomotor system constricts your blood vessels to prepare you for flight. The same thing happens when there is a fall in blood pressure caused by bleeding. The blood vessels are automatically constricted to try to stop the hemorrhage.

VASOPRESSIN (Rx) • **Pitressin.** A hormone normally produced by the body, it prevents the loss of too much water. Vasopressin is used to control frequent urination, increased thirst, and loss of water associated with diabetes insipidus. It is also used to prevent and treat stomach swelling caused by too much gas. Potential side effects include weight gain, chest pain, coma, confusion, tremors, seizures, headache, drowsiness, fever, problems with urination, redness of skin, rash, hives, itching, and swelling of face, feet, hands, or mouth. There may be abdominal cramps, belching, diarrhea, dizziness, increased sweating, increased urge for bowel movements, nausea or vomiting, trembling, wheezing, a white-colored area around the mouth, and pain at the site of injection. This medicine should be taken with one or two glasses of water.

VASOPRESSOR • An agent that constricts the capillaries and arteries and raises blood pressure.

VASOPRINE • *See* Isoxsuprine.

VASOSPASM • A sudden, intense constriction of smooth muscle in vessel walls.

VASOTEC • *See* Enalapril.

VASOXYL • *See* Methoxamine.

VATRONOL NOSE DROPS (VICKS) • *See* Ephedrine.

V-CILLIN K • *See* Penicillin V.

VC-K • *See* Penicillin V.

VCR • *See* Vincristine Sulfate.

VECURONIUM (Rx) • **Norcuron.** A muscle relaxant used as an adjunct (*see*) to general anesthesia. Potential adverse reactions include rapid heartbeat, redness, itching, and respiratory difficulties. Contraindicated in persons allergic to bromides.

VEETIDS • *See* Penicillin V.

VELBAN • *See* Vinblastine Sulfate.

VELNACRINE (Rx) • **Mentane.** A drug to treat Alzheimer's disease; expected to be approved.

VELOSEF • *See* Cephradine.

VELOSULIN • *See* Insulin.

VELSAR • *See* Vinblastine Sulfate.

VELTANE • *See* Brompheniramine.

VENI-, VENO- • Prefixes meaning relating to the veins.

VENLAFAXINE (Rx) • **Effexor.** An antidepressant introduced in 1994. It helps restore the balance of serotonin and norepinephrine in the brain (*see both*). It takes effect within several weeks. Potential adverse effects include sleepiness, dry mouth, dizziness, constipation, nervousness, sweating, weakness, abnormal ejaculation/ orgasm, and loss of appetite. Care should be taken while driving or operating hazardous machinery until the body becomes accustomed to the medication. Has a potential for interaction with MAO inhibitors (*see*). Should be taken with meals.

VENOGLOBULIN • *See* Immune Serum Globulin.

VENOUS • Pertaining to the veins.

VENOUS MUSCLE PUMPS • Skeletal muscular action upon the veins that returns blood to the heart.

VENOUS VALVES • Valves that enable veins to transport blood to the heart by preventing a backward flow away from the heart. They are more numerous in the arms and legs where blood must travel against gravity to reach the heart.

VENTOLIN • *See* Albuterol.

VENTRICLE • A small cavity, such as one of the several cavities of the brain, or one of the lower chambers of the heart.

VENTRICULAR ARRHYTHMIA • Arrhythmia (*see*) in which the electrical impulse originates low in the ventricles of the heart and travels backward to the normal route. The heart may generate little or no pumping action. There may be premature ventricular contractions (PVCs), ventricular tachycardia, and ventricular fibrillation (*see*). *See also* Antiarrhythmics.

VENTRICULAR FIBRILLATION • Random firing of electrical impulses from multiple sites in the ventricles, producing chaotic electrical activity and uncoordinated contraction.

VENUS' HAIR • *See* Maidenhair Fern.

VEPESID • *See* Etoposide.

VERA-A • Homeopathic abbreviation for veratrum (*see*).

VERAPAMIL (Rx) • **Calan. Isoptin. Covera-Hs. Verelan.** An antiarrhythmic drug introduced in 1981 to treat tachycardia (*see*), and to slow ventricular rate in atrial fibrillation (*see*) and flutter. It is also one of the most widely used calcium channel blockers (*see*) for mild high blood pressure. Among verapamil's promoted benefits are that it does not affect total cholesterol, blood sugar levels, kidney function, or electrolytes. Potential adverse reactions include dizziness, headache, fatigue, low blood pressure, congestive heart failure, water retention, constipation, nausea, confusion, impotence, male breast enlargement, loss of balance, blurred vision, hair loss, menstrual disorders, cramps, and liver dysfunction. Verapamil may increase the blood levels of carbamazepine, digitalis, and glycosides (*see all*). It may decrease serum lithium levels. Interaction with propanolol and other beta-blockers (*see*), including the eye medication timolol, may cause heart failure. Used with quinidine, it may cause blood pressure to drop too low. Rifampin may make verapamil less effective. Alcohol may exaggerate the drop in blood pressure. When used with other antihypertensive agents, it will have an additive effect in lowering blood pressure. When used with anesthetics, it may potentiate their activity. This drug may be taken with food. Grapefruit juice may cause potentially dangerous, increased levels of this medication in the blood.

VERATRUM (Rx) (H) • *American Hellebore. Indian Poke. Regroton.* Isolated from the dried rhizome and roots of *Veratrum viride,* which grows in North America. It is used to lower blood pressure. Homeopaths use it to treat memory problems, cough, diarrhea, exhaustion, fever, and vomiting.

VERAZINC (OTC) • *See* Zinc.

VERB • Homeopathic abbreviation for verbascum oil. *See* Mullein.

VERBASCUM THAPSUS • *See* Mullein.

VERBENA • *See* Vervain.

VERCYTE • *See* Pipobroman.

VERELAN • *See* Verapamil.

VERMIFUGE • A medication that kills or expels intestinal worms.

VERMIZINE • *See* Piperazine.

VERMOX • *See* Mebendazole.

VERONICA VIRGINICA • *See* Culver's Root.

VERR–CANTH • *See* Cantharidin.

VERREX–C&M • *See* Podophyllin Resin and Salicylic Acid.

VERRUCA • A wart.

VERSED • *See* Midazolam.

VERTEBRA • Any of the thirty-three bones of the spinal column.

VERTIGO • Dizziness; an illusion of movement.

VERVAIN, EUROPEAN (H) • *Verbena officinalis.* A weed of the verbena family, it is native to Europe and the Far East. A class of medicinal plants used as a flavoring in alcoholic beverages only. Vervain is believed to have been introduced to Rome by the druids. Hippocrates prescribed vervain for wounds, fever, and nervous disorders. In England, vervain was used as a guard against witches. Homeopathic medicine has used it to treat nervous disorders, epilepsy, asthma, whooping cough, hepatitis, and pneumonia. A decoction made from the whole plant is given for eczema and other skin complaints. Vervain should be avoided during pregnancy and in cases of ischemic (*see*) heart disease.

VESANOID (Rx) • An oral formulation of tretinoin (*see*) for the treatment of leukemia that was approved in other countries in 1994 and has been recommended for approval by an FDA expert committee. It is the first retinoic acid approved for a cancer indication.

VESICANT • An agent that causes blistering of the skin.

VESICULATION • The presence or formation of vesicles, or blisters.

VESPRIN • *See* Triflupromazine.

VEXOL • *See* Rimexolone.

V-GAN • *See* Promethazine.

VIABLE • Capable of living.

VIBAZINE • *See* Buclizine.

VIBRA-TABS • *See* Doxycycline.

VIBURNUM EXTRACT (H) • *Caprifoliacea.* **Black Extract. Haw Bark.** Extract of the fruit of a hawthorn shrub. Used in fragrances and in butter, caramel, cola, maple, and walnut flavorings for beverages. Has also been used as a uterine antispasmodic.

VIBURNUM PRUNIFOLIUM • *See* Black Haw.

VICKS FORMULA 44 COUGH CONTROL DISCS • *See* Benzocaine.

VICKS NYQUIL NIGHT-TIME COLD/FLU • *See* Doxylamine.

VICKS SINEX LONG-ACTING NASAL SOLUTION (OTC) • *See* Oxymetazoline.

VICKS SINEX NASAL SOLUTION (OTC) • *See* Phenylephrine.

VICKS VAPORUB (OTC) • *See* Camphor and Eucalyptus.

VICKS VATRONOL NOSE DROPS (OTC) • *See* Ephedrine.

VICODIN (Rx) • **Amacodone. Anodynos-DHC. Bancap HC. Co-gesic. Dolacet. DuocetP. Duradyne DHC. Hydrocet. Hydrogesic. Hyphen. Lorcet HD. Lortab. Norcet. Vapocet. Zydone-W.** All drugs that are a combination of hydrocodone and acetaminophen (*see both*). They are used to relieve mild to moderate pain. Prescribed for those allergic to aspirin but *not* for those who are allergic to acetaminophen or codeine. Vicodin is a stronger pain reliever than codeine. Potential adverse reactions include nausea, vomiting, loss of appetite, dizziness, insomnia, sweating, euphoria, weakness, headache, agitation, incoordination, blurred vision, urinary difficulty, inability to concentrate, reduced sex drive, impotence, itching, rash, anemia, low blood sugar, and yellowing of the skin and eye whites. Should not be used by people with asthma or other breathing problems. Alcohol, tranquilizers, sleeping pills, antihistamines, and other medicines that depress the central nervous system should be avoided when taking vicodin because such combinations can result in respiratory arrest and death. Vicodin may be taken with food.

VIDARABINE MONOHYDRATE (Rx) • **Adenine Arabinoside. Ara-A. Vira-A.** An antiviral drug given intravenously to treat herpes simplex virus encephalitis. It is also used in an ointment to treat viral infections of the eye. Potential adverse effects include anemia, tremor, dizziness, hallucinations, confusion, balance problems, loss of appetite, nausea, vomiting, diarrhea, liver problems, rash, pain at injection site, and weight loss. When used in an eye ointment, it may cause temporary burning, itching, mild irritation, pain, tearing, foreign-body sensation, redness, sensitivity to light, and allergic reactions. Use with allopurinol (*see*) may increase the risk of central nervous system adverse effects.

VIDEX • *See* Didanosine.

VINBLASTINE SULFATE (Rx) • **VLB. Alkaban-AQ. Velban. Velsar. Vincaleukoblastine.** An anticancer drug that arrests cell division, first isolated from periwinkle (*see*), it is used in the treatment of breast or testicular cancer, Hodgkin's disease, non-Hodgkin's lymphoma, choriocarcinoma, lymphosarcoma, neuroblastoma, and some fungal infections. Potential adverse reactions include nausea, vomiting, diarrhea, high blood pressure, depression, a sensation of pins and needles, sore throat, sore mouth, ulcer and bleeding, constipation, loss of appetite, weight loss, abdominal pain, a drop in or absence of sperm, rash, blisters, acute bronchospasm, reversible hair loss, pain in tumor site, and low fever. Mitomycin increases the risk of VLB-caused bronchospasm and shortness of breath. Contraindicated in bacterial infections or in severe lack of white blood cells. Your physician may recommend that you drink more fluids to pass more urine, which will help prevent kidney problems.

VINCALEUKOBLASTINE • *See* Vinblastine Sulfate.

VINCAMINE (Rx) (H) • Isolated from periwinkle (*see*), it is an alkaloid that is used as a blood-vessel dilator.

VINCASAR PFS • *See* Vincristine Sulfate.

VINCRISTINE SULFATE (Rx) • **LCR. Leurocristines. Oncovin. VCR. Vincasar PFS.** An anticancer drug derived originally from periwinkle (*see*), it stops cell division and is used to treat acute lymphoblastic and other leukemias, Hodgkin's disease, lymphosarcoma, reticulum cell sarcoma, neuroblastoma, rhabdomyosarcoma (*see*), Wilms's tumor (*see*), osteogenic sarcoma, and lung and breast cancers. Potential adverse reactions include nausea, vomiting, anemia, nerve damage, wristdrop and footdrop, incoordination, headache, jaw pain, hoarseness, vocal cord paralysis, visual disturbances, muscle weakness and cramps, depression, agitation, insomnia, double vision, drooped eyelid, constipation, cramps, sore mouth, weight loss, trouble in swallowing, urine retention, severe local reaction at injection site, reversible hair loss, and acute bronchospasm. Asparaginase (*see*) may increase its toxicity. Calcium channel blockers (*see*) enhance vincristine's accumulation in cells. Mitomycin may increase the frequency of bronchospasm. Your doctor may ask that you drink extra fluids while taking this medication to lessen the chances of kidney dysfunction.

VINEGAR (OTC) (H) • **Acetic Acid. Massengill Disposable Douches.** Used for hundreds of years to remove lime soap after shampooing. Vinegar is a solvent for cosmetic oils and resins. It is about 4–6 percent acetic acid. Acetic acid (*see*), an important component of vinegar, occurs naturally in apples, cheese, grapes, milk, and other foods. Used in feminine douches. No known toxicity, but may cause an allergic reaction in those allergic to corn.

VINORELBINE TARTRATE • **Navelbine.** An intravenous therapy introduced in 1994 for the treatment of non-small-cell lung cancer, and in combination with cisplatin for the treatment of advanced-stage lung cancer. Under priority review, it took the FDA 15.9 months to approve the medication. It is the first new drug approved in twenty years for the treatment of non-small-cell cancer. Navelbine plus cisplatin (*see*) has shown a median survival benefit of eight to ten weeks over other chemotherapy agents or vinorelbine alone in patients with advanced disease. Side effects—such as nausea, vomiting, and hair loss—were reported as mild to moderate.

VIOFORM • *See* Iodochlorhydroxyquin.

VIOKASE • *See* Pancrelipase.

VIOLET (H) • *Viola odorata.* **Sweet Violet.** The violet is used as a syrup for sore throat, dryness of the upper-respiratory tract, chronic cough, and asthma. It contains saponins, salicylate, alkaloids, flavonoids, and essential oil (*see all*). Also used by herbalists against tumors, to lower blood pressure, and treat urinary-tract infections.

VIOSTEROL • *See* Vitamin D.

VIP • Abbreviation for vasoactive intestinal peptide.

VIRA-A • *See* Vidarabine Monohydrate.

VIRAFERON (Rx) • Approved in the United Kingdom for the treatment of hepatitis C and expected on the United States market soon. *See* Interferon Alfa-2a and Alfa-2b.

VIRAZOLE • *See* Ribavirin.

VIREND • A topical treatment for herpes (*see*) being developed by Shaman Pharmaceuticals, a small company that develops drugs from tropical plants. It is expected, if all goes well, to be on the market in 1996.

VIRIDIUM • *See* Phenazopyridine Hydrochloride.

VIRILON • *See* Methyltestosterone.

VIROPTIC • *See* Trifluridine.

VIRUS • An extremely small structure that has genes and a protein coat, but cannot reproduce by itself. Viruses cannot be seen by standard optical microscopes; they are only visible by using electron microscopes. To reproduce, a virus must enter a cell and use parts of that cell to grow. Viruses can be used to carry genes from one cell to another.

VISCOAT • *See* Chondroitin and Hyaluronate.

VISCOSITY • The thickness of fluids that determines the degree of friction between molecules as they slide by each other.

VISCULOSE • *See* Artificial Tears.

VISINE • *See* Tetrahydrozoline.

VISINE EXTRA EYE DROPS (OTC) • *See* Polyethylene Glycol.

VISKEN • *See* Pindolol.

VISNAGA (H) • *Ammi visnaga.* An erect annual native to the Middle East but cultivated in Europe and South America, its extracts, particularly khellin, are used by herbalists to relieve pain in the urinary tract. It has also been used to treat whooping cough, asthma, and bronchitis. Natural preparations of visnaga have been partly replaced by synthetic khellin, which is used in the treatment of bronchial asthma and angina (*see*). Used in homeopathic medicine, natural khellin dilates blood vessels. Generally nontoxic, but khellin may produce nausea, headache, and insomnia. Khellin accumulates in the body, and visnaga, therefore, should not be used over a long time.

VISTAJECT-25 • *See* Hydroxyzine.

VISTAQUEL • *See* Hydroxyzine.

VISTARIL • *See* Hydroxyzine.

VISTAZINE • *See* Hydroxyzine.

VISTIDE • *See* Cidofovir.

VITA-C CRYSTALS • *See* Vitamin C.

VITACARN • *See* Levocarnitine.

VITACON • *See* Hydroxyzine.

VITAL FORCE • A term used in homeopathy to describe the energy that animates all living things.

VITAMIN A (OTC) • **Acetate and Palmitate. Acon. Aquasol. Oleovitamin A. Retinol. Super D Perles.** A yellow, viscous liquid, insoluble in water. An anti-infective, antixerophthalmic vitamin, essential to growth and development. Deficiency leads to retarded growth in the young, diminished visual acuity, night blindness, and skin problems. Toxic when children or adults receive more than 100,000 units daily over several months. Recommended daily dietary allowance is 1,500 units for infants, 2,000–3,500 units for children, and 4,500 units for adults. Current research seems to indicate that doses of 5,000 units of vitamin A may increase resistance to infection in children and may also help prevent cancers of the lining of organs. Vitamin A is used in lubricating creams and oils for its alleged skin-healing properties. Can be absorbed through the skin. *See* Retinoids, Retin-A, and Xerophthalmia.

VITAMIN A ACID • *See* Tretinoin.

VITAMIN B₁ • *See* Thiamin Hydrochloride.

VITAMIN B₂ • **Riboflavin. Lactoflavin. Riobin.** Formerly called vitamin G. Riboflavin is a factor in the vitamin B complex and is used in emollients. Every plant and animal cell contains a minute amount. Helps to metabolize protein, carbohydrate, and fat, maintains healthy skin and eyes, and aids in the formation of red blood cells and antibodies. Symptoms of deficiency include lesions at the corner of the mouth or cracking around the mouth, skin problems, and eye disorders such as changes in the cornea. It is necessary for respiration, protects the eyes from sensitivity to light, and is used for building and maintaining human body tissues. Recommended daily allowances are: for infants from birth to six months, 0.4 mg; children one to three years, 0.8 mg; four to six years, 1.1 mg; seven to ten years, 1.2 mg; males eleven to fourteen years, 1.5 mg; fifteen to eighteen years, 1.8 mg; nineteen to fifty years, 1.7 mg; fifty-one years and over, 1.4 mg; females eleven to fifty years, 1.3 mg; fifty-one years and over, 1.4 mg; pregnant women, 1.6 mg; lactatimg women, 1.7–1.8 mg. B₂ is used to treat riboflavin deficiency or as an adjunct (*see*) to thiamin treatment for nerve inflammation of lips due to pellagra. In 1992, the FDA proposed a ban on riboflavin in oral menstrual drug products because it had not been shown to be safe and effective as claimed.

VITAMIN B₃ • *See* Niacin.

VITAMIN B₅ • *See* Pantothenic Acid.

VITAMIN B₆ (OTC) • **Pyridoxine Hydrochloride. Beesix. Hexa-Betalin. Hexacrest. Nestrex. Rodex 5. Vitabee 6.** Metabolizes protein, helps produce red blood cells, and maintains proper functioning of nervous system tissue. Vitamin B₆ is believed to act as a partner for more than one hundred different enzymes. A number of the brain chemicals that send messages back and forth between nerves depend upon it for their formation. Vitamin B₆ also reportedly helps rid the body tissues of excess fluid that causes some of the symptoms of premenstrual tension. A deficiency in this vitamin is known to cause depression and mental confusion. The occurrence of seizures in experimental animals in response to vitamin B₆ antagonists has been observed by many. Similar seizures were observed in human infants who were made vitamin B₆ deficient inadvertently when they were fed a commercial infant formula in which the vitamin had not been properly preserved. Certain substances that deplete vitamin B₆ also produce deficiency seizures. Estrogen and cortisone deplete B₆. Storage over a long period of time diminishes the vitamin. Recommended daily allowances are: for newborns and infants to six months, 0.3 mg; children four to six years, 1.1 mg; seven to ten years, 1.4 mg; males eleven to fourteen years, 1.7 mg; fifteen years and over, 2 mg; females eleven to fourteen years, 1.4 mg; fifteen to eighteen years, 1.5 mg;

nineteen years and over, 1.6 mg; pregnant women, 2.2 mg; lactating women, 2.1 mg. Used to treat vitamin B$_6$ deficiency and responsive anemias; also prevents vitamin B$_6$ deficiency during isoniazid (*see*) therapy. Patients are likely to have a deficiency of B$_6$ if they are alcoholics or have burns, diarrhea, heart disease, intestinal problems, liver disease, overactive thyroid, or are suffering the stress of long-term illness or serious injury. Patients on dialysis or who have had their stomachs removed are also probably deficient in the vitamin. Current research seems to indicate that B$_6$ enhances the immune response in the elderly and may alleviate some signs of carpal tunnel (*see*) syndrome. Overdosing on B$_6$ is unwise. A study reported in the *New England Journal of Medicine* in 1983 described the loss of balance and numbness suffered by seven young adults who took from two to six grams of B$_6$ for several months to a year. Other potential adverse reactions include drowsiness and a feeling of pins and needles in limbs. In 1992, the FDA proposed a ban on B$_6$ in fever blister and cold sore treatment products because it had not been shown to be safe and effective as claimed.

VITAMIN B$_9$ • *See* Folic Acid.

VITAMIN B$_{12}$ (OTC)• Cyanocobalamin. Hydroxocobalamin. Alpha-Ruvite. Anacobin. Bedoce. Betalin 12. Bioglan B$_{12}$. Codroxomin. Crystamine. Cyano-Gel. Dodex. Droxomin. Kaybovite. Poyamin. Redisol. Rubesol-1000. Rubramin. Sigamine. Helps form red blood cells and maintains healthy nervous system. Deficiency symptoms include anemia, brain damage, and nervousness. More than one in five older Americans may need to take vitamin B$_{12}$, according to a Tufts University study, to prevent neurological disorders and senility. These people no longer secrete enough stomach acid to absorb the vitamin from foods. The condition, known as atrophic gastritis, affects at least 20 percent of people over the age of sixty. Recommended daily allowances are: neonates and infants to six months, 0.3 mcg; infants six months to one year, 0.5 mcg; children one to three years, 0.7 mcg; four to six years, 1 mcg; adults (both men and women), and children eleven years and over, 2

mcg; pregnant women, 2.2 mcg; lactating women, 2.6 mcg. Potential adverse reactions include blood clots in veins, transient diarrhea, itching, hives, and severe allergic reactions with IV or injection. Aminoglycosides, colchicine, paraminosalicylic acid, and chloramphenicol (*see all*) cause malabsorption of vitamin B$_{12}$.

VITAMIN B COMPLEX FACTOR • *See* Panthenol.

VITAMIN C • Ascorbic Acid. Ascorbicap. Cebid Timecelles. Cetane. Cevalin. Cevi-Bid. Dull-C. Ferancee Chewable Tablets. Fero-Grad 500. Flavorcee. Hemaspan FA. Solucap C. Vita-C Crystals. Helps to form connective-tissue collagen, promotes wound healing, keeps blood vessels strong, and enhances iron absorption. Deficiencies may cause bleeding gums, easy bruising, slow-healing wounds, painfully swollen joints, and impaired digestion. Recommended daily allowances are: for newborns and infants to six months, 30 mg; infants six months to one year, 35 mg; children one to three years, 40 mg; four to ten years, 45 mg; eleven to fourteen years, 50 mg; fifteen years and over, and adults, 60 mg. Vitamin C is used to prevent scurvy, in extensive burns, for wound healing, postoperative wound healing, severe fever, and chronic disease states; also used to prevent vitamin C deficiency in those with poor diet or increased requirement. Current research seems to indicate that vitamin C may reduce the risk of cancers of mouth, esophagus, and stomach, may reduce the risk of cataracts, protect lungs against pollutants, and ease common colds. Higher intakes are associated with higher beneficial high-density cholesterol levels and lower blood pressure. Nobel laureate Linus Pauling caused a run on vitamin C in 1970 by endorsing it as a cold medicine. Although his theories were not widely accepted by the medical community, a great deal of work is now in progress studying vitamin C and immunity. Vitamin C is known to affect the excretion of medications such as barbiturates, and to make them more toxic. Pharmaceutically incompatible with sodium salicylate, sodium nitrate, theobromine, and methenamine. Potential adverse reactions include faintness or dizziness with fast IV administration, diarrhea, heartburn, acid urine, and kidney stones or failure. *See* Ascorbic Acid.

VITAMIN D (OTC) • Calciferol. Calderol. Cholecalciferol. Delta-D. Drisdol. Ergocalciferol. Juper D Perles. Radiostol Forte. Vitamin D$_3$. A pale yellow, oily liquid, odorless, tasteless, insoluble in water. A nutritional factor added to prepared foods. Vitamin D speeds the body's production of calcium and has been found to cause calcium deposits, facial deformities, and subnormal IQs in children of mothers given too much vitamin D. Nutritionists recommend 400 units per day for pregnant women. Some women taking vitamin pills and vitamin-enriched milk and foods consume as much as 2,000–3,000 units daily. Recommended daily allowances for cholecalciferol are: for newborns and infants to six months, 300 IU; infants six months to adults (both male and female) twenty-four years and over, 200 IU; pregnant or lactating women, 400 IU. Used for its alleged skin-healing properties in lubricating creams and lotions. The absence of vitamin D in the food of young animals can lead to rickets, a bone-affecting condition. The vitamin is soluble in fats and fat solvents and is present in animal fats. Absorbed through the skin. Vitamin D$_3$ is used to treat rickets and other vitamin D deficiency diseases; also in the treatment and management of metabolic bone disease associated with chronic renal failure. Potential adverse reactions include vitamin D intoxication, headache, sleepiness, conjunctivitis, photosensitivity, runny nose, nausea, vomiting, constipation, metallic taste, dry mouth, loss of appetite, diarrhea, frequent urination, weakness, and bone and muscle aches. Cholestyramine may impair absorption. Contraindicated in high blood calcium or vitamin D toxicity. Should be used cautiously in patients on digitalis because high levels of calcium may precipitate irregular heartbeat. Mineral oil and cholestyramine resin inhibit the absorption of oral vitamin D. Vitamin D should not be taken in prescription or over-the-counter products without checking first with a physician. Patients taking vitamin D should restrict their intake of magnesium-containing antacids.

VITAMIN E (OTC) • Tocopherols. Alpha Tocopheryl Acetate. Aquasol E. Eprolin. Pertropin Solucap E. Tocopher. Tocophersolan. An antioxidant vitamin that prevents cell-membrane damage, protects red blood cells, and aids in tissue-growth repair. Protects fat in the body's tissues from abnormal breakdown. Experimental evidence shows vitamin E may protect the heart and blood vessels and retard aging. Used as a dietary supplement and as an antioxidant for essential oils, rendered animal fats, or a combination of such fats with vegetable oils. Helps form normal red blood cells, muscle, and other tissues. Recommended daily allowances are: for newborns to six months, 4 IU; infants from six months to one year, 6 IU; children from one to three years, 9 IU; four to ten years, 10 IU; males and females eleven years and over, 12 IU; pregnant women, 15 IU; lactating women, 16 to 18 IU. Vitamin E is used to treat premature infants and patients with impaired fat absorption. Current research indicates that vitamin E may lower risk of cardiovascular diseases (hardening of the arteries, angina, heart attack, and stroke) by reducing oxidation of harmful LDL cholesterol, inhibiting platelet (*see*) activity, and preventing blood clots. Also may enhance immune response in the elderly, prevent toxicity of some drugs, and cut the risk of cancer and cataracts. Mineral oil and cholestyramine resin inhibit GI absorption of oral vitamin E. Harmful effects are rare, but prolonged used of more than 250 mg daily may lead to nausea, abdominal pain, vomiting, and diarrhea. Large doses also may reduce the amounts of vitamins A, D, and K absorbed from the intestines.

VITAMIN G • *See* Riboflavin and Vitamin B$_2$.

VITAMIN H • *See* Biotin.

VITAMIN K (Rx) (OTC) • Recommended daily allowance for adults has not been established, but the safe and adequate daily dietary intake is listed at 0.07 to 0.14 mg. Vitamin K is necessary for blood clotting. Current research seems to indicate that it helps maintain bone mass in the elderly and prevents osteoporosis (*see*). Vitamin K antagonizes the action of anticoagulants and has been used as an antidote in managing overdosages and excessive responses to the latter. The excessive use of vitamin K–containing substances—drugs or dietary items such as green leafy vegetables—should be avoided in patients receiving anticoagulants. *See also* Menadione and Phytonadione.

VITAMIN K₁ • *See* Phytonadione.

VITAMIN K₄ • *See* Menadiol.

VITEX • *See* Chaste Berries.

VITILIGO • **Leukoderma.** Irregular white patches of skin; sometimes, streaks of white or gray hair due to lack of pigment. Usually, there is a family tendency to develop this condition. The white patches are most noticeable when surrounded by deeply tanned skin. It is not a systemic but merely a cosmetic condition.

VIVACTIL • *See* Protriptyline.

VIVARIN (OTC) • A stimulant that contains 200 mg of caffeine (*see*), about the same as two cups of coffee. Use of coffee and other caffeine-containing substances should be limited while taking this medication. Overuse of caffeine may cause nervousness, irritability, sleeplessness, and occasionally, rapid heartbeat. Contraindicated in children under twelve years of age. Vivarin may counteract drugs used to treat heart and blood-vessel ailments, psychological problems, and kidney dysfunction.

VIVELLE (Rx) • An estrogen skin patch introduced in 1995 for the treatment of moderate-to-severe menopausal symptoms. It delivers 17-beta estradiol, the primary estrogen produced by the ovaries, through the skin directly into the bloodstream. The patch comes in four dosages, and a new patch is applied twice weekly. *See* Estradiol.

V-LAX • *See* Psyllium.

VLB • *See* Vinblastine Sulfate.

VM-26 • *See* Teniposide.

VOLATILE OILS • Volatility in oils refers to the tendency to give off vapors, usually at room temperature. The volatile oils in plants such as peppermint or rose produce the aroma. The volatile oils in plants stimulate the tissue with which they come into contact, whether they are inhaled, ingested, or placed on the skin. They can relax or stimulate, irritate or soothe, depending upon their sources and concentrations.

VOLTAREN • *See* Diclofenac Sodium.

VOMITING MEDICATION • *See* Antiemetic.

VOSOL OTIC • *See* Acetic Acid.

VP-16 • *See* Etoposide.

VULNERARY • A substance, usually an herb preparation, applied to wounds to aid healing. Aloe vera and marshmallow root are examples of herbs used for this purpose.

VULVA • External female sex apparatus including the mons pubis, the labia majora and minora, the clitoris, and the opening of the vagina and urethra.

VULVAN • A testosterone (*see*) ointment to treat vulvar dystrophy. Expected to be approved by the FDA.

VULVOVAGINITIS • Inflammation of both the vulva and vagina.

VUMON • *See* Teniposide.

V.V.S. • *See* Sulfabenzamide, Sulfacetamide, and Sulfathiazole.

VX-710 (RX) • A drug produced by Vertex being introduced in the United States to treat multidrug-resistant solid tumors.

VYTONE (Rx) • *See* Iodoquinol and Hydrocortisone.

W

WAHOO • *See* Quassia.

WALL GERMANDER • *See* Germander.

WALNUT, BLACK (H) • *Juglans nigra.* The fruit is used by herbalists to promote strength and weight gain, and to treat skin diseases, including eczema, herpes, and psoriasis. The bark is used to treat constipation. In a six-year study funded by the California Walnut Commission, it was found that frequent consumption of walnuts was associated with a reduced risk of ischemic (insufficient blood supply) heart disease.

WANS (Rx) • *See* Pentobarbital and Pyrilamine.

WARFARIN (Rx) • **Carfin. Coumadin. Panwarfin. Sofarin. Warfilone.** An anticoagulant introduced in 1941 that inhibits vitamin K–dependent activation of clotting factors formed in the liver. Used to treat blood clots to the lung, and in the prevention and treatment of deep-vein blood clots, heart attack, rheumatic heart disease with heart-valve damage, and irregular heartbeat. A combination of warfarin and aspirin is being tested to prevent heart attacks. Warfarin has a narrow margin of safety. Potential adverse reactions include hemorrhage, a drop in white blood cells, intestinal obstruction, diarrhea, vomiting, cramps, nausea, excessive uterine bleeding, rash, hives, loss of hair, and fever. Aspirin and acetaminophen increase bleeding if warfarin is taken over a long period. Also increasing the bleeding potential if taken with warfarin are allopurinol, amiodarone, chloramphenicol, clofibrate, diflunisal, thyroid drugs, heparin, anabolic steroids, cimetidine, disulfiram, glucagon, inhalation anesthetics, metronidazole, quinidine, ethacrynic acid, indomethacin, mefenamic acid, oxyphenbutazone, phenylbutazone, salicylates, influenza vaccine, sulindac, sulfinpyrazone, sulfonamides, and tricyclic antidepressants (*see all*). Cholestyramine, griseofulvin, haloperidol decanoate or lactate, ethchlorvynol, carbamazepine, and rifampin (*see all*) decrease the effectiveness of warfarin. Warfarin is contraindicated in hemophilia, leukemia, open wounds or ulcers, impaired liver or kidney function, severe high blood pressure, and infection of the heart. If you are taking this drug, you should shave with an electric razor and use a soft toothbrush to avoid causing bleeding. Eating leafy green foods high in vitamin K such as broccoli, lettuce, cabbage, and spinach tends to neutralize the effectiveness of warfarin. Eating varying amounts of these vegetables may make the effects of this medication unpredictable. Warfarin should be taken on an empty stomach.

WART OFF • *See* Salicylic Acid.

WARTS • Harmless, small growths on the skin.

WASTING SYNDROME • Any number of conditions, such as anorexia and cachexia (*see both*), that cause loss of body mass, notably protein.

WATER LILY (H) • *Nymphaea alba.* **Candock. Nenuphar. Water Rose.** Cultivated in pools, this beautiful and romantic flower was used in folk medicine to depress sexual function. White and yellow water lilies were used externally to treat various skin disorders such as boils, inflammation, tumors, and ulcers. An overdose can cause adverse effects on the heart.

WBC • Abbreviation for white blood count. If the count is high, infection is suspected.

WEHAMINE • *See* Dimenhydrinate.

WEHLESS • *See* Phenazopyridine Hydrochloride.

WEIGHTROL • *See* Phendimetrazine.

WELEDA AVENA SATIVA (H) • A homeopathic remedy. *See* Oat Fiber.

WELEDA BIDOR (H) • A homeopathic medicine to treat headaches. Contains ferrum sulfa. *See* Iron and Sulfa.

WELEDA PHOSPHORICUM (H) • A homeopathic medicine. *See* Phosphorus.

WELLBUTRIN • *See* Bupropion Hydrochloride.

WELLCOVORIN • *See* Leucovorin.

WESTCORT • *See* Hydrocortisone.

WESTHROID • *See* Thyroid.

WESTRIM LA • *See* Phenylpropanolamine.

WHEALS • *See* Hives.

WHEAT GERM (H) • The golden germ of the wheat, about 2.5 percent of the whole wheat kernel, is high in vitamin E. The germ contains thiamin, riboflavin, and pyridoxine. *See* Tocopherols.

WHEY • The serum that remains after removal of fat and casein from cow's milk. Casein is the principal protein of cow's milk.

WHITE BRYONY • *Bryonia dioica*. A slender herb native to Europe and western Asia and cultivated in moderate zones. Its root is used in homeopathic medicine as a laxative and to treat respiratory ailments, arthritis, and sciatica. In large doses, it can cause bloody diarrhea, and in severe cases respiratory paralysis. Long-term use may lead to kidney dysfunction and to miscarriage.

WHITE COHOSH (H) • *Actaea alba*. A perennial herb native to North America. Its root contains glycosides (*see*). Herbalists use it as a sedative in cases of painful menstruation. It is used in homeopathic medicine to treat arthritis and externally to treat skin inflammation. It is toxic, and an overdose may cause bloody diarrhea, severe vomiting, and hallucinations.

WHITE HELLEBORE (H) • *Veratrum album*. A perennial native to the mountainous regions in Europe and northern Asia. Its rhizome contains alkaloids (*see*). It has been used in homeopathic medicine against scabies and lice and to lower blood pressure and increase sweating. It is highly toxic and is rarely used. *See* Hellebore.

WHITE HOREHOUND • *See* Horehound.

WHITE MINERAL OIL • *See* Mineral Oil.

WHITE PETROLATUM (OTC) • **Caldesene Medicated Ointment. Chapstick Petroleum Jelly Plus. Duolube Eye Ointment. Lacri-Lube NP Lubricant Ophthalmic Ointment. Refresh P.M. Lubricant Ophthalmic Ointment.** A semisolid or liquid mixture of hydrocarbons derived from petroleum. Its chief uses are in mild ointments and eye lubricants. Also used as a laxative.

WHITE POPLAR (H) • *Populus tremuloides* or *P. alba*. The bark of this tree contains glycosides, flavonoids, essential oil, and tannin (*see all*). It is used by herbalists to treat arthritis in which there is much pain and swelling, and to treat colds, fever, cystitis, and diarrhea. Also used to stimulate digestion, particularly where there is a loss of appetite.

WHITE TEA TREE • *See* Cajuput.

WHITE WILLOW BARK (H) • *Salix alba*. The original source of salicin, the forerunner of aspirin. There are more than 130 species of willow, most of them in Europe and North America. White willow bark is mentioned in ancient Egyptian, Assyrian, and Greek literature and was used to combat pain and fever by Galen, Hippocrates, and Dioscorides. Many Native American tribes used it for headache relief, fever, sore muscles, arthritis, and chills. In the mid-1700s, it was used to treat malaria. In the 1800s, salicylic acid was derived from white willow bark, which then led to development of the product we call aspirin. Aspirin was shown to be effective against rheumatic fever, general pain, arthritis, gout, and neuralgia. White willow bark is converted through oxidation to salicylic acid within the body.

WHITFIELD'S OINTMENT (OTC) • Used to treat ringworm of the scalp and athlete's foot. *See* Benzoic Acid and Salicylic Acid.

WHOOPING COUGH • *See* Pertussis.

WIGRAINE • *See* Ergotamine Tartrate.

WIGRETTES • *See* Ergotamine Tartrate.

WILD CARROT (H) • *Daucus carota.* **Lace Flower. Queen Anne's Lace.** This Eurasian herb contains volatile oil and alkaloid (*see both*). Wild carrot is used as a urinary antiseptic by herbalists in the treatment of cystitis and prostatitis. It is also used in the treatment of gout and arthritis. The seeds are used to relieve intestinal gas and colic. Reputed to be effective in breaking up kidney stones.

WILD CHAMOMILE EXTRACT • *See* Matricaria Extract and Oil.

WILD CHERRY (H) • *Prunis serotina. Prunis virginiana.* **Choke Cherry. Wild Black Cherry Bark.** The dried stem bark collected in autumn in North America. Used in cherry flavorings for medicines. Also used medicinally as a sedative and expectorant. It is soothing to the mucous membranes and is widely used in over-the-counter cough medicines. Wild cherry contains hydrocyanic acid and benzaldehyde (*see both*). The American Indians and early settlers were aware that the bark is effective in calming coughs. Wild cherry is still included in the USP (*see*).

WILD GERANIUM • *See* Cranesbill Root.

WILD GINGER (H) • *Asarum heterotropoides. A. canadense.* **Xi Xin.** The root is used by Chinese herbalists to treat menstrual problems and congestion in the lungs and nose. Its warm, pungent action relieves spasms. The American wild ginger is not as strong as the Chinese wild ginger, which can be mildly toxic.

WILD INDIGO (H) • *Baptisia tinctoria.* The root contains alkaloids, glycosides, and resin (*see all*). It is used by herbalists to treat infections of the ear, nose, and throat. Taken both internally and as a mouthwash, it reputedly heals mouth ulcers and sore gums and helps to control pyorrhea. Internally, it is used by herbalists to aid in reducing fevers, constipation, and swollen glands. Externally, in an ointment, it is used to treat infected ulcers and soothe sore nipples. Used in a douche, herbalists say it helps relieve vaginal discharge. Toxic in large doses, it can cause severe diarrhea and violent vomiting and may affect the heart.

WILD LETTUCE (H) • *Lacuca virosa. L. elongata.* **Lettuce Opium.** The dried leaves contain latex, alkaloids, and terpenes (*see all*). It is used by herbalists to treat insomnia, restlessness, and anxiety, especially in children. Also used to treat coughs, colic pains, and painful menstruation, and reputedly eases arthritic pain.

WILD PANSY • *See* Pansy, Wild.

WILD ROSEMARY • *See* Labrador Tea Extract.

WILD THYME (H) • *Thymus vulgaris.* The flowering tops of the plant grown in Eurasia and throughout the United States. The dried leaves are used in emollients and fragrances and as a seasoning in foods. Thyme has also been used as a muscle relaxant.

WILD YAM ROOT (H) • *Dioscorea mexicana. Dioscorea paniculata.* **Chinese Yam. Colicroot. Rheumatism Root.** Japanese researchers in 1936 discovered glycoside saponins of several Mexican yam species from which steroid saponin (*see*), primarily diosgenin, could be derived. These derivatives were then converted to progesterone, an intermediate in cortisone production. Steroid drugs derived from diosgenin include corticosteroids, oral contraceptives, androgens, and estrogens. For more than two centuries, American herbalists used wild yam roots to treat painful menstruation, ovarian pain, cramps, and problems of childbirth. Wild yam root has also been used to treat gallbladder pain and ease the passage of gallstones. Wild yam root can also reputedly lower blood cholesterol and blood pressure. The most widely prescribed birth control pill in the world, Desogen (*see*), is made from the wild yam, confirming what the ancient Mexican women knew all along. They used wild yam as a contraceptive. Long-term use may cool libido. Contraindicated in pregnancy and kidney impairment.

WILLOW BARK • *See* Salicin.

WILLOW LEAF EXTRACT (H) • The extract of the leaves of the willow tree species, genus *Salix*. The willow has been used for pain-relieving and fever-lowering properties since ancient Greece. The American Indians used willow baths to cool fevers, and indeed, the extract of willow contains salicylic acid, a close cousin of aspirin. *See* White Willow Bark.

WILMS'S TUMOR • A malignant tumor of the kidney occurring in children.

WILPOWR • *See* Phentermine.

WINCILLIN-VK • *See* Penicillin V.

WINGEL LIQUID • *See* Aluminum Hydroxide and Magnesium Hydroxide.

WINSTROL • *See* Stanozolol.

WINTERGREEN OIL (H) • *Gaultheria procumbens.* **Checkerberry Extract. Deerberry. Extract and Oil. Methyl Salicylate Extract. Spiceberry. Teaberry.** Obtained naturally from betula, sweet birch, or teaberry oil. Present in certain leaves and bark, but usually prepared by treating salicylic acid with menthol (*see both*). Wintergreen extract is used in root-beer and wintergreen flavorings. Wintergreen oil is an old remedy for rheumatism and rheumatic fever, sciatica, edema, diabetes, bladder disorders, and skin diseases. It contains methyl salicylate (*see*). It is still used for eye lotions, gargles, poultices, antiseptic washes, toothpastes, tooth powders, and perfumes, and in small amounts by herbalists as a diuretic. Large doses cause vomiting. Wintergreen is a strong irritant. Ingestion of relatively small amounts may cause severe poisoning and death. Average lethal dose in children is 10 ml and in adults, 30 ml. It is irritating to the mucous membranes and skin and can be absorbed rapidly through the skin. As with other salicylates, it has a wide range of interaction with other drugs, including alcohol, antidiabetic medications, vitamin C, and tranquilizers. *See also* Periwinkle.

WINTOMYLON • *See* Nalidixic Acid.

WITCH HAZEL (OTC) (H) • *Hamamelis virginiana.* **Hamamelis Water. Tucks Cream. Tucks Premoistened Pads.** A shrub native to eastern states of North America, it grows in damp woods. Both the leaves and bark are astringent, tonic, and sedative. They contain a high level of tannins (*see*). (The commercial product does not contain tannins.) Witch hazel is a soothing, mildly astringent agent used to alleviate irritated skin. It can stop minor bleeding. Internal use is unwise. The oil of this plant contains safrole, a known carcinogen in animals.

WITHANIA (H) • *Withania somnifera.* An herbaceous undershrub native to the Mediterranean region, Africa, Pakistan, and India. The root is used in folk medicine to treat lung and stomach ailments and arthritis. It is also used to treat insomnia. In combination with other plants, it is used in India to treat trigeminal neuralgia (*see*). It is used in eastern Africa as an aphrodisiac. All parts of the plant are toxic.

WITHDRAWAL SYMPTOMS • Physical and mental effects resulting from the withdrawal of addictive substances in patients who have become habituated or addicted to them. The physical symptoms may include vomiting, tremors, abdominal pain, delirium, and convulsions.

WOAD (H) • *Isatis tinctoria.* A biennial widely distributed in Europe, Asia, and North Africa, it is a member of the mustard family. The plant is used to treat St. Anthony's fire (gangrene and inflammation) and for plasters and ointments used to treat ulcers and inflammation.

WOLFINA • *See* Rauwolfia.

WOLF'S-BANE • *See* Aconite and Monkshood.

WOOD BETONY (H) • *Stachys officinalis.* **Betony. Lousewort.** A common herb of eastern North America and the British Isles, it has been used for centuries to treat diarrhea, and as an astringent and sedative. An ingredient in wood betony has been found to be active against tuberculosis. Wood betony has been used by herbalists to treat heartburn, gout, nervousness, cough, bladder and kidney stones, asthma, and fatigue. Also is reputedly good for chronic headaches. The root is both emetic and purgative. The leaves contain mild laxative and astringent agents. A tea brewed from the plant is used in the treatment of stomach disorders.

WOODRUFF (OTC) (H) • *Asperula odorata.* A perennial native to Europe, Asia, and North Africa, it is cultivated in the United States. Woodruff was used in the Middle Ages as a drink for jaundice and liver complaints. Its leaves were laid on open wounds. It was combined with other herbs as a cure for bladder problems, and as a tonic for nervous conditions. Also combined with other herbs in a tea used to treat migraine headache. In 1992, the FDA issued a notice that woodruff had not been shown to be safe and effective as claimed in OTC digestive-aid products. It may cause bleeding.

WOOD SORREL (H) • *Oxalis acetosella.* A delicate perennial, it contains oxalic acid (*see*) and mucilage. A salad of its leaves is eaten as a spring tonic in Europe. In homeopathic medicine, it is used to treat liver and gastrointestinal disorders. It is toxic when ingested in large doses and can cause severe stomach irritation and hemorrhage. Contraindicated in patients predisposed to gout, arthritis, or kidney stones, because oxalic acid can aggravate these conditions. *See* Sorrel Extract.

WOOD SUGAR • *See* D-Xylose.

WORMGRASS • *See* Spigelia.

WORMSEED • *See* Epazote.

WORMWOOD (H) • *Artemisia absinthium.* **Absinthe.** A perennial herb native to the Ural Mountains, taken to Egypt early in recorded history, and listed in Ebers Papyrus as useful for treating headaches and to eliminate pinworm, two uses still prescribed by herbalists. Because it was used to expel tapeworm and other intestinal worms, it was called wormwood. In Europe and North America, it was believed to counteract poi-son. It was recommended for insomnia, jaundice, indigestion, sprains, bruises, and inflammation. Herbalists today recommend an infusion of the leaves and stems to stimulate appetite and soothe stomach pain. In large and/or repeated doses, it is a narcotic poison, causing headache, trembling, and convulsions. Ingestion of the volatile oil or of the liquor absinthe, distilled from wormwood, may cause gastrointestinal symptoms, nervousness, stupor, coma, and death. The use of absinthe is banned in many nations.

WOUNDWORT (H) • *Stachys palustris.* **All-Heal. Clown's Wort. Donkey's Ear. Hedge Dead Nettle.** There are many varieties of woundwort, but all have the same medical action. The leaves of the downy woundwort have been used instead of lint as surgical dressing. They were believed to have a special power in healing the wounds caused by sword thrusts. Woundwort was used by English herbalists for many years to stop bleeding of the lungs and other internal hemorrhages, and to treat severe forms of diarrhea. They claimed that almost any cut or wound would benefit if the newly gathered and washed woundwort leaves were bound to the injury.

WYAMINE • *See* Mephentermine Sulfate.

WYAMYCIN S • *See* Erythromycin.

WYANOIDS (Rx) • A combination of belladonna, ephedrine, bismuth, boric acid, and Peruvian balsam (*see all*), used to relieve symptoms caused by hemorrhoids.

WYCILLIN • *See* Penicillin G.

WYDASE • *See* Hyaluronidase.

WYGESIC (Rx) • *See* Acetaminophen and Propoxyphene.

WYMOX • *See* Amoxicillin.

WYTENSIN • *See* Guanabenz.

X

XANAX • *See* Alprazolam.

XANTH-, XANTHO- • Prefixes for yellow, derived from the Greek word *xanthos,* meaning yellow.

XANTHENE • Colorants are divided into acid and basic groups. Xanthenes are the second-largest category of certified (*see*) coal tar colors. The acids are derived from fluorescein. The quinoid-acid type is represented by FD&C Red No. 3, erythrosine. The phenolic formulations, often called bromo acids, are represented by D&C Red No. 2. The only basic type certified is D&C Red No. 19, also called rhodamine B. Xanthene derivatives are also used as fungicides.

XANTHINE • Occurs in animal organs, blood, urine, yeast, potatoes, coffee beans, and tea. First isolated from gallstones. Xanthines are found in chocolate, coffee, tea, and many drugs such as aminophyllin and caffeine (*see both*). They stimulate the brain, heart, and muscles. They act as diuretics to reduce body fluid and also dilate the heart's blood vessels.

XANTHOMA • A yellowish tumor or slightly raised yellow-colored patch in the skin.

XANTHOMATOSIS • A generalized condition with many deposits of yellowish fatty material in tissues due to abnormal cholesterol and fat metabolism.

XANTHOSIS • A yellowish discoloration of the skin due to eating excessive amounts of carrots or other yellow vegetables, or beta-carotene pills.

XANTHOXYLUM • *See* Zanthoxylum.

XENOTRANSPLANT • Organ transplant between species, for example from pig to human.

XERAC BP-5 • *See* Benzoyl Peroxide.

XERO- • Prefix from the Greek word *xeros,* meaning dry.

XERODERMA • Dry skin.

XERO-LUBE • A saliva substitute.

XEROPHTHALMIA • Dry eyes. Lack of tears may cause infection.

XEROSTOMIA • Dry mouth. Lack of enough saliva.

XI XIN • *See* Wild Ginger.

X-OTAG • *See* Orphenadrine.

X-PREP • *See* Senna.

X-SEB • *See* Salicylic Acid.

X-SEB SHAMPOO • *See* Pyrithione Zinc.

X-SEB T • *See* Coal Tar.

X-SEB T SHAMPOO • *See* Coal Tar, Salicylic Acid, and Ethyl Alcohol.

XYLITOL (OTC) (H) • A sweetener formerly made from birchwood, but now made from waste products of the pulp industry. Xylitol has been reported to have a diuretic effect, but this has not been substantiated. Used in chewing gum and as an artificial sweetener, it has been reported to sharply reduce the incidence of cavities in teeth. The reason is that, unlike sugar, it does not ferment in the mouth. FDA preliminary reports cited xylitol as a possible cancer-causing agent. Xylitol is now used in eleven European countries and the United States and Canada. It is also used in large amounts in the former Soviet Union as a diabetic sweetener. Xylitol was evaluated by the Joint FAO/WHO Expert Committee on Food Additives in Geneva, April 11–20, 1983. On the basis of submitted data, the committee accepted that the adverse effects observed in British studies in which cancer-prone rats were fed large doses of xylitol were species specific and could not be extrapolated to humans. Therefore, no limit on daily intake was set and no additional toxicological studies were recommended. Xylitol can cause stomach upset when taken in large amounts. It may be beneficial to diabetics since metabolism of xylitol does not involve insulin.

XYLOCAINE VISCOUS SOLUTION • *See* Lidocaine.

XYLOMETAZOLINE (OTC) • Chlorohist-LA. 4-Way Long Acting. Neo-Synephrine II. Otrivin. Sine-Off Nasal Spray. Sinex-LA. A nasal decongestant that was changed from Rx to OTC. Potential adverse reactions include rebound nasal congestion or irritation with excessive long-term use, transient burning, stinging, dryness, or ulceration of nasal mucosa, and sneezing. Contraindicated in glaucoma. Should be used cautiously in overactive thyroid, heart disease, high blood pressure, diabetes, and advanced arteriosclerosis, since systemic absorption may occur.

XYLO-PFAN • *See* D-Xylose.

Y

YAM • *See* Wild Yam Root.

YARROW (H) • *Achillea millefolium.* **Milfoil. Soldier's Woundwort.** A strong-scented, spicy, wild herb used in flavorings. Also used in shampoos. Yarrow's astringent qualities have caused it to be recommended by herbalists for greasy skin. According to old herbal recipes, it prevents baldness when used regularly to wash the hair. Used medicinally as an astringent, tonic, and stimulant. Has also been used to treat hemorrhoids, bladder dysfunction, and in weak doses to induce profuse perspiration. It is anti-inflammatory. Yarrow may cause a sensitivity to sunlight and artificial light, in which the skin breaks out and swells. Contraindicated in pregnancy and for those taking anticoagulant medications.

YEAST • A fungus that is a dietary source of folic acid (*see*). It produces enzymes that will convert sugar to alcohol and carbon dioxide.

YEAST INFECTION (VAGINAL) • This condition is caused by an organism called candida, a type of yeast. Even healthy women usually have this yeast on the skin, and in the mouth, digestive tract, and vagina. At times, the yeast can grow quickly. A yeast infection, while it can occur at almost any time of life, is most common during the childbearing years. The infection tends to develop most often in women who are pregnant, diabetic, or taking antibiotics or birth control pills. Symptoms include vaginal itching, a clumpy, white vaginal discharge, vaginal soreness, irritation, or burning, and rash or redness around the vagina.

YE JU • *See* Chrysanthemum.

YELLOW DOCK (H) • *Rumex crispus.* **Curled Dock. Out-Sting.** One of the most common wayside plants, the yellow dock flourishes on wasteland. The herb has antibacterial properties. English children use it as an antidote for nettle sting. It was once used as a primary treatment for scurvy and anemia, probably because of its high iron content. A tincture is used by herbalists to relieve coughs and sore throat. It is also recommended by herbalists for skin diseases, arthritis, piles, bleeding of the lungs, and gallbladder problems. Contains agents similar to those in cascara (*see* Cascara Sagrada). The leaves also contain oxalic acid, which can be toxic.

YELLOW FEVER • An acute, infectious, feverish disease caused by viruses transmitted by the bites of mosquitoes. The disease does not exist in the United States, but travelers to the tropics where yellow fever is endemic require vaccination.

YELLOW FEVER VACCINE (Rx) • **YF-Vax.** Injection of live, attenuated yellow fever virus provides active immunity to yellow fever. Potential adverse reactions include fever, malaise, severe allergic reaction, and mild swelling and pain at site of injection.

YELLOW MERCURIC OXIDE • *See* Mercuric Oxide.

YELLOW OLEANDER (H) • *Thevetia neriifolia.* A shrub native to tropical America and widely grown elsewhere. The seeds contain cardiac glycosides (*see*). Herbalists have used it to treat irregular heart rhythm and as a diuretic to treat edema. Externally, it has been used to treat skin parasites such as scabies and lice. The plant is poisonous.

YELLOW RHODODENDRON (H) • An evergreen shrub native to northern Russia, it is grown as an ornamental in moderate regions. It contains glycoside, arbutin, and tannins (*see all*). The Russians have used to it treat gout and urinary-tract infections. In homeopathic medicine it is used to treat urinary stones and inflammation of the prostate gland. A homeopathic concoction of this plant has reportedly caused poisoning. Symptoms include copious salivation, vomiting, diarrhea, anxiety, dizziness, and skin rash. Honey obtained from the flowers of this plant and related species is toxic, especially to children.

YELLOW ROOT • *See* Goldenseal.

YELLOW SNOWDROP • *See* Adder's-Tongue.

YERBA SANTA FLUID EXTRACT (H) • *Eriodictyon californicum.* **Bear's Weed. Consumptive's Weed. Gordolobo Yerba Tea. Gum Bush. Holy Herb. Mountain Balm.** A fruit flavoring in commercial products derived from evergreen shrubs grown in California. The American Indians smoked or chewed the leaves of this plant as a treatment for asthma. It is still used by herbalists as an expectorant to treat bronchial congestion, asthma, and hay fever. Yerba is also used by herbalists to treat chronic genitourinary-tract inflammations and to mask the bitter taste of drugs. Gordolobo yerba tea has been reported to be toxic to the liver.

YEW (H) • *Taxus baccata.* An evergreen shrub that contains cyanogenic glycosides (*see* Cyan-, Glycosides, and Tannin). Native to Europe and widely cultivated as an ornamental tree elsewhere, it has been used in folk medicine to treat arthritis, respiratory-tract ailments, and urinary problems. In homeopathic medicine, it is employed to treat arthritis, liver, and urinary ailments. Yew is highly toxic.

YF-VAX • *See* Yellow Fever Vaccine.

Y-ITCH • *See* Tetracaine.

YOCON • *See* Yohimbine.

YODOXIN • *See* Iodoquinol.

YOGURT (H) • A fermented, slightly acid, semifluid milk food made of skimmed cow's milk and milk solids to which cultures of two bacteria, *Lactobacillus acidophilus* and *Streptococcus thermophilus,* have been added. According to a report in *Annals of Internal Medicine,* researchers at Long Island Jewish Medical Center, New York, found that women who, for six months, daily ate eight ounces of yogurt containing live cultures of the bacteria *Lactobacillus acidophilus* had a threefold decrease in vaginal yeast infections. *See also* Acidophilus.

YOHIMBINE (Rx) (H) • *Corynanthe yohimbe. Pausinystalia yohimba.* **Aphrodyne. Dayto Himbin. Yocon. Yohimex.** An alkaloid found in Rubiaceae and related trees, such as the African yohimbe. Also in *Rauwolfia serpentina* (*see* Ranwolfia). Its action on blood vessels resembles that of reserpine (*see*), though it is weaker and shorter acting. Widely used in Africa as an aphrodisiac. Although it is not approved for the use, it is prescribed in the United States to increase penile blood flow. Yohimbine is also said to be a stimulant, have a mild antidiuretic effect, and to perhaps increase anxiety. Since yohimbine causes a dilation of the blood vessels, it reduces blood pressure. It is generally not proposed for use in females. Yohimbine readily penetrates the central nervous system and produces complex patterns of response. It is being tested at the University of Medicine and Dentistry of New Jersey as a drug that may help men who experience impotence or a low sex drive. Potential adverse effects of yohimbine are sweating, nausea, and vomiting after injection; dizziness, headache, and skin flushing are reported when it's taken orally. The effective dose is close to the toxic dose. Contraindicated in kidney diseases and in patients sensitive to the drug.

YOHIMEX • *See* Yohimbine.

YOMESAN • *See* Niclosamide.

YUCCA (H) • *Yucca liliaceae. Y. alorfolia.* **Spanish Bayonet.** The southwestern American Indians used this herb for hundreds of years to treat pain and inflammation of arthritis and rheumatism. Yucca can occasionally be purgative and cause some intestinal cramping. In long-term use, it may slow the absorption of fat-soluble vitamins such as A, D, E, and K.

YUMIX • *See* Corn Silk.

YUNAN BAIYAO • *See* Tienchi.

YUTOPAR • *See* Ritodrine.

Z

ZIADIN FORMULA (OTC) • A treatment for persons with moderate psoriasis (*see*). Originally formulated by an Egyptian dermatologist, the active ingredient is salicylic acid (*see*). It also contains camphor and emollients.

ZALCITABINE • DDC. HIVID. The first drug approved for marketing through an accelerated process, zalcitabine was introduced in 1992 for the treatment of AIDS in combination with zidovudine (*see*). Zalcitabine works by inhibiting or reversing the action of transcriptase, a viral enzyme that is critical to the replication cycle of the AIDS virus. It helps to increase immune cells needed to fight the infection. Prescribed for adult patients with advanced HIV infection who are failing to be helped by other drugs including AZT (*see*). Potential adverse reactions include, infrequently, pancreatitis (*see*); moderate or severe nerve damage, which for some patients was clinically disabling, occurred in 17–31 percent of patients treated with zalcitabine in a study.

ZANOSAR • *See* Streptozocin.

ZANTAC • *See* Ranitidine.

ZANTHOXYLUM (H) • **Xanthoxylum. Prickly Ash Bark. Toothache Tree.** A member of the rue (*see*) family, genus *Zanthoxylum.*The dried bark or berries of this tree, which grows in Canada and in the United States, are used to ease the pain of toothache, to soothe stomachache, and as an antidiarrheal medicine.

ZANTHOXYLUM AMERICANUM • *See* Prickly Ash Bark.

ZARONTIN • *See* Ethosuximide.

ZAROXOLYN • *See* Metolazone.

Z-BEC (OTC) • A multivitamin preparation.

ZEASORB-AF (OTC) • *See* Tolnaftate.

ZEFAZONE • *See* Cefmetazole Sodium.

ZEMO (OTC) • An anti-itch lotion containing menthol and bismuth (*see both*).

ZEMURON • *See* Rocuronium Bromide.

ZENATE (OTC) • A multivitamin and mineral preparation.

ZENDOLE • *See* Indomethacin.

ZENTINIC (OTC) • A multivitamin preparation with iron (*see*).

ZENTRON (OTC) • A multivitamin preparation with iron (*see*).

ZEPHIRAN CHLORIDE (OTC) • *See* Benzalkonium Chloride.

ZEPHREX (OTC) • *See* Pseudoephedrine and Guaifenesin.

ZERIT • *See* Stavudine.

ZEROXIN • *See* Benzoyl Peroxide.

ZESTRIL • *See* Lisinopril.

ZETAR (OTC) • *See* Coal Tar.

ZETRAN • *See* Diazepam.

ZIAC (Rx) • *See* Bisoprolol.

ZIDE • *See* Hydrochlorothiazide.

ZIDOVUDINE (Rx) • **Azidothymidine. AZT. Retrovir.** Approved in 1987 to treat patients with AIDS or advanced AIDS-related complex (ARC) who have suffered from *Pneumocystis carinii* pneumonia or a drop in white blood cells. It promotes weight gain and reduces gland swelling. It does not cure AIDS. Potential adverse reactions are severe and include bone-marrow depression, headache, agitation, restlessness, insomnia, confusion, nausea, loss of appetite, rash, itching, fever, chills, muscle pain, lethargy, and fatigue. Must be used with caution in persons with anemia or other blood problems, liver disease, and low amounts of B vitamins in the blood. Zidovudine may interact with a wide range of drugs, increasing the risk of harmful effects. These drugs include any that affect the bone marrow, such as anticancer drugs, and drugs that interfere with the breakdown and elimination of zidovudine, such as trimethoprim, sulfas, and acetaminophen (*see all*). Zidovudine is most effective when taken on an empty stomach, but may be taken with a little food if gastrointestinal upset is a problem.

ZILACTIN • *See* Tannic Acid.

ZILACTIN MEDICATED GEL • *See* Tannic Acid.

ZILADENT ORAL ANALGESIC • *See* Benzocaine.

ZINACEF • *See* Cefuroxime Axetil and Sodium.

ZINC (OTC) • **Orazinc. Sublingual Zinc. Vicon Plus. Z-Bec.** A white, brittle metal, insoluble in water, and soluble in acids or hot solutions of alkalies. A mineral source, it is added to foods as a nutrient. Also widely used as an astringent for mouthwashes. In a study by the Dartmouth College Health Service, use of a zinc lozenge resulted in a 42 percent reduction in the duration of the common cold and reduced symptoms when taken within forty-eight hours of the start of a cold. A number of zinc "cold" lozenges are expected on the market at this writing. Ingestion of zinc salts can cause nausea and vomiting. Zinc can cause contact dermatitis. Taking zinc with bran may make zinc less effective. Zinc interferes with copper absorption and if overused can lead to copper-deficiency anemia.

ZINC ACETATE (OTC) • The zinc salt of acetic acid (*see*), used in medicine as a dietary supplement. In 1992, the FDA proposed a ban on zinc acetate in diaper-rash drug products because it had not been shown to be safe and effective as claimed.

ZINCA-PAC • *See* Zinc Sulfate.

ZINCATE • *See* Zinc Sulfate.

ZINC CAPRYLATE (OTC) • A fungicide. In 1992, the FDA issued a notice that zinc caprylate had not been shown to be safe and effective as claimed in OTC products.

ZINC CARBONATE (OTC) • A crystalline salt of zinc used for coloring. In 1992, the FDA proposed a ban on zinc carbonate in diaper-rash drug products because it had not been shown to be safe and effective as claimed.

ZINC CHLORIDE (OTC) • **Orajel Mouth-Aid.** A zinc salt used as an antiseptic and astringent (*see*). It is also used to help reduce various enzymes and helps to maintain normal growth rates. Also given to improve a deficient sense of taste or smell. Odorless and water absorbing; also a deodorant and disinfectant. Can cause contact dermatitis and is mildly irritating to the skin. Can be absorbed through the skin. In 1992, the FDA proposed a ban on zinc chloride in astringent drug products because it had not been shown to be safe and effective as claimed.

ZINCFRIN (OTC) • *See* Phenylephrine and Benzalkonium Chloride.

ZINC GELATIN (OTC) • **Dome-Paste. Gelucast. Unna's Boot.** Used as a protectant and support to veins that bulge and for similar lesions of the lower limbs.

ZINC GLUCONATE (OTC) • Used as an under-the-tongue wafer to ward off colds and sore throats.

ZINC METALLICUM • Homeopathic name for zinc (*see*).

ZINCON SHAMPOO • *See* Zinc Pyrithione.

ZINC OXIDE (OTC) • **Anusol Ointment. Balmex Baby Powder. Caladryl Clear Lotion. Desitin. Extra Strength Vaseline Intensive Care Lotion. Lassar's Zinc Paste. Nupercainal Suppositories. Pazo Hemorrhoid Ointment.**

Tronolane Hemorrhoidal Suppositories. Zinc oxide, an agent included in sunscreens, aids in skin preparations for painful and itchy conditions such as ulcers, blisters, diaper rash, and hemorrhoids. In 1992, the FDA proposed a ban for the use of zinc oxide to treat insect bites and stings because it had not been shown to be safe and effective as claimed in OTC products, including in astringent (*see*) drug products. *See* Zinc.

ZINC PROPIONATE (OTC) • Derived from propionic acid, it is used as a topical antifungal. In 1992, the FDA issued a notice that zinc propionate had not been shown to be safe and effective as claimed in OTC products.

ZINC PYRITHIONE (OTC) • **Zincon Shampoo.** An antifungal agent used in the treatment of dandruff.

ZINC STEARATE (OTC) • **Zinc Soap.** A mixture of the zinc salts of stearic and palmitic acids. Widely used in cosmetic preparations because it contributes to adhesive properties. Baby powders of 3–5 percent zinc are water repellent and are promoted as preventing urine irritation. Inhalation of the powder may cause lung problems and produce death in infants from pneumonitis with lesions resembling those caused by talc, but more severe. No known toxicity on the skin, but in 1992 the FDA proposed a ban on zinc stearate in astringent (*see*) drug products because it had not been shown to be safe and effective as claimed.

ZINC SULFATE (OTC) • **Bufopto Zinc Sulfate. Clear Eyes ACR Astringent. Eye-Sed Ophthalmic. Op-Thal-Zin. Surbex-750. Visine A.C. Eye Drops. Zinca-Pac. Zincate.** The result of the reaction of sulfuric acid with zinc, it is a mild astringent for the eye and is also used in zinc-supplement preparations. Also used as a styptic, an emetic, and as an aid to wound healing in those deficient in zinc. Irritating to the skin and mucous membranes. May cause eye irritation. Also may cause an allergic reaction. In 1992, the FDA proposed a ban for the use of zinc sulfate to treat fever blisters and cold sores and in astringent (*see*) drug products because it had not been shown to be safe and effective as claimed in OTC drug products.

ZINC UNDECYLENATE (OTC) • **Cruex Antifungal Cream. Desenex Antifungal Cream.** A zinc salt that occurs in sweat; used to combat fungus on the skin. Made by dissolving zinc oxide in diluted undecylenic acid (*see*). Has an odor suggestive of perspiration. No known toxicity.

ZINECARD (Rx) • **Dexrazoxane.** A treatment for women who have received potentially heart-damaging doses of doxorubicin (*see*) for the treatment of breast cancer. During the review, the expert panel struggled with the fact that Zinecard decreased the incidence of congestive heart failure while slightly decreasing doxorubicin's antitumor effects. This did not affect overall survival rates.

ZINGIBAIN • An enzyme in gingerroot that is being studied for use as a digestive aid. *See* Ginger.

ZINGIBER OFFICINALE • *See* Ginger.

ZIRADRYL • *See* Diphenhydramine.

ZIRCONIUM OXIDE (OTC) • In 1992, the FDA issued a notice that zirconium oxide had not been shown to be safe and effective as claimed in OTC poison ivy, poison oak, and poison sumac products, as well as in insect sting and bite products. The FDA also banned zirconium in aerosol antiperspirant sprays.

ZITHROMAX • *See* Azithromycin.

ZIZIPHUS JUJUBA • *See* Jujube Date.

ZOCOR • *See* Simvastatin.

ZOFRAN • *See* Ondansetron.

ZOLADEX • *See* Goserelin.

ZOLICEF • *See* Cefazolin Sodium.

ZOLOFT • *See* Sertraline HCL.

ZOLPIDEM TARTRATE (Rx) • **Ambien.** A sleep aid used in ten countries and introduced in the United States in 1992. A nonbenzodiazepine, it is claimed patients fall asleep within twenty to thirty minutes and there is no evidence of increased wakefulness during the last third of the night. It is used for the short-term treatment of insomnia, and the manufacturer recommends prescriptions should not exceed a one-month supply. Hypnotics are generally limited to seven to ten days of use. Potential adverse effects include drowsiness, dizziness, diarrhea, and drugged feelings and abnormal thinking. It is a central nervous system depressant. Alcohol and other depressants increase zolpidem's central nervous system depression and can cause serious side effects.

ZOLYSE • *See* Chymotrypsin.

ZONE-A (Rx) • *See* Hydrocortisone and Pramoxine.

ZOONOSES • Animal diseases that are transmissible to humans.

ZORPRIN • *See* Aspirin.

ZORVIRAX • *See* Acyclovir.

ZYPREX • *See* Olanzapine.

ZYRTEC • *See* Cetirizine.

BIBLIOGRAPHY

AIDS Medicines: Drugs and Vaccines in Development. 1991 Annual Survey. Washington, D.C.: Pharmaceutical Manufacturers Association.

American Hospital Formulary Service Drug Information 93. Bethesda, Md., 1993.

Berkow, Robert, M.D., editor in chief. *The Merck Manual,* 16th ed. Rahway, N.J.: Merck & Co., Inc., 1992.

Castro, Miranda. *The Complete Homeopathy Handbook.* New York: St. Martin's Press, 1990.

Chilnick, Lawrence, editor in chief. *The Pill Book,* 4th ed. New York: Bantam, 1990.

Clayman, Charles, M.D. *The American Medical Association Guide to Prescription and Over-the-Counter Drugs.* New York: Random House, 1988.

Complete Drug Reference, The. Yonkers, N.Y.: United States Pharmacopeial Convention, Inc., 1992.

Cooley, Donald G. *Family Medical Guide.* New York: Meridith Corporation, 1973.

Drug Facts and Comparisons 1992 Edition. St. Louis: Facts And Comparisons, 1991.

Evashwick, Connie, Sc.D. *Aging and Health: The Role of Self-Medication.* Washington, D.C.: Nonprescription Drug Manufacturers Association, 1991.

Facts & Figures. Washington, D.C.: Nonprescription Drug Manufacturers Association, 1992.

Gordon, Lesley. *A Country Herbal.* New York: Mayflower Books, 1980.

Graedon, Joe. *The People's Pharmacy.* New York: St. Martin's Press, 1986.

Hammons, Christopher, M.B., B.S., L.C.H. *How to Use Homoeopathy.* Australia: Element, 1991.

Harrison, Sheila. *Help Your Child with Homeopathy.* Great Britain: Ashgrove Press Limited, 1989.

Heinerman, John. *Encyclopedia of Fruits, Vegetables and Herbs.* New York: Parker Publishing Co., 1988.

Hensyl, William R., ed. *Stedman's Medical Dictionary,* 25th ed. Baltimore: Williams & Wilkins Co., 1989.

Hoffman, David. *The New Holistic Herbal.* Rockport, Mass.: Element, Inc., 1991.

Kamm, Minnie Watson. *Old-Time Herbs for Northern Gardens.* Boston: Little, Brown & Co., 1938.

Kunz, Jeffrey R. M., M.D., editor in chief. *The American Medical Association Family Medical Guide.* New York: Random House, 1982.

Lacy, Charles, R.Ph., Pharm. D., and Leonard L. Lance, R.Ph. *Quick Look Drug Book.* Baltimore: Williams & Wilkins Co., 1992.

Lieberman, M. Laurence, R.Ph. *The Sexual Pharmacy.* New York: New American Library, 1988.

Loeb, Stanley, ed. *Nursing 92 Drug Handbook.* Philadelphia: Springhouse Corporation, 1992.

Long, James W., M.D. *The Essential Guide to Prescription Drugs 1992.* New York: HarperCollins Publishers, Inc., 1992.

...non, M.A., and Steven Finando, Ph.D. *Alterna-
... Healing.* New York: NAL Books, 1989.

Mindell, Earl, R.Ph., Ph.D. *Earl Mindell's Herb Bible.*
New York: Fireside Books, 1992.

Morgan, Brian, L.G., Ph.D. *The Food and Drug Interaction Guide.* New York: Simon and Schuster, 1986.

Mowrey, Daniel B. *The Scientific Validation of Herbal
Medicine.* New Canaan, Conn.: Keats Publishing, Inc.,
1986.

New Medicines for Women in Development. 1991 Annual
Survey. Washington, D.C.: Pharmaceutical Manufacturers
Association.

*Nonprescription Medicines: A Consumer's Dictionary of
Terms.* New York: Council on Family Health, 1990.

Orphan Drugs in Development. 1992 Annual Survey. Washington, D.C.: Pharmaceutical Manufacturers
Association.

Physicians' Desk Reference, 46th ed. Montvale, N.J.: Medical Economics Data, 1992.

Physicians' Desk Reference for Nonprescription Drugs.
Montvale, N.J.: Medical Economics Data, 1995.

Prous, Joseph, ed. *The Year's Drug News: Therapeutic
Targets.* Barcelona, Spain: Prous Science Publications,
1994.

Public Citizens Health Research Group. *Worst Pills: Best
Pills.* Washington, D.C.: Public Citizens Health Research
Group, 1988.

Quelch, Mary Thorne. *Herbs for Daily Use.* London: Farber & Farber Ltd., 1935.

Sax, Irving N., and Richard J. Lewis, Sr., eds. *Hawley's
Condensed Chemical Dictionary,* 11th ed. New York: Van
Nostrand Reinhold Co., 1987.

Schein, Jeffrey, M.S., and Philip Hansten, Pharm. D. *The
Consumer's Guide to Drug Interaction.* New York: Collier
Books, 1993.

*Self-Medication in the '90s: Practices and Perceptions,
Highlights of a Survey on Consumer Uses of Non-Pre-
scription Medicines.* Washington, D.C.: Nonprescription
Drug Manufacturers Association, 1992.

Talalaj, S., and A. S. Czechowicz. *Herbal Remedies:
Harmful and Beneficial Effects.* Melbourne, Australia: Hill
of Content, 1989.

Tierra, Michael, C.A., N.D. *The Way of Herbs.* New York:
Pocket Books, 1990.

Webster's Third New International Dictionary. Chicago:
G. & C. Merriam Co., 1966.

Weiner, Michael, Ph.D. *Weiner's Herbal 1990 Edition.*
Mill Valley, Calif.: Quantum Books, 1990.

Werbach, Melvyn R., M.D. *Nutritional Influences on Illness.* Conn.: Keats Publishing, Inc., 1987.

Windholz, Martha, ed. *The Merck Index,* 9th ed. Rahway,
N.J.: Merck & Co., Inc., 1982.

Winter, Arthur, M.D., and Ruth Winter. *Eat Right: Be
Bright.* New York: St. Martin's Press, 1988.

Winter, Ruth. *A Consumer's Dictionary of Cosmetic
Ingredients,* 4th rev. ed. New York: Crown Publishers,
Inc., 1994.

———. *A Consumer's Dictionary of Food Additives,* 4th
rev. ed. New York: Crown Publishers, Inc., 1994.